Textbook of
HOSPITAL PSYCHIATRY

DATE DUE

| GAYLORD | #3523PI | Printed in USA |

EDITORIAL BOARD

Textbook of
HOSPITAL PSYCHIATRY

Edited by

Steven S. Sharfstein, M.D., M.P.A.

With Deputy Editors

Faith B. Dickerson, Ph.D., M.P.H.
and
John M. Oldham, M.D., M.S.

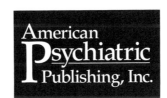

Washington, DC
London, England

Manufactured in the United States of America on acid-free paper
12   11   10   09   08   5   4   3   2   1
First Edition

Typeset in Adobe Kuenstler and Kabel

American Psychiatric Publishing, Inc.
1000 Wilson Boulevard
Arlington, VA 22209-3901
www.appi.org

Library of Congress Cataloging-in-Publication Data
Textbook of hospital psychiatry / edited by Steven S. Sharfstein, Faith B. Dickerson, John M. Oldham. — 1st ed.
    p. ; cm.
    Includes bibliographical references and index.
    ISBN 978-1-58562-322-8 (alk. paper)
1. Psychiatric hospital care—United States. 2. Psychiatric hospitals—United States—Administration.
I. Sharfstein, Steven S. (Steven Samuel), 1942– II. Dickerson, Faith B. III. Oldham, John M.
    [DNLM: 1. Psychiatric Department, Hospital—organization & administration. 2. Hospitals, Psychiatric—organization & administration. 3. Mental Disorders—therapy. 4. Psychology, Medical—organization & administration. WM 27.1 T355 2009]
    RC443.T49 2009
    362.2′1—dc22
                                                                                    2008016936

British Library Cataloguing in Publication Data
A CIP record is available from the British Library.

Dedication

To

Moses Sheppard

and

C. F. Menninger and his sons Karl and Will

—

Founders and Visionaries

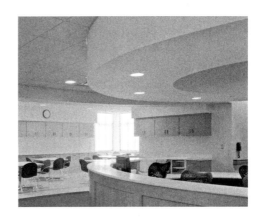

CONTENTS

Part I

Inpatient Practice

Part II

Special Clinical Issues

Part III

The Continuum of Care

Part IV

Structure and Infrastructure

Part V

The Future of Hospital Psychiatry

CONTRIBUTORS

George S. Alexopoulos, M.D.
Professor of Psychiatry, Cornell Institute of Geriatric Psychiatry, White Plains, New York

Donna T. Anthony, M.D., Ph.D.
Associate Professor of Clinical Psychiatry, Weill Cornell Medical Center; Program Director, Psychotic Disorders Continuum at Payne Whitney Westchester, NewYork–Presbyterian Hospital—Weill Cornell Medical Center, White Plains, New York

Joseph C. Blader, Ph.D.
Assistant Professor of Psychiatry, Department of Psychiatry and Behavioral Science, Stony Brook University School of Medicine, Stony Brook, New York

John J. Boronow, M.D.
Medical Director, Adult Services, Sheppard Pratt Hospital; Associate Clinical Professor of Psychiatry, University of Maryland School of Medicine, Towson, Maryland

Harry A. Brandt, M.D.
Director, Center for Eating Disorders, Sheppard Pratt Health System, Towson, Maryland

Francine Cournos, M.D.
Professor of Clinical Psychiatry, Columbia University, New York State Psychiatric Institute, New York, New York

Glenn W. Currier, M.D., M.P.H.
Associate Professor of Psychiatry and Emergency Medicine, University of Rochester Medical Center, Rochester, New York

Kathleen R. Delaney, Ph.D., R.N., P.M.H.–N.P.
Professor of Nursing, Department of Community and Mental Health Nursing, Rush College of Nursing; and Clinical Nurse Coordinator, Children's Inpatient Unit, Rush University Medical Center, Chicago, Illinois

David Ray DeMaso, M.D.
Psychiatrist-in-Chief, Children's Hospital Boston; and Professor of Psychiatry and Pediatrics, Harvard Medical School, Boston, Massachusetts

Faith B. Dickerson, Ph.D., M.P.H.
Director of Psychology, Sheppard Pratt Health System, Baltimore, Maryland; Clinical Associate Professor of Psychiatry, University of Maryland School of Medicine, Baltimore; Head, Stanley Research Program at Sheppard Pratt

Charles C. Dike, M.D., M.P.H., M.R.C.Psych.
Assistant Clinical Professor of Psychiatry, Yale University School of Medicine, New Haven, Connecticut; Medical Director, Whiting Forensic Division of Connecticut Valley Hospital, Middletown, Connecticut

Lisa B. Dixon, M.D., M.P.H.
VA Capitol Network (VISN 5) Mental Illness Research, Education, and Clinical Center (MIRECC), VA Maryland Healthcare System; Department of Psychiatry, Division of Services Research, University of Maryland School of Medicine, Baltimore, Maryland

Mary Ella Dubreuil, R.N., L.C.D.P.
Director of Alcohol and Drug Treatment Services, Butler Hospital, Providence, Rhode Island

Kenneth S. Duckworth, M.D.
Assistant Professor of Psychiatry, Harvard Medical School, Cambridge, Massachusetts; Medical Director, National Alliance on Mental Illness, Arlington, VA; Medical Director, Vinfen Corporation, Dorchester, Massachusetts

Lucy A. Epstein, M.D.
Postdoctoral Clinical Fellow in Psychiatry, Columbia University College of Physicians and Surgeons, New York, New York

Joan K. Feder, M.A., O.T.R./L., C.P.R.P.
Manager of Outpatient Psychosocial Rehabilitation Services, Payne Whitney Manhattan, NewYork–Presbyterian Hospital—Weill Cornell Medical Center, New York, New York

Michael C. Fiori, M.D.
Clinical Assistant Professor of Psychiatry, Department of Psychiatry and Human Behavior, Warren Alpert Medical School of Brown University; and Director, Alcohol and Drug Inpatient Unit, Butler Hospital, Providence, Rhode Island

Carmel A. Foley, M.D., M.H.A.
Assistant Professor of Psychiatry, Albert Einstein College of Medicine of Yeshiva University, Bronx, New York

Jeffrey L. Geller, M.D., M.P.H.
Professor of Psychiatry, Department of Psychiatry, University of Massachusetts Medical School, Worcester, Massachusetts

Ira D. Glick, M.D.
Professor, Psychiatry and Behavioral Sciences, Stanford University School of Medicine, Stanford, California

Judith S. Gonyea, O.T.D., M.S.Ed., O.T.R./L.
Assistant Professor, Occupational Therapy Program, Ithaca College, Ithaca, New York

Gary J. Gosselin, M.D.
Associate in Psychiatry, Children's Hospital Boston; and Instructor in Psychiatry, Harvard Medical School, Boston, Massachusetts

Katherine A. Halmi, M.D.
Director, Eating Disorders Program, NewYork–Presbyterian Hospital—Westchester Division, White Plains, New York

Lisa J. Halpern, M.P.P.
Director, Dorchester Bay Recovery Center, Vinfen Corporation, Dorchester, Massachusetts

Todd Hanson, A.I.A.
Director of Health Services Design, JSA, Portsmouth, New Hampshire

Brian M. Hepburn, M.D.
Executive Director, Mental Hygiene Administration, Maryland Department of Health and Mental Hygiene, Catonsville, Maryland

Margaret E. Hertzig, M.D.
Professor of Psychiatry, Interim Vice Chair, Child and Adolescent Psychiatry, Weill Medical College of Cornell University, New York, New York

Alex Hirshberg, B.A.
Clinical Educator, Adolescent Residential and Partial Hospital Program, McLean Hospital, Belmont, Massachusetts

Kevin Ann Huckshorn, R.N., M.S.N., C.A.P., I.C.A.D.C.
Director, Office of Technical Assistance, National Association for State Mental Health Program Directors, Alexandria, Virginia

Laurie Hurson
St. Joseph's University, Philadelphia, Pennsylvania

Mary E. Johnson, Ph.D., R.N.
Associate Professor of Nursing, Department of Community and Mental Health Nursing, Rush College of Nursing, Evanston, Illinois

Cynthia Kaplan, Ph.D.
Clinical Instructor of Psychiatry, Harvard Medical School, Boston, Massachusetts; Administrative Director, Child and Adolescent Services, McLean Hospital, Belmont, Massachusetts

Dimitris N. Kiosses, Ph.D.
Assistant Professor of Psychology in Psychiatry, Cornell Institute of Geriatric Psychiatry, White Plains, New York

Sibel A. Klimstra, M.D.
Associate Professor of Clinical Psychiatry, Cornell Institute of Geriatric Psychiatry, White Plains, New York

Eugene J. Kuc, M.D.
Associate Professor, Department of Psychiatry and Behavioral Sciences, University of Arkansas for Medical Sciences, Little Rock, Arkansas

Vassilios Latoussakis, M.D.
Research Fellow, Cornell Institute of Geriatric Psychiatry, White Plains, New York

Janice L. LeBel, Ph.D.
Director of Program Management, Commonwealth of Massachusetts, Department of Mental Health, Boston, Massachusetts

Anthony F. Lehman, M.D., M.S.P.H.
Professor and Chair, Department of Psychiatry, University of Maryland School of Medicine, Baltimore, Maryland

Stephanie LeMelle, M.D.
Associate Clinical Professor of Psychiatry, Department of Psychiatry, Columbia University College of Physicians and Surgeons, New York, New York

John R. Lion, M.D.
Private Practice and Clinical Professor of Psychiatry, University of Maryland School of Medicine, Baltimore, Maryland

Richard C. Lippincott, M.D.
Professor, Department of Psychiatry and Behavioral Sciences, University of Arkansas for Medical Sciences, Little Rock, Arkansas

Benjamin Liptzin, M.D.
Professor and Deputy Chair, Department of Psychiatry, Tufts University School of Medicine, Boston, Massachusetts; and Chairman, Department of Psychiatry, Baystate Health, Springfield, Massachusetts

Richard J. Loewenstein, M.D.
Medical Director, Trauma Disorders Services, Sheppard Pratt Health System, Baltimore, Maryland; Associate Clinical Professor, Department of Psychiatry, University of Maryland School of Medicine, Baltimore, Maryland

Francis G. Lu, M.D.
Professor of Clinical Psychiatry, University of California at San Francisco, San Francisco, California

Barbara Roberts Magid, M.B.A.
Director, Division of Professional Services, Sheppard Pratt Health System, Baltimore, Maryland

Andrés Martin, M.D., M.P.H.
Professor of Child Psychiatry and Psychiatry, Child Study Center, Yale University School of Medicine, New Haven, Connecticut

Marlin R. Mattson, M.D.
Professor of Clinical Psychiatry, Weill Medical College of Cornell University, New York, New York

Aaron B. Murray-Swank, Ph.D.
VA Capitol Network (VISN 5) Mental Illness Research, Education, and Clinical Center (MIRECC), VA Maryland Healthcare System; Department of Psychiatry, Division of Services Research, University of Maryland School of Medicine, Baltimore, Maryland

Philip R. Muskin, M.D.
Professor of Clinical Psychiatry, Department of Psychiatry, Columbia University College of Physicians and Surgeons; Chief, Consultation-Liaison Psychiatry, Columbia University Medical Center, New York–Presbyterian Hospital, New York, New York

Michael A. Norko, M.D.
Associate Professor of Psychiatry, Yale University School of Medicine, New Haven, Connecticut; Director of Forensic Services, Connecticut Department of Mental Health and Addiction Services, Hartford, Connecticut

John M. Oldham, M.D., M.S.
Professor and Executive Vice Chair for Clinical Affairs and Development, Menninger Department of Psychiatry and Behavioral Sciences, Baylor College of Medicine, Houston, Texas; Senior Vice President and Chief of Staff, The Menninger Clinic, Houston, Texas

Suzanne Perraud, Ph.D., R.N.
Assistant Professor and Director of Specialty Education, Rush College of Nursing, Chicago, Illinois

Eric M. Plakun, M.D.
Director of Admissions and Professional Relations, The Austen Riggs Center, Stockbridge, Massachusetts; Chair, American Psychiatric Association Committee on Psychotherapy by Psychiatrists

Marilyn Price, M.D.
Clinical Assistant Professor of Psychiatry, Warren Alpert Medical School of Brown University, Providence, Rhode Island

Diana L. Ramsay, M.P.P., O.T.R., F.A.O.T.A.
Executive Vice President and Chief Operating Officer, Sheppard Pratt Health System, Baltimore, Maryland; and past President, National Association of Psychiatric Health Systems (NAPHS), Washington, D.C.

Michael A. Rater, M.D.
Clinical Instructor, Harvard Medical School, McLean Hospital, Belmont, Massachusetts

Patricia R. Recupero, J.D., M.D.
Clinical Professor of Psychiatry, Warren Alpert Medical School of Brown University; and President/CEO, Butler Hospital, Providence, Rhode Island

Robert P. Roca, M.D., M.P.H., M.B.A.
Vice President of Medical Affairs, Sheppard Pratt Health System; Associate Professor of Psychiatry, Johns Hopkins University School of Medicine; Clinical Associate Professor of Psychiatry, University of Maryland School of Medicine, Baltimore, Maryland

Lloyd I. Sederer, M.D.
Medical Director, New York State Office of Mental Health (OMH), New York, New York

Harold I. Schwartz, M.D.
Psychiatrist-in-Chief and Vice President Behavioral Health, Institute of Living/Hartford Hospital, Hartford, Connecticut; Professor of Psychiatry, University of Connecticut School of Medicine, Farmington, Connecticut

Edward R. Shapiro, M.D.
Medical Director and Chief Executive Officer, The Austen Riggs Center, Stockbridge, Massachusetts; Associate Clinical Professor of Psychiatry, Harvard Medical School, Boston, Massachusetts

Marlene I. Shapiro, M.S.W., L.C.S.W.–C.
Program Director, Harry Stack Sullivan Day Hospital, Sheppard Pratt Health System, Baltimore, Maryland

Steven S. Sharfstein, M.D., M.P.A.
President and Chief Executive Officer, Sheppard Pratt Health System, Baltimore, Maryland; Clinical Professor and Vice Chair, Department of Psychiatry, University of Maryland School of Medicine, Baltimore, Maryland

A. Bela Sood, M.D., M.S.H.A.
Professor of Psychiatry, Virginia Commonwealth University School of Medicine, Richmond, Virginia

Bette M. Stewart, B.S.
Department of Psychiatry, Division of Services Research, University of Maryland School of Medicine, Baltimore, Maryland

Anne M. Stoline, M.D.
Staff Psychiatrist, Perry Point VA Medical Center, Perry Point, Maryland

Paul Summergrad, M.D.
Psychiatrist-in-Chief, Tufts–New England Medical Center; and Dr. Frances Arkin Professor and Chairman, Department of Psychiatry, Tufts University School of Medicine, Boston, Massachusetts

Rajiv Tandon, M.D.
Chief of Psychiatry, Mental Health Program Office, State of Florida, Tallahassee, Florida

Howard D. Trachtman, B.S., C.P.S.
Executive Director, Boston Resource Center, Boston, Massachusetts

Susan B. Wait, M.D.
Service Chief, Trauma Disorders Services, Sheppard Pratt Health System, Baltimore, Maryland

Disclosure of Competing Interests

The following authors have competing interests to declare:

George S. Alexopolous, M.D. *Consultant:* Forest; *Grant Support:* Forest, Cephalon; *Speakers' Bureau:* Bristol-Myers Squibb, Cephalon, Forest, GlaxoSmithKline, Janssen, Eli Lilly, Pfizer

Joseph C. Blader, Ph.D. *Grant Support:* Abbot Laboratories

John J. Boronow, M.D. *Speakers' Bureau:* Pfizer, AstraZeneca, Bristol-Myers Squibb

Glenn W. Currier, M.D., M.P.H. *Grant Support:* Pfizer; *Speakers' Bureau:* Bristol-Myers Squibb, Pfizer

Michael C. Fiori, M.D. *Speakers' Bureau:* Reckitt Benckiser

Ira D. Glick, M.D. *Advisory Board:* Janssen, Pfizer, Bristol-Myers Squibb, Solvay; *Speakers' Bureau:* Janssen, AstraZeneca, Pfizer, Bristol-Myers Squibb; *Research Support:* Bristol-Myers Squibb, Shire, Solvay

Janice L. LeBel, Ph.D. *Consultant:* Sheppard Pratt Health System, Hogg Foundation for Mental Health, National Association of State Mental Health Program Directors' Office of Technical Assistance, New Zealand government, Australian government

Benjamin Liptzin, M.D. Associate Medical Director, Health New England

Paul Summergrad, M.D. *Honoraria:* Pfizer, MC Communications

Howard D. Trachtman, B.S., C.P.S. *Grant Support:* AstraZeneca

The following authors have no competing interests to report:
Donna T. Anthony, M.D., Ph.D.; Harry A. Brandt, M.D.; Francine Cournos, M.D.; Kathleen R. Delaney, Ph.D., R.N., P.M.H.-N.P.; David Ray DeMaso, M.D.; Faith B. Dickerson, Ph.D., M.P.H.; Charles C. Dike, M.D., M.P.H., M.R.C.Psych.; Lisa B. Dixon, M.D., M.P.H.; Mary Ella Dubreuil, R.N., L.C.D.P.; Kenneth S. Duckworth, M.D.; Lucy A. Epstein, M.D.; Joan K. Feder, M.A., O.T.R./L., C.P.R.P.; Carmel A. Foley, M.D., M.H.A.; Jeffrey L. Geller, M.D., M.P.H.; Judith S. Gonyea, O.T.D., M.S.Ed., O.T.R./L.; Gary J. Gosselin, M.D.; Katherine A. Halmi, M.D.; Lisa J. Halpern, M.P.P.; Todd Hanson, A.I.A.; Brian M. Hepburn, M.D.; Margaret E. Hertzig, M.D.; Alex Hirshberg, B.A.; Kevin Ann Huckshorn, R.N., M.S.N., C.A.P., I.C.A.D.C.; Laurie Hurson; Mary E. Johnson, Ph.D., R.N.; Cynthia Kaplan, Ph.D.; Dimitris N. Kiosses, Ph.D.; Sibel A. Klimstra, M.D.; Eugene J. Kuc, M.D.; Vassilios Latoussakis, M.D.; Anthony F. Lehman, M.D., M.S.P.H.; Stephanie LeMelle, M.D.; John R. Lion, M.D.; Richard C. Lippincott, M.D.; Richard J. Loewenstein, M.D.; Francis G. Lu, M.D.; Barbara Roberts Magid, M.B.A.; Andrés Martin, M.D., M.P.H.; Marlin R. Mattson, M.D.; Aaron B. Murray-Swank, Ph.D.; Philip R. Muskin, M.D.; Michael A. Norko, M.D.; John M. Oldham, M.D., M.S.; Suzanne Perraud, Ph.D., R.N.; Eric M. Plakun, M.D.; Marilyn Price, M.D.; Diana L. Ramsay, M.P.P., O.T.R., F.A.O.T.A.; Michael A. Rater, M.D.; Patricia R. Recupero, J.D., M.D.; Robert P. Roca, M.D., M.P.H., M.B.A.; Harold I. Schwartz, M.D.; Lloyd I. Sederer, M.D.; Edward R. Shapiro, M.D.; Marlene I. Shapiro, M.S.W., L.C.S.W.-C.; Steven S. Sharfstein, M.D., M.P.A.; A. Bela Sood, M.D., M.S.H.A.; Bette M. Stewart, B.S.; Anne M. Stoline, M.D.; Rajiv Tandon, M.D.; Susan B. Wait, M.D.

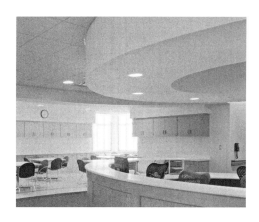

PREFACE

The psychiatric hospital has played essential roles in American psychiatry for more than two centuries. Yet during this time, and especially over the past several decades, hospital psychiatry has seen radical changes. The large rural asylums of the nineteenth century where persons with mental illnesses went for shelter and stayed for years have yielded to the acute psychiatric hospitals of the twenty-first century with lengths of stay measured in days. The stakes have always been high for patients and their families when hospitalization occurs, but the pace of activity during hospitalization and, indeed, the goals of hospitalization have changed profoundly. Today's busy psychiatric inpatient units face extraordinary pressures and complexities, and the stakes are high for all involved. An apt metaphor from Flow Theory is what has been called "being in the zone," which occurs in a wide range of human activities. A person "in the zone" experiences "everything coming together" under extreme pressure to produce a high level of performance. Baseball players "in the zone" describe seeing the stitches on a fastball pitch before they hit a home run; jazz musicians "in the zone" navigate complex chord changes with ease to produce beautiful solos. "In the zone" experiences require a high degree of preparation and technical skill combined with the capacity to relax and focus in real time in order to maximize performance. Modern hospital psychiatry works best "in the zone."

It is difficult to overstate the complexities faced by modern psychiatric hospitals. Because the decision to proceed to hospitalization now is often viewed as a last resort, triggered by significant risk to self or others, the acuity of patients' problems is probably greater than it has ever been. Many patients enter the psychiatric hospital with significant comorbidities, including substance abuse and serious medical problems, that need to be addressed. The array of available effective treatments that can be brought to bear has grown tremendously, but then so have the expectations for quick results. The most effective approaches are interdisciplinary, but these require close coordination among professionals. Critical shortages of mental health professionals from various disciplines abound in many locales. Shortages in community-based services for continued care complicate discharge planning. Further pressures arise from court systems seeking forensic services. Demands for documentation and accountability are rampant. The payers begin to press for rapid discharge as soon as the patient enters the hospital. With all of these pressures, compressed into but a few days, it is no wonder that we hear so many complaints that lengths of stay have become too short to accomplish much more than provision of basic safety during a crisis.

Thus, the launch of this new textbook on hospital psychiatry, with contributions from many leading experts, is timely, occurring when realistic hope and expectations can set a fruitful course for hospital psychiatry in the twenty-first century. Part I of the textbook immediately reveals the many roles of current hospital psychiatry. These hospital programs serve persons across the life span. We see the emergence of units that focus on specific diagnoses, providing specialized care for highly complex subgroups. We see as well the explicit acknowledgment of co-occurring problems, substance abuse, developmental disabilities, and legal entanglements. We see discussion of units focused on ethnic/minority groups, reflecting the ever-growing diversity of our communities. The continuing major roles of public hospitals, both state and federal (Department of Veterans Affairs), reflect the fact that our systems of mental health care still rely heavily on government support, especially with continuing disparities in insurance coverage for mental disorders. The chapters in Part IV (I'll get back to Parts II and III in a moment) underscore the current infrastructure challenges of hospital psychiatry. While many of the topics addressed in these chapters—interdisciplinary staffing, finance, legal and regulatory requirements, discharge and safety, quality indicators, information technology, architecture—would have received coverage in texts on hospital psychiatry 50 years ago, the fact that each now warrants an entire book chapter is telling.

Parts II and III of the book address the broader context of twenty-first-century hospital psychiatry. The chapters in Part III, "The Continuum of Care," highlight the fact that, especially with today's very brief lengths of inpatient stay, hospital-based treatment must be understood within the broader perspective of patients' lives outside the hospital and the services that they need in the community, including mental health clinics, emergency rooms, day hospitals, intensive outpatient treatment, rehabilitation programs, and residential services. The connection of treatment in the hospital with what precedes and follows hospitalization has always been critical, but it is especially so when lengths of stay are so short and the stakes for patients are so high. We know that there are many discontinuities in care. Such discontinuities can be particularly unfortunate, even tragic, when they occur at the interfaces of the hospital and community-based

services. More than ever, hospital psychiatry services must be tightly embedded in a comprehensive continuum of care that does not permit patients to fall through the cracks.

Finally, Part II reflects the newest emerging issues of twenty-first-century hospital psychiatry. The chapters on preventing suicide and improving safety again emphasize the acuity of patients entering the hospital, the pressures created at the convergence of medical necessity and third-party mandates for the shortest possible lengths of stay, accountability, and the critical need to interface with postdischarge community services. Much is at stake. Here we also see the emergence of an age of mental health consumerism and a new spirit of recovery and hope. While chapters on families are not new, the maturing movement toward genuine alliances between families and treatment teams, reflected in this volume, is new. Even newer is the focus on patients' viewpoints and the emerging theme of true collaboration between patients and practitioners in promoting recovery and creating care that is "patient centered." We see in Part II a new emphasis on partnerships—between patients and practitioners, families and practitioners, and hospitals and communities.

In sum, the very brief hospitalizations that characterize twenty-first-century psychiatry can appear as blips in time when viewed across the course of patients' lives. Yet much critical business occurs during these inpatient episodes. Skilled, well-informed inpatient treatment teams must have keen eyes for the significance of the unfolding events, for the opportunities to make critical interventions, and for the connections needed with families and the community-based continuum of care. When such teams are supported by the right system structures, real therapeutic differences can be achieved. For twenty-first-century hospital psychiatry, being "in the zone" can change and save lives.

Anthony F. Lehman, M.D., M.S.P.H.
Professor and Chair, Department of Psychiatry,
University of Maryland School of Medicine

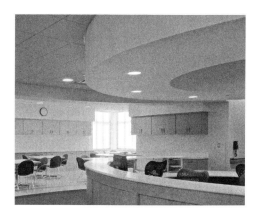

INTRODUCTION

Steven S. Sharfstein, M.D., M.P.A.
Faith B. Dickerson, Ph.D., M.P.H.
John M. Oldham, M.D., M.S.

In the past quarter-century, major changes have occurred in psychiatric treatment. Some of these changes are the result of real progress in the scientific understanding of mental disorders and the development of effective biological and psychosocial treatments. The "evidence base" for psychiatric treatment continues to grow. In addition to scientific progress, there has been a decrease in stigma about receiving psychiatric care. This welcome change has occurred in large part due to the fact that psychiatric treatments work. In addition, consumers and families have increasingly given voice to their experiences and have assumed a stronger role in making decisions about the provision of psychiatric care.

At the same time, there has been some real regression in the care and treatment of persons with mental illness in this country. Cost-driven cutbacks in care as well as faulty and misguided public policies have resulted in the deinstitutionalization of many seriously ill people, with inadequate community services to treat them. These unfortunate trends have resulted in many persons with mental illness becoming homeless or part of the criminal justice system. The scarcity of acute psychiatric beds in this country has reached crisis proportions. Emergency rooms are often in gridlock with acutely ill psychiatric patients stuck with nowhere to go.

This "good news/bad news" scenario has never been more evident than in inpatient care for psychiatric patients, whether in private psychiatric hospitals, in general hospitals, or in the public sector. Acute psychiatric care is focused on crisis stabilization and rapid discharge. Readmissions are common. Intermediate and longer-term care take place primarily in the public sector, often as a result of concerns about public safety. More and more seriously and persistently mentally ill individuals are in jails and prisons.

These unwelcome trends have occurred even as we know more about how to effectively treat and care for people with severe mental illness using a combination of pharmacological and psychosocial treatments in a continuum of care. Psychiatric treatment, especially in the hospital, has become increasingly specialized. Considerable expertise is available for the care of children and adolescents, the very old, and individuals with specific conditions such as eating disorders, post-traumatic stress disorders, psychotic disorders, and brain injuries.

This textbook is all about the "good news" of psychiatric treatment, especially in the delivery of intensive (often lifesaving) care in hospitals. Our hope is that this book will have an impact not only in improving care in hospitals that already provide needed treatment but also in expanding opportunities in new settings, both hospital and nonhospital, to provide available and effective treatments, to do what we can and should do in the context of today's medical marketplace.

Inpatient psychiatric services have declined drastically over the past four decades, and beds have been reduced across public and private settings in a process that has been mainly driven by economics, not clinical science. The downsizing of state- and county-operated mental hospitals has been the most dramatic reason for the large decrease in the total number of inpatient psychiatric beds. In 1970, there were approximately 525,000 psychiatric beds in the United States, with 80% of these beds provided by state or county mental hospitals. By 2002, the total number of psychiatric beds had declined to fewer than 212,000, with 27% of inpatient beds provided by state or county hospitals (Foley et al. 2007). By contrast, in the private sector, growth was most dramatic in the 1970s in general hospitals and in the 1980s in private psychiatric hospitals, which partially offset the decreases in the public sector. However, since the mid-1990s, private-sector downsizing has occurred, adding to the continuing decline in the overall number of inpatient psychiatric beds.

Demand for acute inpatient services was largely stimulated by the needs of patients who were "deinstitutionalized" from state and county hospitals. Insurance coverage through Medicare and Medicaid allowed for the growth of psychiatric beds in the private sector. Prospective payment under Medicare, implemented in 1983, excluded psychiatric hospitals and dedicated inpatient units in general hospitals, fueling the increase in the number of these beds. A peak was hit in 1990 with more than 50,000 beds provided through psychiatric units in general hospitals and 45,000 beds in private psychiatric hospitals. Since that time, however, primarily due to managed care utilization review, these beds have declined in number so that private psychiatric hospital beds today number approximately 25,000 and general hospital beds around 40,000 (Foley et al. 2007). At the same time, emergency department visits for mental disorders have increased from about 1.4 million visits in 1992 to nearly 2.5 million in 2003

(Salinsky and Loftis 2007). Partial hospitalization during this time period fluctuated largely due to shifts in payment policies through the Medicare program. Other potential substitutes for inpatient care have grown some, but these community-based alternatives have been insufficient to truly offset the declines in inpatient psychiatric beds during this time period. A 2006 survey of state mental health authorities revealed that more than 80% of states reported a shortage of psychiatric beds. Among these states, 34 states reported a shortage of acute beds; 16 states, a shortage of long-term-care beds; and 24 states, a shortage of forensic beds. Many states reported longer waiting lists for psychiatric beds. As a result, there is an increased reliance on jails and prisons to address the needs of persons with serious mental illness (National Association of State Mental Health Program Directors 2006).

A recent report on expenditure trends reinforces the findings on the decrease in psychiatric beds. From 1986 to 2003, the proportion of total expenditures for mental health that was spent on inpatient psychiatric treatment fell from 41% to 24%. At the same time, the proportion of total mental health expenditures spent on psychiatric medication grew from 7% to 23% (Mark et al. 2007).

Has the pendulum swung too far from the provision of inpatient care and the financing of that treatment? We hope that this book will be part of a sincere and serious reassessment of the current need for hospital-based level of care and of funding priorities.

Twenty years ago, a textbook entitled *Modern Hospital Psychiatry* was published "to describe the various aspects of inpatient care from admission to discharge and to comment upon various types of hospitals and the role of staff within these institutions" (Lion et al. 1988, p. v). Rereading this textbook underscores the dramatic changes that have occurred in the last two decades. At the time, average lengths of stay in many private psychiatric hospitals as well as inpatient units were three to four times what they are today. The concept of a continuum of care was very rudimentary, and hospital treatment was considered to be a definitive effort to manage the consequences of both acute and chronic mental illness. There was only one chapter on the follow-up to hospitalization. The concept of recovery from serious mental illnesses had not yet been conceived. This volume will hopefully better stand the test of time, but we are sure significant changes will continue to occur in the ever-evolving dynamic of better understanding the basic causes of mental illness and addictions, revisions in diagnostic assessment, even stronger partnerships with consumers and families, and the development of better treatment technologies based on scientific discovery.

Acknowledgments

The editors would like to express their appreciation for the contributions of the editorial board as well as the help of Stephanie Provenza at Sheppard Pratt and Liz Bednarowicz from the Menninger Clinic in the preparation of this manuscript.

References

Foley DJ, Manderscheid RW, Atay JE, et al: Highlights of organized mental health services in 2002 and major national and state trends, in Mental Health, United States, 2004. Edited by Manderscheid RW, Berry JT. Rockville, MD, U.S. Department of Health and Human Services, 2002, pp 200–236. Available at: http://download.ncadi.samhsa.gov/ken/pdf/SMA06-4195/CMHS_MHUS_2004.pdf. Accessed March 2007.

Lion JR, Adler WN, Webb WL (eds): Modern Hospital Psychiatry. New York, WW Norton, 1988

Mark TL, Levit KR, Buck JA, et al: Mental health treatment expenditure trends, 1986–2003. Psychiatr Serv 58:1041–1048, 2007

National Association of State Mental Health Program Directors Medical Directors Council: Parks J, Svendsen D, Singer P, et al. (eds): Morbidity and Mortality in People With Serious Mental Illness, 13th Technical Report. Alexandria, VA, 2006

Salinsky E, Loftis C: Shrinking inpatient psychiatric capacity: cause for celebration or concern? NHPF 823:1–21, 2007

CHAPTER 1

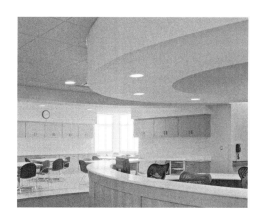

HISTORY OF HOSPITAL PSYCHIATRY AND LESSONS LEARNED

Jeffrey L. Geller, M.D., M.P.H.

The history of American psychiatry, through at least the nineteenth century and early years of the twentieth century, is fundamentally the history of inpatient psychiatry. The founders of the American Psychiatric Association (APA) were founders of an association of medical superintendents, some from state hospitals, others from private psychiatric hospitals. Nine of the original 13 members of the Association of Medical Superintendents of American Institutions for the Insane (AMSAII) had connections with private psychiatric hospitals. Kirkbride had trained at Friends Asylum and was Superintendent of the Pennsylvania Hospital for the Insane. Woodward, Brigham, and Butler had all been associated with the Hartford Retreat; Ray was connected with Butler Hospital; and Earle had associations with both Friends and Bloomingdale Asylums. Two members, Cutter (Pepperell Private Asylum) and White (Hudson Lunatic Asylum) were founders and ran proprietary psychiatric facilities, whereas Bell headed McLean Asylum.

These founders of American psychiatry, and the hospitals with which each was associated, set the course for hospital-based care and treatment to this day. This chapter reviews the history of American psychiatric hospitals and serves as a reference for the other chapters in this book.

The Early Years (The Beginning Through 1920)

Origins of Public Facilities

Public care of persons with insanity began concurrently at multiple levels of government. Prior to the nineteenth century, the care of insane persons was predominantly a local endeavor, took place largely in almshouses, and was generally custodial in nature (Hurd 1916). When states took responsibility for insane paupers in this era, the state would auction these "confessedly undesirable persons" to the *lowest* bidder, because the state had to pay the private family to provide for the basic needs. If no family could be found, jails or strong pens under a relative's supervision were used (Deutsch 1949; Hurd 1916).

In some states, care for the insane poor became organized at the county level. States created state boards of charity to inspect the county establishments that housed insane persons. This system was criticized because local variation was extreme and medical and nursing interventions generally poor (Hurd 1916).

At the outset, "state care" meant a state institution that was established, built, and managed by the state but whose operation was funded by taxpayers and individuals. These were really state-aided facilities. If the patient or family had resources, they paid for care; paupers were the responsibility of the county. Thus, the earliest public facilities—in Williamsburg, Virginia, and Columbia, South Carolina—were established pursuant to this model (Hurd 1916).

State care in which the state was responsible for all insane persons and executed its responsibility through state-managed and -funded hospitals began with Worcester State Hospital in 1833 (Hurd 1916). The development of state care progressed at quite different rates. New Hampshire, for example, did not have an act legalizing state care until 1913 (Hurd 1916).

It was three decades after states began to take responsibility for their insane populations before states began to specifically consider the incurably insane. In 1865, New York State established the first asylum for persons with chronic insanity, the Willard Asylum (Deutsch 1949; Hurd 1916). Not everyone was in favor of such institutions. Amariah Brigham, first superintendent of Utica State Hospital, in a letter to Dorothea Dix in 1866, indicated that he opposed "the establishment of hospitals solely for the incurable insane. They would, in my opinion, soon become objects of but little interest to any one, and where misrule, neglect, and all kinds of abuse would exist and exist without detection" (Deutsch 1949, p. 239).

At this same time, the members of the AMSAII articulated, at their annual meeting, what they believed the states' responsibilities were (Hurd 1916):

1. The state should make ample and suitable provisions for all its insane.
2. No insane person should be treated in any county poorhouse or almshouse.
3. Proper classification is an indispensable element and can only be achieved in facilities specifically constructed for treatment.
4. Curable and incurable persons should not be in separate establishments.
5. States should have asylums placed so that individuals can get treatment near where they reside.

6. Hospitals should have enough wards to treat different classes of insane persons on different wards.
7. Hospitals could have up to 600 patients and properly care for the insane.

In 1868, AMSAII drafted suggested legislation concerning the admittance of patients (Hurd 1916):

1. Insane persons may be placed in a hospital for the insane by their relatives, friends, or legal guardian, but never without the certificate of one or more reputable physicians, after a personal examination, made within 1 week.
2. Insane persons may be placed in a hospital by order of a magistrate, who, after proper inquisition, finds that such persons are at large and dangerous to themselves or others or require hospital care and treatment; the fact of their insanity shall be certified as specified in the preceding section.
3. Insane persons may be placed in a hospital, by order of any high judicial officer, if, on statement in writing of any respectable individual that a certain person is insane, and that the welfare of himself or others requires his restraint, a duly appointed commission finds the person is a suitable case for confinement.

Origins of Private Psychiatric Hospitals

Three facilities began as parts of general medical hospitals. The Institute of the Pennsylvania Hospital started in the general hospital proposed by Benjamin Franklin, with insane persons scattered throughout the hospital, mostly in cellars. A separate wing of the general hospital was then completed, followed finally by a separate structure built in west Philadelphia, some distance from the general hospital, and funded by a colonial grant and subscriptions (Deutsch 1949; Kirkbride 1845).

The Bloomingdale Hospital in New York began as a wing of a general hospital, funded by subscriptions from "philanthropic public spirited" citizens. The locus of care of the insane moved to a separate structure with a grant from the state (Deutsch 1949; Earle 1845).

McLean Hospital in Massachusetts started as part of a general hospital, but services for insane persons were provided in a separate facility from the outset. Initial funding was from bequests, subscriptions, and donations; 3 years after it opened, John McLean of Boston willed $100,000 to the asylum, and the asylum was renamed in his honor (Deutsch 1949; Massachusetts 1845).

Three private psychiatric hospitals began as free-standing institutions funded through different methods. Butler Hospital in Rhode Island resulted from the legacy of a philanthropist, Nicholas Brown, and from a subscription campaign with the major contributions coming from Cyrus Butler at the urging of Dorothea Dix (Deutsch 1949; Ray 1848). The Brattleboro Retreat, which began as the Vermont Asylum for the Insane, was funded through a bequest by the wife of a physician, with additional funds provided by the state (Deutsch 1949). The Hartford Retreat in Connecticut (subsequently named the Institute of Living) resulted from a study by the Connecticut Medical Society that recommended the construction of a freestanding mental institution. The retreat was funded by a state grant, funds from the state medical society, private subscriptions, and a lottery (Connecticut 1845; Deutsch 1949).

Two private hospitals were begun by religious organizations. The Friends Asylum in Pennsylvania was initiated by the Society of Friends. Modeled after the English Quakers' York Retreat, the Friends Asylum was funded by a subscription campaign and in-kind donations. The hospital was established to serve only members of the Society of Friends, but from 1834 to 1845 others were admitted. In 1845, admissions were limited to those connected with the Society of Friends and any others who were former patients (Deutsch 1949; Pennsylvania 1845).

Whereas all of these hospitals were formed under a for-profit model, the Mount Hope Institution in Maryland, which began as Mount Saint Vincent, was based on religious benevolence. Although a Catholic-affiliated institution, it accepted patients of all denominations.

The origins of many of the smaller facilities are much more obscure; many appear to have been set up as a form of private practice. Some that began in the early twentieth century, such as Chestnut Lodge and Austen Riggs, were established as venues to practice certain types of psychiatry (Geller 2006). An interesting thesis for the founding of many nineteenth-century facilities is that physicians who had worked in the public sector needed income-producing ventures later in their careers because there was no public pension or retirement system (Gerald Grob, personal communication, November 2000). A few additional hospitals were created in a fashion similar to the earliest asylums. Moses Sheppard planned for the establishment of a mental institution in Maryland and built a hospital that opened as the Sheppard Asylum. With a subsequent bequest from Enoch Pratt, the facility was renamed Sheppard and Enoch Pratt Hospital (Forbush 1971).

Edward Jarvis, himself an operator of a private facility in Massachusetts, stated in 1860 what he thought was the role of the private facility:

> not to compete with the public institutions in matters of cheapness; but to provide liberally for all the proper wants of their inmates, and charge all for material, time, attention and responsibility, and receive a corresponding reward. Not to receive and treat the violent, the maniacal, the suicidal; but the mild, quiet, and manageable by personal influence. And principally to provide and offer to such patients as can properly enjoy and profit by them, an opportunity of using more of their faculties that are sane, a freer range of occupation and action, more of domestic and social life, more intercourse with the world, and a condition resembling more nearly that of their own homes that can be offered and enjoyed in the public hospitals. (Jarvis 1860, p. 31)

Private–Public Interface

Of the larger private facilities, all but one preceded the state's first public hospital, sometimes by more than 50 years. The private hospitals met a state's need for care of indigent insane persons by admitting "public" patients with varying methods of payment. This arrangement generally continued until the state determined it could provide for those insane who required public support more cost-effectively in state hospitals.

Bloomingdale Asylum was aided by legislative appropriations for its first 30 years; this ended in 1849, and the facility then devoted itself to private patients only (New York 1872). William Rockwell, superintendent of the Vermont Asylum for the Insane (Brattleboro Retreat), proclaimed in 1867 that his hospital could accommodate all insane persons of Vermont who require hospital treatment (Vermont Asylum for the Insane 1868). The Hartford Retreat ended its relationship with the state of Connecticut after 30 years of "receiving such insane patients as were a public charge" (Connecticut 1871). Butler Hospital received an annual appropriation from the state that could be apportioned to specific patients at a fixed annual cap per patient (Butler Hospital for the Insane 1878). This continued even after Butler Hospital sent a large number of the indigent insane patients to the state facility at its opening. Pennsylvania Hospital provided care to a limited number from the state, doing so "without charge of any kind" (Kirkbride 1845).

A social policy evolved in virtually every state that care of its insane citizens would predominantly be a public function. Despite the operation of many private facilities, these accounted for a small percentage of those persons institutionalized by the early twentieth century. On January 1, 1920, there were 232,680 persons in institutions for mental disorders in the United States: 200,109 in state hospitals, 21,584 in county or city facilities, 1,040 in institutions for temporary care, 709 in Public Health Service Hospitals, and 9,238 in private hospitals (Pollock and Forbush 1921). Thus, private facilities accounted for only 4% of persons in psychiatric facilities.

Comparison of Private and Public Facilities

It should come as no surprise that public and private facilities had some common features, because the establishment of many public asylums was directly influenced by the early private asylums. The Friends Asylum and Hartford Retreat influenced the erection and organization of Utica State Hospital; the Hartford Retreat affected the establishment of asylums in Worcester and Boston, Massachusetts; and the Brattleboro Retreat influenced the construction of the state asylum in New Hampshire (Hurd 1913).

At the turn of the twentieth century, the president of the New York State Commission in Lunacy argued that both public and private facilities should be able to admit patients for 48–72 hours on an emergency paper signed by a family physician. "Regular lunacy certification" would follow and thus the use of jails and prisons for the reception of persons "ill of brain disease" could be avoided (Peterson 1902). During the first two decades of the twentieth century, both public and private hospitals had open, unlocked wards, and both were striving to treat patients without the use of seclusion or restraint (Hurd 1916; Page 1904).

Private facilities, like public ones, had issues with overcrowding (Vermont 1890), psychiatrists' violent deaths at the facility ("Death of Dr. George Cook" 1876), unwarranted admissions ("From the Report of the McLean Asylum" 1864), allegations of abuse (Stewart 1874), and stigma (Parsons 1881). Accounts decrying inappropriate admissions and ill treatment can be found from former patients of both public and private facilities (Geller and Harris 1994).

By the 1880s, most psychiatrists agreed that "insane patients can best be managed away from their own homes" (Parsons 1881, p. 586). Some psychiatrists postulated that "well-equipped and well-managed asylums for the insane are among the most important of the outgrowths of modern civilization and benevolence" (Parsons 1881, p. 567).

The private facilities were established for wealthier persons able to pay for more comfort, "suitable medical treatment," and "pursuits and diversions which are most congenial and desirable" ("Private Asylums" 1879, p. 243). Patients were such that when "you encounter persons variously occupied…you find yourself not infrequently quite at a loss to determine whether the persons met with are really the insane, or whether they may be visitors or officials in the establishment" (Wood 1853, p. 212). Private facilities allowed "more judicious social intercourse with the sane," greater personal freedom, more individuation of treatment, closer approximation to family life, greater ratios of physicians and attendants, and less use of "locked and bolted doors, and of barred windows" (Parsons 1881, p. 575).

Public hospitals were entities of state, county, or municipal governments, and by mid-nineteenth century states moved to centralize control and to decrease asylum superintendents' autonomy (Grob 1983). States' oversight over private facilities was extremely variable. By 1910, private facilities came under the oversight of some form of a state board in 16 states. Three other states had alternative methods of oversight. In 11 states, private facilities were required to be licensed (Bureau of the Census 1914), but many were not.

Public institutions sought to lower their censuses even as state hospital populations grew and patients had progressively longer lengths of stay (Grob 1983); private facilities sought patients to maximize their occupancy rates. A fundamental criticism of private facilities was the inherent conflict of interest of the proprietor: "It is not for the interest of the proprietor of a private asylum to cure his patients, and hence they may not make an honest effort to promote their cure" (Parsons 1881, pp. 578–579). Private facilities advertised and were not infrequently endorsed in professional journal editorials ("Two Homes for the Nervous and Insane" 1880). Advertising by private facilities and by physicians was frequent enough that a code for professional advertising was proposed in 1894 ("Provision for Professional Advertising in the Code" 1894).

By the 1880s, some states (e.g., Connecticut, Indiana, Maryland, Massachusetts, New York, Pennsylvania, Rhode Island, and Wisconsin) permitted the commitment of insane persons to private facilities (Board of State Commissioners of Public Charities of the State of Illinois 1885). To relieve crowding at state hospitals, proposals were put forward to "furlough" patients from state hospitals to private facilities in an early version of contemporary "step-down procedures" ("Insane Hospital Annexes" 1880). Similar procedures were recently used in the state of Vermont, for example, for the same reason.

Private hospitals, in contrast to public hospitals, could become quite luxurious. Long Island House, in

Amityville, New York, built a small cottage consisting of a sitting room, bedroom, bathroom, and clothes-press for a single patient in 1900 ("Long Island House, Amityville, NY" 1900). Upham house, at McLean Asylum, included nine suites, each containing a sitting room, bedroom, and bathroom; the house had two private halls, reception rooms, a dining room, a billiard room, and a Turkish bath ("The McLean Asylum for the Insane" 1893).

Greater resources led to remarkably favorable staffing ratios at private hospitals. In the 1850s, Friends Asylum had an attendant for every six patients ("The Asylum" 1851). Both Kirkbride (Pennsylvania Hospital for the Insane 1850) and Jarvis (Association of Medical Superintendents of American Institutions for the Insane 1853) described private attendants for every patient.

In 1851, John Butler, superintendent of the Hartford Retreat, noted both the importance of "mental occupations and amusements" and that many asylums were lacking in the provision of these ("Thirtieth Annual Report of the Officers of the Retreat for the Insane at Hartford, Connecticut" 1855). He repeated this theme 35 years later (Butler 1886). In this early period of inpatient psychiatry, the private facilities offered a remarkable array of activities for amusement and recreation, including baseball, boating, bowling, calisthenics and gymnasiums, concerts, cooking instruction, croquet, exhibitions, fishing, French lessons, golf, horseback riding, lantern slide shows, lectures, medicine ball, museums, pleasure grounds, reading rooms, skating, squash and tennis, stereoscopic views, tea parties, and woodcarving ("At the Pennsylvania Hospital for the Insane" 1852; "Gymnasium for the Insane" 1897; Pennsylvania Hospital for the Insane 1854). Public hospitals did less well in providing amusements but had better developed work programs that were thought to be important to patients' recovery.

Despite all their efforts, private hospitals suffered from the "premature removal of patients" (Butler Hospital for the Insane 1856; "Dr. Butler" 1851; "Dr. Stokes" 1852; Pennsylvania Hospital for the Insane 1854; Sawyer 1879). In 1851, Butler expressed concerns about the outcomes for patients who left the asylum too soon: "Many have relapsed into an incurable state, while others remain half-crazed or nervous invalids, and will probably remain so for life" ("Dr. Butler" 1851, p. 187). Isaac Ray of Butler Hospital called the premature withdrawal of patients "a most disheartening experience of our calling" (Butler Hospital for the Insane 1856, p. 252). The superintendents of the private facilities during this era (unlike public facilities) did not have the

authority to hold patients if family or friends insisted on their discharge ("Dr. Stokes" 1852). Some patients certainly left private facilities due to the inability to pay for further care (Butler Hospital for the Insane 1856; "Dr. Stokes" 1852). Ray, perhaps somewhat cavalierly, exclaimed, "We may indeed be shocked by this balancing of reason, God's greatest gift to man, with a paltry sum of money" (Butler Hospital for the Insane 1856, p. 282). Other patients were removed because family and friends were "impatient for the results" or unwilling to wait until "the disease is fully eradicated" ("Dr. Stokes" 1852, p. 211). Patients who were prematurely discharged from private facilities were not infrequently subsequently admitted to public facilities, due to the lack of an available bed, inadequate financial resources, or the patient's "unmanageable" behavior (Sawyer 1879). Others were concerned that patients discharged before they were medically ready could be a danger to the community from acts of violence (Sawyer 1879).

By the end of the 1880s, there was recognition that "the unparalleled progress in neurology, cerebral anatomy, physiology, pathology and localization of function has enlarged the horizon of our knowledge of disease and of the action of causes" (Andrews 1887, p. 199). This progress "furnished a scientific and positive basis for treatment in many cases of insanity which before was unattainable" (Andrews 1887, p. 199). Inpatient treatments near the end of the nineteenth century included electricity, massage, new medications and more rational prescribing, and oophorectomy (Andrews 1887); enforced rest (Sinkler 1892); hydrotherapy (Niles 1899); and physical training (Channing 1889). These approaches, although suspect in retrospect, represented significant advances for inpatient psychiatric treatment.

Hospitals devised new record-keeping systems to facilitate research ("McLean Hospital, Waverly" 1900); expanded clinical-pathological laboratories ("Psychiatry at the Sheppard and Enoch Pratt Hospital" 1901); focused on such diseases as dementia praecox and syphilis ("Bloomingdale Hospital, White Plains" 1913); and hired physicians with research interests and expertise ("McLean Hospital, Waverly" 1900). The new focus on research is highlighted by a statement by Edward Brush, first superintendent of Sheppard and Enoch Pratt Hospital: "the most important function [of a hospital] is to study disease, its causes, progress, processes, termination and prevention" ("Psychiatry at the Sheppard and Enoch Pratt Hospital" 1901, p. 554).

In the end, however, it was Thomas Kirkbride who made the most prophetic commentary: "So in regard to the support of hospitals for the insane, it will be a sad day for these institutions, and still sadder for the patients in them, when the rivalry of hospitals and their officers shall be, rather to discover for how little their inmates can be kept, than to secure what is best, and most thoroughly promotes the great objects for which they were established" (Kirkbride 1875, p. 99).

The Middle Period (1921–1970)

Changes in American psychiatry between 1921 and 1970 were dramatic and far reaching. In terms of treatment modalities, psychoanalysis was introduced to the inpatient setting in the 1920s. The 1930s witnessed the introduction of the somatic treatments: insulin coma, metrazol shock, and electroconvulsive therapy (ECT) (Kalinowski and Hoch 1946). In the 1940s, attention was directed to establishing milieu therapy in which "all aspects of the patient's life in the hospital were viewed as part of treatment" (Robbins 1966). In the 1950s, the introduction of the first antipsychotic medication, chlorpromazine, fundamentally altered inpatient psychiatry (Smith 1955). And in the 1960s, initial efforts to understand the mechanism of action of psychotropic drugs (Snyder et al. 1970) began efforts that to this day shape our pharmacological armamentarium.

Alternatives to psychiatric inpatient treatment, such as the day hospital, were initiated and promoted. Claims of being the "first day hospital in North America" were made by hospital staff in Boston, Montreal, and Topeka. Psychiatric inpatient treatment based in general hospitals developed during this period (American Hospital Association 1970; Glasscote and Kanno 1965). Psychiatrists attempted to improve diagnostic validity and reliability (Jackson 1970) and to promulgate standards for inpatient psychiatric facilities (American Psychiatric Association 1969). New concepts, such as the rights of mental patients, emerged (Birnbaum 1960), and old nineteenth-century ideas such as "recovery" reemerged (Menninger 1961). Insurances were developed or modified that began to cover the treatment of mental illness—both private and public.

Perhaps the most outstanding change between 1921 and 1970 was the beginning of the shift from hospital-based to non-hospital-based care and treatment of persons with mental illness, a movement retrospectively labeled "deinstitutionalization" but perhaps better characterized as "dehospitalization" (Geller 2000a). The peak year-end inpatient census for all psychiatric patients occurred in 1955.

The falling percentage of patients in public hospitals in the 1930s and 1940s was due to the creation and expansion of veterans' hospitals and in the 1960s was due, in part, to the expanding role of the general hospitals. From the 1930s through the 1960s, the percentage of the total psychiatric inpatients accounted for by the private psychiatric hospitals was steady and small. The transfer of care from public inpatient setting to "the community" during the 1950s and 1960s contributed to the decline in utilization of state hospital beds.

1920s–1930s

In 1920, the National Committee for Mental Hygiene surveyed institutions for persons with mental diseases, mental deficits, epilepsy, alcoholism, and drug addiction and found 625 institutions in the United States, 388 public and 237 private. Thirty-two states had private institutions for mental patients, but their total census accounted for only 4% of the 232,680 persons with mental disorders actually in psychiatric hospitals.

Institutions to treat persons with mental illness continued to open throughout the 1920s, whereas some private hospitals closed. In a 1923 report by the U.S. Census Bureau, there were 267,617 patients in 526 (55% public) hospitals. This rate of 242 resident patients per 100,000 general population was an increase from the 1880 rate of 82. This change was attributed to both an actual increase in the rate of mental diseases and a greater use of hospitals (Pollock 1925).

During the 1920s, psychoanalysis was introduced to hospitals. Occupational therapy, long used in public hospitals, became of greater interest to private hospitals. It was stressed that "therapeutic occupation" should be conducted off the wards in an "occupational building" (Haas 1924)—early "psychosocial rehabilitation malls."

In 1932, mental institutions represented 10% of the total number of all registered hospitals but accounted for nearly 50% of the patient population in hospitals ("Hospitals for Nervous and Mental Patients" 1933). Most patients were in public hospitals; private hospitals had just under 1% of all psychiatric inpatients ("Nineteen Hundred Thirty-Six Censuses of Mental Patients" 1938). Whereas public hospitals were struggling with limited resources for ever-expanding patient populations—420,553 nationwide in 1938—private hospitals had rather impressive staffing ratios, with 1 physician for every 17 patients ("Hospitals for Nervous and Mental Patients" 1933), 1 nurse per 3 patients, and 1 attendant per 4 patients (Grimes 1934).

Private sanatoriums, often located near large cities, were run for profit, emphasizing "comfort, hygiene, sanitation, beauty, and pleasure" (Grimes 1934). Public hospitals were generally constructed away from population centers and sometimes replaced if an urban center spread too close to the institution.

The sanatoriums were often owned by physicians, wholly or in part (Grimes 1934). The ratio of physicians to patients at sanatoriums was 1:17. The nurse-to-patient ratio was about the same, whereas the attendant-to-patient ratio was 1:3.5 ("Hospitals for Nervous and Mental Patients" 1933).

In the 1930s, somatic treatments moved from endocrine replacement therapy to narcosis, insulin convulsive therapy, metrazol shock, and electroshock therapy (Kalinowski and Hoch 1946). Other treatments included medication, hydrotherapy, psychotherapy, occupational therapy, physical therapy, and even surgery. Recreation was deemed important. Psychotherapy focused on extending patients' insight and available affective expression (Menninger 1936). Patients discharged as recovered or improved represented 65% of the total number of patients admitted (Grimes 1934).

There were also rest homes in the 1930s. These provided primarily custodial care for persons with some financial means who needed "mental medicine." Activities were limited, discharge of patients was slow, and many patients with chronic mental diseases lived their lives out in these rest homes (Grimes 1934).

New loci of treatment opened during the 1930s: the psychopathic hospital (Campbell 1930) and psychiatric ward in the general hospital (Heldt 1939). Although the presence of these psychiatric units was small (only 112 of 4,309 general hospitals had "departments for mental patients" in 1932), general hospitals were rapidly adding psychiatric units. Such units were not always welcomed by hospital medical staff, who were concerned that "noisy, destructive, violent or suicidal patients" would disrupt the general hospital (Young 1939).

The stigma of mental illness and of hospitalization were prominent no matter what the type of hospital. In 1936, the *American Journal of Psychiatry* commented on "the worry over the 'disgrace' of having been a patient in a mental hospital" ("The 'Stigma' of Mental Illness" 1936, p. 476). This editorial sadly opined that "psychosis as an illness to be considered and treated as a medical issue like other forms of disability" would do little to destigmatize the patient or the psychiatrist. Psychiatric patients organizing their own services and advocating for themselves has its modern roots in the 1930s (Friedman 1939).

1940s–1950s

The 1940s represent the nadir of America's public mental hospitals. Care of the mentally ill was described as substandard and a national disgrace. Deficiencies of state hospitals are well documented in the pages of professional journals such as *Mental Hygiene* (Klapman 1944). Exposés were available in books (Deutsch 1948), magazines (Maisel 1946), and fictionalized accounts (Ward 1946). In 1945, *The Modern Hospital* noted, "the sorriest spectacle in hospital service to-day is the treatment accorded the psychiatric patient" ("Modern Hospital Announces Prize Competition" 1945, p. 530). Private mental hospitals could not fill the need because they were just too costly. In 1945, the per capita annual expenditure in state, county, and city hospitals was $391 and in private hospitals was $2,000 ("Costs of Long-Term Mental-Hospital Care" 1949). The middle class could simply not avail themselves of private inpatient treatment. This meant that those with moderate incomes had no choice but the public hospital (Sherman and Hoffman 1950).

Attempts were made to improve inpatient treatment through the promulgation of principles and standards, such as those put forward by the Division of Mental Hygiene of the U.S. Public Health Service, the National Committee for Mental Hygiene, and the APA's Committee on Psychiatric Standards and Policies, and through surveys (Liebman and French 1949). One such survey found that of inpatient facilities with fewer than 101 patients, 44 of 46 (96%) were private; of facilities with 101–1,000 patients, 10 of 40 (25%) were private; and of facilities with more than 1,000 patients, 0 of 99 were private (Liebman and French 1949). A 1947 survey of private mental institutions found that the total number of beds for mental illness (excluding mental retardation, epilepsy, and alcohol and drug abuse) in private sanatoriums, rest homes, and psychiatric units in general hospitals was 21,956. There were 10 states and territories with no beds in these categories of hospitals; 6 had fewer than 100, 26 had 100–999, and 6 had 1,000 or more beds. States in the last category were, in descending order of number of beds, New York, Pennsylvania, California, Illinois, Maryland, and Connecticut (Sherman and Hoffman 1950).

Although there was relatively little hospital construction during the 1940s (Liebman and French 1949), the federal government became involved in the provision of inpatient psychiatric services in ways it had not done previously (Felix 1947). Much of the federal effort was directed to the public sector, but the Hill-Burton Bill funded the construction of psychiatric units in general hospitals, and the National Mental Health Act supported research and training in private psychiatric facilities.

In the 1950s, attention turned to understanding the psychiatric hospital as a social system (Greenblatt et al. 1957). There was general agreement on the objective of any mental hospital (which sounds quite contemporary) "to effect maximum improvement of the individual patient as rapidly as possible. This should mean assisting him to return to the community as a contributing member of society" (Myers and Smith 1956, p. 6). If this objective could not be met, the hospital was to work out "the best adjustment possible for the patient within or without the hospital setting, with a persistent and continuous effort to improve the adjustment" (Myers and Smith 1956, p. 6).

Private hospitals accounted for less than 3% of the total mental hospital beds, but they accounted for 25%–40% of the annual admissions to all mental hospitals (Reed 1958). Rapid turnover of patients was accomplished through a four-decade trend of maintaining fewer "hard core" patients, those hospitalized beyond 3 years' length of stay (Morris and Brunt 1957). Long-term patients were the responsibility of the state. Many psychiatrists running private psychiatric hospitals expressed concern about these hospitals' viability (Otis and Robinson 1951). The medical director of McLean Hospital stated at the 1950 APA Institute (in another quite modern-sounding refrain), "The time when you could run a private hospital as a hospital and make money has gone. Operating expenses have so increased that it is almost impossible to collect the cost from our patients" (Otis and Robinson 1951, p. 161).

Although some new private hospitals opened in the 1950s, other long-established, private mental hospitals went bankrupt, such as Norway Foundation in Indiana and Butler Hospital in Rhode Island (Reed 1958). (Butler Hospital reopened 1 year after it closed in response, in part, to public support.) The demise of these two hospitals was attributed to expanding competition from general hospital psychiatric units (Dunn 1951), the inability to charge patients what they could afford and be able to meet expenses (Reed 1958), decaying physical plants, and staff dissatisfaction (Reed 1958). Health insurance coverage that excluded mental disorders (Bennett 1959) made matters worse.

The absolute shortage of psychiatrists impacted negatively on all inpatient psychiatry. Despite an increase of 57% (from 5,534 psychiatrists in the United States to 8,713) between 1950 and 1956, there was "only one psychiatrist for every 19,200 citizens" ("Care and Treatment" 1957). Between 1948 and 1957, during most of which the public hospital census was increasing, the state hospitals improved their psychiatrist-to-patient ratio from 1:259 to 1:161. This 37.6% improvement still left them far from the APA minimum standard of 1:30 (Tallman 1960). It was estimated at the end of the decade that an additional 12,000 psychiatrists were needed (Squire 1961).

Innovations did emerge during this dark era for inpatient psychiatry, a period made worse by the burden World War II placed on these hospitals. Such innovations include the sending of follow-up questionnaires to discharged patients ("Post-Release Questionnaire" 1951), formation of ex-patient organizations ("Club Formed for Patients, Ex-Patients, and Relatives" 1950), desegregation of psychiatric hospitals (Stevens 1952), evaluation of long-term intensive inpatient psychotherapy with psychotic patients, greater emphasis on rehabilitation ("Rehabilitation of the Mentally Ill" 1954), and development of day hospitals (Hayman 1957). Somatic treatments initiated prior to 1950 continued to be used during the decade: frontal lobotomy (Freeman 1957), insulin shock therapy (Brannon and Graham 1955), and ECT (Wolfe 1955).

The beginning of modern psychopharmacology was perhaps the greatest change in inpatient psychiatry in the 1950s. Treatment with chlorpromazine was reported from both public and private hospitals (Bennett et al. 1956; Kinross-Wright 1955). Research and development expanded during the later 1950s to include promethazine (Erwin 1957), thioridazine (Cohen 1958), and imipramine (Azima and Vispo 1958).

1960s

In the 1960s, opinions about private psychiatric hospitals varied from "I doubt if many private mental hospitals will survive the next ten years" (Barton 1962, p. 661) to "The private mental hospital will continue to be the central or primary resource supplying the psychiatric needs of the community" (Jones 1964, p. 336). One private hospital attending psychiatrist proclaimed, "It is the role of the private psychiatric hospital to be the leader, the pilot, on all fronts, in exploring new areas in the prevention and treatment of mental illness, in setting and maintaining standards, in fostering true multidisciplinary cooperation and activity, and in serving the community" (Bernard 1964, p. 22). Identified advantages of private hospitals included creating a microcosm of the community at large (Wayne 1961); providing patient-centered treatment (Bernard 1964; Wayne 1961); better integrating inpatient services into longitudinal treatment of the patient (Myers 1961); better serving first admissions (Bernard 1964; Wayne 1961); treating patients for shorter lengths of stay (Garber 1961); maintaining a better-trained staff with less administrative interference with clinical practice (Bernard 1964; Myers 1961); and providing treatment in a less stigmatizing environment (Garber 1961).

Inpatient psychiatric hospitalization outside of state hospitals became more available as health insurance for hospitalization expanded to include psychiatric treatment (Coordinating Committee on Professional Standards in Psychiatry 1961). Early efforts to include psychiatric treatment were made by the Federal Employees Health Benefits Program in 1962 (Anster 1969), the United Auto Workers and the automobile industry in 1965 (Anster 1969), the Health Insurance Plan of Greater New York in 1965 (Goldensohn et al. 1969), Medicare in 1966 ("The Effect of Medicare on the Accreditation of Psychiatric Hospitals" 1966), and Blue Cross/Blue Shield nationally in 1969 (Anster 1969). Problems due to the perceived misuse of insurance for hospitalization for mental illness were already recognized in the 1960s. To remedy these, proposed interventions included peer review (Anster 1969), reimbursement for partial hospitalization and other alternatives to inpatient treatment (Felix 1965), and national health insurance (Gorman 1969). "Dumping" and "cost shifting" emerged as part of the everyday life of inpatient psychiatry. As one public hospital superintendent lamented, "Most Blue Cross plans cover mental illness for only 21 days. So the patient goes to a private institution for three weeks. If he gets well, he goes home, saved from disgrace. If he fails to get well, he comes to us. Result: we get the failures, plus the blame for having failures" (Davidson 1964, p. 280).

During the 1960s, the public sector became focused on psychotropic drugs' effects on state hospital utilization (Brill and Patton 1962) and the simultaneous use of two or more "tranquilizers," already referred to in the 1960s as "polypharmacy" (Merls et al. 1970). University departments of psychiatry and private hospitals were examining comparisons of the usefulness of the different phenothiazine derivatives (Casey et al. 1960), mechanisms of action of antidepressant medications (Schildkraut et al. 1971), and the merits of unilateral rather than bilateral ECT (Whiteborn and Betz 1960). Hospitals, especially private ones, were interested in refining the roles of the psychiatrist (Whiteborn and

Betz 1960), the nurse (Payne 1966), the social worker (Pinsky and Levy 1964), the psychiatric aide (Bernstein and Herzberg 1970), and the "multidisciplinary team" (Howard 1960). Psychiatrists grappled with understanding such concepts as therapeutic community (Gralnick and D'Elia 1969) and countertransference in milieu treatment (Wesselius 1968); improving intensive rehabilitation (Howard 1960); and understanding the effects of social competence on prognosis (Rosen et al. 1968).

Much happened in the 1960s that influences American inpatient psychiatry to this day: American presidents such as Kennedy (1964) and Johnson ("President Johnson Signs Comprehensive Health Planning Bill" 1967) showing a greater interest in mental health; members of the American bar advocating that committed psychiatric patients had a *right* to treatment (Bazelon 1969; Birnbaum 1965); new public funding streams for psychiatric treatment (Gibson 1967); and new standards for psychiatric facilities, including those defined by *Wyatt v. Stickney* (1971).

In 1966, Lawrence Kubie forecasted the necessary expansion of the private psychiatric hospital into a "treatment center" with "residential, vocational, educational and recreational" components; with "simple and natural" pathways in and out of the hospital; with intensive inpatient treatment, "night-care," and "daycare centers"; and with an expanded array of tasks and activities never previously thought to be functions of the private psychiatric hospital. Kubie (1968) doubted that the community could ever serve the needs of patients without psychiatric hospitals. Many of Kubie's thoughts echo those of his nineteenth-century predecessors.

The Modern Era (1971–2007)

It was in 1969–1970 that the Survey and Research Branch of the National Institute of Mental Health, and subsequently the Center for Mental Health Services, began to regularly collect data on all providers of mental health services. The National Association of Psychiatric Health Systems collects data annually on its membership. Other data sources include the American Hospital Association; the National Mental Health Facility Study, funded by the National Institute of Mental Health, and publishing results circa 1988; the APA and the National Association for Mental Health conjointly as the Joint Information Service; the National Association of State Mental Health Program Directors; and others.

Considering all sources of data, it is clear the total number of inpatients in the United States declined steadily from 1970 to 2000. The number of inpatient beds and percentage of the total that belonged to state hospitals declined steadily from 1970 to 1998; private hospitals showed an increase of both until a decline began after 1990; and general hospitals showed a generally steady increase in both. In 1970, the bed distribution was state hospitals, 78.7%; private hospitals, 2.7%; and general hospitals, 4.3%. By 1998, the percentages were 24.3%, 12%, and 20.7%, respectively.

The number of facilities and number of occupied beds show a similar pattern. In 1969, there were 310 state and county hospitals with 309,969 patients; private hospitals numbered 150, with a year-end census of 10,963; and the 604 general hospital psychiatric units had 17,808 beds. By 1998, the numbers had shifted: 229 state and county facilities had 56,955 patients; 348 private psychiatric hospitals had 21,478 patients; and 1,593 general hospitals had 37,002 patients. In 2000, for the first time in three decades, the number of facilities decreased in all three categories.

The total number of admissions increased progressively from 1969 through 1998, as did the percentage of admissions accounted for by private psychiatric hospitals. In the 1990s, private hospitals had small increases in the number of admissions; there were decreasing numbers of state hospital admissions generally compensated for by increased admissions to general hospitals. From the 1960s through the 1990s, the private and general hospitals consistently had a greater percentage of admissions than they did percentage of beds, reflecting shorter lengths of stay than at state and county hospitals.

The work settings and caseloads for inpatient psychiatrists shifted substantially from 1976 to 1998. In 1976, there were 45 patients per psychiatrist in public facilities, 8 per psychiatrist in private hospitals, and 5 per psychiatrist in general hospitals. Over the two decades that followed, the burden on the public psychiatrist improved, that of the private hospital psychiatrist worsened, and that of the general hospital psychiatrist experienced little change. By 1998, psychiatrists' caseloads were 20 patients in public hospitals, 12 in private hospitals, and 4.5 in general hospitals.

Expenditures per civilian population between 1969 and 2000 decreased steadily for the public hospitals, peaked for the private hospitals in 1990, and increased for the general hospitals until 1994. These expenditures for the private hospitals were 345% higher in 1990 than in 1969 but were 23% *lower* in 1994, 55% lower in 1998, and 63% lower in 2000 than in 1990.

1970s

In the 1970s, states were contemplating phasing out state hospitals ("California Announces Plans to Close State Hospital" 1973; "Massachusetts Study Proposes Phase-Out of State Mental Hospitals" 1974), and general hospital psychiatric units were becoming more of a presence (Flamm 1979). In 1971, the average number of beds in a general hospital psychiatric unit was 35 (median 28), representing about 9% of the hospital's total beds; the average length of stay was 11 days (Greenhill 1979). The expanding role of general hospital psychiatry drew caution from some who warned general hospital staff "to be on guard against some growing efforts to convert general hospital units into miniature state hospitals" (Flamm 1979, p. 191).

In the early 1970s, little attention was paid to improving the private sector's capacity for, and integrating the private sector into, the treatment of persons with the most debilitating psychiatric illnesses (Kanno 1971). However, private psychiatric hospitals began undergoing a fundamental change in the 1970s. In the 1960s, "long-term inpatient care was thought to be the best treatment money could buy" (Stone 2003); hospitals provided psychoanalytically oriented treatment at a "leisurely pace that involved months or years of hospitalization" (Hirschowitz 1974, p. 730). Declining numbers of individuals willing or able to pay for such treatment and more readily available third-party coverage led to private hospitals admitting patients of different socioeconomic and ethnic backgrounds and keeping them for shorter lengths of stay. For some, this shift was not made easily (Hirschowitz 1974).

At the end of the 1970s, the president of Pennsylvania Hospital opined on the major problems facing psychiatrists in American hospitals: 1) rising health care costs, 2) planning and coordinating of health services for the good of all segments of the community, 3) "costly," "confusing," "onerous," "duplicative," and "counterproductive regulations," 4) growing demand to collect data and provide survey information, and 5) questions about the best manner in which to govern hospitals (Cathcart 1979).

1980s

In 1982, an article published in *Hospital and Community Psychiatry* predicted private hospitals would increasingly be owned by large corporations, whereas sole-proprietorship and individual hospitals would decrease (Pottash et al. 1982). This became true, and more quickly than the authors might have imagined.

Expansion in the private sector in the 1980s was both remarkable and not distributed across the United States based on need. Distribution favored those states with the fewest regulations. By the end of the 1980s, states without "certificate of need" laws had an average of 33% more for-profit psychiatric beds than did regulated states (Sharkey 1994). About two-thirds of payments came from patients' fees in the 1980s, but Medicaid and state mental health agencies began to become more prominent payers as the 1980s progressed.

The 1980s presented a real opportunity for the growth of private psychiatric hospitals (Dorwart and Schlesinger 1988; Levenson 1982). Private corporations were ready to seize this opportunity to realize huge profits in the "psychiatric hospital industry" (Levenson 1982; Schlesinger and Dorwart 1984; Sharkey 1994). For-profit psychiatry, especially with its control of a large percentage of psychiatric beds, created its own set of problems. For-profit hospitals were the least likely to treat the most functionally disabled; would treat few, if any, patients who could not pay; usually had poorer staff-to-patient ratios than nonprofit hospitals; failed to provide education to students and professional trainees; failed to contribute adequately to research; provided a lower quality of care overall (Eisenberg 1984; Levenson 1982); were disengaged from the communities in which they were located (Dorwart et al. 1989); and hired away graduating residents from academic and public-sector jobs with higher salaries (Brodie 1983). Evidence accumulated by mid-decade did not support the belief, much to the surprise of many, that for-profit hospitals were more efficient (Schlesinger and Dorwart 1984). Nonetheless, state governments began embracing privatization of state mental health services (Dorwart et al. 1989).

In 1979, there were 7 psychiatric hospital chains (Levenson 1982). By 1982, most of the proprietary psychiatric beds were owned by chains, and the chains' power and influence rose. In 1983, there were 25 psychiatric hospital chains. By 1984, there were 75 such chains. By 1983, the for-profit psychiatric chains were dominated by four corporations: Hospital Corporation of America (HCA) in Nashville, Tennessee, with 3,162 beds; Charter Medical Corporation in Macon, Georgia, with 2,422 beds; National Medical Enterprises, Inc., in Los Angeles, California, with 1,952 beds; and Community Psychiatric Centers in Pomona, California, with 1,838 beds. The growth and revenues of these for-profit psychiatric hospital chains throughout the 1980s can only be called astounding. By the mid-1980s, the four major providers of private psychiatric hospitals/beds controlled 85% of the market (Sharkey 1994).

Proponents of psychiatric chains claimed that they were poised to take on the public sector: "By the end of the decade, the private sector will have replaced most of the psychiatric services currently provided by federal, state and local governments" (Kuntz 1981, p. 90). Although this point was never reached, innovations that could affect private–public partnerships were explored and in some instances implemented (McNeil et al. 1980).

In the early 1980s, there was a debate throughout the United States as to which sectors of psychiatric inpatient treatment should be responsible for involuntary admissions and/or difficult-to-manage patients. In 1980, the Massachusetts Psychiatric Society disseminated a position paper on involuntary psychiatric admissions to general hospitals, asserting 1) there should be separate locked and unlocked units; 2) general hospitals should not be required to lock units; 3) involuntary patients should be staffed as though they required "psychiatric intensive care"; 4) not all involuntary patients could be treated in a general hospital; 5) unresolved legal issues impeded implementation of involuntary treatment; 6) specially designed units would be required; 7) adequate reimbursement would have to be established; 8) the general hospital must be able to control its admissions and discharges; 9) partial hospital programs must be developed; and 10) there could not be "arbitrary governmental mandates" (McNeil et al. 1980).

Psychiatric hospitalization was becoming progressively more expensive, especially for the major payers: business and the federal government. Evidence emerged that private psychiatric hospitals were attempting to maximize the use of reimbursable days. A study of more than 120,000 persons ages 13–22 years showed that as days in hospital were approved at 7-day intervals, so too was there a pattern of peaks of discharge at 7-day intervals (Sharkey 1994). In a study of 32,240 discharges from private psychiatric hospitals, those discharges covered by Medicare showed a ratio of Medicare-covered days to total inpatient days near 1:1.

To counteract escalating costs, employers began to adopt mechanisms to control psychiatric hospitalizations in the late 1980s (Sharkey 1994). Early efforts, such as prospective, concurrent, and retrospective utilization review, were quickly supplemented by prospective payment, capitation, insurance deductibles, copayments, and annual limits on inpatient days. Managed care companies specializing in psychiatric services management sprang up and almost as quickly consolidated to provide a range of "products" to control costs (Geller 1998). Some of these companies were accused of overly restricting access because at-risk contracts provided them a financial incentive to do so. Monitoring a patient's progress and refusing to pay once the patient could be taken out of the hospital to less expensive alternative care was not new to this era. Similar processes had been used by cities and towns when they bore the expenses for hospitalization of their residents at asylums in the nineteenth century (Grob 1983).

The 1980s did not lack for interest in what was occurring *in* psychiatric hospitals, such as who was being treated, by what methods they were treated, and what the staff's and patients' perceptions of treatment were. A study at Highpoint Hospital in New York showed that when comparing the 1980s with the 1960s, inpatients in the 1980s were younger (mean age dropped from 38 to 25 years); less likely to be diagnosed with a schizophrenic disorder and more likely to be diagnosed with an affective disorder; considerably more likely to have a substance use disorder; less likely to be referred by a physician (a drop from 90% to 50%); and likely to have a length of stay half as long (a drop from 2 years to 1 year) (Gralnick and Caton 1992).

Researchers at the Menninger Foundation conducted a study of staff perception of difficult inpatients. Their findings indicated "withdrawn psychoticism" was the variable most related to perceived difficulty. The next most related factor was character pathology. The "suicide–depressed" and "violence–aggression" factors were less related to perceived difficulty. The authors speculated that the false notion "violence looms large" in the perception of difficulty is secondary to administrative concerns and episodic concerns about violent patients (Colson et al. 1985).

McLean Hospital staff studied patients' satisfaction with their hospital treatment 3 months after discharge. Rated as having the greatest degree of satisfaction was the high quality of the staff (especially paraprofessionals and nurses); rated as lowest was the cost of treatment. Patients were also quite dissatisfied with the information they received regarding their treatment and progress (Eisen and Grob 1982).

1990s

Throughout the 1990s, the total and average number of beds per private hospital decreased, as did the average length of stay (National Association of Private Psychiatric Hospitals 1991, 1992; National Association of Psychiatric Health Systems 1993, 1994, 1995, 1996, 1997, 1999, 2000, 2002, 2003). In the early 1990s, the practices the chain hospitals had used to fill beds were

called into question, based in part on U.S. Department of Justice intelligence regarding fraud by private hospital chains (Sharkey 1994). Hospital chains began experiencing major losses, as high as $201.9 million in 1994. Assets were falling and lawsuits were flourishing, with settlements in the hundreds of millions of dollars ("NME to Provide $2.5 Million in Free Patient Care as Part of Settlement Agreement in Texas Lawsuit" 1992; Sharkey 1994; "Tenet Agrees to Pay Patients $100 Million in Malpractice Claims" 1997).

Several phenomena affected the fate of all psychiatric hospitals in the 1990s. First among these is managed care. By 1990, the provision of utilization management (i.e., preadmission certification, concurrent utilization review and case management) had become a major industry in and of itself. Although utilization management might have some beneficial effects, Sharfstein (1990) pointed out in 1990 that "the vast majority of utilization management...has as its objective cost containment pure and simple" (p. 965).

The loss of the psychiatrist's autonomy and treatment decision-making authority produced widespread consternation (Schlesinger et al. 1996; Sharfstein 1990; Wickizer et al. 1996). In a survey of 2,541 psychiatrists with active hospital affiliations, almost two-thirds reported needing prior approval from insurance companies for admission and more than three-quarters indicated some pressure from insurance companies to discharge patients earlier than they thought clinically appropriate (Schlesinger et al. 1996). Analysis of 2,265 utilization management cases revealed an overreliance on treatment protocols and evidence that almost all cases received prior approval for the same number of days despite a wide range of diagnoses (Wickizer et al. 1996).

The fact that cost benefits were examined from the perspective of the insurer but little account was taken of the hospitals' costs in executing repeated requests for extensions of stay was particularly burdensome for psychiatric hospitals (Sharfstein 1990; Wickizer et al. 1996). In the same analysis of the 2,265 cases just mentioned, investigators found that 70% of patients were approved for one or more treatment extensions and 40% of patients with extended stays had had three or more requests (Wickizer et al. 1996).

Managed care did decrease length of stay, and it appeared to do so progressively through the decade. Shorter lengths of stay meant increased pressure on private and general hospitals to keep beds filled and increased pressure on patients. One study found that close scrutiny by insurance companies became a major stressor to patients: insurance review became a focus of treatment; staff felt pushed into demanding improvement at a rate patients could not reasonably meet; and the more adversarial and irrational the review process, the more likely it was to feed into patients' and families' preexisting psychopathology (Gabbard et al. 1991).

Psychiatric hospital staff were generally dissatisfied with utilization management firms. In findings reported from a 1990 survey of 136 hospitals, 51% of hospitals indicated that patients left against medical advice after a reviewer said that treatment would not be covered; 49% reported that patients did not receive appropriate follow-up treatment because it was not covered; 47% said that preadmission review prevented patients' hospitalizations; 48% reported that utilization management firms lacked specific psychiatric criteria; 56% indicated difficulty making telephone contact with these firms; and 82% said that reviewers were unfamiliar with local resources ("Private Psychiatric Hospitals Report Wide Dissatisfaction With Managed Care Reviews" 1990). Hospitals were particularly concerned about these firms' lack of understanding of the relationship between psychiatric symptoms and social support systems. Hospital staff were taxed by spending an average of 63 hours per week on utilization management issues ("Managed Care Survey Finds Improvements, But Problems Remain" 1991).

By 1993, a survey of 141 private psychiatric hospitals showed improvements had been made. Reviewers were more often clinicians (70% of respondents), and these reviewers usually had experience in psychiatric or substance abuse treatment (65%). However, complaints remained about preadmission reviews preventing admissions (71%), reviews requiring discharges too early (89%), and discharges against medical advice when coverage was denied (51%) (National Association of Psychiatric Health Systems 1993).

The 1990s saw the privatization of public mental health services (Dorwart and Epstein 1993) in what could be considered a return to the early-nineteenth-century utilization of private hospitals for public patients. Medicaid, Medicare, and state funds were directed to the private sector to greater degrees (Dorwart et al. 1991). States assisted freestanding private hospitals in obtaining waivers of the IMD (Institution for Mental Diseases) rule (Geller 2000a) to become Medicaid eligible (Geller 1998) and developed public-sector managed care contracts, sometimes bypassing the state's department of mental health entirely (Geller 2000b).

Evidence emerged that the private psychiatric hospitals were not equally welcoming to all public-sector patients. In national data sets (Dorwart et al. 1991; Olfson and Mechanic 1996), and in data from Maryland (Minkin et al. 1994) and Massachusetts (White et al. 1995), for example, consistent variables emerged that distinguished public from private admissions: behavioral history, diagnoses, and insurance. A greater reliance on the private system for those formerly treated in the public system precipitated many unintended consequences, including inpatient treatment farther from one's home community (Geller 1991), less continuity of inpatient treatment and associated longer lengths of stay (Geller et al. 1998), new loci and patterns of recidivism (Geller et al. 1998), and an ongoing debate about quality of care in private versus public settings (Dorwart et al. 1991). One measure of quality of care, staffing ratios (Dorwart et al. 1991), showed a narrowing of the difference between public and private facilities as the ratio of psychiatrists to patients improved in the public sector.

The concept of treatment in the "least restrictive alternative" affected all inpatient settings. An ill-defined concept, such treatment nonetheless was used to justify many alternatives to inpatient settings. The general and private hospitals were seen as less restrictive than the public hospitals for not entirely clear reasons (Geller 1991), but all manner of alternative service arrangements were seen as less restrictive than *any* hospital for acute or longer-term care and treatment (Geller 2000b; Sledge et al. 1996).

2000–2007

In 2001, the United States had 5,558 nonfederal hospitals, of which 479 were psychiatric hospitals. These hospitals had a total of 88,762 beds and 25,078,529 inpatient days. Of 4,728 general hospitals, there were 1,778 (37%) with psychiatric inpatient care. Inpatient psychiatry in the United States had become a *business*. As one observer noted, "Madness has become an industrialized product to be managed efficiently and nationally in a timely manner as it passes through the hands of clinic workers" (Donald 2001, p. 435).

In a meta-analysis comparing for-profit and nonprofit psychiatric inpatient care between 1980 and 2001, the major finding was the "performance superiority of the nonprofit psychiatric providers compared with the for-profit providers...the overwhelming majority of the studies undermine a performance rationale for public policy decisions to expand for-profit inpatient healthcare" (Rosenau and Linder 2003, p. 186). Nonetheless, that is what state governments continued to do. Downsizing state workforces appeared to take precedence over other considerations.

The practice of psychiatry appears to have shifted in response to shorter lengths of stay. A study at McLean Hospital in 2002 comparing inpatient antipsychotic medication use in 1989, 1993, and 1998 showed that the chlorpromazine-equivalent final total dosage of all antipsychotic medications used at discharge in 1998 was 29.3% greater than in 1993 and 46.1% greater than in 1989. The average time from admission to first antipsychotic dose decreased precipitously from 6.8 days in 1989 to 1.5 days in 1993 and 0.9 days in 1998. Two or more antipsychotic medications were used during 20% of inpatient days in 1998, 4 times the use in 1993 and more than 10 times the use in 1989 (Centorrino et al. 2002).

Since 2000, more attention has been paid to managed care's effects on inpatient utilization, and the voices of critics have not quieted. One critic lamented, "These managed care algorithms represent more than they claim, for they do not represent an advance in scientific knowledge of the Natural world of mental illness so much as they reproduce a moral ideology and actively encourage a notion of personhood and a psychiatric science more suitable to business and consumer culture" (Donald 2001, p. 435).

Much of the financial news of the early years of the twenty-first century bodes poorly for psychiatric hospitals. Although overall health care spending increased by 15.7% between 1992 and 1999, mental health and substance abuse spending decreased by 17.4%. Behavioral health care spending went from 7.2% of total private health insurance spending to 5.1% during this same time period (National Association of Psychiatric Health Systems 2003b).

These changes are impacting all psychiatric hospitals. Total and per-capita expenditures for services in private hospitals are falling disproportionately to lower inpatient utilization. Between 1994 and 2000, utilization decreased by 32% whereas expenditures decreased by 56%. The public hospitals did not fare as poorly: beds decreased by 25% and expenditures by 29%. The general hospital units actually had a lower decrease in expenditures (13.5%) than in beds (23%). Although inpatient occupancy rates rose in the private hospitals (there are fewer hospitals), hospitals offering partial programs or those offering outpatient services dropped by 20%–25% between 2000 and 2001 (National Association of Psychiatric Health Systems 2003a). Reimbursement rates have fallen such that they often do not even meet the total costs of care and treatment (Frank et al. 2003). As reimbursement rates fall, costs to deliver treatment increase, attributable to workforce shortages, increasing professional

liability insurance, escalating pharmaceutical costs, and more regulatory requirements (National Association of Psychiatric Health Systems 2003b).

Oversight is increasing. As one example, the Office of the Inspector General of the Department of Health and Human Services has stepped up its investigation of inpatient Medicaid claims for 21- to 64-year-olds who were patients in freestanding psychiatric hospitals (Office of Inspector General 2002, 2003) while criticizing the Centers for Medicare and Medicaid Services for conducting an inadequate number of surveys and for being too reliant on the findings of the Joint Commission on Accreditation of Healthcare Organizations. The Office of the Inspector General recommended a minimum number of facility reviews per cycle and a coordination of efforts of all external reviewers.

Public hospitals also face uncertain economic times. Medicaid's progressive decrease of disproportionate share payments to public mental hospitals (Office of Inspector General 2002) is stressing some states' ability to operate their public system at its pre-2000 scale.

The landscape of American inpatient psychiatry, both private and public, is changing dramatically in the first decade of the twenty-first century. In 2001, the five private psychiatric hospitals remaining in Maryland were having financial problems. More than 50% of their admissions were publicly funded, and reimbursement was about $100 per day less than costs (Taylor 2001). One of these hospitals, Taylor Manor, sold its license to operate inpatient and adolescent residential beds to Sheppard Pratt Health System. Another, Chestnut Lodge, closed its doors in April 2001 after 90 years in operation; it was bankrupt, and a public effort to save it was unsuccessful. In the spring of 2000, the Menninger Clinic of Topeka, Kansas, needed a dramatic fix. The previous year the clinic had had 2,238 admissions to its 143 beds but lost $2.9 million. Menninger Clinic transferred its 48-bed acute program to another hospital in Topeka and moved the rest of its operation to Houston, Texas (Petterson 2002).

In the public sector, state actions are all over the place. States, counties, and municipalities continue to close public hospitals even in the face of negative press about alternatives (Bonner 2007; Sullivan and Seligman 2003). Pennsylvania continued to downsize its public bed supply, closing several hospitals. North Carolina was building a new hospital to replace two hospitals in the Raleigh area; Massachusetts was doing the same in the central part of the state. Vermont has plans to close its 50-bed state hospital and partner with the University of Vermont to build a new hospital. Oregon is replacing its aging state hospital in Salem with two new facilities. Nevada has opened two state hospitals since 2000. California built a 1,500-bed facility for forensically committed individuals, representing the first new California facility in more than 50 years. New Jersey replaced Greystone Park Psychiatric Hospital. The list goes on.

States continue to operate their public hospitals under two distinct models: those that take acute patients (mostly the uninsured, underinsured, publicly insured, or behaviorally out-of-control) and those that direct all acute admissions to the private sector, reserving the state hospitals for the longer-term patients. Most states have seen the percentage of forensically committed patients climb dramatically (Bloom 2006; Texas Department of State Health Services 2006) despite concurrent transinstitutionalization to jails and prisons. The state hospital situation has raised more concerns about staff safety than have been heard for decades and led one medical director to quip, "We used to be civil."

Conclusion

Inpatient psychiatry started out with the best of intentions, awash in "magnificent beneficence" (President Franklin Pierce's description), with asylums reporting cure rates approaching 100%. All too soon the powerful scourge that insanity proved to be simply overwhelmed available resources. Take Danvers State Hospital in Massachusetts, for example. It opened in May 1878 amidst public admiration that it was "light, airy, cheerful...with magnificent arrangements" ("Opening of the Hospital" 1878). The facilities were such that persons might not even know they were in an asylum, and hence the cutlery was stamped only "Danvers," not "Danvers Asylum" or "Danvers Hospital" ("Opening of the Hospital" 1878). At the turn of the twentieth century, the hospital's caliber of professional care and treatment was such that no restraint or seclusion was used (Page 1904). Yet the hospital's superintendent was soon lamenting, "It may be asserted that the lunatic hospital, per se, is not a remedy for insanity. In fact, as generally regarded by its inmates, it provokes inimical effects and in some cases aggravates the mental disease.... The physician may render some important service, but he is greatly in the dark as to the actual requirement" (Ramseur 2005, p. 103). By 1946, conditions were simply frightening. On September 13 of that year, there were nine staff persons to cover 13 wards with a census of 2,300 patients (Ramseur 2005).

In the first decade of the twenty-first century, inpatient psychiatry appears to be in a position to move back toward its roots of enlightened care and treatment. To do so, and to avoid descending into a state like the abyss that followed World War II, all aspects of inpatient psychiatric treatment should be under review. Hence this book.

Psychiatric hospitals are shrinking, growing, being torn down, and being newly built all at the same time. Debates are ongoing as to the actual effect of public-sector managed care (Domino et al. 2004) and the misutilization of jails and prisons as substitutes for psychiatric hospital beds (Banks et al. 2000; Domino et al. 2004). Persons in need of inpatient treatment, be it acute or longer term, find themselves at a loss because the beds do not exist (Bloom 2006). Beds may not exist or be accessible because the size of the network's providers is limited as a means of controlling cost, and/or reimbursement rates are lower than the hospital's expenditures (Appelbaum 2003). As if that is not enough, the Centers for Medicare & Medicaid Services is phasing in the prospective payment system for inpatient psychiatry; armed forces returning from Iraq and Afghanistan are putting new demands on the mental health system (Hoge et al. 2004); and some fear that privatization of formerly public inpatient services means less oversight, with risks to persons with serious mental illness (Holcomb and Heyman 2002). However, none of these problems is insurmountable. All persons involved in the design, implementation, funding, and monitoring of hospital psychiatry need to recognize the fundamental role hospital psychiatry plays in our health care system.

As the future of hospital psychiatry evolves in this century, perhaps we would do well to keep in mind the sage advice Edward Jarvis gave to the AMSAII in the mid-nineteenth century:

> The wise manager of the insane carefully analyzes the condition of his patients, and ascertains what elements are diseased and what are sound. Having determined this, he cautiously respects and avoids all interference with every power and faculty, every principle, opinion, emotion, taste or desire, that is in good health, and applies his influence only to such as are not in good condition, and this he does in such a way as not to disturb the others. He therefore, so far as is consistent with the patient's recovery or best progress, applies no restraint, opposes no purpose, denies no indulgence, contradicts no opinions that are not disordered, and do not minister to the disease. Thus he sustains as great an amount of healthy

mental and moral constitution as possible, by means of which he hopes to overcome the disturbance in those which are diseased. (Jarvis 1860, p. 28)

References

American Hospital Association: Mental Health Services and the General Hospital: A Guide to the Development and Implementation of Mental Health Service Plans. Chicago, IL, American Hospital Association, 1970

American Psychiatric Association: Standards for Psychiatric Facilities. Washington, DC, American Psychiatric Association, 1969

Andrews JB: The distribution and care of the insane in the United States. Am J Insanity 44:192–211, 1887

Anster SL: Insurance coverage for "mental and nervous conditions": developments and problems. Am J Psychiatry 126:698–705, 1969

Appelbaum PS: The "quiet" crisis in mental health services. Health Aff 22:110–116, 2003

Association of Medical Superintendents of American Institutions for the Insane: Proceedings of the Eighth Annual Meeting of the AMSAII. Second day—morning session. Am J Insanity 10:74–79, 1853

At the Pennsylvania Hospital for the Insane. Am J Insanity 9:183–185, 1852

Azima H, Vispo RH: Imipramine: a potent new anti-depressant compound. Am J Psychiatry 115:245–246, 1958

Banks SM, Stone JL, Pandiani JA, et al: Utilization of local jails and general hospitals by state psychiatric center patients. J Behav Health Serv Res 27:454–459, 2000

Barton WE: Administration in Psychiatry. Springfield, IL, Charles C Thomas, 1962

Bazelon DL: The right to treatment: the court's role. Hosp Community Psychiatry 20:129–135, 1969

Bennett AE: Problems establishing and maintaining psychiatric units in general hospitals. Am J Psychiatry 115:974–979, 1959

Bennett AE, Ford FC, Turk RE: Clinical investigation of chlorpromazine and reserpine in private psychiatric practice. Am J Psychiatry 112:782–787, 1956

Bernard RI: The position of the private psychiatric hospital. Ment Hosp 15:19–22, 1964

Bernstein S, Herzberg J: Small group experience with psychiatric aides. Ment Hygiene 54:113–117, 1970

Birnbaum M: The right to treatment. Am Bar Assoc J 46:499–505, 1960

Birnbaum M: Some comments on "the right to treatment." Arch Gen Psychiatry 13:34–45, 1965

Bloom JD: Civil commitment is disappearing in Oregon. J Am Acad Psychiatry Law 34:534–537, 2006

Bloomingdale Hospital, White Plains. Am J Insanity 70:536–537, 1913

Board of State Commissioners of Public Charities of the State of Illinois: Eighth Biennial Report of the Board of State Commissioners of Public Charities of the State of Illinois. Springfield, IL, H.W. Rokker, 1885

Bonner L: Scarcity of mental-health care traps patients in vicious cycle. News and Observer, March 4, 2007, p 1

Brannon EP, Graham WL: Intensive insulin shock therapy: a five-year survey. Am J Psychiatry 111:659–663, 1955

Brill H, Patton, RE: Clinical-statistical analysis of population changes in New York State mental hospitals since introduction of psychotropic drugs. Am J Psychiatry 119:20–35, 1962

Brodie HKH: Presidential address: psychiatry—its locus and its future. Am J Psychiatry 140:965–968, 1983

Bureau of the Census: Insane and Feeble-Minded in Institutions, 1910. Washington, DC, Government Printing Office, 1914

Butler Hospital for the Insane: Report of the trustees and superintendent of the Butler Hospital for the Insane. Am J Insanity 12:280–285, 1856

Butler Hospital for the Insane: Report of the Butler Hospital for the Insane, 1877. Am J Insanity 34:548, 1878

Butler JS: The individualized treatment of the insane. Alienist Neurol 7:435–460, 1886

California announces plans to close state hospital. Hosp Community Psychiatry 24:249, 1973

Campbell CM: The work of the psychopathic hospital. Ment Hygiene 14:883–900, 1930

Care and treatment. Ment Hygiene 41:589, 1957

Casey JF, Laskey JJ, Klett JC, et al: Treatment of schizophrenic reactions with phenothiazine derivatives: a comparison study of chlorpromazine, trifluoperazine, mepazine, prochlorperazine, perphenazine and phenobarbital. Am J Psychiatry 117:97–105, 1960

Cathcart HR: Issues facing American hospitals. Hosp Community Psychiatry 30:193–194, 1979

Centorrino F, Eakin M, Bahk WM, et al: Inpatient antipsychotic drug use in 1998, 1993, and 1989. Am J Psychiatry 159:1932–1935, 2002

Channing W: Physical training of the insane. Am J Insanity 46:166–175, 1889

Club formed for patients, ex-patients, and relatives. APA Mental Hospital Services Bulletin 1:6, 1950

Cohen S: TP-ZI, a new phenothiazine. Am J Psychiatry 115:358, 1958

Colson DB, Allen JG, Coyne L, et al: Patterns of staff perception of difficult patients in a long-term psychiatric hospital. Hosp Community Psychiatry 36:168–172, 1985

Connecticut. Retreat for the Insane. Am J Insanity 2:66–68, 1845

Connecticut. Forty-fifth and forty-sixty annual reports of the officers of the Retreat for the Insane at Hartford, Conn: 1869 and 1870. Am J Insanity 27:326, 1871

Coordinating Committee on Professional Standards in Psychiatry: Report of the Coordinating Committee on Professional Standards in Psychiatry. Am J Psychiatry 117:757–760, 1961

Costs of long-term mental-hospital care. Ment Hygiene 33:155–156, 1949

Davidson HA: The snake pits hiss back: a letter to the APA from a hospital superintendent. Am J Psychiatry 121:279–280, 1964

Death of Dr. George Cook. Am J Insanity 33:132–135, 1876

Deutsch A: The Shame of the States. New York, Harcourt, Brace, 1948

Deutsch A: The Mentally Ill in America. New York, Columbia University Press, 1949

Domino ME, Norton EC, Morrissey JP, et al: Cost shifting to jails after a change to managed mental health care. Health Serv Res 39:1379–1402, 2004

Donald A: The Wal-Marting of American psychiatry: an ethnography of psychiatric practice in the late 20th century. Cult Med Psychiatry 25:427–439, 2001

Dorwart RA, Epstein SS: Privatization and Mental Health Care: A Fragile Balance. Westport, CT, Auburn House, 1993

Dorwart RA, Schlesinger M: Privatization of psychiatric services. Am J Psychiatry 145:543–553, 1988

Dorwart RA, Schlesinger M, Horgan C, et al: The privatization of mental health care and directions for mental health services research, in The Future of Mental Health Services Research (DHHS Publ No ADM-89-1600). Edited by Taube CA, Mechanic D, Hohmann AA. Washington, DC, U.S. Government Printing Office, 1989

Dorwart RA, Schlesinger M, Davidson H, et al: A national study of psychiatric hospital care. Am J Psychiatry 148:204–210, 1991

Dr. Butler of the Hartford Retreat for the Insane. Am J Insanity 8:187–188, 1851

Dr. Stokes, Eighth Annual Report of the Mount Hope Institution, near Baltimore, for 1850. Am J Insanity 8:209–212, 1852

Dunn WH: Mental-health opportunities in the general hospital. Ment Hygiene 35:190–198, 1951

Earle P: Historical and descriptive account of the Bloomingdale Asylum for the Insane. Am J Insanity 2:1–12, 1845

Eisen SV, Grob MC: Measuring discharged patients' satisfaction with care at a private psychiatric hospital. Hosp Community Psychiatry 33:227–228, 1982

Eisenberg L: The case against for-profit hospitals. Hosp Community Psychiatry 35:1009–1013, 1984

Erwin HJ: Clinical observations on the use of promethazine hydrochloride in psychiatric disorders. Am J Psychiatry 113:783–787, 1957

Felix RH: The National Mental Health Act. Ment Hygiene 31:363–374, 1947

Felix RH: Improving health insurance coverage for psychiatric illness. Am J Psychiatry 121:731–735, 1965

Flamm GH: The expanding roles of general-hospital psychiatry. Hosp Community Psychiatry 30:190–191, 1979

Forbush B: The Sheppard and Enoch Pratt Hospital, 1853–1970: A History. Philadelphia, PA, JB Lippincott, 1971

Frank RG, Goldman HH, Hogan M: Medicaid and mental health: be careful what you ask for. Health Aff 22:101–113, 2003

Freeman W: Frontal lobotomy 1936–1956: a follow-up study of 3,000 patients from one to twenty years. Am J Psychiatry 113:877–886, 1957

Friedman JH: An organization of ex-patients of a psychiatric hospital. Ment Hygiene 23:414–420, 1939

From the report of the McLean Asylum. Am J Insanity 21:235–238, 1864

Gabbard GO, Takahashi T, Davidson J, et al: A psychodynamic perspective on the clinical impact of insurance review. Am J Psychiatry 148:318–323, 1991

Garber RS: The private hospital's responsibility for leadership. Ment Hosp 12:16–17, 1961

Geller JL: Any place but the state hospital: examining assumptions about benefits of admission diversion. Hosp Community Psychiatry 42:145–152, 1991

Geller JL: Mental health services for the future: managed care, unmanaged care, mismanaged care, in Humane Managed Care? Edited by Schamess G, Lightburn A. Washington, DC, National Association of Social Workers, 1998, pp 36–50

Geller JL: Excluding institutions for mental diseases from federal reimbursement for services: strategy or tragedy. Psychiatr Serv 51:1397–1403, 2000a

Geller JL: The last half-century of psychiatric services as reflected in Psychiatric Services. Psychiatr Serv 51:41–67, 2000b

Geller JL: Avoiding extinction: successful private psychiatric hospitals in the opening decade of the twenty-first century. Psychiatr Q 77:251–271, 2006

Geller JL, Harris M: Women of the Asylum. New York, Anchor Books, 1994

Geller JL, Fisher WH, McDermeit M, et al: The effects of public managed care on patterns of intensive use of inpatient psychiatric services. Psychiatr Serv 49:327–332, 1998

Gibson RW: Title XIX: psychiatric provisions and limitations. Hosp Community Psychiatry 18:88–91, 1967

Glasscote RM, Kanno CK: General Hospital Psychiatric Units: A National Survey. Washington, DC, American Psychiatric Association and National Association for Mental Health, 1965

Goldensohn SS, Fink R, Shapiro S: Referral, utilization, and staffing patterns of a mental health service in a pre-paid group practice program in New York. Am J Psychiatry 126:689–697, 1969

Gorman M: National Health Insurance: an idea whose time has come. Am J Psychiatry 126:708–711, 1969

Gralnick A, Caton CLM: Long-term hospital treatment: a 25-year study. Psychiatr Q 63:199–208, 1992

Gralnick A, D'Elia F: A psychoanalytic hospital becomes a therapeutic community. Hosp Community Psychiatry 20:144–146, 1969

Greenblatt M, Levinson DJ, Williams RH: The Patient and the Mental Hospital. Glencoe, IL, Free Press, 1957

Greenhill MH: Psychiatric units in general hospitals: 1979. Hosp Community Psychiatry 30:169–182, 1979

Grimes JM: Institutional Care of Mental Patients in the United States. Chicago, IL, Author, 1934

Grob GN: Mental Illness and American Society, 1875–1990. Princeton, NJ, Princeton University Press, 1983

Gymnasium for the insane. Am J Insanity 53:626–627, 1897

Haas LJ: The backbone of an occupational building for mental and nervous patients. Ment Hygiene 8:737–752, 1924

Hayman M: A unique day therapy center for psychiatric patients. Ment Hygiene 41:245–249, 1957

Heldt TJ: Psychiatric services in general hospitals. Am J Psychiatry 95:865–871, 1939

Hirschowitz RG: Two psychiatric hospitals in transition: studies in staff behavior. Hosp Community Psychiatry 25:730–733, 1974

Hoge CW, Castro CA, Messer SC, et al: Combat duty in Iraq and Afghanistan, mental health problems, and barriers to care. N Engl J Med 351:13–22, 2004

Holcomb J, Heyman M: Closing a state hospital. Psychiatr Serv 53:1179–1180, 2002

Hospitals for nervous and mental patients. JAMA 100:895–897, 901–910, 1933

Howard BF: An optimistic report on total rehabilitative potential of chronic schizophrenics. Arch Gen Psychiatry 3:345–356, 1960

Hurd HM: Three-quarters of a century of institutional care of the insane in the United States. Am J Insanity 69:469–481, 1913

Hurd HM (ed): The Institutional Care of the Insane in the United States and Canada. Baltimore, MD, Johns Hopkins Press, 1916

Insane hospital annexes. Alienist Neurol 1:558, 1880

Jackson B: The revised Diagnostic and Statistical Manual of the American Psychiatric Association. Am J Psychiatry 127:65–73, 1970

Jarvis E: On the proper functions of private institutions or homes for the insane. Am J Insanity 17:19–31, 1860

Jones CH: Discussion. Ment Hosp 15:336, 1964

Kalinowski LB, Hoch PH: Shock Treatments and Other Somatic Procedures in Psychiatry. New York, Grune & Stratton, 1946

Kanno CK: Eleven Indices: An Aid in Reviewing State and Local Mental Health and Hospital Programs. Washington, DC, Joint Information Service, 1971

Kennedy JF: Message from the President of the United States relative to mental illness and mental retardation. Am J Psychiatry 120:729–737, 1964

Kinross-Wright V: Chlorpromazine treatment of mental disorders. Am J Psychiatry 111:907–912, 1955

Kirkbride TS: A sketch of the history, building, and organization of the Pennsylvania Hospital for the Insane. Am J Insanity 2:97–114, 1845

Kirkbride TS: Pennsylvania. Report of the Pennsylvania Hospital for the Insane, 1874. Am J Insanity 32:95–99, 1875

Klapman JW: Public relationships of the mental hospital. Ment Hygiene 28:381–396, 1944

Kubie L: The future of the private psychiatric hospital. Int J Psychiatry 6:419–433, 1968

Kuntz E: Hospital chains grab psychiatric business from government facilities. Mod Healthc 11(11):90, 1981

Levenson AI: The growth of investor-owned psychiatric hospitals. Am J Psychiatry 139:902–907, 1982

Liebman S, French RL: Patient population distribution in mental hospitals in the United States. Am J Psychiatry 105:489–493, 1949

Long Island House, Amityville, NY. Am J Insanity 57:403, 1900

Maisel AQ: Bedlam 1946. Life 20:102–118, 1946

Managed care survey finds improvements, but problems remain. Hosp Community Psychiatry 42:964–965, 1991

Massachusetts. McLean Asylum for the Insane. Am J Insanity 2:55–58, 1845

Massachusetts study proposes phase-out of state mental hospitals. Hosp Community Psychiatry 25:492–493, 1974

McLean Hospital, Waverly. Am J Insanity 57:397–399, 1900

McNeil DN, Stevenson J, Longabaugh RH: Short-term inpatient care and readmission rates: the CMHC approach versus the private approach. Hosp Community Psychiatry 31:751–755, 1980

Menninger K: The course of illness. Bull Menninger Clin 25:225–240, 1961

Menninger WC: Psychiatric hospital therapy designed to meet unconscious needs. Am J Psychiatry 93:347–360, 1936

Merls S, Sheppard C, Collins L, et al: Polypharmacy in psychiatry: patterns of differential treatment. Am J Psychiatry 126:1647–1651, 1970

Minkin EB, Stoline AM, Sharfstein SS: An analysis of the two-class system of care in public and private psychiatric hospitals. Hosp Community Psychiatry 45:975–977, 1994

Modern Hospital announces prize competition. Ment Hygiene 29:530–531, 1945

Morris HH, Brunt MY: Disposition of first admissions to a private psychiatric hospital, 1920–1951. Am J Psychiatry 113:1024–1029, 1957

Myers JM: Experiences at the Institute of the Pennsylvania Hospital. Ment Hosp 12:39–40, 1961

Myers JM, Smith LH: The organization of a mental hospital. Ment Hosp 7(6):6–10, 1956

National Association of Private Psychiatric Hospitals: 1990 Annual Survey. Final Report. Washington, DC, National Association of Private Psychiatric Hospitals, 1991

National Association of Private Psychiatric Hospitals: 1991 Annual Survey: Final Report. Washington, DC, National Association of Private Psychiatric Hospitals, 1992

National Association of Psychiatric Health Systems: 1992 Annual Survey: Final Report. Washington, DC, National Association of Psychiatric Health Systems, 1993

National Association of Psychiatric Health Systems: 1993 Annual Survey: Final Report. Washington, DC, National Association of Psychiatric Health Systems, 1994

National Association of Psychiatric Health Systems: Trends in Psychiatric Health Systems: A Benchmarking Report. National Association of Psychiatric Health Systems 1995 Annual Survey Report. Washington, DC, National Association of Psychiatric Health Systems, 1995

National Association of Psychiatric Health Systems: Trends in Psychiatric Health Systems: A Benchmarking Report. National Association of Psychiatric Health Systems 1996 Annual Survey Report. Washington, DC, National Association of Psychiatric Health Systems, 1996

National Association of Psychiatric Health Systems: Trends in Behavioral Healthcare Systems: A Benchmarking Report. National Association of Psychiatric Health Systems 1997 Annual Survey Report. Washington, DC, National Association of Psychiatric Health Systems, 1997

National Association of Psychiatric Health Systems: Trends in Behavioral Healthcare Systems: A Benchmarking Report. National Association of Psychiatric Health Systems 1998 Annual Survey Report. Washington, DC, National Association of Psychiatric Health Systems, 1999

National Association of Psychiatric Health Systems: Trends in Behavioral Healthcare Systems: A Benchmarking Report. National Association of Psychiatric Health Systems 2000 Annual Survey Report. Washington, DC, National Association of Psychiatric Health Systems, 2000

National Association of Psychiatric Health Systems: Trends in Behavioral Healthcare Systems: A Benchmarking Report. National Association of Psychiatric Health Systems 2001 Annual Survey Report. Washington, DC, National Association of Psychiatric Health Systems, 2002

National Association of Psychiatric Health Systems: Trends in Behavioral Healthcare Systems: A Benchmarking Report. National Association of Psychiatric Health Systems 2002 Annual Survey Report. Washington, DC, National Association of Psychiatric Health Systems, 2003a

National Association of Psychiatric Health Systems: Challenges Facing Behavioral Health Care: The Pressures on Essential Behavioral Healthcare Services. Washington, DC, National Association of Psychiatric Health Systems, 2003b

New York. Report of the Bloomingdale Asylum, 1871. Am J Insanity 28:549, 1872

Niles HR: Hydrotherapy in the treatment of mental diseases. Am J Insanity 55:443–447, 1899

Nineteen hundred thirty-six censuses of mental patients. Ment Hygiene 22:340, 1938

NME to provide $2.5 million in free patient care as part of settlement agreement in Texas lawsuit. Hosp Community Psychiatry 43:852–853, 1992

Office of Inspector General: Review of Medicaid Inpatient Psychiatric Claims for 21- to 64-Year-Old Residents of Private Psychiatric Hospitals That Are Institutions for Mental Diseases in California During the Period July 1, 1997 through January 31, 2001. Washington, DC, U.S. Department of Health and Human Services, 2002

Office of Inspector General: Review of Medicaid Claims for 21- to 64-Year-Old Residents of Private Psychiatric Hospitals in Texas That Are Institutions for Mental Diseases. Washington, DC, U.S. Department of Health and Human Services, 2003

Olfson M, Mechanic D: Mental disorders in public, private nonprofit and proprietary general hospitals. Am J Psychiatry 153:1613–1619, 1996

Opening of the hospital. Danvers Mirror, May 18, 1878

Otis WJ, Robinson GW: Private hospitals, in Mental Hospitals 1950. Edited by Overholser W. Washington, DC, American Psychiatric Association, 1951, pp 159–171

Page CW: Mechanical restraint and seclusion of insane persons. Boston Med Surg J 151:590–595, 1904

Parsons RL: On the private care of the insane. Alienist Neurol 2:564–588, 1881

Payne SM: The evolution of therapeutic care and clinical specialization in psychiatric nursing. Perspect Psychiatr Care 4:12–19, 1966

Pennsylvania. Asylum for the relief of persons deprived of the use of their reason. Am J Insanity 2:147–151, 1845

Pennsylvania Hospital for the Insane: Report of the Pennsylvania Hospital for the Insane for the year 1849. Am J Insanity 6:322–329, 1850

Pennsylvania Hospital for the Insane: Report of the Pennsylvania Hospital for the Insane for the year 1853. Am J Insanity 11:186–188, 1854

Peterson F: Twentieth century methods of provision for the insane. Am J Insanity 58:405–415, 1902

Petterson JL: Topeka's Menninger Clinic to create partnership, move to Houston. The Kansas City Star, December 5, 2002

Pinsky S, Levy ES: Social group work in a private hospital. Ment Hosp 15:516–524, 1964

Pollock HM: Book Review: Report of Census of Institutions for Mental Disease, U.S. Census Bureau. Washington, DC, Government Printing Office, 1925

Pollock HM, Forbush EM: Patients with mental disease, mental defect, epilepsy, alcoholism and drug addiction in institutions in the United States, January 1, 1920. Ment Hygiene 5:139–169, 1921

Post-release questionnaire. APA Mental Hospital Services Bulletin 2:5, 1951

Pottash ALC, Gold MS, Bloodworth R, et al: The future of private psychiatric hospitals. Hosp Community Psychiatry 33:735–739, 1982

President Johnson signs comprehensive health planning bill. Hosp Community Psychiatry 18(1):59, 1967

Private asylums. Boston Med Surg J 101:243, 1879

Private psychiatric hospitals report wide dissatisfaction with managed care reviews. Hosp Community Psychiatry 41:938, 941, 1990

Provision for professional advertising in the Code. Alienist Neurol 15:135–137, 1894

Psychiatry at the Sheppard and Enoch Pratt Hospital. Am J Insanity 57:553–558, 1901

Ramseur M: Haunted Palace: Danvers Asylum as Art and History. South Harwich, MA, ARTSHIP Publishing, 2005

Ray I: The Butler Hospital for the Insane. Am J Insanity 5:1–24, 1848

Reed PB: The role of the private psychiatric hospital. Ment Hosp 9:34–35, 1958

Rehabilitation of the mentally ill. Mental Hygiene 38:692–693, 1954

Robbins LL: Reflections 1940–1966. Bull Menninger Clin 30:190–206, 1966

Rosen B, Klein DF, Levenstein S, et al: Social competence and posthospital outcome. Arch Gen Psychiatry 19:165–170, 1968

Rosenau PV, Linder SH: A comparison of the performance of for-profit and non-profit U.S. psychiatric inpatient care providers since 1980. Psychiatr Serv 54:183–187, 2003

Sawyer JW: Rhode Island. Report of the Butler Hospital for the Insane: 1878. Am J Insanity 35:584–586, 1879

Schildkraut JJ, Winokur A, Draskocy PR, et al: Changes in norepinephrine turnover in rat brains during chronic administration of imipramine and protriptyline: a possible explanation for the delay in onset of clinical antidepressant effects. Am J Psychiatry 127:1032–1039, 1971

Schlesinger M, Dorwart R: Ownership and mental-health services. N Engl J Med 311:959–965, 1984

Schlesinger M, Dorwart RA, Epstein SS: Managed care constraints on psychiatrists' hospital practices: bargaining power and professional autonomy. Am J Psychiatry 153:256–260, 1996

Sharfstein SS: Utilization management: managed or mangled psychiatric care? Am J Psychiatry 147:965–966, 1990

Sharkey J: Bedlam, Greed, Profiteering, and Fraud in a Mental Health System Gone Crazy. New York, St. Martin's, 1994

Sherman IC, Hoffman HR: Facilities in private mental institutions in the United States and Canada. Am J Psychiatry 106:268–269, 1950

Sinkler W: Diseases and conditions to which the rest treatment is adapted. J Nerv Ment Dis 17:321–338, 1892

Sledge WH, Tebes J, Wolff N, et al: Day hospital/crisis respite care versus inpatient care, part II: service utilization and costs. Am J Psychiatry 153:1074–1083, 1996

Smith K: Chlorpromazine and Mental Health. Philadelphia, PA, Lea & Febiger, 1955

Snyder SH, Taylor KM, Coyle JT, et al: The role of brain dopamine in behavioral regulation and the actions of psychotropic drugs. Am J Psychiatry 127:199–207, 1970

Squire MB: Open-staff policy opens the door to improved psychiatric therapy. Hospitals 35:64–67, 1961

Stevens RB: Interracial practices in mental hospitals. Ment Hygiene 36:56–65, 1952

Stewart WF: Maryland. Forty-Third Report of the Maryland Hospital for the Insane: 1872–1873. Am J Insanity 31:101–102, 1874

Stone AA: Reel Life: Girl Interrupted. Clinical Psychiatric News, August 2003, pp 61–62

Sullivan K, Seligman K: S.F. mental ward is budget victim: critics decry "unethical" discharge of severely ill patients. San Francisco Chronicle, April 27, 2003, p A1. Available at: http://www.sfgate.com/cgi-bin/article.cgi?file=/chronicle/archive/2003/04/27/MN146527.DTL. Accessed April 16, 2007.

Tallman FK: The state mental hospital in transition. Am J Psychiatry 116:818–824, 1960

Taylor B: Psychiatric hospitals experience hard times. Maryland Psychiatrist 27:3–4, 2001. Available at: http://www.mdpsych.org/SP01_bTaylor.htm. Accessed April 5, 2007.

Tenet agrees to pay patients $100 million in malpractice claims. Psychiatr Serv 48:1216–1217, 1997

Texas Department of State Health Services: Joint Hearing of Senate Health and Human Services and Senate State Affairs. Joint Interim Charge #3. August 23, 2006. Austin, TX, Texas Department of State Health Services, 2006. Available at: http://www.dshs.state.tx.us/legisla-tive/presentations/082306HHSStateAffairsJoint.ppt#260,1,JointHearingofSenateHealthandHumanServicesandSenateStateAffairs. Accessed April 9, 2007.

The asylum near Frankford, in Pennsylvania. Am J Insanity 8:179–181, 1851

The effect of Medicare on the accreditation of psychiatric hospitals. Hosp Community Psychiatry 17:18–19, 1966

The McLean Asylum for the Insane. Alienist Neurol 14:142, 1893

The "stigma" of mental illness. Am J Psychiatry 93:476–478, 1936

Thirtieth annual report of the officers of the Retreat for the Insane at Hartford, Connecticut. April 1, 1854. Am J Insanity 11:257–261, 1855

Two homes for the nervous and insane. Alienist Neurol 1:391, 1880

Vermont. Am J Insanity 46:434, 1890

Vermont Asylum for the Insane: Thirty-first annual report of the officers of the Vermont Asylum for the Insane. Am J Insanity 24:420, 1868

Ward MJ: The Snake Pit. New York, Random House, 1946

Wayne GJ: The case for the psychiatric hospital. Ment Hosp 12(3):5–10, 1961

Wesselius LF: Countertransference in milieu treatment. Arch Gen Psychiatry 18:47–52, 1968

White CL, Bateman A, Fisher WH, et al: Factors associated with admission to public and private hospitals from a psychiatric emergency screening site. Psychiatr Serv 46:467–472, 1995

Whiteborn JC, Betz BJ: Further studies of the doctor as a crucial variable in the outcome of treatment with schizophrenic patients. Am J Psychiatry 117:215–223, 1960

Wickizer TM, Lessler D, Travis KM: Controlling inpatient psychiatric utilization through managed care. Am J Psychiatry 153:339–345, 1996

Wolfe GE: Electric shock treatment: a "must" for chronic patients in mental hospitals. Am J Psychiatry 111:748–750, 1955

Wood GB: History of the Pennsylvania Hospital for the Insane. Am J Insanity 9:209–213, 1853

Wyatt v. Stickney, 325 F. Supp. 781, 784 (M.D. Ala. 1971)

Young GA: Experiences with psychiatric departments in the general hospitals of Omaha. Am J Psychiatry 96:69–75, 1939

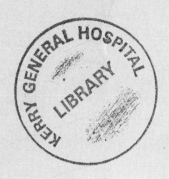
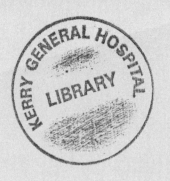

Part I

INPATIENT PRACTICE

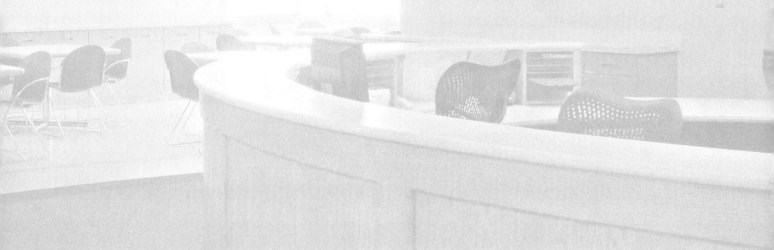

CHAPTER 2

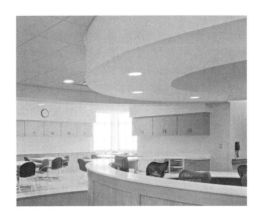

THE ACUTE CRISIS STABILIZATION UNIT FOR ADULTS

Ira D. Glick, M.D.
Rajiv Tandon, M.D.

With the introduction of a range of effective psychopharmacological therapies in the 1950s, the function of psychiatric hospitalization changed from humane long-term care to active treatment. Whereas short-term psychiatric hospitalization back then referred to hospital stays of less than 1 year, during the 1970s the average length of short-term psychiatric hospitalization decreased from 1 month to 2 weeks and has now been reduced to less than 1 week on average (Glick and Hargreaves 1979; Glick et al. 2003; National Association of Psychiatric Health Systems 2000; Sederer and Rothschild 1997). At the same time, the number of admissions has risen steadily, as has the severity of illness of the patients admitted to inpatient psychiatry units. Both patient turnover and the acuity of illness on the inpatient unit have in-

creased very significantly; this fact is supported by the greater severity of illness required to meet "medical necessity criteria" to "qualify" for hospitalization and the greater severity of illness at the time of discharge. These trends are not unique to the United States and are seen in countries across the world (Glick et al. 2003; Lelliott 2006; Ruud et al. 2006; Walsh 2006).

Settings in which acute inpatient psychiatric care may be provided vary substantially and include psychiatry units in a general hospital, specialized private or public psychiatry hospitals, crisis stabilization units that may or may not be attached to a hospital, and short-term residential treatment facilities (Geller 2006; Lipsitt 2003; Walsh 2006). Of the approximately 150,000 psychiatric inpatient beds in the United States today, approximately one-third are in general

We appreciate reviews and critiques by Rose Marie Sime, M.D., and Michael D. Jibson, M.D., Ph.D. We thank Grady Carter, M.D., for his contribution to an earlier version of this chapter.

hospitals, one-third in state psychiatric hospitals, and the remainder in freestanding psychiatric hospitals and crisis stabilization units. It is astounding that almost one-fourth of all stays in U.S. community hospitals for patients 18 years of age and older—7.6 million of nearly 32 million stays—involved depression, bipolar disorder, schizophrenia, and other psychiatric disorders or substance use–related disorders in 2004, according to a new report by the Agency for Healthcare Research and Quality (2004). There are considerable differences in the staffing and scope of services that can be provided at each of the types of psychiatric hospital settings, and the licensing and other regulatory elements vary as well. Although each of these settings currently experiences stress from a different set of fiscal and competitive pressures, the settings share several common attributes and challenges.

Inpatient treatment is both the most expensive and most restrictive station of psychiatric care. The imperatives of treating patients in the least restrictive setting and of cost containment, particularly fueled by managed care, have led to a perception that admission to an inpatient psychiatric setting represents a failure of treatment and is best avoided. This perception is in sharp contrast to the traditional view of the inpatient psychiatry setting as an opportunity to provide necessary intensive diagnostic and/or therapeutic services that can dramatically improve the trajectory of an individual's mental illness. We believe that this latter perspective remains valid, although it needs to be specifically operationalized in view of current realities; this is the focus of our chapter.

Model of the Adult Inpatient Unit, Circa 2008

In this chapter, we share our experiences from short-stay (5–10 days) general psychiatric units from across the country and review studies on inpatient psychiatric care. Evolving from an asylum model emphasizing containment in the absence of effective therapies, the current model is more akin to a modern medical-surgical intensive care unit, with rapid diagnosis and psychopharmacological intervention as its foundation. Although most patients will be acutely stabilized and discharged within 3–10 days of a hospital stay, there is a bimodal curve in length of stay in that approximately 20% of patients require longer lengths of stay (14–21 days) because of symptom acuity, treatment-resistant illnesses, or the lack of safe discharge options in the community. We provide a framework and guidelines

for treatment for clinicians, focusing on the following functions of the hospital unit:

1. *Safety:* Keeping a patient safe (medically and from harming self) and keeping others safe from the patient (aggression and other destructive behavior)
2. *Diagnosis and triage:* Providing an opportunity for intensive monitoring and diagnostic assessment that might, for example, enable a clinical outpatient impasse to be broken, and thereby changing posthospital readmission patterns
3. *Treatment:* Implementing or initiating a rigorous treatment strategy aimed at changing the course of the illness
4. *Respite:* Providing education and respite to caregivers and outpatient treatment providers, although this arguably might be viewed as a luxury

Admission Criteria and Objectives of Hospitalization

This model is predicated on the realities of inpatient practice in the United States in 2007. Average stays vary from 3 to 5 days to 1 month depending on the population served and funding available. Whereas general admission criteria are based on symptom acuity and safety considerations, specific admission criteria depend on the nature and location of the inpatient unit, available acute psychiatric care alternatives, and funding sources. Although specific admission criteria vary depending on payer and health care system factors, all admission criteria include an emphasis on dangerousness and the absence of less restrictive alternatives (Constantine et al. 2006; Warner 1995). A patient can arrive on the inpatient unit as a transfer from another unit or hospital, as an emergent admission from the hospital's emergency department or a central receiving facility, or as an urgent "direct" admission from an outpatient clinical facility. The focus of intervention is always the acute patient. Having said that, we should make explicit that the role of the hospital for the chronic psychiatric patient, hospitalized for both psychiatric and nonpsychiatric reasons (usually varying amounts of suicidal ideation and/or behavior, homelessness, or substance abuse), is still unsettled and problematic. Management of such patients varies from state to state depending on bed availability and other community resources available.

Regardless of setting or length of stay, the objectives of the hospital admission are to rapidly gather relevant history, make a diagnosis, set goals focused on the presenting problem, and promptly initiate appropriate treatment. Table 2–1 details a day-by-day plan for hospital treatment.

Whereas the ultimate goal for most patients is to change the long-term life trajectory in a positive direction, the proximate objective is to change the patient's condition in order to enable the patient to successfully return to his or her community or other less restrictive setting; however, the extent of funding for hospital treatment constrains what can be done. In most cases, the funding is controlled by managed care administrator-clinicians who are not directly involved in treatment. The dilemma is that the unit physician has the legal responsibility for the patient but is not the ultimate decision maker about the length of stay that will be reimbursed.

The single guiding principle of inpatient psychiatric treatment is crisis stabilization, with *crisis* broadly defined to include issues such as dangerousness to self or others, acute decline in function, and a therapeutic impasse. It should be emphasized that the primary clinician must think this through with each patient and the patient's family (or the caseworker if no family is available) at each hospitalization. It is critical that the inpatient treatment episode be viewed as one important step in a continuum of care and not as the entirety of care that can completely "fix" the problem or illness.

Hospitalization for psychiatric disorders has evolved in a manner similar to that of hospitalization for other medical and surgical conditions: the hospital is a setting where patients are admitted when they are acutely ill so that the treatment team can make one, or at most two, interventions to change the trajectory of the illness or problem. An analogy to an intensive care unit may be appropriate in that although the inpatient psychiatric intervention is crucial to the overall treatment, it is one station in a continuum of care.

The Family as Partner on the Treatment Team

Given the acuity of the illness in the context of short hospital stays and the fact that persons admitted to a psychiatric unit may have cognitive impairment, working with families of psychiatric inpatients becomes mandatory. If there is no family, a case manager is almost always a necessity. In our experience, almost every patient has some significant other; the critical task is to find that person, which may involve some extra work by both the medical and social work staff. In this context, Haru and Drury (2007) have written an important guide for inpatient clinicians that includes the rationale for involving families at admission (and after discharge), a working model of inpatient treatment, important skills to assess and treat families (with multiple case examples), and a discussion of impediments, barriers, and legal issues. In order to successfully treat the kinds of patients now being hospitalized, the treatment team must include not only the impaired patient but also the patient's outside support system. The individuals in the support system not only serve as diagnostic informants but also provide a transition to the community for the patient and offer a means to integrate knowledge of the patient from outside of and within the hospital setting.

Diagnostic Workup

It is critical that the specific objective or objectives of a particular inpatient episode be spelled out early in the course of hospitalization and that resources be principally directed toward addressing those objectives. The necessary focus of an inpatient episode is formulated by understanding the presenting complaint in the context of the psychiatric multiaxial diagnosis and life circumstances, including recent stressors. The key element in defining these focal objectives and developing a useful treatment plan is answering the following question: Why is this patient here at this time? To answer this question, the clinician needs input not only from the patient but also from the outpatient provider, the family or other caregiver, and the admitting source such as the psychiatric emergency department or consultation–liaison service. In conjunction with other stakeholders, the inpatient team formulates a specific strategy for addressing the focal problem.

How can one expeditiously define these individualized objectives? On the inpatient units with which we are most familiar, the tasks of defining individualized objectives and reallocating resources are explicitly prioritized in order to address this function. We accomplish this function by expanding the roles that the staff members play in liaison and coordination with outpatient settings and helping staff members develop specific expertise in managing behavioral emergencies, psychopharmacology, and discharge planning. We have also attempted to achieve an optimal balance between the seemingly conflicting objectives of defining the focal problem accurately and doing so expeditiously. Because time is at a premium, we require that the focal problem be formulated within 24 hours of hospitalization, even on weekends, and that a strategy

TABLE 2–1. Adult psychiatry inpatient unit crisis stabilization pathway based on a 5-day length of stay

	Day 1—Assessment and crisis management	Day 2—Completion of assessment and initiation of "focused treatment"	Day 3—Continuation of focused treatment	Day 4—Assessment of safety and discharge readiness	Day 5—Discharge with smooth handoff
Assessment	**Conduct assessment and needs evaluation**				
	Physician: History, examination, formulation, order laboratory tests, consultations	Finalize presumptive diagnosis, evaluate laboratory results	Assess physical health and psychopathology	Assess patient safety and physical/mental health	Carefully assess patient safety
	Nursing: Assess safety and other needs	Define mental/physical health needs, reevaluate safety	Monitor safety, vital signs, self-care, sleep	Assess adequacy of self-care and support needs	Repeat physical and mental examination
	Social work: Contact outpatient team/collateral informants, determine legal status and resources	Monitor safety, vital signs, sleep, nutrition, self-care	Review progress toward defined target outcomes	Evaluate response of target symptoms and needs	Repeat structured assessments, including rating scales
		Complete assessment of legal issues, living and financial needs		Assess extent to which focal problem has been addressed	
	BEGIN TO DEFINE THE FOCAL PROBLEM: *Why admission here, now?*	CLEARLY DEFINE THE FOCAL PROBLEM			
Treatment	**Establish safety and plan focused intervention**	**Finalize and begin definitive interventions**			
	Continue outpatient medications as appropriate	Initiate new medication treatment and taper of prior medication as appropriate	Continue to implement medication plan	Complete implementation of medication plan	Review safety plan
	Implement safety precautions/monitoring as indicated	Use as-needed medications for specific target symptoms as appropriate	Continue individual and group therapy as indicated	Prepare discharge prescriptions	Review postdischarge plan with patient and family
	Plan family/network interventions as appropriate	Implement individual/group therapeutic interventions as appropriate	Evaluate effectiveness of and response to interventions	Continue to assess response to various interventions	Continue various interventions as appropriate
	Orient patient to the unit	Implement family and other network interventions	Continue family and other network interventions as required	Evaluate learned coping strategies	Dispense postdischarge medications with education
	Plan individual therapy as feasible and indicated	Implement individualized safety and behavioral/cognitive plan	Implement medication and other patient education	Assess patient and family understanding	

TABLE 2–1. Adult psychiatry inpatient unit crisis stabilization pathway based on a 5-day length of stay *(continued)*

	Day 1—Assessment and crisis management	Day 2—Completion of assessment and initiation of "focused treatment"	Day 3—Continuation of focused treatment	Day 4—Assessment of safety and discharge readiness	Day 5—Discharge with smooth handoff
Discharge planning	**Assessment of aftercare needs and resources** Assess follow-up and living arrangements Assess financial stability and need for assistance Assess employment or educational issues Conduct safety evaluation in likely postdischarge setting Assess other specific needs and issues	**Define aftercare needs and develop a plan to address them** Address specific postdischarge needs: legal, living, care, fiscal Define approximate length of stay on inpatient unit	**Concretize postdischarge plan** Begin to arrange outpatient appointments Identify likely discharge date Coordinate other postdischarge arrangements as necessary	Identify tentative return-to-work/school date and complete necessary paperwork Complete discharge paperwork Confirm appropriate postdischarge living and care arrangements	Reconfirm and document postdischarge follow-up arrangements Complete all aftercare arrangements Review follow-up plan and confirm patient and family understanding DISCHARGE PATIENT

for addressing the problem be developed at the same time. This process requires adequate staffing at all times; psychiatrists must be available to make diagnoses and treatment plans even during nights and weekends, just as in an intensive care unit.

The patient's preadmission course of psychiatric illness and pattern of mental health service utilization can be instructive (Bowers 2005; Ionescu and Ruedrich 2006). Is this a first-time admission with or without a previous history of mental health treatment? If the person has previously received psychiatric treatment, is treatment discontinued or ongoing? Does the recent course of illness suggest progressive gradual decompensation or a rapid acute deterioration?

A specific initial task is to make as accurate a diagnosis as possible in a very short period of time, usually 1 day. This task fits nicely with mandates from the Joint Commission and state regulatory agencies that require clinicians to expeditiously perform comprehensive assessments for inpatients. A comprehensive diagnosis, as described in the multiaxial formulation in DSM-IV-TR (American Psychiatric Association 2000), consists of five parts:

1. A phenomenological Axis I diagnosis of psychopathology based on DSM-IV-TR (e.g., bipolar disorder, currently depressed with psychotic features, recurrent)
2. An Axis II personality disorder diagnosis (if present). This could also include an assessment of maladaptive personality features or defense mechanisms that do not meet criteria for a personality disorder. Importantly, a "personality disorder" can be primary (i.e., lifelong and starting at a young age) or secondary to an Axis I disorder (e.g., a mood disorder).
3. Diagnosis of any somatic medical conditions that may be present
4. A systems diagnosis focusing on the patient's support system. This corresponds to Axis IV, which encompasses psychosocial and environmental problems.
5. An assessment of the patient's overall level of functioning

We mention all five axes because clinicians may forget one or another axis that may represent a crucial problem area to address.

The first priorities for the clinician should be to determine the nature of the disorder(s) and how this relates to the presenting problem: Why is the patient here now? Next, the clinician needs to determine what kinds of resources the patient and support system have to support the treatment that needs to be delivered. It is also important to identify the immediate stressors that have upset the balance in the patient's life and precipitated the admission and try to alleviate them as feasible. Specific questions that clinicians should ask as part of the assessment include

1. Why is this patient being admitted?
2. Is the admitting diagnosis correct?
3. Were the medications prescribed prior to admission correct for the patient's symptomatology (which may be different from the medications being correct for the diagnosis)? Were the medications prescribed in the correct dosage and of adequate duration? Were the medications being taken as prescribed?
4. Is the patient or immediate family member receiving some type of psychotherapy? What has been the course of the psychotherapy? Have there been any recent changes in the circumstances of the psychotherapy? For example, is the therapist currently on vacation?
5. Has the patient's social support system changed or failed? Does the patient, correctly or incorrectly, anticipate a change in his or her social system, which includes the outpatient psychiatric clinicians?

One critical element in the diagnostic process is ruling out delirium or another psychiatric disorder secondary to substance use or a general medical illness. This can often be done most efficiently while the patient is hospitalized and laboratory testing, imaging, and consultants in other medical specialties are readily available. To be efficient and efficacious, specific clinical protocols must be individualized for the specific setting for each of the most common disorders treated. This is all the more important given the life-threatening nature of some of the medical disorders (e.g., head injury or seizure disorder) that can cause psychiatric symptoms. If a patient has a psychiatric diagnosis, physicians are often too ready to attribute all of the patient's symptoms to that diagnosis, while they may minimize or not conduct a serious workup for medical conditions.

It is also now incumbent on psychiatric physicians to assume responsibility for some of the primary medical care during an inpatient stay, no matter how short the stay. In addition to a comprehensive physical examination (including body mass index and extensive neurological evaluation), all patients must receive a basic laboratory workup that includes a complete blood count, basic renal and hepatic functions (blood urea nitrogen, creatinine, alanine transaminase, aspartate aminotransferase, bilirubin), hemoglobin A_{1C}, lipid profiles, and a toxicology screening. Additional laboratory and radiological evaluations may be required as individually appropriate. Other medical consultations should be expeditiously obtained if necessary.

Because patients may have difficulty providing a coherent history, another important diagnostic task is to gather collateral information. The patient's account of the events leading up to admission must always be supplemented with accounts from family members, friends, and especially other providers. We recognize that family and other significant others may not be available because of alienation or schedule conflicts. However, given the illness acuity plus the short length of stay involved in most admissions, we believe it is mandatory that, just as in intensive care, staff members make every effort to contact the patient's immediate family, doctor, and caseworker.

Hospitalization allows a variety of professionals with different perspectives, including physicians, nurses, occupational therapists, and psychologists, to observe and evaluate the patient. The inpatient unit traditionally has significant resources that are relevant to the diagnostic task. Given decreasing lengths of stay and a focus on acute stabilization, clinicians are often tempted to defer definitive diagnosis in favor of a "not otherwise specified" diagnosis. However, we believe that this does the patient a disservice because it can lead to effective treatment being deferred, and symptoms may be overlooked that need attention. Instead, a "most likely" diagnosis or set of diagnoses should be formulated, with necessary caveats, and appropriate treatment should be promptly initiated.

The legal status of the patient and his or her competence and ability to understand the nature of illness and treatment alternatives should be ascertained. Informed consent is the bedrock of treatment. If the patient is unable to fully participate in this process, this should be ascertained at the time of admission or prior to it if a scheduled admission. Appropriate steps should be taken to address the situation, such as approaching the court to seek authorization for necessary treatment, family involvement, and/or appointment of a guardian advocate. Delays in initiating appropriate treatment on account of the inability of the patient to provide valid informed consent should be minimized (details vary by state).

By the end of the evaluation, the treatment team should have determined the likely clinical diagnosis or diagnoses, identified the set of circumstances that necessitated the current hospitalization, elucidated the immediate stressors and current resources, and ascertained specific patient vulnerabilities and system factors that affect treatment.

Therapies

The master treatment plan is developed by next answering the question "What needs to happen in order to solve this focal problem or problems?" (Harper 1989). It is most efficacious if the focal problem is one that the inpatient psychiatry unit can better address than another type of setting such as a medical unit. Is it possible to develop objectives that are specific to the needs of the patient and have some possibility of modifying the course of the illness and yet are modest enough to be attainable? Our broad strategy is designed to address the specific circumstances of the inpatient episode in the context of the functions that an inpatient unit performs best.

Case Vignette

A 19-year-old female student is admitted to an inpatient unit on account of a drug overdose that followed the breakup of a significant relationship. The patient is in outpatient treatment and has a diagnosis of a recurrent depressive disorder and borderline personality disorder. Her inpatient treatment must address safety needs, a diagnostic reevaluation, possible changes in the therapeutic plan, and respite to allow resolution of the trauma of the breakup.

How this patient should be treated is discussed next, and later in this chapter the vignette will continue.

Goals of Treatment

After diagnosis, the next task is to identify the goals of the treatment. One must always ask patients what their goals are for the hospital stay. It is important to ask patients what they would like to see happen for them in the course of this hospital stay. Equally important is to ask family members the same question. It must be recognized that the goals that patients, families, or even outpatient therapists express may be different from those identified by the inpatient team. Finally, treatment goals should be discussed among and with the outpatient treatment team. Chances for good treatment outcome improve to the extent that a consensus on diverse objectives can be achieved. As noted earlier, the most important tasks include identifying and alleviating, if possible, the stresses that upset the patient's balance and interfere with his or her ability to live outside the hospital; decreasing symptoms;

changing the posthospital life trajectory from the pre-hospital downward course; and beginning the process of educating the patient and family.

Specific Treatment Interventions (Therapies)

DETOXIFICATION FROM SUBSTANCES

Substance use disorders are highly comorbid with other psychiatric diagnoses, and problems related to substance abuse frequently precipitate or substantially contribute to the admission. Rapid detoxification is among the tasks that can best be accomplished in the hospital. Although some general psychiatry inpatient units still perform this function, specialized substance abuse detoxification units perform this function in many settings.

FAMILY INTERVENTION

It is very important to evaluate the patient's support system. Even during a very short stay, it is virtually mandatory to have at least one session with the people who are most important to the patient. This allows the clinical team to gather information, provide education about the patient's illness and its treatment, and undertake other interventions specific to the situation. The importance of education in leading to a better outcome is underrecognized (Glick et al. 1994). As noted earlier, the involvement of the family is also invaluable in obtaining the needed consent for both information gathering and treatment.

INDIVIDUAL PSYCHOTHERAPY

Given the short length of stay now predominant, hospital staffs often forget to talk to the patient. Regardless of how long the patient stays in the hospital, basic principles of individual therapy should be followed. These include establishing an alliance; providing support, hope, and education; and even, on occasion, making an interpretation, if it would advance the aims of the hospitalization. In fact, a 2007 study documented the effectiveness of adding both brief and intensive psychotherapy plus pharmacotherapy for depressed inpatients (Schramm et al. 2007).

INITIATION OR MODIFICATION OF PSYCHOPHARMACOLOGICAL TREATMENT

Medication management is usually central to the treatment regimen (Glick et al. 1991; Kingbury et al. 2001;

Tandon et al. 2006). The crucial first step is to make an accurate diagnosis and identify target symptoms. An early decision point is whether to continue outpatient medications. To make this decision rationally, the clinician needs to undertake a significant amount of investigation in order to gather a medication history that includes dosages, duration, rationale for use, and, most important, prior therapeutic response and side effects. This labor-intensive task is essential in effectively and quickly developing an appropriate treatment plan. Taking a patient off medications is often as helpful an intervention as starting new medications, particularly given issues related to drug interactions and potent clinical effects of treatment discontinuation.

In our inpatient units we tend to take a twofold approach. First, we select a primary medication for the patient's psychiatric illness (e.g., an antipsychotic or a mood stabilizer, or an antidepressant) and titrate it rapidly to a therapeutic dosage. Because antipsychotics, mood stabilizers, and antidepressants all take days or weeks or months to achieve their full effectiveness, we treat symptoms such as agitation aggressively with as-needed medication (usually benzodiazepines) to provide patients with some short-term relief. One of the most common, although understandable, mistakes can be to attempt to speed up response by giving higher doses of the primary medication when what is mostly needed is an understanding of the normal course of response and patience on the part of the clinician. Such a mistake is often made based on the unrealistic hope that the patient will be asymptomatic at the time of discharge rather than having the realistic expectation that the patient's symptoms will be sufficiently reduced to allow continuation, and fine-tuning, of treatment in another setting.

We also recommend making only one change in medication at a time, if possible. This strategy is often difficult given short lengths of stay, but our practice after making a diagnosis is to determine what is the most effective medication with which to start and its initial target dosage. Ideally, this is carried out concurrently with tapering of the patient's previous medications that, by history, seemed to be ineffective or inappropriate for the diagnosis. The hospital psychiatrist must identify the benefits versus the costs of each medication. By cost, we mean not just financial cost but more importantly the costs in terms of side effects and medication interactions. The pros and cons of discontinuing a previous medication must also be carefully considered. Although pharmacotherapy must be individualized, evidence-based guidelines can provide useful guidance (Tandon et al. 2006).

It is important not to undermedicate the patient. Finding the best possible dosage in 3–10 days is a very difficult objective to achieve. Although there is considerable heterogeneity among patients with regard to the optimal dosage, we recommend rapidly achieving the average target dosage for the situation and making short-term adjustments only if absolutely necessary. The dosage selection needs to factor in diagnosis, age, stage of illness, prior response, and concurrent medical conditions as much as possible.

As a rule of thumb, we recommend using fewer rather than more medications. It is important not to get fixed in the practice of prescribing what may be described as the "usual cocktail" (e.g., an antipsychotic plus a mood stabilizer, an antidepressant plus a benzodiazepine plus a sleeping pill) (Kingbury et al. 2001). It is important to remember that once a patient is discharged from an inpatient facility, the outpatient clinician is likely to continue this treatment regimen indefinitely, because the clinician may fear that changing the regimen may lead to worsening symptoms or a downward course.

Although we advocate using the minimum number of medications, we also recommend not temporizing when considering adding a medication because of an acute situation such as escalating agitation. The usual mistake is to delay until an adverse event occurs, such as the patient becoming acutely agitated or assaultive. This situation arises more often when treating patients with schizophrenia or bipolar disorder mania, but it also occasionally occurs in treating patients with major depressive disorder or even severe personality disorder associated with substance abuse. The usual approach is to use a short-acting benzodiazepine (e.g., lorazepam) or diphenhydramine or increase the dosage of a sedating antipsychotic.

Nonadherence to medication treatment is a major problem that often leads to repeated hospitalizations. To improve patient adherence to treatment, we suggest working with significant others during the hospital stay, striving to minimize adverse effects, and focusing on patient and family education. If the treatment team is in doubt about a patient's willingness to take medication, team members should not hesitate to consider and prescribe a long-acting injectable medication, if an appropriate medication is available, to ensure compliance. We do not routinely recommend obtaining medication blood levels, because they are both hard to obtain in a timely fashion and costly. It may also be useful to ask patients frankly if they take all their medications all the time.

With regard to discharge medications, we recommend not making downward dosage adjustments immediately prior to discharge because lowering the dosage at this point may lead to an exacerbation of symptoms just at the time the patient must leave the hospital. Instead, it is better to have the outpatient physician regulate the dosage. Close coordination with the outpatient team is crucial; this entails ensuring a smooth handoff to the aftercare clinic or other setting where the patient will continue in treatment. Timely transmission of necessary clinical information to the outpatient team to facilitate an effective transfer of care is a very high priority. This builds on coordination of care with the outpatient team from the time of admission throughout the course of inpatient treatment. Time constraints can make such coordination challenging (Boyer et al. 2000), but it is one of the most important elements in ensuring good outcomes. It is usually necessary both to make verbal contact with the outpatient team and to actually transmit written documents, including the treatment goals and medications.

We have found rating scales to be extremely useful in measuring the response of defined target symptoms to prescribed psychopharmacological treatment. Although a lengthy battery of instruments is not desirable and may be cumbersome, the use of simple and reliable scales as individually appropriate is strongly recommended. The Clinical Global Impression Severity and Improvement scales and the Brief Psychiatric Rating Scale are useful instruments to track overall illness severity and psychopathology (Tandon et al. 2006).

To summarize, here are some basic guidelines. As a rule of thumb,

- Don't diagnose patients with "NOS" (not otherwise specified); make a working diagnosis as is done in the rest of medicine.
- Do initiate treatment promptly.
- Don't practice polypharmacy; less is more.
- Don't underdose; prescribe no more or less than needed.
- Do select treatment based on a comprehensive history of previous treatment response.
- Don't repeat a failed treatment; if it did not work the first time, it usually will not work the second.
- Don't assume that patients have no significant others (broadly defined); almost everyone has some significant other, even the homeless.
- Don't delay initiating treatment, but don't overmedicate either.
- Do track response with the use of reliable rating scales.

Milieu Management

The structure and setting of the inpatient unit are central to its function, and the unit milieu is of critical therapeutic importance. The locations of patient rooms, group activity rooms, the nursing station, the meal room, and other elements of unit geography significantly affect the ability of the treatment team to effectively carry out unit functions. An explicit stable daily routine, along with a clear set of unit procedures and rules that are consistently implemented, facilitates a predictable and safe environment. Such an environment provides the context for effective therapy. Nursing professionals play the key role in the creation and maintenance of such a unit milieu. With the changing nature of the patient population on an inpatient psychiatry unit, the function of acute inpatient psychiatric nursing has continued to evolve (Bowers 2005; Deacon et al. 2006; Lamb and Weinberger 2005). Nursing personnel maintain safety on the unit and manage the unit environment, collect and communicate information about patients, provide personal care, manage disturbed behavior, and give and monitor treatment. Nursing personnel also may lead a variety of therapeutic groups, such as psychoeducational groups focusing on a disorder, substance abuse, or compliance.

The role of recreational and leisure activities ("activity therapy") during an acute psychiatric hospitalization continues to evolve. There has been a continuing reduction in the use of such activities in the context of cost containment, very short hospital stays, and the changing role of a short-term psychiatric unit in a continuum of care. The use of focused patient therapy groups, such as dialectical behavior therapy or cognitive-behavioral therapy, or family support groups depends on the specific setting, the resources of the inpatient unit, and the population that it serves. Inpatient psychoeducation for both patients and family members is strongly recommended. Here we suggest daytime groups for patients and evening groups for significant others around topics discussed earlier. Referral to consumer groups such as the National Alliance on Mental Illness are usually very helpful over the long run.

Management of Suicidal and Aggressive Behavior

One basic role of the inpatient unit is to keep patients safe. On our units, about 50% of patients are admitted involuntarily—that is, they are judged to be a danger to themselves or others or are unable to care for themselves and often do not wish or see the need for hospitalization. Hospitalization serves the dual functions of maintaining safety until the risk of harm is reduced while actively reducing the risk of such harm. Specific expertise to perform these functions includes effective court liaison, violence and suicide management, and the ability to perform thorough risk assessments. This remains an inexact science—but the best prediction remains a past history of severe attempts. The issue here for the inpatient staff is to have trained personnel available to evaluate (and document) risk because outside stressors as well as mental status will change during the course of even a brief hospitalization.

Individualized assessment of risk and of the precipitants of aggressive behavior should be performed at the time of admission (Serper et al. 2005). A careful history and evaluation to assess the risk of suicidal behavior are essential components of the initial clinical workup. Staff members should be trained in appropriate techniques to manage aggressive behavior (Morrison 2003). Although seclusion and restraint should be utilized infrequently, if at all, staff members need to be trained in their safe and appropriate use (Sailas and Wahlbeck 2005).

Another important clinical issue is the situation of a patient on an inpatient unit who has attacked or who threatens to kill the treating psychiatrist or other staff members. The most appropriate response is to take the threatening behavior at face value, as though it could happen, rather than simply interpreting or ignoring it. One should assume that the behavior is part of the patient's acute symptomatology. A second step is to attempt to determine from referral sources if there is a history of threats or of actual violence. Third, it is prudent to reevaluate the medication regimen and consider increasing the dosage of medication for that particular illness and/or adding a benzodiazepine, if indicated. It may also be advisable to transfer the patient to another physician or another unit, especially if the treating staff are uncomfortable working with such a patient.

Discharge Planning

The next task, if time allows, is to help the patient and family change the posthospital trajectory, because the patient is usually on a downward slope during the acute illness. The objective is to make one or at most two interventions to change life for both the patient and family after the hospital stay, targeting the types of psychosocial and environmental problems rated on

Axis IV. This strategy can be the most important part of a hospitalization and has the potential to significantly change the course of a patient's illness. Inpatient education programs focused on surviving outside the protected hospital setting are helpful; this may include multiple structured small-group meetings focusing on education about the illness and coping strategies.

We try to link the patient to an outpatient psychiatrist and other services as needed; typically, an outpatient appointment is scheduled for the patient within 1 week of hospital discharge. In today's environment, patients may also need help with other services such as case management and housing; one should at least begin the process of meaningfully addressing these needs while the patient is still hospitalized. Effectiveness of inpatient/outpatient handoffs is a primary index of quality inpatient psychiatric treatment (Joint Commission 2008).

Case Vignette (continued)

Let us revisit the inpatient stay of the 19-year-old female student who was admitted to our inpatient unit on account of a drug overdose that followed the breakup of a significant relationship. As previously noted, the patient was in outpatient treatment and had a diagnosis of a recurrent depressive disorder and borderline personality disorder. After initial detoxification and life-supportive monitoring and therapy, an individualized safety plan was developed with the patient, and she learned coping skills in an individual and unit group setting. In view of nonresponse to an adequate trial of the current antidepressant, the agent was switched and a low dosage of a sedating antipsychotic added in view of symptoms of paranoia and insomnia. Three friends who reside in the same dormitory as the patient and constitute her immediate support system (they had accompanied the patient to the emergency department from which she was admitted to the inpatient unit) participated in two meetings with the patient and her inpatient social worker. Following discussion with the outpatient therapist, the patient was referred to a dialectical behavior therapy program.

We also routinely recommend referral to appropriate consumer organizations such as the National Alliance on Mental Illness and Alcoholics Anonymous in order to improve posthospital outcome (Glick and Dixon 2002).

Conclusion

In summary, the following steps are involved in an inpatient episode: defining the focal problem, making a diagnosis, formulating specific goals for the admission, determining which treatments to prescribe, reinforcing or rebuilding the patient's support system, and establishing outpatient care. The role of the family and significant others is central. Key tasks to be performed by the inpatient unit include liaison and coordination with multiple groups (e.g., outpatient team, psychiatry emergency services, the court system, family members, other caregivers, community mental health agencies, various social and governmental agencies); rapid comprehensive assessment (e.g., descriptive and diagnostic, medical, personality, system); maintenance of patient safety and a therapeutic environment (Boyer et al. 2000); and smooth and expeditious transfer to another residential and treatment system.

This concept of the acute inpatient psychiatric unit as a provider of focused, individualized, intensive short-term care necessitates a reconsideration of the optimal use of staff and other resources. From a staffing perspective, one needs to evaluate how resources can be best utilized within local constraints to address the objectives of the program. New educational programs for staff are usually necessary to adequately train clinicians of all disciplines. The organization of the inpatient treatment team needs careful attention. Different team members have defined and differentiated roles that must be effectively coordinated. The unit psychiatrist or service chief plays a key role as the team leader. It is important to emphasize that treatment is shaped not only by how much a psychiatrist knows but also by his or her attitudes and knowledge about the model of inpatient treatment. It is important to remember that although managed care and its reviewers can suggest treatment, the inpatient psychiatrist and team have the ultimate responsibility for treatment decisions. Therefore it is advisable not to make medication changes or dosage adjustments or add medications if data for the change are lacking. Receiving additional authorized days from the managed care company is not a good rationale for making particular treatment decisions.

The contradictions between the theory and practice of inpatient work are apparent to anyone who has worked on an inpatient psychiatric unit. Current short stays necessitate urgency, although given the slow pace of symptom response, patience is also a necessary virtue. Likewise, the acuity of symptoms mandates a rapid response, yet the need for a thorough workup that takes time requires slowing things down. The kind of multimodal treatment we are recommending requires a multidisciplinary staff that can be difficult to maintain in the face of economic pressures. Each inpatient unit will need to make the appropriate compromises, depending on local conditions, in order to deliver the best treatment possible given the reality of fiscal constraints. In addition, in order to succeed and deliver competent care, every inpatient service must have an outpatient service link. Without such a link, the patient is more likely to be discharged without adequate aftercare plans, and the risk of rehospitalization increases.

The approach to inpatient psychiatry we propose focuses on creating patient-specific objectives that are congruent with the functions that inpatient psychiatry units can best perform. The highlights of this approach include making an accurate diagnosis, delivering effective medication, involving the patient's support system, and coordinating care with outpatient providers. These are all things that can be accomplished or at least started during a relatively short hospital stay. It should be emphasized that the inpatient unit is one station in a continuum of care that plays a specific role in this continuum. Because it is the most expensive component on this continuum, optimal and efficient utilization of this resource is essential.

The inpatient psychiatry system still has an extremely important role to play in the treatment of psychiatric illness. Its principal function is that of crisis stabilization. Rather than being preoccupied with how much could be accomplished in earlier periods, inpatient providers can be enthusiastic about their clearly defined tasks in this new era of treatment. In addition, payers and utilization reviewers can be assured of meaningful and efficient inpatient stays from which patients are likely to benefit maximally. Finally, it is important to maintain a mechanism for assessing how well a particular inpatient unit or system is accomplishing its objectives over time. This assessment should include both objective measures of assessing treatment outcome (measured against admission goals) and the commonly used patient and family satisfaction measures.

References

Agency for Healthcare Research and Quality: Care of Adults With Mental Health and Substance Abuse Disorders in U.S. Community Hospitals (Publ No 07-0008). Washington, DC, Agency for Healthcare Research and Quality, 2004

American Psychiatric Association: Diagnostic and Statistical Manual of Mental Disorders, 4th Edition, Text Revision. Washington, DC, American Psychiatric Association, 2000

Bowers L: Reasons for admission and their implications for the nature of acute inpatient psychiatric nursing. J Psychiatr Ment Health Nurs 12:231–236, 2005

Boyer C, McAlpine DD, Pottick KJ, et al: Identifying risk factors and key strategies in linkage to outpatient psychiatric care. Am J Psychiatry 157:1592–1598, 2000

Constantine R, Kershaw M, Robinson P: Florida's Mental Health Acute Care/Crisis Services: Background and Strategies for Reform. Tampa, University of South Florida, 2006

Deacon M, Warne T, McAndrew S: Closeness, chaos, and crisis: the attractions of working in acute mental health care. J Psychiatr Ment Health Nurs 13:750–757, 2006

Geller JL: A history of private psychiatric hospitals in the USA: from start to almost finished. Psychiatr Q 77:1–41, 2006

Glick ID, Dixon L: Patient and family support organization services should be included as part of treatment for chronic psychiatric illness. J Psychiatr Pract 8:63–69, 2002

Glick ID, Hargreaves WA: Psychiatric Hospital Treatment for the 1980s: A Controlled Study of Short Versus Long Hospitalization. Lexington, MA, Lexington Press, 1979

Glick ID, Burti L, Suzuki K, et al: Effectiveness in psychiatric care, I: a cross-national study of the process of treatment and outcomes of major depressive disorder. J Nerv Ment Dis 179:55–63, 1991

Glick ID, Burti L, Okonogi K, et al: Effectiveness in psychiatric care, III: psychoeducation and outcome for patients with major affective disorder and their families. Br J Psychiatry 164:104–106, 1994

Glick ID, Carter WG, Tandon R: A paradigm for treatment of inpatient psychiatric disorders: from asylum to intensive care. J Psychiatr Pract 9:395–402, 2003

Harper G: Focal inpatient treatment planning. J Am Acad Child Adolesc Psychiatry 28:31–37, 1989

Haru AM, Drury LM: Working With Families of Psychiatric Inpatients. Baltimore, MD, Johns Hopkins University Press, 2007

Ionescu D, Ruedrich S: Inpatient treatment planning: consider six preadmission patterns. Curr Psychiatry 5:23–31, 2006

Joint Commission: Performance Measurement Initiatives: Hospital-Based, Inpatient Psychiatric Services (HBIPS) Candidate Core Measure Set, last updated February 15, 2008. Oakbrook Terrace, IL, The Joint Commission, 2008. Available at: http://www.jointcommission.org/PerformanceMeasurement/PerformanceMeasurement/Hospital+Based+Inpatient+Psychiatric+Services.htm. Accessed April 22, 2008.

Kingbury SJ, Yi D, Simpson GM: Rational and irrational polypharmacy. Psychiatr Serv 52:1033–1036, 2001

Lamb HR, Weinberger LE: The shift of psychiatric hospital inpatient care from hospitals to jails and prisons. J Am Acad Psychiatr Law 33:529–534, 2005

Lelliott P: Acute inpatient psychiatry in England: an old problem and a new priority. Epidemiol Psichiatr Soc 15:91–94, 2006

Lipsitt DR: Psychiatry and the general hospital in an age of uncertainty. World Psychiatry 2:87–92, 2003

Morrison E: An evaluation of four programs for the management of aggression in psychiatric settings. Arch Psychiatr Nurs 17:146–155, 2003

National Association of Psychiatric Health Systems: Annual Survey Report: Trends in Behavioral Healthcare Systems. A Benchmarking Report: Length of Stay Declines as Patient Numbers Rise. Washington, DC, National Association of Psychiatric Health Systems, 2000

Ruud T, Lindefors N, Lindhardt A: Current issues in Scandinavian acute psychiatric wards. Epidemiol Psichiatr Soc 15:99–103, 2006

Sailas E, Wahlbeck K: Restraint and seclusion in psychiatric inpatient wards. Curr Opin Psychiatry 18:555–559, 2005

Schramm E, van Calker D, Dykiereth P, et al: An intensive treatment program of interpersonal psychotherapy plus pharmacotherapy for depressed inpatients: acute and long-term results. Am J Psychiatry 164:768–777, 2007

Sederer LI, Rothschild AJ: Acute Care Psychiatry: Diagnosis and Treatment. Baltimore, MD, Williams & Wilkins, 1997

Serper MR, Goldberg BR, Herman KG, et al: Predictors of aggression on the psychiatric inpatient service. Compr Psychiatry 46:121–127, 2005

Tandon R, Targum SD, Nasrallah HA, et al: Strategies for maximizing clinical effectiveness in the treatment of schizophrenia. J Psychiatr Pract 12:348–363, 2006

Walsh D: Coming in from the cold: from psychiatric to general hospital. The Irish experience. Epidemiol Psichiatr Soc 15:95–98, 2006

Warner R: Alternatives to the Hospital for Acute Psychiatric Treatment. Washington, DC, American Psychiatric Press, 1995

CHAPTER 3

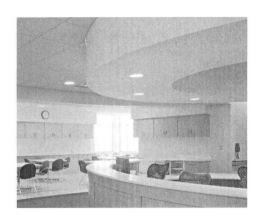

THE CHILD UNIT

Joseph C. Blader, Ph.D.
Andrés Martin, M.D., M.P.H.
A. Bela Sood, M.D., M.S.H.A.
Carmel A. Foley, M.D., M.H.A.

Admission Criteria

The indications for the admission of children to acute inpatient psychiatric care resemble those that apply currently to other age groups—that is, hospitalization may be appropriate when an individual exhibits behavior that warrants placement in a highly regulated and supervised environment because that behavior

1. Poses danger to oneself or others;
2. Impairs functioning and exceeds the capacity of less restrictive available resources to manage it effectively; or
3. Represents a symptom pattern so atypical or alarmingly quick to develop that the inpatient setting offers best chances for prompt, thorough assessment and resolution.

By emphasizing severity rather than forms of behavioral disturbance, these indications inherently encompass a broad range of clinical problems. Nevertheless, among children there seem to be several specific

patient presentations that instantiate these criteria most of the time.

Dangerous Behavior

The harmful behavior that preadolescents admitted to acute inpatient psychiatric care most commonly display involves intermittent rageful episodes during which the child is highly aggressive and combative. For the most part, the incidents that catalyze admission to hospital represent an *escalation* of chronic aggression toward more harmful behavior. Long-standing difficulties with impulse control and emotional volatility are common in these youngsters' developmental histories. These problems in turn set the stage for extensive histories of both self-directed aggression and aggression that manifests as angry, uncontrolled outbursts of physical and verbal assaultiveness and damage to property. The precipitants of these behaviors are typically real or perceived frustrations, impediments to the child's preferred activities, disagreements, or other relatively minor provocations that peers handle with composure. The events that lead to admission, therefore, seldom represent the onset of violent behavior in a previously well-controlled individual. Rather, the episode usually involves a major increment in dangerousness (e.g., use of a sharp object, aggression directed toward a baby or toddler, hurling of objects like classroom chairs, threats) that caregivers can no longer handle in a less restrictive setting.

Children at risk of harming themselves often present as a psychiatric emergency that warrants admission. Fortunately, intentional self-injury occurs infrequently among children relative to adolescents, and suicide is rare (Kloos et al. 2007; Peterson et al. 1996). It is more often children's verbal statements about wanting to die that elicit concern. In one common scenario, remarks about "being better off dead" or "maybe I should just kill myself," or even brandishing a knife or wrapping material around one's own neck, arise as a result of extreme frustration in children for whom a "meltdown" reflects the intensity of their distress rather than suicidal or homicidal intent. When the acute explosion has passed, the child's overall satisfaction with life may quickly rebound. However, the event often leaves parents distraught, concerned for their child's safety, and feeling guilty. Likewise, such behavior also ratchets up the concern of school personnel and community practitioners, making referral to inpatient care more likely. Very rarely, a single violent act of aggression may warrant admission to acute care for evaluation.

Another scenario that warrants inpatient care to reduce the risk for intentional self-harm develops when children who experience sustained dysphoria dwell on death as a solution to their chronic psychic pain. Major depression, maltreatment, severe family conflict, or other stressors are often the backdrop for these problems. The children may have kept these ruminations to themselves for some time. As such, it is their disclosure to adults, rather than symptom or functional change per se, that often motivates admission.

Impairments Inadequately Treated in Outpatient Care

Psychiatric symptoms may produce serious impairments that prior treatment has not adequately alleviated. Even if these symptoms do not entail imminent danger, inpatient treatment may be sought so that interventions can be introduced at a higher intensity and frequency than is otherwise possible. For example, children who refuse to leave home to attend school often do so with outpatient treatment that emphasizes management of anxiety and family processes to promote attendance. However, a few children become violent when pushed to go to school in the face of severe

anxiety. These youngsters might require hospital treatment to disrupt a pattern that may have culminated in several months of nonattendance.

Some disturbances involve disruptive behavior that poses no genuine physical danger but nonetheless exceeds the capability of the child's family or educational milieu to manage it effectively. Animosity, frustration, hopelessness, or strains on family functioning may have so negatively impacted relationships that typical outpatient interventions would have practically no chance to succeed. Hospital admission may present the most viable means to provide reprieve, hopefulness for families, and the implementation of interventions to promote behavioral stability.

Sudden, Medically Complicated, or Perplexing Symptoms

Outpatient and emergency department clinicians may seek the monitoring and evaluative services that inpatient settings afford when they encounter children who display a sudden change in mental status, developmental skills, or bizarre behavior. Pediatric specialties at times seek to admit or transfer patients whose physiological symptoms, such as persistent vomiting, encopresis, pain, or nonepileptic seizures ("pseudoseizures"), appear to have no medical etiology, and clinicians suspect significant psychosocial influences on their emergence. Compared with pediatric wards, psychiatric settings have more restrictive visiting policies and engage children in a broader array of activities. Therefore, the potential to observe the child closely both with and apart from the family appears to be a reasonable approach to address these concerns.

Poor adherence to treatment for established chronic illnesses, especially among youngsters with a comorbid psychiatric disorder, may also be an impetus to seek inpatient care. Psychiatric expertise and a well-controlled milieu may leverage behavior change and perhaps identify the emotional issues suspected to underlie noncompliance.

There are some disturbances for which specialized hospital settings exist only in a few major centers in the United States; for affected children in many communities the "general" child psychiatric unit may be the only available resource. For example, some youngsters present with severe, repetitive self-injurious behavior that develops in the context of developmental disabilities. Youngsters who resist nutrition include those with early onsets of the "classical" eating disorders (anorexia and bulimia) and those with feeding disorders who are older than the age range for which pediatric management is more typical (infancy to age 3 years).

Other Situations

Family courts and child welfare authorities may refer children to psychiatric inpatient facilities for evaluations. Their goal is to obtain input on disposition recommendations that will address the youth's behavior (e.g., unmanageability in the community) or care needs (e.g., suitability of current living arrangements). It is best to have clarity from the outset that the *agency* is, in fact, the one seeking professional services, much like any other forensically oriented assessment. That clarity may come in the form of a standing contract with the facility or a court order. Problems arise when an agency prompts a family to initiate a voluntary admission for their child in the expectation that the agency will receive professional opinions that address its own agenda (such as removal of the child from parental custody). The agency's goals are then apt to conflict with the hospital's primary allegiance to the child and family's therapeutic needs and confidentiality, which only concerns about child endangerment can supersede in nonforensic situations.

Evolution of Inpatient Services for Children

Although confinement of adults with severe mental illness was a common practice for centuries, the presence of children in such facilities seems to have been rare. Neuropsychiatric inpatient services for children originated in U.S. urban areas in the early twentieth century, chiefly to provide custodial care for youngsters with postencephalitic impairments acquired during the era's infectious epidemics. By midcentury, inpatient settings for children developed to treat behavioral disturbances that were not accompanied by major "organic" or neurodevelopmental problems. The prevailing psychoanalytic approaches embraced a developmental model that rooted many forms of mental illness in unfavorable events and relationships in early life. Therefore, the placement of a child who had already begun to experience psychiatric symptoms in a special caretaking environment seemed to offer an opportunity for "corrective" experiences that would offset earlier pathogenic influences. Naturally, there was no expectation that this would be a rapid process, and long stays in hospitals and residential treatment settings were common.

By the late twentieth century, three trends, each 20–30 years in the making, crystallized and combined to alter significantly children's psychiatric inpatient services. First, *developments in psychiatric practice*,

notably evidence for the efficacy for children of selected pharmacotherapies and of focused, practically oriented psychosocial interventions, had at least two important effects: 1) they changed the time horizon for therapeutic efforts to gain traction from years to months or weeks; and 2) they helped to upend the view that improvement in seriously disturbed children's well-being necessitated long-term separation from their families. Second, a broad societal movement toward *reduced reliance on institutional settings* for individuals of all ages with severe mental illness in favor of enhanced community-based systems of care was generally successful. A parallel movement that strove to meet the needs of psychiatrically ill children and their families without separating them for long periods highlighted the poignancy and grief of children and parents separated before there was an opportunity to attempt less drastic interventions (Knitzer 1982; Knitzer and Cooper 2006). In the absence of evidence that long periods in treatment settings apart from their families offered any countervailing advantages for the majority of youths, the desirability of supporting families to manage a child's disturbance in the least restrictive setting possible became the guiding principle for both mental health systems planning and individual care determinations.

A third trend was developments in the *financing of mental health services* that emphasized the containment of costs. Lengths of stay declined markedly between the early 1990s and 2004, and reimbursements to hospital facilities also declined (Blader and Carlson 2007; Case et al. 2007; Ringel and Sturm 2001). Nonetheless, overall annual population-adjusted rates (i.e., percentage of individuals in the general population) of psychiatric hospitalizations for children and adolescents have actually increased (Blader and Carlson 2007).

In effect, then, these three trends brought into alignment optimism about the potential for scientifically based advances in treatment to alter the course of mental illness, the moral imperative of providing care through community-based services when possible to minimize separations of families, and economic interests in less costly care. The results for psychiatric inpatient care of children have been to reorient its mission toward crisis stabilization; comprehensive (if not definitive) assessment of a child's difficulties and longer-term needs; and arrangement of resumption of appropriate care in a less restrictive setting. It therefore occupies a specific niche within, ideally, a coordinated system of care that calibrates services to current need by including an array of supportive interventions that include home-based therapies, "wraparound services," enhanced outpatient and day treatment programs, help managing periodic flare-ups in disturbances, and respite care for families. At present, however, these services remain unevenly available, and demand exceeds supply in many localities. Priority for intensive community-based services often goes to youths deemed to be at risk for out-of-home placement. As a practical matter, such risk is quite often demonstrated by prior hospitalization, and we have noted that rates of admissions have not declined among young people.

In summary, although resources devoted to inpatient care have constricted and admission requires greater justification, it appears doubtful that the compensatory supports to help children get and stay well in their own communities have flourished to the extent hoped for.

Case Vignette

Leon, age 11, was admitted for his fifth psychiatric hospitalization. The precipitant was a new burst of unbridled anger and aggression directed at both his parents, resulting in a significant knee injury to his father. Other severe acts of aggression in the recent past included swinging a hammer at his older brother and breaking a window in the family home. In addition, he had threatened to kill himself on several occasions, but this was invariably in the context of angry moments, and he had taken no self-injurious actions.

The night before the aggressive episode that led to admission, Leon was extremely oppositional and unruly at bedtime, and his parents were sufficiently intimidated that they gave him 3 mg of clonazepam all at once. He was, of course, very sleepy the following morning, and it was being readied for school that triggered the aggressive episode that culminated in his hospitalization.

Pharmacotherapy just prior to admission comprised olanzapine (30 mg daily in three divided doses). He was also prescribed risperidone 0.5 mg in the morning and evening, divalproex sodium (1,000 mg extended-release at bedtime), and benztropine (1 mg twice daily).

Leon was adopted from an Asian country at age 14 months by a married couple in their 40s. Nothing is known of his biological relatives or the rearing environment during his first year of life. He walked by 20 months and was considered slow to develop language. Nevertheless, he did not attend any school program until he was 6 years old, when school enrollment became mandatory. Arriving in first grade, the teacher quickly expressed concerns about his short attention span, inability to sit still, tendency to wander around the classroom, and general disruptiveness in that setting. By now, the parents recognized that the high level of activity and poor impulse control that he displayed at home were developmen-

tally inappropriate and therefore accepted the school's effort to provide special services, but they did not seek other treatment for these difficulties.

Despite his difficult start in life, Leon was a healthy boy with no medical illnesses. Psychological testing revealed him to be of average intelligence, with mild weaknesses in expressive language and fine motor coordination, both of which were being addressed within his school program. Several placements within the local school district, in ascending levels of restrictiveness, were not helpful. However, by the fifth grade, Leon began an out-of-district privately run special education day school. The parents were quite pleased with this setting, and although there were disruptions and altercations in the school context, the program was well equipped to help him regain self-control.

His first psychiatric hospitalization occurred at age 6 years because of aggressive, disruptive, and unmanageable behavior at home. The initial diagnosis was attention-deficit/hyperactivity disorder (ADHD), and stimulant treatment was undertaken, although the parents could not later recall accurately the exact agents, dosages, durations, and outcomes of these trials. During this admission, Leon became notably less volatile, and he was discharged to family with recommendations for outpatient services. However, soon after returning home, his behavior dangerously worsened, and he was readmitted. This pattern recurred yet a third time. Following this third hospitalization, he was referred to a group residence in the community. The parents were initially relieved with this option, and an interim plan was established that included extensive outpatient support as well as home-based instruction provided by his school district. Nonetheless, a month later, these services had not been implemented, and Leon was not enrolled in any school and had received no meaningful tutoring or treatment.

Understandably, Leon had become quite unruly in what for him was an entirely boring environment. This resulted in yet another hospitalization, and the agency that oversaw the group residential program closed his case. This disillusioned the parents, who were now untrusting of any out-of-home placement. The social services system provided an intensive case manager who was well regarded by the parents because she was available to them for emotional support by telephone, visited them regularly, and provided practical assistance such as travel vouchers and some respite care. However, this did nothing to solve the ongoing "meltdowns" in the home.

Disenchanted with treatment by a variety of private practitioners and community mental health agencies, the parents transferred his care to the psychiatric outpatient clinic of a large tertiary care medical center in the year prior to the current admission. By now they had been informed that Leon had bipolar disorder. Despite his father's admonitions, he persisted in accessing pornography on the Internet. The parents represented this to the admitting clinicians as evidence of hypersexuality. There was no history of other sexually inappropriate behaviors or evidence of abuse or neglect since coming to the United States. The parents seemed ambivalent about Leon's current treatment, conveying on the one hand that they thought his medication regimen was helpful yet readily acknowledging on the other hand that his overall functioning remained quite impaired and in any event had not prevented the current hospitalization.

At the time of admission, the parents spoke at length of their conviction that Leon had Asperger's syndrome. They had been alerted to this condition by friends and had begun to read up on the subject, persuading themselves that the child definitely met criteria for this condition.

Dramatically, following admission, Leon was calm and cooperative, showing no evidence of a sustained mood disorder. Apart from his brittle frustration tolerance that one might construe as rigidity, he displayed none of the core abnormalities of a pervasive developmental disorder.

This case exemplifies many of the challenges that children's inpatient psychiatric services currently confront. These services lie at the conjunction of the urgent need to address acutely disturbing behavior that nonetheless is part of a chronic set of difficulties. Immense family strain and desperation both promote and derive from serial hospitalizations. Because the quality of community-based psychiatric services (when available) may be suboptimal, pharmacotherapeutic situations as troubling as that described are not uncommon (e.g., using concurrent antipsychotics, switching medications abruptly to deal with situational crises, enabling high-dose benzodiazepine use for behavioral dyscontrol at parental discretion). Many of the most severe problems in child psychiatry elude wide diagnostic consensus, so that families receive cacophonous messages from clinicians. Potentially useful supportive services are unevenly available, which leads to gaps in care that may precipitate readmissions. Finally, inpatient settings often face the quandary of keeping in hospitals minimally symptomatic children who nonetheless are very likely to destabilize after discharge. Mindful of these difficult contextual issues, we turn to the programmatic and operational elements of the inpatient service itself as it strives to fulfill its contemporary mission.

Diagnostic Workup

Clinical Assessment at Admission

The overriding goal of inpatient psychiatric treatment for patients of all ages is restoration of functioning so they can resume care in less restrictive environments.

One corollary is that the clinician has to be simultaneously *comprehensive* in obtaining sufficient information to characterize the nature, course, and context of the individual's disturbance and *focused* on the specific behaviors and events that culminated in the person's need for intensive psychiatric intervention *at this time*. Conducting such an evaluation for children has distinct elements.

First, the principal informant is rarely the patient him- or herself but rather adult caregivers. For the most part, these are the child's parents. History must be a composite "best estimate" of parent and child information. Children are more likely to provide accurate information about their subjective experiences of anxiety and mood problems, whereas parents more accurately convey details of overt behavior, especially conduct problems ("externalizing" behaviors). However, children in nonparental care account for a fair proportion of those admitted to inpatient services (dosReis et al. 2001; McMillen et al. 2004; Pottick et al. 2005). The evaluation's thoroughness and accuracy may suffer from the vagaries of agency record keeping, staff turnover, and incomplete familiarity with the child's early years by the current caregivers.

Second, standardized rating scales, such as the Child Behavior Checklist (Achenbach and Rescorla 2000) and the Behavior Assessment System for Children (Reynolds and Kamphaus 2002) provide norm-referenced scores for a number of areas of clinical concern. There are versions for both parent and teacher completion, and the same child's scores from these two settings are often very informative, especially when there are discrepancies. Beyond characterizing the child's own behavior, caregivers can furnish details of family history. Besides these broad-spectrum scales, other tools may be useful in specific situations. For instance, the Child Mania Rating Scale (Pavuluri et al. 2006) and Children's Depression Rating Scale (Poznanski and Mokros 1995) may aid differential diagnosis in their respective domains by guiding the clinician's attention toward evaluating symptoms in a developmentally sensitive manner and yielding a percentile that reflects severity.

Third, a *developmental perspective* is an important element of any child psychiatric assessment. This expectation seems to intimidate some clinicians, for whom it conjures the complexity of remembering a long list of milestones and normal acquisition of skills from birth onward. In truth, a straightforward approach focused on major areas of practical significance, preferably aided by a protocol of standard questions, will yield the most relevant clinical information.

One should learn about any major pre-, peri-, or neo-natal insults and toxic exposures. To the extent possible, a description of early temperament, emphasizing interest in other people, soothability, activity level, and overall emotional tone, is helpful to obtain. Disruptions in caregiving arrangements, especially when associated with parental incapacitation or familial conflict, are important to document, along with other unusual or traumatic events. Significant problems or delays in physical growth, sensory functions, and basic skills acquisition (language, motor, academic) that evoked concern or needed intervention are critical to identify and naturally lead to questions about current functioning and services in the affected areas.

The child's early experiences in preschool and school settings provide crucial data about behavioral development, socialization, readiness for development of academic skills, and handling of separations from home. The trajectory of school experiences warrants thorough questioning, particularly special services or individualized evaluations that arise from behavioral or scholastic difficulties. The quantity and quality of peer relationships are significant indices of functioning. Visits with, and activities involving, other kids outside of school may reflect both major problem areas and potential strengths. It is not uncommon that a child shows markedly better functioning and adjustment outside of home than within the family, or vice versa, and this has clear implications for treatment planning.

Fourth, contextual factors hold particular relevance for the severity of a child's psychiatric disorder. Changes in school setting, family composition, parental illness, peer-related events (real or perceived victimization, volatile relationships), and so on deserve inquiry as stressors. We could also include here changes in the child's treatment regimen, including pharmacotherapies. Of course, even without differences in prescribed treatment, altered adherence may produce unwelcome clinical change. Children on extended visits to a different household (e.g., vacation time with the parent in whose home they do not otherwise reside) may modify treatment, owing to inadvertent confusion or skepticism about its value.

Accessory Assessments

Common laboratory assessments of metabolic, hematological, and endocrine parameters as well as electrocardiography are nearly universal in hospital settings. If a child's preadmission treatment included agents for which therapeutic drug monitoring is standard, these should be part of admitting orders. Nonstandard tests should be considered as the clinical situation suggests (e.g., ammonia for a child treated with valproate accompanied by marked behavior change). Currently, the chief role of laboratory tests among child psychiatric patients is to rule out alternative medical etiologies and screen for other illnesses that may need intervention rather than to aid in differentiation among psychiatric diagnoses.

Psychological testing, once administered with psychodiagnostic goals in mind, is now rarely routine. Cognitive and neuropsychological evaluations have come to play a larger role but are still requested sparingly given their expense and time constraints on acute care admissions. Their potential to elucidate learning or developmental deficits in a child whose difficulties were attributed to a primary behavior disorder, however, can offer tangible benefits to the patient and be particularly useful in postdischarge planning, including appropriate school placement.

The attending psychiatrist should request consultation from the relevant pediatric specialty for children who received treatment for a general medical condition prior to admission. The inpatient assessment may also involve pediatric consultation to aid diagnosis. Pediatric neurology may be called, for instance, to evaluate for potential seizures or neurodegenerative diseases, which can manifest as "phenocopies" of some psychiatric conditions. The consultant will order or recommend further tests as needed and provide guidance for management while the child is in the hospital.

Observation

The opportunity for experienced personnel to observe a child's behavior, mood, and interactions with peers and family is the singular strength of the inpatient setting. These observations permit more direct assessment that bypasses some of the distortions that secondhand reports of children's psychiatric symptoms inevitably carry. One can more readily (although not always) distinguish truly manic "grandiosity" from socially inappropriate bragging, weepiness secondary to unipolar depression from the frustrated crying that comes and goes with episodic rages, reluctance to bathe that is related to anxiety rather than oppositionality, and so forth. On the other hand, the change in environment may at times itself lead to a temporary reduction of symptoms or a "honeymoon" (Blader et al. 1994). These instances pose a risk of identifying the presenting problem as situation bound, especially when short stays preclude symptom resurgence in the hospital. The opportunity to observe family interactions beyond the limited contexts that the outpatient office affords is extremely important, given the salience of interpersonal factors for the development and the treatment of the most common psychiatric disorders of childhood (disruptive, anxiety, and mood disorders).

Therapies

Medication Treatments

ORGANIZATIONAL ASPECTS OF HOSPITAL-BASED PHARMACOTHERAPY

Children admitted to inpatient care most often come with medication regimens. Ideally, the safety of the inpatient setting affords the opportunity to reexamine prior treatment with an eye to the potential for behavioral toxicity to emerge idiopathically from some medications or their combinations. Judicious tapering may afford the opportunity to reduce treatments that may be superfluous or that were initiated on the premise that the child had a problem that inpatient assessment does not confirm. Children with limited prior medication treatment can start therapy in a setting whose intensive monitoring permits vigorous titration but whose structure and safety also permit a more patient approach, avoiding the unwarranted dosage escalations that problematic behavior in less secure outpatient settings may elicit. By the same token, however, this high degree of supervision should not instill a false sense of security that leads one to titrate, taper, or substitute agents with undue haste.

Cost containment efforts that emphasize ongoing review of hospital course may exert a countervailing influence on best practices (e.g., Bronfman 1999). When payers scrutinize therapeutic maneuvers every 2 days or so, clinicians' behavior may veer toward more aggressive pharmacotherapy to demonstrate they are doing "something." This in turn militates against trials that are long enough to establish a regimen's value. Unfortunately, the evidence base for the optimal care of children with illness refractory to initial treatment steps is very sparse. Psychopharmacology for children admitted to inpatient settings is therefore especially vulnerable to assuming a rather improvisational character.

The transition between inpatient and community clinicians is another possible organizational influence on pharmacotherapy and patient outcomes. The limited data available suggest that medication regimens at discharge are often modified by outpatient providers (Blader 2006a). It is unknown to what extent changes in pharmacotherapy are consequences of the course of the child's illness, the waning of a treatment's tolerability and efficacy, or the proclivities of individual clinicians.

PRINCIPLES, STRATEGIES, AND TACTICS

We noted earlier that aggressive and uncontrolled behaviors are the principal reasons for the psychiatric hospitalization of preadolescents, yet these behaviors develop in the context of diverse forms of psychopathology that may warrant distinct approaches to pharmacotherapy (Connor 2002). To determine which approach or algorithm may be appropriate for a child, therefore, the clinician has to discern the relative contributions of potential sources of impairment (e.g., impulse-control deficits, affective instability, cognition, sensory disturbance [Blader and Jensen 2007]).

Overall, the principle espoused in available guidelines is to treat the "primary disorder" first (Pappadopulos et al. 2003). For instance, current guidelines for the pharmacotherapy of aggressive behavior in the context of a primary disruptive disorder and comorbid ADHD recommend stimulant treatment (with behavioral intervention) first, leveraging the large effects of stimulant monotherapy on impulse control for this patient group. Cotherapy with an antipsychotic agent or a mood stabilizer might then be considered for aggression that is refractory to optimal stimulant treatment (Pliszka et al. 2006), although the evidence base for sequential treatment of this sort remains meager (Blader et al. 2007). Severe agitation developing in the context of psychosis obviously warrants antipsychotic treatment first. Behavioral explosiveness seen when others interfere with the compulsive behavior of a child with obsessive-compulsive disorder would likewise be suitable for treatment that aims to attenuate the youngster's anxiety disorder.

Recent expert consensus panels endeavor to provide clinicians with evidence-based guidance on the management of aggressive behavior that does not respond adequately to pharmacotherapy for the child's primary condition (Jensen et al. 2007; Schur et al. 2003). In particular, these guidelines highlight the evidence base for antipsychotic and mood-stabilizing medications and emphasize the "start low, go slow" approach to titration.

Whichever disorder or target symptom is the focus of pharmacotherapy, quantitative assessment of outcomes is strongly advised. Memory and review of chart notes, even if they were infallible indices of a patient's true clinical condition, are very hard to correlate accurately with changes in treatment. Resources may constrain such efforts, but ideally one would have fairly frequent rating-scale scores that reflect target symptoms, other related areas of difficulty, and the child's functioning. These areas may change desynchronously (e.g., attention better, aggression same, peer involvement worse), so that global assessments might obscure important aspects of clinical response. One useful brief rating scale that tracks several domains of behavioral difficulties is the Child Behavior Rating Form (Kolko 1993).

DRUG–DRUG INTERACTIONS

Interactions between agents might vitiate efficacy or risk toxicity. Pharmacodynamic interactions arise when joint administration of two drugs markedly increases their separate risks for adverse effects on the same physiological system or organ. For instance, oral preparations of α_2-adrenergic agonists are short acting, particularly clonidine. Some patients may experience hypertensive rebound after the drugs' direct pharmacological hypotensive effect subsides. The sympathomimetic action of psychostimulants may exacerbate rising blood pressure if administration coincides with such rebound (Regino et al. 2000).

Pharmacokinetic interactions occur when one agent's presence alters the absorption, distribution, metabolism, or excretion of other compounds (Flockhart and Oesterheld 2000; Vinks and Walson 2003). Administration of bupropion, for example, inhibits a cytochrome P450 isoenzyme, 2D6 (Kotlyar et al. 2005), that is important to the metabolism of the antipsychotic risperidone (Shin et al. 1999). Compensatory mechanisms may offset a potential "shortage" of the key enzyme when they are coadministered. However, a bottleneck in metabolic activity may expose some individuals (e.g., low producers of a particular cytochrome or of alternative pathways) to supratherapeutic levels of a drug or its metabolites. These situations may necessitate dosage reductions to maintain efficacy and tolerability. By the same token, *discontinuation* of an agent may hasten the metabolism of the other drug, possibly leading to subtherapeutic bioavailability given the same oral dose. Symptom resurgence, therefore, might not necessarily demonstrate that the discontinued drug was effective but perhaps that the remaining agent is now, in essence, underdosed.

Psychotherapies

Most child inpatient programs incorporate the triad of individual, family, and group psychotherapies.

INDIVIDUAL PSYCHOTHERAPY

As with outpatients, the specific content of individual psychotherapy with hospitalized children varies considerably as a function of the youngsters' developmental level and presenting problems. Insight-oriented therapy that relies on introspection, verbal expression, and linking of problematic behavioral patterns to core emotional conflicts is seldom fruitful and in any event is regarded as more suitable for longer-term care than acute inpatient stays afford. A more concrete, essentially cognitive-behavioral, approach rooted in recent events may be productive for many children. Praise and recognition for behaviors that reflect therapeutic progress (e.g., handling provocation or frustration with composure, appropriately interacting more with peers, talking about feelings rather than acting impulsively on them) is worthwhile. Likewise, reviewing difficult moments in a nonconfrontational way that helps the child to develop and rehearse alternative reactions, and to see an incident from different perspectives, is also appropriate. Interactions during family visits are further grist for the mill in helping the child identify feelings that lead to agitated behavior. Time can also be well spent observing the child in social interaction and facilitating appropriate involvement.

Many hospitalized children have experienced more than a fair share of misfortune, if not outright trauma. Such early life events include shuttling between caregivers, maltreatment, inadequate care, family discord, exposure to violence and destruction, chronic illness, and losses that include parental incapacitation, incarceration, terminal illness, and death. Although children typically prefer to avoid discussing these topics, empathy and support are important. It may be appropriate for the clinician to let the child know of his or her awareness and understanding of these adversities and to seek to alleviate the shame, self-blame, fear, and hopelessness to which these ordeals often give rise. Helping the child anticipate and be hopeful about how things will turn out after discharge may provide needed support that is otherwise unavailable. The conversation may end up being rather one sided. Clinicians whose prior experience has been principally with adults may find this disconcerting at first. They may benefit from supervision that reassures them that their efforts are worthwhile. Well-intentioned efforts to prod a reticent child into expressing his or her feelings may be more aversive and frustrating for the child than helpful.

FAMILY THERAPY

Family therapy on acute care inpatient settings has rather practical goals, given the time constraints. For the majority of children, this will tend to emphasize development of behavioral support strategies that are more likely to promote more cooperative behavior and better-modulated responses to upset. As the situation may warrant, other foci may include developing parental responses to, for instance, a child's dysphoria, worries, and severe avoidant behavior, along with recognition that certain parent–child interactions may inadvertently reinforce a child's resorting to these maladaptive reactions to stress.

The quality of the parent–child relationship is reflected in warmth, positive involvement, appropriate discipline, and concern that is genuine but not overbearing. Cultivating these may be particularly important for long-term outcome (Blader 2004, 2006b). The agenda for family treatment often also needs to address many adversities that impact on the caregivers' well-being and capacity to handle their child's psychiatric illness adequately. These include conflict between caregivers, antagonisms between the family and other service providers and schools, limited resources, parental illness, and so forth. Prioritizing these concerns, taking both urgency and tractability into account while maintaining alliance with the family, is a significant challenge for acute care settings.

GROUP PSYCHOTHERAPY

It is customary for direct care staff, with or without other clinical staff, to meet with all children together once or twice a day. Although their agenda may seem "administrative" (discussing the schedule for the day, introducing new patients, offering good wishes to those set for discharge), these meetings can be a forum for children to help one another by encouraging peer praise, eliciting solutions to common difficulties, or offering feedback on how one's behavior has influenced others. Therapies that address children's social skills, anger control, and problem solving, among other things, have shown value among outpatients (Lipman et al. 2006; Lochman et al. 2006; Sukhodolsky et al. 2000). Group adaptations for children provide opportunities for skill practice and modeling. Some of these interventions are designed to follow a sequence that builds on earlier sessions. Implementing such treatments contends with the discontinuities that short stays and shifting group membership produce. Clinicians often improvise by adapting these treatments into more self-contained components. One could see these adaptations as dilutions of evidence-based treatments. On the other hand, inpatient settings offer opportunities for prompting and coaching in the use of specific skills to address real-life situations as they occur on the unit.

Patient and Family Education

Family therapy often involves psychoeducation, but some services endeavor to provide support and knowledge through additional outreach to families. One common format is a clinician-moderated group for parents that offers presentations on a variety of topics related to mental health issues and advocacy. Attending families provide one another with assistance and support. Parents may be invited to participate after the child's discharge as well. Family resource centers located on or near the unit can provide families with informational materials about children's mental health and community resources.

Clinicians customarily discuss pharmacotherapeutic options with families, and doing so ideally also serves to educate and empower families. The conversation should clarify the treatment's rationale, risks, manner of evaluating outcomes, and time frame for judging usefulness and encourage questioning and voicing of concerns. The dialogue should be summarized via progress notes in the medical record. Separate consent-to-treat documents for each therapeutic maneuver are seldom necessary, and the standard hospital forms at admission usually fulfill medicolegal requirements for routine treatments. More formal consent procedures in most jurisdictions pertain to certain treatments that are relatively unusual in child psychiatry (e.g., electroconvulsive therapy, clozapine) or to situations in which children are under the guardianship of a public agency.

In communities where multilingualism is common, hospitals typically offer interpreter services. Information in psychiatric settings, however, tends to be far more personal, detailed, and in some ways nuanced than in other hospital areas. Psychiatric services may need to evaluate whether the hospitalwide resources offer the confidentiality protections and quality required.

Older children in particular often harbor confusion over what admission to a psychiatric inpatient service means for their emerging identities, have concerns about stigma, and are ambivalent about treatment. As unit composition permits, groups for these youngsters, who are usually developmentally further along than most child inpatients, can provide needed mutual support and psychoeducation. Otherwise, these are appropriate emphases for individual therapy.

Rehabilitation and Recreational Therapies

In most settings, children's education continues throughout their stays on inpatient psychiatric services, at least when school is in session in the community. Participation in a hospital's school setting also provides clinicians with enormously helpful information about the child's functioning, both academic and behavioral. Some acute care units have dedicated classrooms in which children spend a full school day, and the activities and structure unmistakably resemble a "regular" school. Other units may have a teacher who provides individualized tutoring and gives assignments and materials to the patients, devoting relatively fewer hours of the day to academic involvement. Teachers most often have a special education background and are employees of the public educational jurisdiction for the hospital's environs. A few psychiatric facilities operate their own accredited schools and endeavor to recover tuition costs from patients' home school districts. Teachers' perspectives and expertise make their input on patients' functioning and clinical progress an important resource.

Another critical program component is structured activities for children's recreation and socialization. Staff specialists responsible for these services are typically from the facility's rehabilitation, child life, activities therapy, or other similar departments. Personnel are often occupational therapists and from other related disciplines. In the best of situations, patients can have some choice about which of a few concurrent activities to attend. This helps keep the group sizes more manageable and enables more meaningful interaction. Off-unit spaces (e.g., playgrounds or swimming pools) and off-grounds trips can be important experiences that counteract the institutionalizing effects of longer-term stays.

Milieu Management

The admission process usually culminates in an orientation of children and their families to the unit's program, routines, and rules. Parents appreciate clear verbal and written explanations of how cooperative behavior is recognized and how poor rule adherence is addressed. This information helps establish appropriate expectations for how staff will interact with the child and comfort that discipline is not arbitrary. Similarly, rules specifically for parents will often identify which items are not permitted on the unit, that visiting times are not merely "guidelines," the circumstances under which staff may direct parents to leave the unit, and so on.

On children's units, milieu-based programs based on behavior modification principles are nearly ubiquitous. They are often called "level," "point," or "token economy" systems. At their core, these programs define specific behaviors to promote or discourage and

apply staff feedback and consequences accordingly. Because these procedures are core elements of many interventions for children's behavioral disorders (e.g., Kazdin 1997), these milieu programs play a significant role in treatment for the large number of children admitted for conduct disturbances. In addition, these systems provide a form of structure and governance by codifying basic rules and how infractions will be addressed. Because these systems often include some quantification of behavioral adjustment, in the form of points and such, they can also furnish a means of plotting clinical progress.

As with any good behavioral therapy program, the consistency of feedback is paramount, especially praise and recognition, which should be abundant but sincere. This would in many cases accompany assignment of points or tokens for achieving the positive behavioral goals of the activity or time of day, which is well defined. In some versions, each patient also has a few individualized goals for which he or she obtains praise, encouragement, or correction as well as points earned. The actual privileges or rewards toward which points accrue can involve some that are earned daily (video game time) and some that are based on accumulation over several days (privilege level). The former enable the patient to begin each day with a new start and to benefit accordingly.

The shortcomings of these approaches chiefly stem from their potential to be rigid and from their emphasis on the application of consequences to shape behavior (Mohr and Pumariega 2004). Individual variation in what triggers displays of behavioral disturbance and, for that matter, what constitutes a "reward" can in some cases place the therapeutic value of unit-wide behavioral systems at odds with their role in "governance." Perhaps a child's resistance to staff direction may be reduced by a period of gentle, affable engagement beforehand, while the typical consequences for noncompliance (warnings, time-outs, loss of points) most often lead to escalating agitation. "Time out" from an activity may be a consequence that many children are motivated to avoid, but for others it may function as an escape from an undesired activity or a means to gain attention.

To overcome these problems, most settings do manage to incorporate program modifications as needed for individual patients. Individualized assessment of the situational *context* that gives rise to behavior and the *function* that behavior serves in fulfilling some need, albeit maladaptively, is an important facet of behavior therapy (e.g., O'Neill et al. 1997). This type of individualized planning within a milieu setting can be complicated by constraints on staffing and difficulties in convincing children that apparent inequities in staff responses do have an underlying fairness. As interventions involving many staff over several shifts and hospital areas become more diverse and nuanced, they risk reintroducing the inconsistencies and idiosyncrasies in staff. These issues may be surmountable, however, and several facilities are evaluating implementations of these approaches (Greene and Ablon 2006; Greene et al. 2006; Martin et al., in press). Ways to minimize staff "drift," "regression to the behavioral mean," and "one size fits all" approaches to patient care can include frequent cross-disciplinary communication, preferably blended into existing unitwide structures (such as team meetings) rather than in separate standalone meetings; standalone meetings organized on a periodic or ad hoc basis, particularly during times of transition or staff turnover or after critical incidents; and scheduling and documentation templates that incorporate best practices, individualized plans, and iteratively updated information.

Staffing Patterns

Staffing ratios should be ideally calculated based on national benchmarks for each discipline. However, it is usually in the discipline of nursing that such benchmarks are frequently available. Generally a 1:3 staff-to-patient ratio for acutely ill patients and 1:5 for longer-term patients meet national standards. Full-time equivalents are calculated based on data such as average daily census, number of work shifts, and skill mix. However, patient acuity, which varies based on multiple factors including seasonal variations, is rarely taken into account when full-time equivalents are calculated. This often produces a perception of burnout and compassion fatigue in the caregivers of acutely ill patients. Management of staffing is crucial to the smooth operations of an inpatient unit.

Management and Prevention of Suicidal and Aggressive Behaviors

Acute Management

ENHANCED MONITORING

Patients thought to pose increased risk to themselves or others may be considered for more vigilant observation to enable prompt intervention and support when early signs of faltering composure arise. One version involves constant supervision by a specifically designated staff member who keeps a written log of the patient's status at frequent intervals ("one-to-one observation," or "1:1"). Currently, many if not most hospital psychiatric settings do not receive additional personnel when 1:1 is deemed necessary. In these cases, the rest of the service makes do with reduced staffing. Variations include orders for 1:1 assignment only outside of structured activities where the additional surveillance may be redundant with existing oversight. The necessity for these measures is usually reassessed on a daily basis and orders renewed or discontinued accordingly.

DE-ESCALATION STRATEGIES

In few occupations does one more regularly encounter agitated, upset, belligerent, and, at least temporarily, irrational individuals than in providing direct care to inpatients in psychiatric settings (Nijman et al. 2005). The ability to help the overwrought child handle upsets without disruptive or destructive impact is particularly vital for staff on children's units. Recent federal regulations now require formal training, demonstrated competence, and periodic retraining in early identification and nonphysical intervention with patients whose behavior might place them at risk for severe escalation (Centers for Medicare and Medicaid Services 2006). Several resources to inform such staff development are currently available (American Psychiatric Association et al. 2003; Cowin et al. 2003; Grenyer et al. 2004).

Techniques for nonphysical crisis management or de-escalation in psychiatric settings share some general principles. Many approaches emphasize detection of early warning signs for growing agitation. Children are perhaps less likely to show a period of sulkiness, brooding, pacing, and glares that, for older persons, often signals simmering upset that further provocation can bring to boil. Rather, quick, overtly combative, or oppositional reactions to feeling thwarted or offended are more likely among highly impulsive youngsters. Nonetheless, the child who seems to be in a generally bad mood may be at higher risk on a given day, so extra attention and support are, of course, both compassionate and useful in reducing risk.

When the fuse is lit but harm has yet to occur, the situation is ideally handled when the adults display calm, concern, and confidence. Hasty staff reactions that convey agitation, threats, hostility, and anxiety may further inflame the situation. Therefore, the optimal approach is for staff to adopt a nonthreatening posture and seek clarification for what appears to be troubling the child. Empathizing and offering suggestions or choices for constructive engagement in dealing with the situation provide the individual with control and avert the sense of being "cornered." An available staff member with whom the child has a particularly good relationship may be most successful at engaging him or her at such affectively charged times. A chorus of adults, however well intended, may be too stimulating and counterproductive, and a better outcome may result if others linger in the background to intervene only if things deteriorate. Of course, if the situation de-escalates by virtue of the child's participation, then all can exuberantly express their admiration to the child for "making good decisions" and "doing a great job being in charge of your own behavior."

The presence of other patients may make the child's acquiescence less likely if he or she feels that doing so would be humiliating. The incident may also become dangerous or upsetting to other children. When practical, it is best to help the child to voluntarily leave a group setting or at times to relocate the other patients.

PHARMACOLOGICAL INTERVENTION

Medications may be administered to hasten the resolution of a specific episode of severe behavioral agitation that is under way or imminent. A common context for doing so is when concurrent standing treatments to improve the patient's emotional volatility, impulsivity, distorted judgment, or other psychopathological processes driving dyscontrol have yet to yield the intended effects. In general, the use of medications in this fashion (i.e., *pro re nata* [prn] or *statim* [stat] use) is disfavored for children in all but extreme situations, for reasons that derive from both practical pharmacological and regulatory considerations.

As a practical matter, children admitted to the hospital with aggressive behavior commonly receive antipsychotic medication as part of their regular treatment, and the introduction of an ad hoc dose or a different compound (several atypical antipsychotics currently lack immediate-release injectable preparations that highly uncooperative patients may require) to the standing regimen carries risks. Benzodiazepines may increase disinhibition and aggression (Bond 1992) and are disfavored for treating childhood aggression outside of acute use in psychosis or mania. Antihistamines are considered fairly safe in this context, although their true pharmacological effect, relative to the impact on the child of intramuscular administration per se, is questionable (Vitiello et al. 1991).

Regulations with the broadest nationwide applicability are those that the federal government issues as conditions of participation for hospitals to receive funds from Medicare and, in effect, from all other revenues authorized by the Social Security Act, including Medicaid. These regulations address when a pharmacological intervention constitutes a form of "restraint," in which case administration is controlled by a number of restraint-related provisions, including prohibition of prn use (Centers for Medicare and Medicaid Services 2006). Practitioners must be mindful of these and other regulatory requirements governing the use of medications to assist in alleviating severe behavioral agitation.

PHYSICAL SECLUSION AND RESTRAINT

The mental health codes of most North American jurisdictions permit the application of involuntary constraints on a person's mobility by hospital personnel as a last resort in true emergencies. The isolation of a person in a room with insuperable barriers to his or her voluntary exit is *seclusion*. The application to one's body of physical force or a device (or, in circumstances noted earlier, medications) to restrict movement is *restraint*.

Governmental regulations specify many of the procedures to be followed in these situations. These require the facility to establish a written protocol for handling nascent crises to avert the need for physical interventions and the criteria for judging that these interventions have not been successful before proceeding to apply the more restrictive alternatives. In addition, the decision-making process, staff training, forms of documentation, specific methods or devices applied, observation, monitoring of vital signs, duration of the intervention, and so forth also must adhere to the standards set by governmental and accrediting bodies. In the United States, federal regulations establish basic nationwide standards through the conditions of participation they promulgate for Medicare and Medicaid. State and local laws may establish requirements that are more stringent than federal ones (e.g., shorter permitted periods of seclusion or restraint). Indeed, states can prohibit them either altogether or for specific patient groups. Where localities have separate departments for mental health and developmental disabilities, there may be separate regulations that apply to those with mental retardation.

All of these provisions cover children, and it is only recently that maximum durations for each restraint/seclusion order differ by age (e.g., 8 years and younger, 1 hour; 9–17 years, 2 hours; 18 years and older, 4 hours; local requirements may authorize even shorter periods) (Centers for Medicare and Medicaid Services

2006). Nonetheless, all incidents involving minors receive special scrutiny owing to their greater overall vulnerability and dependence, increased susceptibility to the physical and psychological harms the interventions may themselves produce, and, often, the view that children's limited size and strength should render them seldom necessary. Of perhaps more relevance to children is the practice of staff physically holding a child to prevent mobility for relatively brief periods (physical as opposed to "mechanical" restraint). Facilities routinely have policies for training, implementation, and review of their use. Tragically, incidents involving physical restraint of this type have accounted for the most child fatalities due to asphyxiation (Joint Commission on Accreditation of Healthcare Organizations 1998; Nunno et al. 2006).

Having exhausted nonphysical methods to reduce the threats an individual's behavior poses, seclusion and restraint interventions are often implemented in a stepwise fashion; that is, seclusion is thought to be less invasive and may be undertaken first. If the child endangers him- or herself during seclusion, the team may consider restraint as the next step. There are concerns that the physical coercion these procedures involve, especially restraint, may be particularly disturbing to children with histories of trauma or abuse (Cotton 1989).

Both applicable laws and institutional regulations delineate monitoring procedures for patients during the period of seclusion or restraint. At a minimum, these procedures require constant observation of the patient (in some jurisdictions achievable via closed-circuit television). Monitoring serves two purposes. The first is to ensure that an individual is not subject to these interventions for longer than is necessary. Staff members performing observation therefore record at frequent intervals the patient's behavior, efforts at communicating after some period of relative calm, and periodic physician's assessments. The second purpose is to guarantee the patient's safety given the risks these procedures pose, including tragic outcomes involving injury or death. Consequently, periodic assessments of vital signs, respiration rates, needs for nourishment and voiding, adequate "slack" where devices contact the body, and so on are required and must be documented clearly. Pulse oximetry has been proposed as a direct measurement of blood oxygenation during prolonged episodes of restraint. Currently, the approach does not constitute an accepted or even widely used standard of care, and some critics have opposed it on the grounds that it may "sanction" the use of restraint by focusing on how safe the practice is rather than on

ways to minimize its use or its duration. Moreover, there is no evidence that the use of pulse oximetry decreases restraint-related fatalities. The best approach to such serious, if rare, events may be in decreasing the overall use of restraints.

It bears emphasizing that these approaches are last-resort crisis interventions and should not be construed, or justified, as treatments for psychiatric illness as such. The use of interventions whose putative efficacy is predicated on the experience of discomfort, pain, or humiliation is unacceptable as elements of routine treatment for individuals with mental illness. Unusual circumstances that might justify their short-term use to avoid an even more dire outcome remain highly controversial.

Prevention

High-quality, well-supervised, and developmentally appropriate unit programming is obviously important for children in hospital settings. It is also beneficial for minimizing the sorts of episodes that can culminate in harmful behavior. Times of day during which behavioral escalations are frequent require scrutiny, especially when seclusion and restraint often occur. These may coincide with periods of major transitions, suboptimal staff-to-child ratios, free-play times that degenerate into a free-for-all, and so forth. Certain routines that require high staff assistance (e.g., getting dressed, getting ready for bed, doing homework) may benefit from staggering to involve smaller groups of youngsters at a time. A single bedtime for children of diverse developmental levels may also contribute to chaos when the overtired children become overstimulated whereas the far-from-tired ones dread lengthy confinement to bed before they are biologically ready for sleep. The conclusion of visiting hours may be stressful for children as family departs, and the whole period terribly so for children whom no adult comes to see. Extra care and something to look forward to at these times may be essential. There are also, of course, situations in which particular staff members, whatever their other professional assets, may inadvertently contribute to the instability of a particular phase of unit activity.

Children with whom staff interventions have come to include high utilization of seclusion or restraint will often require modification to their care plans. Ideally, these are rooted in a functional assessment of what appears to trigger the youngster's difficulties, whether there are feasible environmental changes that can mitigate them, and what steps can meet the child's needs more adaptively. It is tempting to defer reassessment of a child's treatment plan and pin all hopes on a change in pharmacotherapy that will pay off with vastly improved behavioral adaptability. Unfortunately, by the time a child's severe dyscontrol has become persistent in the hospital, he or she will likely have already experienced numerous interventions, and the prospects that the additional maneuver will have fast and robust payoff may be slim. There is the further risk that frequent application of physical interventions to control behavior degrades the child's relationships and expectations of others so that the pattern becomes self-sustaining and possibly less responsive to pharmacotherapy.

Medicolegal and Risk Management Considerations

Because children are a particularly vulnerable population, their treatment on an inpatient service incurs a few protective and regulatory obligations beyond those that pertain to psychiatric care in general. Parents are empowered in most jurisdictions to provide consent for their child's treatment throughout childhood. States differ in the age at which parental consent alone is no longer sufficient for a voluntary admission, and the patient's consent to admission and treatment becomes necessary between the ages of 14 and 16. Separation agreements and divorce decrees may apportion medical decision making apart from emergency situations to one parent. In some instances, one parent's rights have been terminated, and there might even be court orders limiting or prohibiting a parent's contact with the child. It is recommended that copies of these documents be obtained early in admission.

State laws also differ in the threshold required to establish the need for involuntary commitment, but most allow temporary detention of minors through certification of dangerousness to self or others after a face-to-face evaluation by a mental health clinician. Usually the brief period of being detained in a psychiatric facility allows observation, assessment, and—most importantly—the development of a safety plan. A commitment hearing with a judge must occur within a specified time period to determine disposition: continued inpatient level of care, outpatient care, or no care at all.

Inpatient settings can also serve to uncover abuse: physical, emotional, or sexual. Any clinician who suspects the abuse must report to the state child protective services, and if the perpetrator is the primary caregiver or lives within the same household as the child,

the child must not be returned to that primary caregiver's home until the suspicion is ruled out through investigation.

Informed consent must be obtained from parents for any child for whom psychopharmacological intervention is being considered. In many states, use of prn medications may be interpreted as chemical restraints. As noted earlier, practitioners must be aware of the state human rights laws specifically pertaining to seclusion and restraint.

Discharge Planning

Involvement of Community Providers, Resources, and Significant Others

A postdischarge care plan that leverages extended familiarity with a child and family's needs is one of the major goals of hospitalization. In acute care settings with diminishing lengths of stay, however, planning for continuing care needs in the community practically needs to begin at admission. This requires the engagement of community clinicians and others to learn firsthand their perceptions of the main impediments to the child's doing well at home and whether they have specific questions about the child's difficulties they would like hospital-based assessment to address. In the absence of laboratory or radiological tests to provide objective support or refutation of diagnostic beliefs, the hospital clinician's credibility will depend on the quality of communication and its responsiveness to what the community provider needs to know. Perfunctory discharge summaries that recite medications and dosages, often without clear statements of their rationales and textured descriptions of response, are unlikely to serve this function well. This bidirectional communication can only take place if the family consents to it, so hesitations the family may harbor about doing so should be broached at admission. If families wish to go elsewhere for follow-up care, the appropriate linkages should start sooner rather than later.

Much the same applies to collaborating with the child's home school district, given the large proportion of child inpatients who receive special education services prior to admission. Schools and clinicians may differ on the appropriate setting, especially for the child who was highly disruptive before hospitalization. Some districts contemplating a more restrictive setting for a child may be willing to have the child return to the prior program before discharge to see for themselves, as it were, how well the clinician's claims of improvement generalize even for a short period outside the unit. In any event, a child's community teachers often find the unit's schoolteachers' reports of the child's current status particularly credible, and predischarge contact between them is often useful to facilitate. At one time it was common for a behaviorally stable child to stay in the hospital for additional time so that school authorities could devise an appropriate service plan rather than discharge a child with no appropriate educational setting. Financial pressures to shorten lengths of stay to what is absolutely vital to stabilize the patient's clinical condition have largely eliminated this option. It therefore behooves all parties to secure appropriate services expeditiously.

Various forms of enhanced community-based services beyond routine outpatient care have been developed with the psychiatrically hospitalized child in mind. These include home-based services, respite care for families, case management to help coordinate the multitude of services families often require, and other services to support families.

A perennial source of complications for discharge planning, not to mention heartbreak, is the large number of hospitalized children residing in surrogate care arrangements before admission. Foster parents are often heroic figures intensely devoted to the children in their homes despite limited support from agencies. There are instances, however, in which hospitalized children cannot return to these homes. Sometimes the agency's goal is to reunite siblings, or a biological parent may be on the cusp of regaining custody. A number of youngsters, however, have serially resided in several homes because the severity of their disorder has exceeded caregivers' capacities.

Transition to Next Level of Care

Acute care units at times play a pivotal role in a child's admission to a residential treatment service or to subacute inpatient psychiatric care. This can be a lengthy process and often necessitates a good deal of conferencing of hospital staff with potential facilities and the social service officials who, as the usual source of funding, are also involved. Some states have "single point of entry" arrangements whereby the governmental authority receives the relevant clinical material and then deals directly with potential residential centers. Hospital staff may have to advocate strenuously for an interim discharge plan so the child does not languish in the hospital unnecessarily. There are also financial pressures that arise when it is determined that a child no longer needs the acute hospital setting, because payers may reimburse the hospital at a reduced rate, corresponding to a so-called alternative level of care. Payers may apply this rate retrospectively (i.e., after discharge).

From a clinical standpoint, it will often fall to hospital clinicians to help the child avoid succumbing to two risks. The state of limbo can understandably give rise to despondency or apathy, exacerbated by prolonged time in a small setting designed for short stays, which can become mind-numbingly tedious. This gives rise to a second hazard, institutionalization, that may make adaptation to more normal environments difficult and anxiety provoking.

Specialty Day Hospital

Day treatment programs for children are usually a melding, in varying emphases, of special education and psychiatric care. At one end, there are specialized schools for those with social–emotional impairments that have some therapeutic component or a psychiatric consultant, and at the other are true day hospitals with primary psychiatric emphasis and specialized education services as a major adjunct.

Day treatment programs have in the past cared for youth over fairly long periods, not unlike day hospitals for adults with chronic severe psychiatric illness. This has changed somewhat, and many day treatment or partial hospitalization programs are now conceived to provide medium-term subacute care (i.e., weeks to months, rather than years) as a station on the road toward full community reintegration.

In another emerging model, the "partial hospital," a child is discharged to home but continues to participate in weekday schooling and rehabilitation activities on the inpatient unit for 1 or more weeks. This can be a less costly alternative for children whose postdischarge needs are not entirely clear or when there is a lag until an appropriate school setting becomes available. Families often value the continuity of care. However, in many areas the family has to provide transportation for this service when schools do not have the willingness or the administrative agility to implement the arrangements promptly.

Conclusion

Inpatient services for children have changed markedly over the past 20 years. Once conceived as a therapeutic modality that could bring about major changes in disturbances of behavior and personality development, the mission of psychiatric hospitalization now is chiefly to help temporize major crises that arise from dangerously volatile behavior or worrisome changes in mental status. Most inpatient services are therefore not in themselves "solutions" to the major psychiatric disorders of childhood, whose courses are typically chronic, but rather are a component within a continuum of care to be used sparingly. Currently, referrals to these services often harbor a hope that specialists in severe childhood psychiatric illness will clarify diagnosis, arrive at an effective treatment regimen, and plan aftercare services that will improve the prospects for successful development. The evidence base to support these functions, however, remains limited: definitive diagnoses for many very ill youngsters are elusive and sometimes determinable only after years of observation and treatment; treatments for this patient group have little or no evidence of their value, because the study of interventions for children who have gained little relief from first-line treatments lags well behind that of adults; and prognostic judgments and estimation of treatment needs lack an empirical basis and remain at best inspired guesswork. At the same time, it seems uncertain that almost 20 years of greater attention to alternatives that might avert psychiatric admissions for children have had widespread impact. These enhanced outpatient services are unevenly available, embrace a variety of service models, and after all this time remain for many regions within the realm of "demonstration projects" rather than a fully functioning accessible part of routine care.

The coming years, therefore, present new challenges for children's inpatient services. The importance of relevant research to anchor the evaluative and treatment functions of hospitalization is immense. Mental health systems of care for children are still evolving; reduced lengths of stay and greater hurdles to access have saved money, whereas the outpatient alternatives that would really reduce overall admissions are tentative. For many families, quality child psychiatric services are barely available. These systems factors exert pressures on inpatient settings that are mandated to discharge youngsters quickly despite a shortage of adequate outpatient services.

Within the inpatient service itself, programming and staff morale strive to consolidate a sense of mission in light of these changes. It remains unclear how best to reconcile the potential for these unique settings to profoundly alter the life course of a child with psychiatric illness with recent trends that accord them a merely palliative role.

References

Achenbach TM, Rescorla LA: Manual for ASEBA School-Age Forms and Profiles. Burlington, VT, Research Center for Children, Youth, and Families, 2000

American Psychiatric Association, American Psychiatric Nurses Association, National Association of Psychiatric Health Systems: Learning From Each Other: Success Stories and Ideas for Reducing Restraint/Seclusion in Behavioral Health. Washington, DC, American Psychiatric Association, 2003

Blader J: Symptom, family, and service predictors of children's psychiatric rehospitalization within one year of discharge. J Am Acad Child Adolesc Psychiatry 43:440–451, 2004

Blader JC: Pharmacotherapy and postdischarge outcomes of child inpatients admitted for aggressive behavior. J Clin Psychopharmacol 26:419–425, 2006a

Blader JC: Which family factors predict children's externalizing behaviors following discharge from psychiatric inpatient treatment? J Child Psychol Psychiatry 41:1133–1142, 2006b

Blader JC, Carlson GA: Increased rates of bipolar disorder diagnoses among US child, adolescent, and adult inpatients, 1996–2004. Biol Psychiatry 62 (suppl):107–114, 2007

Blader JC, Jensen PS: Aggression in children: an integrative approach, in Lewis' Child and Adolescent Psychiatry: A Comprehensive Textbook, 4th Edition. Edited by Martin A, Volkmar FR. Baltimore, MD, Lippincott Williams & Wilkins, 2007, pp 467–483

Blader JC, Abikoff H, Foley C, et al: Children's behavioral adaptation early in psychiatric hospitalization. J Child Psychol Psychiatry 35:709–721, 1994

Blader JC, Schooler NR, Jensen PS, et al: Efficacy of adjunctive divalproex sodium for stimulant-refractory aggression among children with ADHD. Presented at the 160th Annual Meeting of the American Psychiatric Association, San Diego, CA, May 2007

Bond AJ: Pharmacological manipulation of aggressiveness and impulsiveness in healthy volunteers. Prog Neuropsychopharmacol Biol Psychiatry 16:1–7, 1992

Bronfman ET: Inpatient child mental health treatment: strategies used to manage treatment, in The Traumatic Bond Between the Psychotherapist and Managed Care. Edited by Weisgerber K. Northvale, NJ, Jason Aronson, 1999, pp 123–136

Case BG, Olfson M, Marcus SC, et al: Trends in the inpatient mental health treatment of children and adolescents in US community hospitals between 1990 and 2000. Arch Gen Psychiatry 64:89–96, 2007

Centers for Medicare and Medicaid Services: Medicare and Medicaid programs; hospital conditions of participation: patients' rights: final rule (42 CFR 482). Fed Regist 71:71378–71428, 2006

Connor DF: Aggression and Antisocial Behavior in Children and Adolescents: Research and Treatment. New York, Guilford, 2002

Cotton NS: The developmental-clinical rationale for the use of seclusion in the psychiatric treatment of children. Am J Orthopsychiatry 59:442–450, 1989

Cowin L, Davies R, Estall G, et al: De-escalating aggression and violence in the mental health setting. Int J Ment Health Nurs 12:64–73, 2003

dosReis S, Zito JM, Safer DJ, et al: Mental health services for youths in foster care and disabled youths. Am J Public Health 91:1094–1099, 2001

Flockhart DA, Oesterheld JR: Cytochrome P450-mediated drug interactions. Child Adolesc Psychiatr Clin North Am 9:43–76, 2000

Greene RW, Ablon JS: Treating Explosive Kids: The Collaborative Problem-Solving Approach. New York, Guilford, 2006

Greene RW, Ablon JS, Martin A: Use of collaborative problem solving to reduce seclusion and restraint in child and adolescent inpatient units. Psychiatr Serv 57:610–612, 2006

Grenyer BF, Ilkiw-Lavalle O, Biro P, et al: Safer at work: development and evaluation of an aggression and violence minimization program. Aust N Z J Psychiatry 38:804–810, 2004

Jensen PS, Youngstrom EA, Steiner H, et al: Consensus report on impulsive aggression as a symptom across diagnostic categories in child psychiatry: implications for medication studies. J Am Acad Child Adolesc Psychiatry 46:309–322, 2007

Joint Commission on Accreditation of Healthcare Organizations: Preventing restraint deaths, in Sentinel Event Alert (Issue 8). Oakbrook Terrace, IL, Joint Commission on Accreditation of Healthcare Organizations, 1998, pp 1–2

Kazdin AE: Parent management training: evidence, outcomes, and issues. J Am Acad Child Adolesc Psychiatry 36:1349–1356, 1997

Kloos AL, Collins R, Weller RA, et al: Suicide in preadolescents: who is at risk? Curr Psychiatry Rep 9:89–93, 2007

Knitzer J: Unclaimed Children: The Failure of Public Responsibility to Children and Adolescents in Need of Mental Health Services. Washington, DC, Children's Defense Fund, 1982

Knitzer J, Cooper J: Beyond integration: challenges for children's mental health. Health Aff 25:670–679, 2006

Kolko DJ: Further evaluation of inpatient child behavior ratings: consistency across settings, time, and sources. Journal of Emotional and Behavioral Disorders 1:251–259, 1993

Kotlyar M, Brauer LH, Tracy TS, et al: Inhibition of CYP2D6 activity by bupropion. J Clin Psychopharmacol 25:226–229, 2005

Lipman EL, Boyle MH, Cunningham C, et al: Testing effectiveness of a community-based aggression management program for children 7 to 11 years old and their families. J Am Acad Child Adolesc Psychiatry 45:1085–1093, 2006

Lochman JE, Powell NR, Jackson MF, et al: Cognitive-behavioral psychotherapy for conduct disorder: The Coping Power Program, in Conduct Disorders: A Practitioner's Guide to Comparative Treatments. Edited by Nelson WM III, Finch AJ Jr, Hart KJ. New York, Springer, 2006, pp 177–215

Martin A, Krieg H, Esposito F, Stubbe D, Cardona L: Restraint and seclusion reduction through collaborative problem solving: a five-year prospective inpatient study. Psychiatr Serv (in press)

McMillen JC, Scott LD, Zima BT, et al: Use of mental health services among older youths in foster care. Psychiatr Serv 55:811–817, 2004

Mohr WK, Pumariega AJ: Level systems: inpatient programming whose time has passed. J Child Adolesc Psychiatr Nurs 17:113–125, 2004

Nijman H, Bowers L, Oud N, et al: Psychiatric nurses' experiences with inpatient aggression. Aggress Behav 31:217–227, 2005

Nunno MA, Holden MJ, Tollar A: Learning from tragedy: a survey of child and adolescent restraint fatalities. Child Abuse Negl 30:1333–1342, 2006

O'Neill RE, Horner RH, Albin RW, et al: Functional Assessment and Program Development for Problem Behavior: A Practical Handbook, 2nd Edition. Pacific Grove, CA, Brooks/Cole Publishing, 1997

Pappadopulos E, Macintyre JC II, Crismon ML, et al: Treatment recommendations for the use of antipsychotics for aggressive youth (TRAAY), part II. J Am Acad Child Adolesc Psychiatry 42:145–161, 2003

Pavuluri MN, Henry DB, Devineni B, et al: Child Mania Rating Scale: development, reliability, and validity. J Am Acad Child Adolesc Psychiatry 45:550–560, 2006

Peterson BS, Zhang H, Santa Lucia R, et al: Risk factors for presenting problems in child psychiatric emergencies. J Am Acad Child Adolesc Psychiatry 35:1162–1173, 1996

Pliszka SR, Crismon ML, Hughes CW, et al: The Texas Children's Medication Algorithm Project: revision of the algorithm for pharmacotherapy of attention-deficit/hyperactivity disorder (ADHD). J Am Acad Child Adolesc Psychiatry 45:642–647, 2006

Pottick KJ, Warner LA, Yoder KA: Youths living away from families in the US mental health system: opportunities for targeted intervention. J Behav Health Serv Res 32:264–281, 2005

Poznanski EO, Mokros HB: Children's Depression Rating Scale–Revised. Los Angeles, CA, Western Psychological Services, 1995

Regino R, Baren M, Connor DF, et al: Patterns of use of clonidine alone and in combination with methylphenidate, in Ritalin: Theory and Practice, 2nd Edition. Edited by Greenhill LL, Osman BB. Larchmont, NY, Mary Ann Liebert, 2000, pp 401–404

Reynolds CR, Kamphaus RW: The Clinician's Guide to the Behavior Assessment System for Children (BASC). New York, Guilford, 2002

Ringel JS, Sturm R: National estimates of mental health utilization and expenditures for children in 1998. J Behav Health Serv Res 28:319–333, 2001

Schur SB, Sikich L, Findling RL, et al: Treatment recommendations for the use of antipsychotics for aggressive youth (TRAAY), part I: a review. J Am Acad Child Adolesc Psychiatry 42:132–144, 2003

Shin J-G, Soukhova N, Flockhart DA: Effect of antipsychotic drugs on human liver cytochrome P-450 (CYP) isoforms in vitro: preferential inhibition of CYP2D6. Drug Metab Dispos 27:1078–1084, 1999

Sukhodolsky DG, Solomon RM, Perine J: Cognitive-behavioral, anger-control intervention for elementary school children: a treatment outcome study. Journal of Child and Adolescent Group Therapy 10:159–170, 2000

Vinks AA, Walson PD: Pharmacokinetics I: developmental principles, in Pediatric Psychopharmacology: Principles and Practice. Edited by Martin A, Scahill L, Charney DS, et al. New York, Oxford University Press, 2003, pp 44–53

Vitiello B, Hill JL, Elia J, et al: Prn medications in child psychiatric patients: a pilot placebo-controlled study. J Clin Psychiatry 52:499–501, 1991

CHAPTER 4

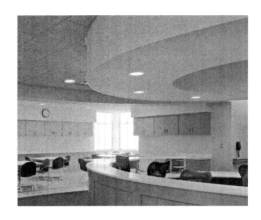

THE ADOLESCENT UNIT

Gary J. Gosselin, M.D.
David Ray DeMaso, M.D.

Inpatient psychiatry programs are the intensive care units of the adolescent mental health service system. They are meant to address the serious risks and severe impairments caused by the most acute and complex forms of mental illness that cannot be managed effectively at any other level of care. Inpatient hospitalization is a consultative and collaborative systems-based endeavor geared to produce rapid clinical stabilization that allows for an expeditious, safe, and appropriate treatment transition to a less intensive level of mental health care (Pottick et al. 2001).

Hospital admission should not be a default substitute for absent or underdeveloped community-based mental health programs that could provide clinically appropriate, less restrictive, and more economical mental health care to families and adolescents (Bartlett et al. 1999; Mansbach et al. 2003). The current national health care environment has produced significant service shortages at all levels of mental health care for adolescents. These shortages are reflected in the substantial demands faced by inpatient units that must provide effective, economical, and ethical care (Case et al. 2007; Dickey et al. 2001; Geller and Biebel

2006). This chapter presents an overview of the adolescent inpatient psychiatry unit through descriptions of admission criteria, assessment, treatment, milieu management, management of aggressive and suicidal behaviors, and discharge planning.

Admission Criteria

High levels of illness severity and significant functional impairments are the dual markers that signal a need for inpatient psychiatry admission. Clinical criteria for admission must include significant signs and symptoms of active mental illness. Functional indicators for admission usually include a significant risk of self-harm and/or harm to others. In some cases, there might be an inability to meet basic self-care or health care needs that jeopardizes the well-being of an adolescent. Serious emotional disturbances that prevent participation in family, school, or community life can also rise to a level of global impairment that can only be addressed on an inpatient basis. Scales and instruments to rate illness severity and functional impairments are available to identify clinical markers for inpatient care and enhance the reliability of treatment monitoring during the hospital course. Rating tools relevant to level-of-care screening include the Child Global Assessment Scale and the Child and Adolescent Level of Care Utilization System/Child and Adolescent Service Intensity Instrument (Fallon et al. 2006; Shaffer et al. 1983).

Every hospital admission has specific legal requirements. Voluntary or involuntary civil commitment criteria must be satisfied. Consent to admission is often required from parent and adolescent, especially for adolescents approaching the age of majority. Joint custody arrangements present a requirement that both custodial parents reach agreement about the admission decision. Due process notifications related to legal rights and status must also be provided to patients and parents as part of the admission process. Practitioners should be thoroughly familiar with the specific state mental hygiene legal standards governing their location of inpatient practice.

Assessment

General Strategies and Methods

The diagnostic workup is a systematic screening and assessment process prioritized to identify dysfunction that places the patient at greatest risk. The principles and practices outlined in the "Practice Parameters for the Psychiatric Assessment of Children and Adolescents" are applicable to the inpatient assessment process (American Academy of Child and Adolescent Psychiatry 1997). Multiple sources of information from collateral contacts such as outpatient clinicians, pediatricians, community service providers, and school personnel should be utilized to cross-check and verify assessment findings. Consents to contact collateral information sources are needed at the outset of the admission.

Diagnostic evaluations must take into account the range of developmental phenomena possible during the adolescent years, a period spanning the end of late childhood to the start of the young adult years. A determination of the concordance or discrepancy among the domains of physical, emotional, social, behavioral, cognitive, and adaptive functioning is particularly salient in assessing the impact of severe mental illness on developmental status. Failure to attain expected or loss of attained developmental milestones requires that a developmental disorder or neurodegenerative process be ruled out.

High-risk screening is an important part of the diagnostic evaluation aimed at identifying and addressing potential sources of imminent harm in a case. It covers past and current instances of significant physical illness, suicide, self-injury, violence as victim or perpetrator, fire setting, sexual abuse as victim or perpetrator, risky sexual behavior, and substance intoxication, abuse, or dependence. Results of the high-risk screening are used to prioritize the clinical interventions necessary to establish and maintain patient safety. Risk is subsequently reassessed prospectively over the course of hospitalization to maintain safety, evaluate intervention effectiveness, and gauge readiness for discharge.

The use of structured instruments to record findings provides systematic organization and reliability to the screening and assessment process (Hughes et al. 2000). The rapid pace and high volume of work on inpatient units are best served by rating instruments that allow for accurate, reliable, and efficient administration (Table 4–1). Structured rating forms for interviews, such as the Brief Psychiatric Rating Scale for Children, that prompt clinicians to elicit and record specific clinical findings build consistency of diagnostic coverage and establish a standard systematic approach that guards against errors of omission (Hughes et al. 2001; Lachar et al. 2001). Questionnaires for parents and teachers are useful to collect and organize relevant clinical data. Computer-based assessment tasks continue to emerge as a clinically useful diagnostic modality (Cawthorpe 2001).

Clinical Interview

The clinical interview remains the cornerstone of psychiatric assessment and diagnosis. It is where clinician and patient meet, rapport is established, the patient gains voice, cooperation is fostered, mental status is examined, the history is obtained, and the therapeutic relationship takes shape. Interviews are performed with the patient individually, with the parents separate from the patient, and with the patient and parents together.

Adolescents are commonly seen separately from their parents early in the admission so that their view of the current crisis can be heard and so that they can share sensitive yet crucial information that they often would not speak about while in the presence of a parent. Confidentiality conditions for a patient's interview disclosures involve a delicate balancing of an adolescent's privacy interests with a parent's right to know about assessment findings and treatment planning. This situation comes into vivid relief when central features of a case involve matters pertaining to re-

TABLE 4–1. Selected brief rating scales and diagnostic instruments for adolescent inpatient unit

Descriptive symptom profile or global functioning

Brief Psychiatric Rating Scale, Child Version (Hughes et al. 2001)

Clinical Global Impressions (Guy 1976)

Children's Global Assessment Scale (Shaffer et al. 1983)

Specific target symptoms

Children's Depression Inventory (Kovacs 1985)—depression

Children's Yale-Brown Obsessive Compulsive Scale (Goodman et al. 1991)—obsessions and compulsions

Conners Rating Scales—Revised (Conners et al. 1998)—attention, hyperactivity

Modified Overt Aggression Scale (Kay et al. 1988)—aggression

Revised Children's Manifest Anxiety Scale (Reynolds and Richmond 1985)—anxiety

Young Mania Rating Scale (Young et al. 1978)—mania

Side-effect measures

Barnes Akathisia Scale (Barnes 1989)

Abnormal Involuntary Movement Scale (Guy 1976)

productive health and substance abuse, both areas often considered by public health laws to be the adolescents' protected health information when care is delivered to them in outpatient settings. Careful analysis of the unique aspects of each case must be done to determine what constitutes a necessary disclosure to prevent harm and what adverse effects might result from a confidentiality breach. It is here that clinical, ethical, and legal analyses should pull together.

Substance Abuse Screening

Substance abuse risk looms significantly in adolescent mental health populations and must be addressed in every case (Hovens et al. 1994). The CRAFFT substance abuse test (Table 4–2) is a tool that provides an effective and efficient screening approach to this problem (Knight et al. 2002). Positive screening results on this test indicate that closer assessment of drug treatment needs is warranted. Care must be taken to identify substance dependence and risks for substance withdrawal. Intoxicated patients should be given time to clear in a medically supervised setting before they are admitted for psychiatric treatment. Their clinical condition can change markedly during this period as their intoxication resolves or withdrawal signs emerge.

Reproductive Health Services

Reproductive health services are a core component of adolescent medicine practice. These services should be available to address matters related to sexuality, pregnancy, and sexually transmitted diseases. There should

be capacity to address the needs of sexual assault victims who have been referred for admission. This entails close coordination with emergency services to ensure that timely collection of physical evidence, antiviral prophylaxis, and emergency pregnancy prevention have been initiated as needed prior to admission.

Medical History, Physical Examination, and Laboratory Testing

Medical clearance starts with a careful and thorough medical history and physical examination that are performed by a qualified pediatric or adolescent medicine practitioner. When child and adolescent psychiatrists are called on as the primary practitioner to complete medical clearances, they must have maintained their knowledge of appropriate health screening and examination skills to meet national standards of practice for the physical evaluation of adolescents. Care must be taken to ensure that medical evaluation is not shortchanged due to the presentation of the patient with acute behavioral and emotional issues. Significant physical illness comorbidity rates have been noted in adolescent populations receiving psychiatric services (Warner 2006). A body map of injury patterns, including scars, bruises, cuts, and abrasions, should be completed as part of the admission physical assessment. Injury mapping provides baseline information about findings that might be pertinent to child protection matters, and they are also key checkpoints in tracking of patterns of self-injury that might happen over the course of treatment. The medical clearance of

TABLE 4–2.   The CRAFFT Substance Abuse Screening Test for adolescents

C	Have you ever ridden in a **C**AR driven by someone (including yourself) who was "high" or had been using alcohol or drugs?
R	Do you ever use drugs or alcohol to **R**ELAX, feel better about yourself, or fit in?
A	Do you ever use alcohol or drugs while you are **A**LONE by yourself?
F	Do you ever **F**ORGET about things you did while using alcohol or drugs?
F	Do your **F**AMILY or **F**RIENDS ever tell you that you should cut down on your drinking or drug use?
T	Have you ever gotten into **T**ROUBLE while you were using alcohol or drugs?

Scoring: 2 or more Yes answers indicates a problem needing follow-up.

Source.   Center for Adolescent Substance Abuse Research at Children's Hospital Boston.

overdoses usually requires a period of preadmission prospective monitoring of blood levels and clinical status to verify physical stability.

Nutritional status should be screened routinely. Risk for cardiovascular and metabolic complications related to obesity must be identified and managed. Body mass index (BMI) should be recorded and trended across treatment settings, as there is a secular U.S. trend of increasing adolescent BMI. Weights below 75% ideal body weight often indicate a need for inpatient admission to address factors contributing to significant nutritional compromise in the context of an eating disorder or another severe neurovegetative disturbance. Immunization status and tuberculosis exposure and screening history must be checked and updated. Tuberculin skin testing should be performed if it is not current, particularly in individuals admitted from high-exposure-risk locations. The need for isoniazid treatment should be ascertained early in the hospital course because decisions about medication selection and dosage will be affected if isoniazid is prescribed.

Common baseline laboratory tests and their rationales are outlined in Table 4–3.

Imaging and Electroencephalography

Brain imaging in the absence of focal neurological findings produces low yield in detection of central nervous system findings in clinical populations with primary psychiatric disorders, yet severe, unremitting psychopathology in the form of psychosis or mood symptoms can provide reason to pursue imaging for possible occult lesions (Santosh 2000). Similar arguments can be made for electroencephalography or functional brain imaging as part of the workup for patients presenting with severe, persistent symptoms if disruption of brain activity has not been ruled out. A

significant history of head trauma also is a relative indication to pursue imaging. Cognitive decline, disorientation, and the presence of focal findings suggest a stronger need to pursue neurological consultation and workup that are likely to include studies of brain structure and function.

Psychological Testing

Psychological consultation can aid the diagnostic process in several valuable ways. Standardized measures of cognitive and adaptive functioning are useful to evaluate suspected deficits in these developmental domains. A personality assessment such as the Minnesota Multiphasic Personality Inventory, Adolescent Version, can generate information about psychopathology and an individual's relative strengths and weaknesses (Janus et al. 1998). Projective techniques can provide a perspective on significant alterations in thinking that might not be readily discernible during a clinical interview. Psychological consultation is invaluable in the interpretation of existing psychometric data obtained from collateral contacts. Behavioral psychologists can contribute operational assessment of behaviors and effective contingency plans. Psychological consultation is not indicated in every case. Given the availability of limited provider resources, it should be accessed judiciously based on the specific demonstrated individualized needs of each patient.

Treatment

Biopsychosocial Formulation and Treatment Planning

Assessment data are incorporated into a biopsychosocial formulation of the causal factors contributing

TABLE 4-3. Common laboratory tests and monitoring rationale for adolescents facing inpatient psychiatry hospitalization

Test	Monitoring rationale
Serum electrolytes	Baseline health measure
	Elevated bicarbonate level associated with vomiting
Blood urea nitrogen	Renal function measure, hydration status
Serum creatinine	Renal function measure, drug elimination
Serum phosphate	Indicator of nutritional status
	Critical shifts in refeeding syndrome
Complete blood count	Baseline health measure, medication side effects
Liver function tests	Baseline health measure, medication side effects
Pregnancy test	Baseline health measure relevant to multiple aspects of care
Serum prolactin	Hypothalamic pituitary function baseline, neuroleptic effects
Urine toxicology screening	Detection of illicit drug ingestion
Urinalysis	Baseline health measure, renal function, hydration status
Serum drug levels	Therapeutic monitoring, management of overdose
Glucose, triglycerides, and serum lipids	Metabolic syndrome risk, medication side effects
Electrocardiography	Cardiac baseline, medication side effects

Note. Specific laboratory testing is governed by the clinical circumstances of each case.

most directly to the need for admission. The treatment plan is tailored to meet the most acute needs and tap into the strengths of each patient and family (Harper 1989). The goals set in the treatment plan must be realistically attainable and consistently oriented toward functional adaptation and the restoration of health and safety. Treatment plans and clinical documents should be written in language that is understandable to adolescent patients and their families. The use of a patient's or parent's terms, phrases, themes, and metaphors adds personal relevance and power to the treatment planning process. Patients and parents should be invited to join treatment planning sessions as significant collaborators with the most extensive knowledge of and investment in the life of the patient and family. Community-based providers are essential treatment planning resources and should be invited to participate in treatment planning sessions. Conference calls and speakerphones are effective technologies to support coordination and continuity of care with community service providers during treatment planning sessions. Patients can benefit from the continuity of care and clinical contact that occur when existing community-based providers are able to meet with the patient in the hospital as a member of the treatment team.

The interventions of the treatment plan should address the most impairing symptoms and have some evidence of effectiveness when applied to similar cases. Interventions are multimodal and are likely to include medication, psychotherapy, educational services, activity therapy, therapeutic recreation, case management, and discharge planning.

Medication

Medication treatment is one component of a balanced multimodal intervention plan informed by a formulation of the biological, psychological, and social factors that contributed most immediately to the need for inpatient admission. Psychopharmacology is symptom-based and directed to address the most severe and impairing dimensions of active psychopathology. The main foci of inpatient medication interventions are to select or adjust appropriate agents, establish dose tolerability to treatment initiation or change, and coordinate with outpatient providers to maintain continuity of clinical management from preadmission through postdischarge phases of treatment. Rating scales will help to structure tracking of signs and symptoms, treatment response, and side effects.

Medication selection should target the most impairing symptom dimensions of mental illness. When multiple disorders are present, shared symptom dimensions of anxiety, agitation, insomnia, thought disorder, or mood disturbance are treated with the simplest effective medication strategy. Bostic and Rho (2006) posited a model for dimensional treatment and symptom targeting that is well suited to the inpatient setting, where clinical presentations are complex and multiple disorders frequently overlap. Shaw and DeMaso (2006) also provided an example of target symptom prescribing that is concordant with these principles (Table 4–4).

Inpatient practitioners are asked to evaluate and adjust medication combinations with limited scientific data available to support their clinical decision making, particularly when addressing drug combinations in patients with very complex and treatment-resistant conditions (Duffy et al. 2005; Safer et al. 2003). There should be a close working relationship with pharmacy services to evaluate potential drug interactions and gather relevant drug information to inform treatment decisions.

Because the time frames of inpatient care are often shorter than the known dose–response effects of many medications, coordination with referring and follow-up providers to plan in-hospital adjustments and to map postdischarge monitoring of treatment is necessary to complete drug trials. The handoff of inpatient care should communicate a clear monitoring plan to the receiving clinician, because treatment effects and side effects can emerge from weeks to months after changes are made.

Of particular note is the need to maintain vigilance for emerging suicide risk when treating depression with or without antidepressant medications. When suicidality is present, consideration should be given to the potential ameliorating role of antidepressant therapy. Conversely, the potential exacerbating effect of antidepressant therapy must be considered if suicidality worsens during a course of antidepressant treatment. The reader is advised to be aware of the recent controversies surrounding U.S. Food and Drug Administration regulations requiring that all antidepressants carry a "black box" warning about possible increased risk for suicide when they are used to treat depression in all children and adolescents.

Medication decision making and consent procedures on an adolescent unit are triangulated between patient, parents, and clinician. Parental consent and patient assent are always required for medication treatment unless there are emergency exceptions or a legal basis exists for treatment over objection. Emergency

TABLE 4–4. Target symptom approach to medication selection

Target symptom	Medication considerations
Aggression	Selective serotonin reuptake inhibitor
	Selective norepinephrine reuptake inhibitor
	Atypical or typical antipsychotic
	Benzodiazepine
	Mood stabilizer
	Alpha agonist
	Beta blocker
	Stimulant
Agitation	Atypical or typical antipsychotic
	Benzodiazepine
	Diphenhydramine (younger children)
Anxiety	Benzodiazepine
	Antidepressant
	Buspirone
	Gabapentin
	Alpha agonist
Depression	Selective serotonin reuptake inhibitor
	Serotonin–norepinephrine reuptake inhibitor
Inattention	Stimulant
	Atomoxetine
	Bupropion
Insomnia	Diphenhydramine
	Benzodiazepine
	Trazodone
	Hypnotic (e.g., zolpidem, zaleplon)
	Amitriptyline
	Mirtazapine
Mania	Atypical or typical antipsychotic
	Mood stabilizer
Psychosis	Atypical or typical antipsychotic
	Benzodiazepine
Withdrawal	Clonidine
	Benzodiazepine

Source. Adapted from Shaw and DeMaso 2006.

conditions for medication treatment entail an acute risk of harm if immediate treatment is not provided to address physiological compromise such as acute dystonic reactions or intolerable distress that is unresponsive to nonmedication interventions. The emergency conditions and the rationale for such emergency medication use in such situations should be well documented, and the parent should be informed of the situation in a timely manner.

Adolescents in treatment are forging lasting attitudes about the role that medication will play in their lives. Evidence demonstrates increased susceptibility of young persons to antipsychotic side effects at higher dosages (Chakos et al. 1992; Zhang-Wong et al. 1999). Around puberty, adolescents can be exquisitely sensitive to any changes in bodily appearance or function that is perceived to be related to illness or treatment. The relationship of sexual side effects of drug treatments to sexual maturation, treatment outcomes, patient attitudes, and participation in care has yet to be rigorously evaluated and merits investigation.

Psychotherapies

Inpatient psychotherapy programs incorporate individual, group, and family therapy modalities to identify and support existing adaptive strengths of an adolescent and family as they attempt to come to terms with and manage the signs and symptoms of an acute mental illness. Psychotherapy aids the acquisition of new knowledge and coping skills. The psychotherapeutic frame of inpatient work is decidedly short term, with an emphasis on establishing and maintaining continuity in previous and future therapies. Admission of a client to an inpatient unit provides an opportunity for consultation when there is already ongoing psychotherapeutic work in the community.

People enter inpatient treatment with diverse needs and capacities for therapeutic engagement. This requires an adaptable psychotherapy program with individual, family, and group components that can be adjusted to meet the unique requirements of each clinical situation. The specific therapeutic techniques and orientations available on a unit will tap into the psychotherapy training and skills of the staff.

When available, evidence should be used to guide treatment selection. For example, evidence exists for the efficacy of cognitive-behavioral, interpersonal, and family therapies in the treatment of adolescent depression (Mufson et al. 2004; Weersing and Brent 2006). Some psychosocial interventions can be considered potentially effective in the treatment of various clinical symptoms or syndromes (Table 4–5).

TABLE 4–5. Psychosocial treatment modality selection based on clinical indication

Clinical indication	Treatment modality
Depression	Cognitive-behavioral therapy
	Interpersonal therapy
	Psychodynamic psychotherapy
	Family therapy
Bipolar disorder	Cognitive-behavioral therapy
	Family-focused treatment
Emotional dysregulation	Cognitive-behavioral therapy
	Dialectical behavior therapy
Stress and trauma	Cognitive-behavioral therapy
	Trauma systems interventions
	Psychodynamic psychotherapy
Psychosis	Social skills training
	Supportive psychotherapy
	Family therapy
Anxiety	Cognitive-behavioral therapy
	Exposure
	Modeling
	Family therapy
Eating disorders	Family therapy
	Multidisciplinary team collaboration
	Motivational interviewing
Disruptive behavior	Behavioral systemic therapy
	Multisystemic therapy
	Cognitive-behavioral therapy
	Functional family therapy
Substance abuse	Motivational interviewing

Therapeutic alliances between clinicians, adolescents, and families are needed to support and sustain the clinical work to be done during the hospital admission. Alliance formation is fostered when a patient's and family's concerns are heard, appreciated, and addressed in the clinical work. Motivation to join in the therapeutic work will vary substantially among adolescents and their families. Motivational interviewing techniques are evolving as potentially useful tools to help adolescents participate as active agents in their health care decision making (Erickson et al. 2005).

Every effort is needed to have the work proceed in a collaborative spirit that is free from coercion. This is a most challenging task to accomplish in situations involving involuntary commitment or in the presence of significant disagreements among treatment participants. A reframing of treatment orientation in terms of health and safety priorities can help to build consensus in such difficult situations. Sometimes participants must "agree to disagree" as outside dispute resolution such as involuntary commitment hearings is pursued. Navigation of these delicate scenarios requires thoughtful integration and compassionate application of clinical, ethical, and legal perspectives.

Younger adolescents sometimes benefit from access to interactive play therapy techniques as developmental adaptations to aid their participation in the treatment (Russ 2004). Expressive therapy modalities such as music, art, movement, and drama can provide entry points to the psychotherapeutic process for kids who are not ready or able to engage through talk. Visual aids such as sticker plans or behavior charts are particularly helpful with younger adolescents.

INDIVIDUAL THERAPY

Individual psychotherapy emphasizes therapeutic elements of relaxation training, stress reduction, anger management, self-monitoring, safety planning, communication building, symptom management, treatment planning, and patient education. This is an area in the work where new skills or approaches can be introduced that might be practiced in session and then generalized to group therapy or family therapy encounters during the hospital stay.

Individual therapy provides a partially sheltered psychotherapeutic venue for the adolescent. The scope of confidentiality for the individual therapy process must be explicitly delimited at the outset of treatment. Boundaries of confidentiality usually end in the face of impending danger when unit staff must act to preserve safety. Care must also be taken to explain the role of treatment team members who will hear about the individual therapy sessions in team meetings or treatment planning sessions.

FAMILY THERAPY

Inpatient family therapy work identifies and supports existing family strengths, enhances effective communication, resolves conflicts, negotiates consensus, establishes safety, provides information, and plans for the transition to the next setting of care (Strickland-Clark et al. 2000). Family members usually need various forms of support to help them cope with the anxieties and uncertainties surrounding the adolescent's admission. Existing sources of support can be accessed within the family's relationships, cultural practices, spiritual beliefs, and community resources. The family sessions are also a central location for support through information sharing that enhances collaboration and choice making in the treatment process. Family therapy also seeks to build consensus on the aims of inpatient treatment. It is here that conflicts are addressed, differences resolved, and compromises negotiated in the service of the adolescent's care.

Family interventions will involve time spent alone with the parents or guardians to take history and plan treatment. Shapiro et al. (2006) defined five types of parent work, including assessment and monitoring of change, help for parents in understanding their child, parent training, parent guidance, and parent counseling. Siblings, grandparents, or other significant family members might also be included in the family work as indicated by the specifics of the family's circumstances. Preparation of agenda, rehearsal of presentations, communication practice, and general attitudinal and emotional readiness for family therapy sessions are frequently worked on in separate parent and individual sessions with the adolescent. The family work also provides a venue to present findings and recommendations related to assessment and treatment.

GROUP THERAPY

Group therapy modalities draw on interpersonal dynamics, perspective sharing, collective support, and consensus building as therapeutic processes. Adolescent peer group members can provide powerful and enlightening feedback to teenagers that would have little impact when spoken by adults or authority figures (Cramer-Azima and Richmond 1989). Group process with adolescents must be shaped by therapists trained to do group work. Although the adolescents are the most visible actors in the group setting, the therapists must continuously keep the process moving in a constructive direction. The tone and the atmosphere of groups must be calm, orderly, and respectful. There should be a consistent set of rules and expectations that are reviewed at the start of each group. Printed versions of the rules can be posted near the meeting place and distributed to group members for their information. Group formats should accommodate for the frequent shifting of membership and the possibility that patients might only be present for a single session. This is addressed by having clear instructions and expectations for participation available at the start of the group to help members participate (Malekoff 2004). Having a record or manual of effective group procedures, structures, and activities also serves to maintain the continuity of the programming as therapists join or leave the unit.

Therapy groups can focus on specific therapeutic areas and skills such as anger management, relaxation training, social skills, hygiene, and grooming. They might have a health education orientation that focuses on matters of reproductive health, substance abuse, smoking cessation, or medication treatment. Single-gender girls' or boys' groups can be used to address issues related to identity formation and gender-based developmental issues. There are also task-oriented groups such as community meetings and goals groups. Group tasks can be supported by individual work that helps patients to prepare goals and agenda items for presentation in goals groups and community meetings. Goals prepared and presented by someone in a morning goals group should state a goal for the day that maintains relevance with his or her individual treatment goals. Closure groups are commonly conducted in the evening to follow up on the work that was done toward goals throughout the day.

Acting-out behavior can spread quickly in groups. It must be monitored, prevented, and contained rigorously by staff interventions in a seemingly effortless and calm way. Individuals at risk to act out and disrupt groups are best identified well before the start of a group session to assess whether they can be helped to prepare for the group or require more individualized programming away from the group setting. The following vignette illustrates this approach.

> Betty and Wilma, two 15-year-old girls, had exchanged hostile words about each other's close family members in a squabble at breakfast. Staff separated them immediately. After breakfast, Betty was frowning, avoiding eye contact, and pacing anxiously. Wilma was observed mumbling under her breath and staring at Betty. The unit's daily community meeting was about to begin. Both girls soon would be expected to join the group and as a result be in close proximity. Unit staff noted the ongoing hostile and defensive tone of interaction between the girls manifested through their states of physical tension, facial expressions, and muttered verbal communication. Each girl was approached by a staff member who shared a good rapport and alliance with her. Quiet conversations were started individually with each girl as staff walked with them to their rooms, while the rest of the unit assembled for community meeting. In her conversation with staff, Betty reported that she had grown intimidated by Wilma's frequent attempts to sit near her over the prior 2 days. She revealed a need to defend herself with aggressive words and, if necessary, physical violence. Wilma revealed that she felt disrespected by Betty, who seemed to shun her attempts to befriend her. Each girl privately indicated a desire to reach a peace settlement mediated by staff. In the ensuing mediation session, both girls were able to share how they could give and receive mutual respect. The conflict was resolved, and a public group confrontation was avoided. The girls were able to save face and rejoin the milieu without further incidents.

Group therapy sessions offer significant exposure, desensitization, and practice opportunities for kids who are having difficulties joining and participating in social situations. They are excellent settings to make naturalistic observations pertinent to clinical and functional assessment. Multifamily groups can be welcome sources of support where families learn about the treatment process, acquire parenting skills, identify community resources, or just find time to get together and share constructive diversion in a game or leisure activity. Many units hold parents' nights or family nights for this purpose.

Patient and Family Education

Family empowerment is strongly rooted in the teaching and learning that occur between family members and the treatment team. At its finest, it is a mutual learning process where the treatment team gains knowledge about how to best help the family and the family learns the information needed to make informed decisions and be fully engaged in the care. An initial assessment of communication and learning capacities will identify needs for adaptive communication devices, language translation, or cultural interpretation that must be addressed before authentic learning can occur.

Teaching efforts during the admission process should be sensitive to the needs of patients and families as they grapple with the uncertainties and stresses of hospitalization and the implications of acute, serious mental illness in a young family member. Meetings with unit staff, photographs of the unit, a printed unit guide, and a preadmission tour of the unit can be effective aids to provide information, allay worries, and help families to understand the nature and purpose of hospitalization. Materials and information to support learning might include Web sites, pamphlets and flyers about adolescent health risks, medication information sheets, diagnosis-specific information, parenting skills, and developmental topics (DeMaso et al. 2002).

School

Every unit should have a classroom program with a teacher who provides instruction and coordinates educational planning with local schools to identify potential learning needs and help patients maintain continuity of academic work between the community and hospital settings. The unit classroom provides an excellent location to observe a patient's functional status in a naturalistic setting. Review of a student's daily schoolwork can reveal much about how he or she is concentrating, completing assignments, following directions, and meeting the myriad demands that exist in a classroom setting. Records of attendance on the unit often can be transmitted to the community home school to maintain credit status.

Rehabilitation and Recreational Therapies

Rehabilitative principles are focused to reduce impairments caused by mental illness or comorbid physical disabilities. Rehabilitative emphasis is placed on the practice of activities of daily living, personal hygiene, symptom management, or development of social skills. Physical therapy might be indicated when motor or musculoskeletal deficits are noted. Occupational therapy might be needed to address sensory integration deficits. Speech and language specialists should be available to participate in the care of persons with sensory deficits or communication disorders.

Leisure activities should be structured and well monitored in designated areas. Active involvement of patients by milieu staff in age-appropriate leisure activities that are enjoyable and interesting is more likely to keep patients constructively engaged while eliminating potential for boredom-inspired mischief. Opportunities for physical exercise and fresh air are needed to support the physical needs of growing youth (Curran 1939). Leisure planning exercises can be done to help adolescents learn to organize and structure their time.

Nutritional Intervention

Hospitalized teenagers often require nutritional interventions. Some psychotropic medication treatments have been causally associated with weight gain (Correll and Carlson 2006). Of note, hospitalization has been associated with increased BMI (Putnam et al. 1990). Patients with eating disorders will need specialized meal programs and nutritional restoration plans. Weight loss due to appetite disturbance secondary to physical illness or medication side effects might need to be addressed through meal plan adjustments.

Religious and Cultural Needs

Patients' spiritual needs continue when they are admitted to the hospital. Availability of chaplaincy for various faiths should be maintained to support patients and families if they wish to maintain religious and spiritual observance (Moncher and Josephson 2004). A unit must also find and maintain connections with its local community to develop and maintain culturally informed awareness for the needs of the people it serves.

Milieu Management

The unit milieu is a safe 24-hour treatment setting with client-centered programming built from therapeutic and social components. All milieu interactions between unit staff and clients carry therapeutic potential and should be shaped and informed by sound psychotherapeutic principles. The tone and philosophy of a unit flow from the core human values that are embraced and transmitted by the staff, patients, and families involved in the life of the place. All persons participating on the unit should be invited to make a durable commitment to the values of safety, health, human rights, mutual respect, nonviolence, fairness, and personal integrity. Adolescents who are developmentally primed to explore the ethical and philosophical aspects of their lives and relationships usually resonate with a values-based milieu approach. These core values can be codified in a set of unit rules that are transmitted in writing and posted in a prominent location. All persons on the unit are expected to follow the unit rules, and all members of the milieu should be encouraged to help each other learn and follow the rules.

Unit scheduling and routines should convey a sense of predictability, planning, and order. There should be a daily schedule available to view in a prominent location. Changes in the schedule should be anticipated and announced in a timely fashion. Transitions within a program are previewed with patients, and clear instructions about how to change locations should be given. Patients should not be left in unsupervised areas. Unit point or level systems should be commensurate with the needs of the population served. Level systems on short-stay units must be simple, quick to learn, and effective in motivating adolescents to participate. Well-designed inpatient behavioral interventions are valuable tools that structure treatment with components that can be applied in postdischarge settings to maintain adaptive function.

The environmental design and management of the unit must guard against excessive visual, auditory, or tactile stimulation that might cause undue patient anxiety and distress. Control of the environment also requires surveillance for potentially harmful objects and substances. Belongings checks are done by staff when patients enter the unit on admission and upon return from therapeutic passes.

Media access and content must also be closely monitored to prevent untoward exposure to questionable materials. Allowed content should be consonant with the core values that form the basis for unit rules. Content should be vetted by staff and families. There should be clinical awareness of media content as potential triggers for signs and symptoms of disorders. The selection of movies, television programming, video games, magazines, and books provides a golden opportunity for engagement of adolescents in discussions of core human values.

The acuity level of a unit's patient population will have a profound effect on the milieu. Patients requiring a high level of direct individual care can have broad impact on a milieu by diverting staff from performance of more general milieu management functions. The acuity mix and staff ratios must be monitored and adjusted continuously to ensure that patient safety and care quality can be maintained. As a general rule, as unit acuity rises, the staff-to-patient ratio must also rise.

An inpatient milieu is supported by the collaborative work of a multidisciplinary team that might include child and adolescent psychiatrists, psychologists, nurses, milieu counselors, social workers, expressive arts therapists, occupational therapists, nutritionists, recreational therapists, utilization review staff, teachers, administrative managers, clerical staff, and ancillary support staff. The guiding principle of unit staffing is to meet the individualized clinical needs of each patient admitted while maintaining cohesive program functioning. Role definition and function of each member of the milieu team, regardless of discipline, will be defined by credentialing, experience, training, and areas of competence. The mix of disciplines available to staff a unit will be limited by local workforce availability and the significant national shortage of practitioners with expertise to provide mental health services to adolescents.

Management of Aggressive and Suicidal Behaviors

Significant risks of aggression and/or suicide are common indications for referral and admission to inpatient treatment settings (Olfson et al. 2005). The process of identifying and managing risks of harm from aggression begins with the first contact of the referral and admission process. Patient safety and effective clinical coordination are well served by an initial screening to evaluate patient safety needs prior to transfer and admission. Early contact between referrers and inpatient staff provides a preliminary opportunity to provide information to the patient and family and engage them in the referral and transfer process. Having specific information about what will happen can allay anxiety and prevent frustration that can further fuel emotional crises.

At the time of admission, a strengths-based assessment to evaluate effective coping strategies and sources of support presents an excellent opportunity to start alliance building and identify interventions that might help a patient avert acute behavioral or emotional crises (LeBel et al. 2004). The early identification of vulnerabilities to crises such as escalation triggers, fears, anxieties, frustrations, and concerns can help the clinical team and the patient work together on a plan to establish and maintain safety during the admission.

The safety planning process introduces a patient to staff members and forms working alliances that form a basis of support for the patient during the admission (Beauford et al. 1997; Green et al. 2006). It identifies and strengthens the patient's current adaptive coping skills and provides a blueprint for the development of new coping skills to reduce stress and build calmness. The plan identifies and provides safe locations on the unit for the patient to use for the application or acquisition of coping skills. Medication use might also be indicated to reduce distress, aid relaxation, and help a patient participate in the acquisition of the cognitive, emotional, and behavioral skills needed to participate in the safety plan.

A key element of crisis prevention requires knowledge of the patient, including the stresses he or she is facing and the behavioral warning signs of impending crises of frustration, agitation, or aggression.

Anticipation of difficult phone calls, therapy sessions, or interpersonal interactions can aid staff in being available and prepared to help the patient during such difficult moments. Special attention to proper maintenance of interpersonal space must be individualized to meet the needs of each patient. Traumatized youth are particularly vulnerable to triggers that echo previous abuse such as physical touch or invasion of boundary space. Kids with processing difficulties such as language-based learning disabilities or sensory impairments can interpret neutral stimuli as hostile (Rutter et al. 2006). Explicit and understandable communication must be established to prevent defensive reactions leading to behavioral escalation.

A safe and effective crisis management approach continually aims to minimize the frequency, duration, and severity of behavioral crises to eliminate self-directed or interpersonal violence and implement the safest and least restrictive clinical interventions that do not require the application of physical force. Physical restraint, either mechanical or chemical, is an intervention of last resort. It should be used most sparingly and only to prevent immediate bodily harm. If and when restraint is used, the staff involved must have specialized training, function as a team under the direction of a designated team leader, and employ sound principles of physical management that minimize the opportunity for physical injury of all involved (Masters and Bellonci 2002). When patients are in seclusion or restraint, they must be constantly monitored to ensure that they are physically safe. Ongoing clinical monitoring of a patient in restraint or seclusion should track a patient's level of alertness, orientation, responsiveness, body position, airway, respirations, body temperature, circulation, and motor-sensory status. If available, pulse oximetry can be an additional technology to monitor blood oxygenation and augment detailed clinical monitoring.

Debriefings of the patient, parents, and staff for each restraint episode should assess the impact of the restraint on the patient, their family, the other patients on the unit, and the unit staff. Strategies to identify safer effective alternatives to potential future crises should be explored. Review of any difficulties or lack of coordination in the crisis response team should be identified and addressed through collaboration, practice, and training. Staff debriefings should be used as a place for analysis, problem solving, and staff support. The stressful nature of involvement in restraint episodes and aggression management exacts a toll on patients and staff. Reverberations will be felt throughout the unit following a restraint episode, and staff must be prepared to address patient concerns as they work to restore the milieu's therapeutic equilibrium.

Consistently implemented, safe physical management skills require active staff training and practice at the individual and team levels. Mock codes or case simulations combined with classroom learning should be scheduled regularly. Ad hoc review and practice are also helpful to prepare for risky situations as they occur. The effectiveness of crisis management protocols requires ongoing evaluation to characterize and track event rates, intervention outcomes, and results of staff training. The clinical characterization and management of aggressive episodes can be aided by instruments such as the Modified Overt Aggression Scale (Collett et al. 2003; Kay et al. 1988; Sorgi et al. 1991). Ratings of episode duration, severity, and behavioral specifics can be tracked and trended at the individual, caseload, and unit level using computers.

Effective suicide prevention requires the establishment and maintenance of communication between the adolescent and a support network that is likely to include parents, family, school personnel, outpatient providers, and the inpatient team. Once communication is established, work can be done to help develop the self-monitoring skills of the patient and the monitoring capacities of support network members. The therapeutic work will emphasize core symptom reduction contributing to suicide risk and the identification and practice of safe alternative coping strategies (Brent 1997; Miller et al. 2007). A means reduction component might be needed as part of a safety plan that helps family members to eliminate or limit access to dangerous objects and substances in the community setting. Imminently suicidal inpatients will likely need constant monitoring in a safe location of the unit until imminent risk of self-harm or suicide subsides. In self-injurious patients, injury patterns should be recorded at the time of admission and rechecked periodically at points during the admission to assess clinical progress.

Discharge Planning

Discharge planning begins at the time of admission when efforts are made to coordinate care with services and resources that are already in place for the adolescent in the community. The patient and parents must be engaged continuously in planning aftercare throughout the hospital stay. Utilization management personnel support the treatment and discharge planning process by identifying appropriate aftercare resources, communicating with families about options, and coordinating care with external case managers. Stepdown care might be needed in partial hospital or residential settings if integrated services in a single location remain indicated after sufficient clinical stabilization occurs (Daniel et al. 2004). Informational materials can help families and patients learn about options in residential, partial hospital, or other community programs. Therapeutic passes can be used to phase a patient back into the home and community settings while assessing the effects of exposure to environmental stress and readiness for discharge.

Impediments to discharge include a pervasive lack of appropriate services at lower levels of care. Adolescents approaching the age of majority face major difficulties transitioning care to young adult or adult services due to lack of services and lack of integration between adolescent and adult systems of care. Major shortages exist in aftercare services for adolescents with dual diagnoses of mental illness and developmental disabilities or substance abuse. Adolescents recovering from substance abuse disorders and addictions might benefit from referral to 12-Step recovery programs. Return to the educational environment will need to be coordinated between hospital and school, often in the form of a school reentry meeting. Patients and parents often want guidance on how to discuss the inpatient admission with peers, family members, and school staff.

Transition from the hospital entails active coordination, collaboration, and communication with aftercare service providers. In best-case scenarios, aftercare providers working within a system of care with inpatient units will already know the patient and will have been actively involved in processes of admission referral, inpatient treatment planning, and arrangement of discharge in a seamless integration that provides minimal disruption in care and function for the benefit of patients and families.

Conclusion

Inpatient psychiatry units will continue to provide the most intensive treatment role within an evolving system of adolescent mental health services. The essential inpatient work of rapid assessment, treatment planning, clinical stabilization, and effective transitioning of treatment to less intensive levels of care will remain in place. To perform their essential functions effectively and efficiently, inpatient programs will need the advocacy of families, community providers, agencies, lawmakers, and professional organizations

to ensure that the current unmet mental health needs of adolescents are addressed by establishing sufficient resources to support care outside the hospital setting.

Several trends will continue into the foreseeable future. Identification of clinically meaningful outcome measures will loom as a challenge to the design, evaluation, and delivery of effective inpatient care. Training, recruitment, and retention of staff with the specialized skills for inpatient work will persist as a significant unmet human resource need. Efforts to reduce coercion in treatment settings will accompany a growing awareness of the physical and psychological risks associated with exposure to force or threats of force. Inpatient and outpatient services will be blended via community-based teams to assist families during the transition of care from the hospital to the home. There will be new ways for families and guardians to participate on units via leadership and caregiving roles. Most optimistically, the collaboration of providers with patients and families will shape a future for inpatient care that is scientifically based, ethically informed, human rights–oriented, and delivered with compassion.

References

American Academy of Child and Adolescent Psychiatry: Practice parameters for the psychiatric assessment of children and adolescents. J Am Acad Child Adolesc Psychiatry 36 (suppl):4S–20S, 1997

Barnes TR: A rating scale for drug induced akathisia. Br J Psychiatry 154:672–676, 1989

Bartlett C, Evans M, Holloway J, et al: Markers of inappropriate placement in acute psychiatric inpatient care: a five hospital study. Soc Psychiatry Psychiatr Epidemiol 34:367–375, 1999

Beauford JE, McNiel DE, Binder R: Utility of the initial therapeutic alliance in evaluating psychiatric patients' risk of violence. Am J Psychiatry 154:1272–1276, 1997

Bostic JQ, Rho Y: Target symptom psychopharmacology: between the forest and the trees. Child Adolesc Psychiatr Clin N Am 15:289–302, 2006

Brent DJ: The aftercare of adolescents with deliberate self-harm. J Child Psychol Psychiatry 38:277–286, 1997

Case BG, Olfson M, Marcus SC, et al: Trends in the inpatient mental health treatment of children and adolescents in US community hospitals between 1990 and 2000. Arch Gen Psychiatry 64:89–96, 2007

Cawthorpe D: An evaluation of a computer-based psychiatric assessment: evidence for expanded use. Cyberpsychol Behav 4:503–510, 2001

Chakos MH, Mayerhoff DI, Loebel AD, et al: Incidence and correlates of acute extrapyramidal symptoms in first episode of schizophrenia. Psychopharmacol Bull 28:81–86, 1992

Collett BR, Ohan JL, Myers KM: Ten-year review of rating scales, VI: scales assessing externalizing behaviors. J Am Acad Child Adolesc Psychiatry 42:1143–1170, 2003

Conners CK, Sitarenios G, Parker, JD, et al: Revision and restandardization of the Conners Teacher Rating Scale (CTRS-R): factor structure, reliability, and criterion validity. J Abnormal Child Psychol 26:279–291, 1998

Correll CU, Carlson HE: Endocrine and metabolic adverse effects of psychotropic medications in children and adolescents. J Am Acad Child Adolesc Psychiatry 45:771–791, 2006

Cramer-Azima FJ, Richmond LH: Adolescent Group Psychotherapy. Madison, CT, International Universities Press, 1989

Curran FJ: Organization of a ward for adolescents in Bellevue psychiatric hospital. Am J Psychiatry 95:1365–1386, 1939

Daniel SS, Goldston DB, Harris AE, et al: Review of literature on aftercare services among children and adolescents. Psychiatr Serv 55:901–912, 2004

DeMaso DR, Ginnis K, Sinclair C, et al: Helping With Your Child's Psychiatric Hospitalization: A Practical Guide for Parents. Boston, MA, Children's Hospital Boston, 2002. Available at: http://www.childrenshospital.org/clinicalservices/Site1908/Documents/parentguide.pdf. Accessed April 28, 2007.

Dickey B, Normand SL, Norton EC, et al: Managed care and children's behavioral health services in Massachusetts. Psychiatr Serv 52:183–188, 2001

Duffy FF, Narrow WE, Rae DS, et al: Concomitant pharmacotherapy among youths treated in routine psychiatric practice. J Child Adolesc Psychopharmacol 15:12–25, 2005

Erickson SJ, Gerstle M, Feldstein SW: Brief interventions and motivational interviewing with children, adolescents and their parents in pediatric health care settings: a review. Arch Pediatr Adolesc Med 159:1173–1180, 2005

Fallon T, Pumariega A, Sowers W, et al: A level of care instrument for children's systems of care: construction, reliability and validity. J Child Family Stud 15:143–155, 2006

Geller JL, Biebel K: The premature demise of public child and adolescent inpatient psychiatric beds, part II: challenges and implications. Psychiatr Q 77:273–291, 2006

Goodman WK, Price LH, Rasmusen SA, et al: Children's Yale-Brown Obsessive Compulsive Scale (CY-BOCS). New Haven, CT, Department of Psychiatry, Yale University School of Medicine, 1991

Green RW, Ablon JS, Martin A: Innovations in child and adolescent psychiatry: use of collaborative problem solving to reduce seclusion and restraint in child and adolescent inpatient units. Psychiatr Serv 57:610–612, 2006

Guy W: Abnormal Involuntary Movement Scale, Clinical Global Impressions, ECDEU Assessment Manual for Psychopharmacology, Revised Edition. Rockville, MD, National Institute of Mental Health, 1976

Harper G: Focal inpatient treatment planning. J Am Acad Child Adolesc Psychiatry 28:31–37, 1989

Hovens JG, Cantwell DP, Kiriakos R: Psychiatric comorbidity in hospitalized adolescent substance abusers. J Am Acad Child Adolesc Psychiatry 33:476–483, 1994

Hughes CW, Rintelmann J, Mayes T, et al: Structured interview and uniform assessment improves diagnostic reliability. J Child Adolesc Psychopharmacol 10:119–131, 2000

Hughes CW, Rintelmann J, Emslie GJ, et al: A revised anchored version of the BPRS-C for childhood psychiatric disorders. J Child Adolesc Psychopharmacol 11:77–93, 2001

Janus MD, de Groot C, Toepfer SM: The MMPI-A and 13-year-old inpatients: how young is too young? Assessment 5:321–332, 1998

Kay SR, Wolkenfeld F, Murrill LM: Profiles of aggression among psychiatric patients, I: nature and prevalence. J Nerv Ment Dis 176:539–546, 1988

Knight JR, Sherritt L, Lydia A, et al: Validity of the CRAFFT substance abuse screening test among adolescent clinic patients. Arch Pediatr Adolesc Med 156:607–614, 2002

Kovacs M: The Children's Depression Inventory (CDI). Psychopharmacol Bull 21:995–998, 1985

Lachar D, Randle SL, Harper RA, et al: The brief psychiatric rating scale for children (BPRS-C): validity and reliability of an anchored version. J Am Acad Child Adolesc Psychiatry 40:333–340, 2001

LeBel J, Stromberg N, Duckworth K, et al: Child and adolescent inpatient restraint reduction: a state initiative to promote strength-based care. J Am Acad Child Adolesc Psychiatry 43:37–45, 2004

Malekoff A: Group Work With Adolescents: Principles and Practice, 2nd Edition. New York, Guilford, 2004

Mansbach JM, Wharff E, Austin SB, et al: Which psychiatric patients board on the medical service? Pediatrics 111:693–698, 2003

Masters KJ, Bellonci C: Practice parameter for the prevention and management of aggressive behavior in child and adolescent psychiatric institutions with special reference to seclusion and restraint. J Am Acad Child Adolesc Psychiatry 40:1356–1358, 2002

Miller AL, Rathus JH, Linehan MM, et al: Dialectical Behavior Therapy With Suicidal Adolescents. New York, Guilford, 2007

Moncher FJ, Josephson AM: Religious and spiritual aspects of family assessment. Child Adolesc Psychiatr Clin N Am 13:49–70, 2004

Mufson L, Dorta KP, Moreau D, et al: Interpersonal psychotherapy for depressed adolescents. Arch Gen Psychiatry 61:577–584, 2004

Olfson M, Gameroff MJ, Marcus SC, et al: National trends in hospitalization of youth with intentional self-inflicted injuries. Am J Psychiatry 162:1328–1335, 2005

Pottick KJ, Barber CC, Hansell S, et al: Changing patterns of inpatient care for children and adolescents at the Menninger Clinic, 1988–1994. J Consult Clin Psychol 69:573–577, 2001

Putnam D, Williams RA, Weese D, et al: The effect of inpatient psychiatric hospitalization on weight gain in children and adolescents. Psychiatr Hosp 21:119–123, 1990

Reynolds CR, Richmond BO: Revised Children's Manifest Anxiety Scale. Los Angeles, CA, Western Psychological Services, 1985

Russ SW: Play in Child Development and Psychotherapy: Toward Empirically Supported Practice. Mahwah, NJ, Lawrence Erlbaum, 2004

Rutter M, Kim-Cohen J, Maughan B: Continuities and discontinuities in psychopathology between childhood and adult life. J Child Psychol Psychiatry 47:276–295, 2006

Safer DJ, Zito JM, DosReis S: Concomitant psychotropic medication for youths. Am J Psychiatry 160:438–449, 2003

Santosh PJ: Neuroimaging in child and adolescent psychiatric disorders. Arch Dis Child 82:412–419, 2000

Shaffer D, Gould MS, Ambrosini P, et al: A children's global assessment scale (CGAS). Arch Gen Psychiatry 40:1228–1231, 1983

Shapiro JP, Friedberg RD, Bardenstein KK: Child and Adolescent Therapy: Science and Art. Hoboken, NJ, Wiley, 2006

Shaw RJ, DeMaso DR: Clinical Manual of Pediatric Psychosomatic Medicine: Mental Health Consultation With Physically Ill Children and Adolescents. Washington, DC, American Psychiatric Publishing, 2006

Sorgi P, Ratey JJ, Knoedler DW, et al: Rating aggression in the clinical setting: a retrospective adaptation of the Overt Aggression Scale: preliminary results. J Neuropsychiatry Clin Neurosci 3:S52–S56, 1991

Strickland-Clark L, Campbell D, Dallos R: Children's and adolescent's views on family therapy. J Family Ther 22:324–341, 2000

Warner LA: Medical problems among adolescents in US mental health services: relationship to functional impairment. J Behav Health Serv Res 33:366–379, 2006

Weersing VR, Brent DA: Cognitive behavioral therapy for depression in youth. Child Adolesc Psychiatr Clin N Am 15:939–957, 2006

Young RC, Biggs JT, Ziegler VE, et al: A rating scale for mania: reliability, validity and sensitivity. Br J Psychiatry 133:429–435, 1978

Zhang-Wong J, Zipursky RB, Beiser M, et al: Optimal haloperidol dosage in first episode psychosis. Can J Psychiatry 44:164–167, 1999

CHAPTER 5

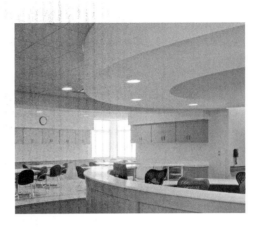

THE GERIATRIC UNIT

Sibel A. Klimstra, M.D.
Vassilios Latoussakis, M.D.
Dimitris N. Kiosses, Ph.D.
George S. Alexopoulos, M.D.

Compared with younger adults, geriatric (older than 64 years) psychiatry patients are almost twice as likely to be treated in hospital settings (Colenda et al. 2002). Common diagnostic categories are mood disorders—particularly depressive disorders—and dementias (Blank et al. 2005; Blixen et al. 1997; Weintraub and Mazour 2000; Zubenko et al. 1997). Less frequent inpatient diagnoses include primary psychotic disorders (10%; Zubenko et al. 1997), bipolar disorder (8%–10%; Depp and Jeste 2004), substance use disorders (6.8%), and delirium (4.7%) (Blank et al. 2005). Of note, inpatient primary Axis II disorders are rare, at least in part due to some decline in personality disorder frequency with aging (Abrams and Bromberg 2006). Comorbid personality disorder rates are not as rare and appear to be highest in depressed hospitalized elderly (6%–24%; Kunik et al. 1994), but they may be underrecognized due to the acuity of Axis I disorders and medical comorbidities.

Although, for most geriatric patients, inpatient length of stay has shortened considerably (Weintraub and Mazour 2000), there is a subset of patients who have protracted hospital stays. Factors associated with increased length of stay include electroconvulsive therapy (ECT), higher Brief Psychiatric Rating Scale positive symptoms scores, falls, pharmacology complications, multiple previous psychiatric hospitalizations, court proceedings for continued inpatient stay or treatment, consultation delay, and lack of ECT on weekends (Blank et al. 2005).

Admission Criteria/Considerations

Geriatric inpatients are admitted from a variety of settings—the medical inpatient unit, assisted living or skilled nursing facilities, or directly from the community. Broad criteria for admission parallel those used for general adults. However, in the geriatric population, there is an emphasis on suicide risk and inability to care for self. The elderly have the highest suicide risk of all age groups. Currently they represent 13% of the population but account for 18% of completed suicides (Arias et al. 2003), and the elderly suicide rate for those 75 years and older is 1.5 to 2 times that of the general population (Kochanek et al. 2004). Elderly white males largely account for these rates. Although elderly persons attempt suicide less frequently than younger adults, their attempts are more often lethal (Conwell et al. 2002a). Risk of geriatric suicide is highly correlated with depression severity (Alexopoulos et al. 1999; Simon and VonKorff 1998). Additional factors that increase suicide risk include psychotic depression, alcoholism, abuse of sedative-hypnotic medication, bereavement or recent loss, and disability development (Alexopoulos et al. 2001). Presence of a firearm in the home is independently associated with suicide risk (Conwell et al. 2002b). Geriatric delusional depression is often optimally treated in an inpatient setting due to the elevated suicide risk and the likely need for ECT or combination drug strategies requiring close monitoring (Meyers and Chester 1994), especially in frail elderly persons with medical comorbidities.

Elderly psychiatric patients have frequent coexistence of cognitive impairment and medical comorbidities. Elderly patients with dementia are often admitted for uncontrolled aggression or severe behavioral disturbances. Inability of a community-dwelling older person to care for him- or herself may trigger an admission referral. These patients may be malnourished, dehydrated, and inadvertently nonadherent to medication regimens. Due to physical frailty and medical comorbidities or cognitive deficits, outpatient evaluation and psychotropic medication stabilization may be unsafe (Rabins et al. 1997). Medically ill or medically high-risk patients requiring inpatient psychiatric treatment may be admitted to a combined medical geriatric unit that offers more integrated monitoring and treatment (Folks and Kinney 2002) or to a psychiatric unit within a general medical hospital.

Diagnostic Workup

Evaluation requires a systematic approach, incorporating fundamental aspects of adult evaluation as well as attending to factors specific to the older adult. Psychiatric disorders in the elderly often occur in the context of medical and neurological illness. Geriatric psychiatry inpatients have an average of five or six active medical problems, which is comparable with geriatric medical inpatients (Zubenko et al. 1997). The psychiatrist needs to conduct a thorough history of psychiat-

ric, neurological, and physical signs and symptoms, including any decline in cognition, nutritional status, and functioning, as well as careful inquiry into all medical conditions and medications. Attention should be given to potential misuse or abuse of alcohol and over-the-counter and prescription drugs, such as opiate analgesics and benzodiazepines. These substances are more commonly used by the elderly than are illicit substances of abuse (Bartels et al. 2005), may cause mood or cognitive disorders, and place patients at risk for withdrawal syndromes. Because of potentially poor insight due to psychiatric illness or cognitive deficits, detailed information from family and caregivers is critically important (Rabins et al. 1997). The clinician separately considers psychiatric, medical, and neurological differential diagnoses and then resynthesizes the case, considering the interplay of comorbidities with the presenting signs and symptoms. For example, an elderly patient presenting with depression in the context of a worsening chronic pain syndrome may have depression-driven intensification of preexisting pain. This integrated approach is a key element in successful diagnosis and treatment of the elderly.

Past psychiatric history should attempt to differentiate early- versus late-onset disorders because these may have distinct characteristics or prognostic significance. Past history of substance use, including prescription medications and alcohol, should be probed for. Family history should include familial or genetic factors of affective and cognitive illnesses, medical/neurological illness manifesting as psychiatric syndromes, and attempted or completed suicide. An age-appropriate social history should focus on social support/isolation, including whether involved family members live locally or distantly; financial status and retirement issues; the ability to perform basic and instrumental activities of daily living (ADLs); and recent losses, including bereavement issues.

Mental status assessment should always include a cognitive assessment. The Mini-Mental State Examination (MMSE) is one of the most widely used, global standardized cognitive assessments. It is brief, easy to administer, and assesses domains of orientation, memory, concentration, language, and constructional ability (Folstein et al. 1975). The MMSE is not sensitive in assessing executive function that may be impaired in dementias and geriatric depression. A brief and clinically relevant assessment for this cognitive domain is the Clock Drawing Test, which can reveal executive dysfunction in depressed elderly (Woo et al. 2004) and in elderly patients with a normal MMSE result (Juby et al. 2002). The Mini-Cog is a brief and effective tool for dementia detection (Borson et al. 2003). It combines a three-item recall question and the Clock Drawing Test and performs at least as well as the MMSE in multiethnic elderly populations (Borson et al. 2005). When dementia is suspected or diagnosed prior to admission, it is important to confirm the type of dementia (e.g., Alzheimer's disease, vascular dementia, dementia with Lewy bodies) and, if necessary, to order targeted neuropsychological examinations to aid in differential diagnosis.

A comprehensive physical and neurological examination is necessary. It is important not to confuse normal age-related neurological changes—such as head/neck tremor, muscle atrophy of the hands, nonspecific gait disturbance, impaired conjugate upgaze, and reduced ankle vibratory sense—with neurological disease (Mancall 2006).

Admission assessment of nutritional and functional status, including gait assessment and fall risk, should be made. On an inpatient geropsychiatric unit, the presence of cardiac arrhythmias, Parkinson's disease, dementia diagnosis, and use of ECT or mood stabilizers are associated with increased fall risk (de Carle and Kohn 2001). Postural hypotension is also a significant fall risk (Tinetti et al. 2006), and sitting/standing blood pressures should be a routine part of vital sign assessment.

Laboratory tests not only aid in differential diagnosis—possibly elucidating medical factors contributing to or causing psychiatric signs and symptoms—but also help assess safety factors for medication or ECT administration. Admission laboratory screening, similar to that done in younger adults, may include electrolytes, blood urea nitrogen/creatinine, fasting blood glucose, liver function tests, thyroid function tests, lipid profile, complete blood count, urinalysis, urine toxicology, and possibly blood alcohol level. Serum drug levels for nortriptyline, desipramine, lithium, valproic acid, and digoxin, as well as prothrombin time/international normalized ratio if warfarin is present, should be ordered. Chest X ray may be part of a delirium workup. Electrocardiography is often ordered (Vergare et al. 2006). Standard laboratory tests for dementia include serum chemistries; renal, liver, and thyroid function tests; vitamin B_{12} level; and complete blood count. Syphilis serology, urinalysis, erythrocyte sedimentation rate, heavy metal and toxicology screening, HIV testing, chest X ray, electroencephalograms, electrocardiograms, and lumbar puncture may be ordered based on historical or examination findings (Boyle et al. 2006). Structural neuroimaging with magnetic resonance imaging or noncontrast computed tomography is recommended for initial dementia evaluations (Knopman et al. 2001) or when focal neurological lesions are suspected (Rabins et al. 1997). The clinical use of functional neuroimaging is limited to special circumstances. In particular, Medicare coverage allows positron emission tomography as a differential diagnosis tool in patients with clinical symptoms of frontotemporal dementia.

Medication Treatments

Common geriatric inpatient psychiatric syndromes include severe depressive disorders and cognitive disorders. This section emphasizes treatment in these domains. Treatment of geriatric bipolar disorder, delirium, and schizophrenia is also discussed. The primary goals of inpatient treatment are to initiate safe and effective acute-phase therapies while managing medical comorbidities, maintaining the patient in a supportive environment, and providing sound aftercare referral and treatment recommendations.

Geriatric Depression

MAJOR DEPRESSIVE DISORDER

DSM-IV-TR (American Psychiatric Association 2000) describes major depressive disorder, with or without psychotic features, that can be severe and may require inpatient treatment. Geriatric major depression can be challenging to diagnose because elderly persons underreport depressive mood symptoms (Gallo and Rabins 1999) and more frequently focus on anhedonia and the physical complaints of poor sleep, low energy, and appetite and weight loss. These latter symptoms may overlap with and therefore incorrectly be attributed to comorbid medical and dementing illnesses. However, in many cases, physical symptoms experienced by depressed elderly persons have root causes in medical illness with intensification by the depressive illness (Alexopoulos et al. 2002a).

Symptoms of sad mood, frequent tearfulness, and recurrent thoughts of suicide and death are more reliable in establishing major depression in the elderly population (Alexopoulos et al. 2002c). Additional symptoms of anhedonia, social isolation, hopelessness, helplessness, worthlessness, nondelusional guilt, psychomotor agitation or retardation, and impairment in decision making and daily planning of activities can help establish the diagnosis (Alexopoulos et al. 2002c).

The current DSM classification system fails to incorporate the cognitive impairments that are often present in elderly depressed patients without dementia (Alexopoulos 1990). These include deficits in attention, mental processing speed, and executive function (Elderkin-Thompson et al. 2003; Kindermann et al. 2000; Lockwood et al. 2002). Interestingly, despite remission of depression, these cognitive impairments may persist in an attenuated state.

Major depressive disorder with psychotic features occurs in approximately 36%–45% of all inpatient depressed elderly persons (Meyers 1995). Across all age ranges, about 25% of inpatient psychotic depression is misdiagnosed, primarily due to lack of psychosis recognition (Rothschild et al. 2008). Delusions are more common than hallucinations and are often characterized as somatic, guilty, nihilistic, persecutory, or, less commonly, jealous in nature (Alexopoulos 2004).

ADDITIONAL LATE-LIFE DEPRESSIVE SYNDROMES

Additional syndromes of late-life depression outside the current DSM classification that have clinical significance for treatment and/or prognosis are described below.

Depression with reversible dementia. Depression with reversible dementia—formerly referred to as *pseudodementia*—is a significant risk factor for irreversible dementia. A subset of depressed elderly patients (18%–57%) develop a dementia that remits with depression remission, although some cognitive deficits usually persist (Emery 1988). Approximately 40% of these patients with reversible dementia develop an irreversible dementing illness within the proceeding 3 years (Alexopoulos et al. 1993).

Vascular depression. The vascular depression hypothesis characterizes cerebrovascular disease as predisposing, precipitating, or perpetuating a subtype of depression (Alexopoulos et al. 1997b; Krishnan et al. 1997). Data that support this include the high comorbidity of vascular disease and depression as well as awareness that vascular lesions can lead to specific behavioral symptoms. Vascular depression has its own phenotype. Elderly patients with this syndrome have increased apathy, psychomotor retardation, and poor insight but less guilt and agitation compared with elderly patients without vascular disease risk factors (Alexopoulos et al. 1997a; Krishnan et al. 1997). These patients also have greater disability and cognitive impairment, particularly in the domains of verbal fluency and object naming (Alexopoulos et al. 1997a).

Awareness of this depression subtype may lead to different treatment strategies. For example, treating vascular disease or its risk factors may ameliorate the risk for or course of vascular depression. Similarly, antidepressants with dopaminergic or noradrenergic properties that facilitate ischemic recovery may be superior to those with α-adrenergic–blocking properties that inhibit ischemic recovery (Alexopoulos et al. 1997b).

Depression–executive dysfunction syndrome. Some elderly depressed patients have frontostriatal dysfunction as suggested by neuroimaging and neuropathological studies. Fronto-striatal-limbic system dysfunction in this subset of patients has been described and termed the *depression–executive dysfunction syndrome* (Alexopoulos 2001). Phenotypically, these patients have psychomotor retardation, a relative paucity of vegetative symptoms, decreased interest in activities, suspiciousness, and impaired instrumental ADLs. Patients with this syndrome respond less well to antidepressants, including selective serotonin reuptake inhibitors (SSRIs; Alexopoulos et al. 2002b, 2005b; Potter et al. 2004), but one study indicates they respond well to problem-solving therapy (Alexopoulos et al. 2003).

EARLY- VERSUS LATE-ONSET ILLNESS

In an effort to explore contributing factors of geriatric depression—including an association of neurological disease with late-life depression—attempts have been made to differentiate depressed patients according to time of onset. However, this classification has not been particularly useful from either a clinical or theoretical standpoint. Time of onset can be difficult to determine, and early depressive episodes may affect neurological functioning over time (Alexopoulos 2004). The putative mechanism for this involves depression-driven increases in stress that lead, through intracellular mechanisms, to reduction of neurotrophic factors, causing decreased survival or functioning of neurons over time (Duman et al. 1997).

ACUTE-PHASE INPATIENT TREATMENT OF LATE-LIFE DEPRESSION

The "Expert Consensus Guideline Series: Pharmacotherapy of Depressive Disorders in Older Patients" (Alexopoulos et al. 2001) outlines acute-phase treatment strategies for depression. The guideline methodology uses quantitative survey data from experts based on clinical knowledge and literature review to answer practical clinical questions for which other evidence-based studies do not exist. Although not covered here, continuation- and maintenance-phase treatment strategies are also well described in this guideline. The inpatient clinician should be familiar with these strategies and communicate them to the outpatient psychiatric treater for optimal continuity of care.

Severe unipolar major depressive disorder without psychotic features. The treatment of choice is combination pharmacotherapy and psychotherapy, with another first-line option being pharmacotherapy alone. Treatment of geriatric depression should consist of single antidepressant trials, with adequate dosages for adequate duration. If there is no response, monotherapy with another antidepressant should follow. If there is partial response, augmentation strategies should be initiated. SSRIs are the antidepressants of choice because they are equally efficacious as the older tricyclic antidepressants, are safer in overdose, and have a more favorable side-effect profile, including lack of quinidine-like cardiovascular effects. The clinician should be aware of SSRI risks pertinent to the elderly. A large population-based study of older adults (age > 50 years) found daily SSRI use was associated with increased risk of falls and double the risk of fragility fractures (Richards et al. 2007). There has also been concern that SSRIs may confer an increased risk of suicide. Compared with other antidepressants, one study reported almost a fivefold increased risk of elderly suicide—but only during the first month of SSRI initiation. The absolute suicide risk was low (1 in 3,353 SSRI-treated patients), and many of these deaths were likely due to depressive illness and not medication. SSRI treatment benefits appear to outweigh this small risk (Juurlink et al. 2006). Monitoring suicidality over the course of treatment is always prudent but is especially so during the first month after antidepressant initiation.

Serotonin–norepinephrine reuptake inhibitors (SNRIs) are other first-line agents. The clinician needs to pay attention to potential but uncommon supine diastolic blood pressure elevations, established as dose dependent in the elderly for immediate-release venlafaxine (Staab and Evans 2000; Thase 1998) and reported in unspecified age populations for extended-release preparations in daily doses ranging from 37.5 to 225 mg. The relationship to dosage is currently unclear (Thomson 2007). Bupropion and mirtazapine are alternative treatment strategies, as are tricyclic antidepressants in patients without cardiac conduction defects. To minimize side effects, preferential use of nortriptyline or desipramine is recommended, and doxepin, imipramine, and amitriptyline should be avoided. Trazodone for antidepressant use in the elderly should be avoided.

Choosing among various antidepressant agents can be a challenging task for the inpatient psychiatrist. Interestingly, the STAR*D study supports the idea that for patients who fail to respond to a single antidepressant trial (citalopram in the study), basing subsequent trials on differing versus similar pharmacological classes of medication or putative mechanism of action does not affect treatment outcome. It also provides evidence for use of itemized symptom measures rather than global impression to detect improvement and effectiveness of both triiodothyronine (T_3) and lithium augmentation (Rush 2007).

ECT is an alternative treatment strategy to pharmacotherapy. ECT has been shown to be effective in the elderly (Tew et al. 1999) and safe in patients with comorbid medical conditions (Alexopoulos 2004). Failure of two adequate trials of antidepressants, acute suicide risk, and medical comorbidity complicating antidepressant medication treatment are reasons to consider use of ECT.

Unipolar major depressive disorder with psychotic features. Expert opinion has stated that the treatment of choice for geriatric delusional depression is either combination antidepressant and atypical antipsychotic or ECT (Alexopoulos et al. 2001). Preferred antidepressants include SSRIs and SNRIs, although this awaits direct empirical testing in the elderly. However, in the first randomized efficacy study in elderly delusional depression, combination nortriptyline and perphenazine, although well tolerated, provided no additional therapeutic benefit to nortriptyline alone (Mulsant et al. 2001). A multicenter randomized, prospective, double-blind trial funded by the National Institute of Mental Health is under way to examine—in both geriatric and younger adults—the acute efficacy of combination therapy with olanzapine and sertraline versus monotherapy with olanzapine (Andreescu et al. 2007).

Dementia/Delirium

Elderly persons are particularly susceptible to delirium due to the increased prevalence of dementia, multiple medical and neurological comorbidities, and polypharmacy. Delirium, with its broad symptom profile, may create diagnostic confusion with other common psychiatric syndromes such as dementia, depression, hypomanic and manic states, schizophrenia, and substance use disorders. Delirium is frequently missed, especially in patients who are not hyperactive or agitated and thus not a behavioral problem (Armstrong et al. 1997; Johnson et al. 1992). When in doubt, it is prudent to assume the diagnosis of delirium, which should be viewed as a medical emergency and, unless treated, may lead to significantly worsened outcomes, including greater mortality (McCusker et al. 2002) and morbidity, prolonged hospital stays, and increased rates of institutionalization. Key features include the acute or subacute development of disturbances in attention and orientation, sleep–wake cycle, and psychomotor functions. Psychomotor disturbances may give rise to hyperactive states, mixed states, or (less commonly in the elderly) hypoactive states (Armstrong et al. 1997; Johnson et al. 1992). A systematic workup must then proceed while safety issues of the delirious patient are attended to. A careful history and physical and neurological examination may guide the selection of more tailored workups. Three points need to be stressed in the search of possible etiologies of delirium:

1. Delirium is often multifactorial (Meagher et al. 2006).
2. The admission assessment may have already identified delirium risk factors that could guide further workup.
3. Common causes of delirium in the elderly are frequently not central nervous system–related and include polypharmacy, infections such as urinary tract infection, and dehydration (Young and Inouye 2007).

Medical and/or neurology consultation may be warranted while the basic workup (complete blood count, electrolytes, liver and renal function tests, glucose, electrocardiogram, urinalysis, chest X ray, and erythrocyte sedimentation rate) is being completed. Further patient-specific tests may be warranted. Management should proceed concurrently with diagnostic assessment. Environmental manipulations should always be considered and include 1) correction or optimization of sensory deficits (e.g., use of glasses, hearing aids, and dentures; adequate lighting; noise reduction); 2) measures promoting familiarity or orientation to surroundings (a visible clock and calendar, presence of a relative or family photos, frequent reality orientations); and 3) a reassuring and clear communication style by staff and family members (American Psychiatric Association 1999; Inouye et al. 1999).

The pharmacological management of delirium mainly involves antipsychotic medications. Benzodiazepines have limited usefulness, except in alcohol or benzodiazepine withdrawal. Haloperidol, administered orally or intramuscularly, is helpful in the majority of cases. More recently, atypical antipsychotics are emerging as alternative options, but further study is needed prior to advocating their use (Seitz et al. 2007; Young and Inouye 2007).

NEUROPSYCHIATRIC AND BEHAVIORAL DISTURBANCES ASSOCIATED WITH DEMENTIA

Neuropsychiatric and behavioral disturbances associated with dementia include psychosis and a range of agitated behaviors (including aggressive, physically nonaggressive, and verbal/vocal agitated behaviors). Inpatient psychiatric admission is primarily reserved for those elderly patients with dementia whose behavior is a danger to themselves or others or has led to a notable decline in functioning. It is critical to identify and track specific targeted treatment symptoms during the course of the hospitalization. The etiology of the behavioral disturbances is often multifactorial, and careful assessment is required. Common causes of agitation in dementia patients include superimposed delirium, depression, and psychosis. Additional important causes include dysuria, dyspnea, abdominal discomfort from constipation, and pruritis (Alexopoulos et al. 2004, 2005a). Yet there are a number of patients with "idiopathic" agitation syndromes, perhaps due to behavioral disinhibition caused by impairment of frontal and/or parietal structures.

NONPHARMACOLOGICAL APPROACHES

Environmental over- or understimulation, space restriction, a sudden decline in a patient's ability to communicate, and problems in caregiver approach to the patient are common and perhaps easily reversible causes of disruptive behaviors in the elderly patient with dementia (Alexopoulos et al. 2004; Cohen-Mansfield 2001). Although frequently overlooked, environmental manipulations—such as reducing overstimulation; speaking in a soft, supportive tone; optimizing hearing and vision; improving communication through nonverbal means; or attending to a patient during calm periods—may be beneficial.

PHARMACOLOGICAL APPROACHES

The clinician must first rule in or out delirium and treat appropriately. When agitated depressive symptoms are present, an SSRI trial is indicated. Expert consensus states that antipsychotics are the preferred treatment choice when delusions are present and are even favored in nondelusional patients (although they may not be as efficacious as when delusions are present) (Alexopoulos et al. 2004). However, antipsychotic use has come under increased scrutiny in the elderly. In April 2005, the U.S. Food and Drug Administration issued a public health advisory and required all manufacturers of atypical antipsychotics to add a "black box" warning to their labeling describing a 1.6- to 1.7-fold mortality increase, primarily due to cardiac-related events or infections, in elderly patients with dementia and behavioral disturbances (U.S. Food and Drug Administration 2005). An independent meta-analysis of randomized, controlled studies of atypical antipsychotics echoed these concerns. Death occurred slightly more frequently with atypical antipsychotics versus placebo (3.5% vs. 2.3%; Schneider et al. 2005).

In a large retrospective mixed-diagnosis study, elderly patients on antipsychotic medication 180 days or less had a higher risk of death with conventional antipsychotics versus atypical antipsychotics (relative risk, 1.37; Wang et al. 2005). More recently, the double-blind, placebo-controlled National Institute of Mental Health–sponsored Clinical Antipsychotic Trial of Intervention Effectiveness—Alzheimer's Disease (CATIE-AD) study examined ambulatory outpatients with Alzheimer's disease and behavioral problems such as psychosis, agitation, or aggression (Schneider et al. 2006). Patients randomly received treatment with olanzapine, quetiapine, risperidone, or placebo and were followed for up to 36 weeks. Time to treatment discontinuation for any reason did not differ significantly among the medication and placebo groups. Median time to discontinuation due to lack of efficacy was significantly longer with olanzapine (22.1 weeks) or risperidone (26.7 weeks) than with quetiapine (9.1 weeks) or placebo (9.0 weeks). Discontinuation rates due to intolerance, adverse effects, or death were 24% with olanzapine, 18% with risperidone, 16% with quetiapine, and 5% with placebo. However, these findings from an ambulatory population may not be applicable to the inpatient dementia population with likely more severe behavioral problems.

Clinicians should exercise judgment in the use of all antipsychotics—both conventional and atypical—for severe behavioral disturbances in dementia. When inpatient antipsychotic use is necessary, the clinician needs to be aware of diagnostic differences in antipsychotic response time. Although an antimanic response may be seen within 2–4 days and an antipsychotic response in schizophrenia within 1 week, dementia-related behavioral and antipsychotic response may take several weeks. Therefore, there is a danger for clinicians to generalize their experiences,

which may lead to overdosing and serious side effects. A useful inpatient strategy is initiation and maintenance of a low-dosage atypical neuroleptic using time-limited, low-dosage benzodiazepines administered at fixed time intervals rather than on an as-needed basis (with heightened fall precautions) to symptomatically treat dementia-related agitation until the therapeutic effects of antipsychotics are established. Agitated and aggressive behaviors in patients with Alzheimer's disease have responded to risperidone at a dosage of 1 mg/day or olanzapine at a dosage of 5–10 mg/day (Sink et al. 2005; Wang et al. 2005). Antipsychotic risk, including the risk of metabolic syndrome, cerebrovascular accidents, or even death, should be discussed with the family. Clinicians should document their rationale for choosing an antipsychotic, including other approaches considered or attempted first and the risk–benefit ratio. Documentation should include risk of withholding antipsychotic treatment.

Although not useful in the acute control of behavioral disturbances in inpatients with dementia, cognitive enhancers such as cholinesterase inhibitors or memantine may be helpful for long-term management because they have been shown to improve not only cognitive but also behavioral, emotional, and psychotic symptoms (Beier 2007; Cummings et al. 2000, 2004; Tariot et al. 2004; Trinh et al. 2003). Similarly, SSRIs can be considered for dementia-related behavioral disturbances, although they may be more useful in preventing future episodes than in treating the current ones. Nevertheless, in at least one study citalopram outperformed placebo in the acute (less than 3 weeks) treatment of psychotic symptoms and behavioral disturbances in nondepressed inpatients with dementia (Pollock et al. 2002).

Bipolar Disorder

Compared with elderly persons with unipolar depression, elderly bipolar patients are about four times as likely to have had an inpatient psychiatric admission over the previous 6 months (Bartels et al. 2000) and have a greater (non-suicide-related) mortality rate (Shulman et al. 1992). The prevalence of bipolar disorder in community populations decreases with increasing age. Older bipolar patients have less comorbid substance use disorders compared with younger bipolar patients. They probably do not have more mixed episodes or a poorer treatment response compared with younger bipolar patients (Depp and Jeste 2004). Despite their lower substance use disorder comorbidities compared with younger bipolar patients, elderly bipolar patients have greater functional and cognitive impairment (Depp et al. 2005), including more confusion and disorientation (McDonald 2000).

EARLY- VERSUS LATE-ONSET ILLNESS

Elderly patients with early-onset manic symptoms are more likely than those with late-onset illness to be medication nonadherent (58% vs. 34%) and aggressive or threatening (66% vs. 37%) prior to psychiatric inpatient admission and to require emergency petition for hospitalization (37% vs. 14%) (Lehmann and Rabins 2006).

Vascular disease is a potential etiology or risk factor for late-onset bipolar disorder. Late-onset bipolar disorder is associated with a greater degree of neurological disease and possibly less bipolar family history (Depp and Jeste 2004). Additionally, compared with age-matched bipolar patients with early-onset mania, those with late-onset (age 47 years and older) mania have greater vascular risk factors or disease (hypertension, cerebrovascular accidents, coronary artery disease, atrial fibrillation, diabetes mellitus, hypercholesterolemia, or hyperlipidemia) (Cassidy and Carroll 2002). Elderly bipolar patients have increased frontal deep white matter signal hyperintensities compared with age-matched community members, and data suggest that severity of right frontal signal hyperintensities may be associated with late-onset mania (de Asis et al. 2006).

DIFFERENTIAL DIAGNOSIS

For geriatric patients presenting with late-onset manic symptoms, the inpatient clinician should evaluate carefully for *secondary mania,* a term describing mania due to general medical conditions or substances (Krauthammer and Klerman 1978). As described earlier, patients with late-onset mania are more likely to have vascular disease, pointing to the need to concomitantly assess and potentially treat conditions such as hypertension, vascular heart disease, diabetes, and stroke (Sajatovic et al. 2005). Common medications associated with mania include antidepressants, benzodiazepines, sympathomimetics, dopaminergic drugs used to treat Parkinson's disease, and corticosteroids (Van Gerpen et al. 1999). Interestingly, higher dosages of corticosteroids rather than age itself are associated with increased risk (Ganzini et al. 1993; Van Gerpen et al. 1999).

TREATMENT

Older bipolar patients (age > 65 years) have twice the psychiatric inpatient length of stay as younger bipolar patients (Brown 2001; Depp and Jeste 2004), which may reflect a longer time for comorbid medical or psychiatric symptom resolution (Depp and Jeste 2004). The American Psychiatric Association's (2002) *Practice Guideline for the Treatment of Patients With Bipolar Disorder* provides some treatment guidance. An evidence-based review for late-life bipolar pharmacotherapy treatment finds that lithium and divalproex are the two most common antimanic agents studied, and uncontrolled studies suggest that they are efficacious. However, there are little geriatric evidence-based data for therapeutic concentration ranges or adequate duration of dosing for acute treatment with antimanic agents. No systematic drug treatment studies for geriatric bipolar depression were found. Likewise, there are no geriatric bipolar treatment studies comparing ECT and pharmacotherapy (Young et al. 2004). A retrospective study found no difference among lithium, valproic acid, and carbamazepine treatment in terms of length of geriatric inpatient stay or Global Assessment of Functioning score improvement (Sanderson 1998). More definitive treatment efficacy answers should emerge soon. A multicenter randomized, double-blind, prospective trial funded by the National Institute of Mental Health is under way to assess the acute treatment efficacy of lithium versus divalproex in geriatric mania. Meanwhile, current strategies are as follows (Young et al. 2004):

1. The treatment of choice in geriatric mania is monotherapy with a mood stabilizer. Initial target range for serum lithium concentrations is 0.4–0.8 mEq/L, but patients may require levels in the range of 0.8–1.0 mEq/L. Divalproex sodium may be given with target serum concentrations used for younger adults. Carbamazepine should be considered a second-line treatment. For partial monotherapy mood stabilizer responders, the addition of an atypical antipsychotic or a second mood stabilizer may be considered.
2. For geriatric bipolar depression, monotherapy with lithium may be given. Lamotrigine should be considered using similar dosing strategies as for younger adults. If necessary, an antidepressant may be added.
3. ECT may be considered in either phase of geriatric bipolar disorder. General rationales for ECT use include the severely ill or deteriorating patient for whom rapid response is critical, pharmacotherapy trials involving relatively greater risk than ECT, pharmacotherapy-refractory illness, and inability to tolerate pharmacotherapy side effects (Weiner

2001), which is often seen in the frail, medically compromised elderly patient.

Schizophrenia

EARLY- VERSUS LATE-ONSET ILLNESS

In schizophrenia, even the age at which the term "late onset" applies is in dispute, with some requiring onset after age 40 years and others at 45 or even 60 years (Andreasen 1999; Howard and Rabins 1997). DSM-IV-TR does not distinguish between late- and early-onset schizophrenia. Nevertheless, there are clinical, neuropsychological, neuroimaging, and genetic differences:

1. In late-onset schizophrenia, symptomatology tends to be milder and negative symptoms, thought disturbances, and first-rank Schneiderian symptoms are less common. Delusions and hallucinations are common to both groups.
2. Neurocognitive deficits exist in both chronic and late-onset schizophrenia. There is disagreement as to whether patterns of cognitive impairments are similar (Almeida 1999) or markedly different, with cognitive decline and dementia occurring earlier (within 5 years) in the late-onset schizophrenic group.

INPATIENT TREATMENT

For newly diagnosed late-onset schizophrenia, it is important to first rule out other causes and treat accordingly. The mainstay of geriatric schizophrenia treatment is antipsychotic pharmacotherapy. Elder-specific concerns include an increased risk of cerebrovascular adverse events, and even death. Most, if not all, of those risks were observed in dementia patients with behavioral disturbances, and it is unclear whether they pertain to other elderly clinical samples. In a recent mixed-age study, there was similar effectiveness (a measure of efficacy and tolerability) between atypical and typical antipsychotics (Schneider et al. 2006). Required antipsychotic dosages for elderly schizophrenic patients are intermediate to those for younger schizophrenic patients and dementia patients (Alexopoulos et al. 2004). Elderly patients with schizophrenia will need psychosocial services upon discharge.

Drug–Drug Interactions

Psychoactive medication use in late life should be approached with extra care. The number of medications used in the elderly, including those admitted to an inpatient psychogeriatric unit, is larger compared with younger populations. Normal aging is associated with physiological changes that alter the pharmacokinetics of various substances, leading to variable clearances, free concentrations, and volume of distributions (Pollock 1998). Aging also leads to pharmacodynamic alterations. Furthermore, aging is associated with increased prevalence of medical and neurological comorbidities (e.g., renal or heart failure, liver disease, Parkinson's disease) that confer extra vulnerabilities. Finally, the consequences of drug-induced adverse events may be more serious in the elderly. An exhaustive list of potential drug–drug interactions is beyond the scope of this chapter; instead, we provide guiding principles and common examples of interactions involving psychoactive medications:

1. Dose initiation and speed of titration need to be individualized. Chronological age is only one factor to be considered. Knowledge of physical health status, including comorbid illnesses, is essential. The elderly often have side effects at lower dosages than younger adults. In light of this knowledge, "start low and go slow" may apply differently to different patients.
2. Psychoactive substances should be prescribed for specific psychiatric diagnoses and target symptoms. Criteria for initiating or terminating a trial should be planned. Adequate target dosing is critical and may depend on diagnosis or type of medication used. For example, compared with younger adults, elderly persons require the same target dosage of SSRIs and SNRIs. For neuroleptics, the target dosage in elderly patients is diagnosis dependent. Compared with younger adults, elderly patients require lower target dosages of neuroleptics for schizophrenia and lower dosages still for dementia-related psychosis and behavioral disturbances (Alexopoulos et al. 2004; Madhusoodanan et al. 2007). In light of this, we propose that the "start low and go slow" injunction should be revised to "start low, go slow, but get there."
3. On admission and before addition of a new medication, concurrent medications need to be scrutinized for potential drug–drug or disease–drug interactions. A number of online drug information databases (Clauson et al. 2007) as well as software programs for handheld devices (Mattana et al. 2005) are available to assist in the detection of drug–drug interactions. Their routine use should be considered in clinical practice.
4. The use of psychotropic medications on an as-needed basis should be minimized and reviewed regularly. As-needed use can lead to inappropriate accumulation of plasma levels. Frequently, such use

clouds the clinical picture and results in knee-jerk reactions guided by fleeting symptoms rather than a targeted treatment plan. Table 5–1 lists examples of various mechanisms of drug–drug interactions of particular clinical importance in the elderly.

Psychotherapies

Due to the time-limited nature of acute psychiatric hospitalization, traditional psychotherapy models are applicable to only a minority of patients. Awareness of basic treatment principles can guide discharge recommendations. Within geriatric psychiatry, the best-studied psychotherapy application is for the treatment of major depression. Combination psychotherapy and psychopharmacology is the optimal acute treatment strategy for geriatric depression (Alexopoulos et al. 2001; Arean and Cook 2002). Cognitive-behavioral therapy (Gallagher and Thompson 1982; Thompson et al. 2001), interpersonal therapy (IPT; Reynolds et al. 1999; Schneider et al. 1986), and problem-solving therapy (PST; Alexopoulos et al. 2003; Arean et al. 1993) are the three therapies best shown to have efficacy in geriatric major depression (Frazer et al. 2005). Modified cognitive therapy techniques have been described specifically for elderly depressed inpatients (Casey and Grant 1993).

A significant proportion of elderly depressed patients have comorbid cognitive impairment (Alexopoulos et al. 2002c), and therefore current psychotherapies have addressed this patient population. PST has shown efficacy in depressed elders with mild executive dysfunction (Alexopoulos et al. 2003). IPT and PST have been modified for depressed elderly persons with moderate cognitive impairment, but no efficacy data have yet been published (Kiosses 2007; Miller and Reynolds 2007). IPT-CI (IPT for cognitive impairment) addresses role conflicts by incorporating caregiver needs along with those of the cognitively impaired depressed patient (Miller and Reynolds 2007). PST-CD (PST for cognitively impaired, disabled elders) incorporates compensatory strategies to bypass behavioral limitations associated with cognitive deficits and invites caregivers to participate in therapy when the patients cannot follow the problem-solving stages alone (Kiosses 2007). Both IPT-CI and PST-CD may be useful discharge treatment recommendations to this population and their caregivers.

Psychotherapeutic approaches to reducing agitation need further research. In a large randomized, placebo-controlled clinical trial, caregiver behavioral training, haloperidol (mean dose, 1.8 mg/day), trazodone (mean dose, 200 mg/day), and placebo produced comparable modest reductions in agitation in patients with Alzheimer's disease (Teri et al. 2000).

Patient and Family Education

Patient and family assessment begins prior to admission with understanding the patient's living circumstances, whether any caregivers exist, and what expectations the patient and family have for discharge arrangements. Ideally, the geriatric social worker will establish patient and family contact within the first 24 hours of admission. Psychosocial assessment encompasses safety of current living arrangement, including driving and ability to function alone, any presence of emotional and/or physical elder abuse, and the physical and mental ability of the caregiver to function in his or her role, including the presence of caregiver cognitive impairment or depression and the degree of social support (Thompson et al. 2006).

Caregiver assessment, particularly caregiver abilities and any caregiver depression, should be emphasized. Almost one-third of primary caregivers to community-dwelling patients with moderate to advanced dementia experience significant depressive symptoms. Relationship to patient (wife or daughter), increased time spent caregiving, and impairment in physical functioning are all caregiver-influenced factors associated with increased caregiver depression. Younger age, lower education, white or Hispanic ethnicity, increased ADL dependency, and behavioral disturbance are patient-influenced factors associated with increased caregiver depression (Covinsky et al. 2003).

Depending on the patient's physical and cognitive state, family member roles can vary widely, ranging from supportive to surrogate decision making. Inpatient psychoeducation may emphasize increased caregiving skills and resource awareness. Factors correlated with degree of family involvement during geropsychiatric hospitalization include complexity and awareness of the patient's needs and altered caregiver role on discharge (Owens and Qualls 2002).

Patients admitted from a nursing home often have severe behavioral dyscontrol, and transfer can happen quickly, leaving the patient and family little time to process this change. Social workers educate family members about the patient's disease processes and resultant cognitive, mood, and behavioral changes. The entire treatment team assesses for environmental triggers and behavioral strategies to manage agitated, ag-

TABLE 5–1. Examples of age-related changes in pharmacokinetics and pharmacodynamics

Process	Aging effects	Clinical examples
Distribution	Decreased volume of distribution for hydrophilic drugs	Lithium toxicity
	Increased volume of distribution for hydrophobic drugs	Diazepam accumulation with repeated dosages
Phase I metabolism (general effect)	Decreased hepatic blood flow leading to reduced hepatic metabolism	Accumulation of various psychotropics (e.g., tertiary tricyclic antidepressants)
Phase I metabolism	Decline in cytochrome P450 (CYP) 1A2 activity	Clozapine toxicity, especially in an elderly patient who quits smoking
	Decline in CYP3A activity	Toxicity involving several different psychotropic medications (e.g., antidepressants, antipsychotics), especially in the presence of a CYP3A inhibitor (e.g., certain antibiotics, antifungals, nefazodone)
Pharmacodynamics	Increased vulnerability to orthostatic hypotension	Risk of falls when an α-blocker is combined with a low-potency antipsychotic
	Increased vulnerability to anticholinergic activity	Risk of delirium when cimetidine is combined with a tricyclic antidepressant

gressive states. In addition, social workers teach caregivers, both professional staff and family, successful patient-specific behavioral strategies. For example, noise-related sleep deprivation is a common environmental cause of agitation in the nursing home and relatively easy to modify. Social workers are also integrally involved in discharge plans. Patients who are treated on specific geriatric psychiatry inpatient units receive more appropriate referral to age-specific aftercare (Yazgan et al. 2004).

Rehabilitation and Recreational Therapies

Activity programs ideally offer a blend of physical and mental tasks and encourage patients to perform them as independently as possible. Benefits to geriatric patients include the physical, cognitive, emotional, spiritual, and social domains. Specific activities are described in the book *Activities for the Elderly: A Guide to Quality Programming* (Parker et al. 1999). Recreational group activities need to be adaptable to those who are physically impaired. Occupational therapy may emphasize group ADL skills with the dual purpose of social activity and individual skill assessment and intervention. Geriatric occupational therapy also uses rehabilitation models of functional status and

emphasizes physical skills such as strengthening and positioning (Inventor et al. 2005). To accommodate most levels of physical skill, group activity can be modified to include either seated or standing exercise.

Cognitive stimulation techniques are used with geriatric inpatients, although they may be of limited benefit for dementia patients, who can experience frustration (Rabins et al. 1997). Groups focusing on current events are used for memory and orientation enhancement. Wellness groups for higher-functioning patients focus on themes of stress and anger management, social activity, and healthy living choices, including exercise and nutrition; time management skills may be less pertinent to retired elderly.

Music therapy as an intervention for dementia patients with agitation and aggressive behaviors in long-term-care settings (Gerdner 2005) may be used on inpatient geriatric units. Pet therapy is also being used on inpatient geriatric units. Preliminary research suggests it may reduce ECT-associated fear (Barker et al. 2003) and dementia-related irritability (Zisselman et al. 1996).

Geriatric Milieu Management

There is significant benefit to specialized geriatric psychiatry inpatient units as opposed to mixed-age units.

Compared with elder care on general psychiatric units, elderly patients on specialized geriatric psychiatry units are more likely to receive thorough medical and structured cognitive assessments, psychotropic side-effect and blood-level monitoring, and aging-sensitive aftercare referral (Yazgan et al. 2004). The clinical utility of mental health assessment protocols and multidisciplinary teamwork within a geriatric psychiatry unit has been described (Ngoh et al. 2005). In a study of 31 inpatient psychiatry units across the country, geriatric professionals were surveyed to understand what practices were adopted for optimal care. Physical modifications included handrails; tub lifts; specialized furniture such as movable geri-chairs, recliners, lowered and/or electric beds and hospital beds; wheelchair accessibility; specialized flooring; and increased walking areas. Safety emphasis included restraint reduction, fall prevention plans with protocols and screening, and monitoring of physical signs and symptoms such as pain, dysphagia, and oral intake. Increased family contact was encouraged. More than 75% of all specialized geriatric units provided reminiscence groups, family and patient education, exercise and music groups, and recreational/leisure activities. Fifty-five percent of the units used nurse-led groups. Challenges to care included nursing staffing shortage, lack of staff training in geriatric psychiatry, patient medical acuity, balancing of restraint/seclusion regulations with fall prevention, and discharge placement difficulties. Excellence in multidisciplinary care (67% of respondents) was the factor most commonly identified for a successful unit. Additional factors included availability of geriatric medicine physicians and on-unit services (Smith et al. 2005). Readily available on-unit geriatric medicine and neurology consultation services are optimal, given the high degree of medical comorbidity.

The adaptation of successful geriatric psychiatry inpatient care within existing mixed-age frameworks is an alternative milieu model to an independent geropsychiatry unit that, although perhaps ideal, may not be feasible for administrative or financial reasons. Faced with these limitations, one study describes an inpatient "geropsychiatric unit without walls." A "Senior Team Program" for geropsychiatric inpatients was created within an existing adult inpatient unit of a general hospital. Geriatric patients were clustered together, physical modifications were made, and staff received geriatric care training. Remarkably, over the first 14 months of the program, the elderly "fall" rate was reduced, and no geriatric patient required restraints (Nadler-Moodie and Gold 2005). Additional geriatric milieu management requires awareness that

cognitive impairment may limit psychotherapy; the use of "behavior as communication" becomes critical. Tolerance of wandering behaviors, while monitoring safety, is encouraged (Inventor et al. 2005).

Management of Suicidal and Aggressive Behaviors

Among elderly patients admitted to a psychiatric inpatient unit, more than 50% of suicides occur within the first week of admission or discharge (Erlangsen et al. 2006). Once the decision to hospitalize occurs, immediate and ongoing assessment of the elderly inpatient's suicidal risk and potential risk of harm to others should be made, and an appropriate observational status should be ordered. Geriatric inpatient suicide risk assessment parallels adult risk assessment and includes such factors as history of attempts, active suicidal ideation with lethal plan, and psychosis. A study of mixed-age psychiatric inpatients who completed suicide highlighted the importance of implementing continuous one-to-one observation of the high-risk patient (as opposed to 15-minute checks) and targeting severe anxiety/agitation as a means of improving suicide risk assessment and intervention (Busch et al. 2003). The use of lithium for bipolar disorder patients and clozapine for patients with schizophrenia or schizoaffective disorder has been shown to decrease suicidality in mixed-age or young adult outpatient populations (Meltzer and Baldessarini 2003; Meltzer et al. 2003; Tondo et al. 2001) and may be a reasonable strategy for reducing chronic suicide risk.

Management of Aggressive Behaviors

Up to 30% of all elderly psychiatric inpatients manifest violent or assaultive behavior over a 3-day period, and these events significantly prolong hospital stay (Patel and Hope 1992). The presence of "organic mental disorders" predicts violence. Aggressive behaviors in this diagnostic group are also more likely to persist. Compared with younger psychiatric inpatients, fellow patients, as opposed to professional staff, are the more common assault victims of the elderly patient (Cooper and Mendonca 1991; Miller et al. 1993; Wystanski 2000). Evaluation and treatment algorithms for this diagnostic group were described earlier in the section "Neuropsychiatric and Behavioral Disturbances Associated With Dementia." The clinician should ascertain whether there is an underlying pattern to the aggressive outbursts (e.g., occurring at times of care or only with a specific staff member). Environmental interventions should always be tried first. If there is a specific syndrome present (psychosis, depression, or mania), appropriate psychotropic trials should be initiated. Acute management of an assaultive geriatric patient may require treatment with atypical antipsychotics and/or benzodiazepines. It is critical to note that in the elderly, dementia-related aggressive behaviors frequently respond to lower dosages of antipsychotics than violence associated with primary psychotic and mood disorders. Benzodiazepines are associated with a risk of falls and increased confusion. Agents such as lorazepam that lack primary hepatic metabolites are preferred.

Seclusion and Restraint

Avoidance of restraints is particularly important in the elderly, who are often frail and have significant medical comorbidities. Acute problematic behaviors in elderly patients with dementia often de-escalate through stimulation reduction and behavioral techniques such as distraction. Use of two- and four-point restraints should be rare. Devices such as geri-chairs, tabletops, vest restraints, and side rails are more common restraint types seen on geriatric inpatient units. Fall-prevention monitoring devices, such as chair and bed alarms, are not restraints. They alert staff when patients at increased risk of falls attempt to transfer independently.

Discharge Planning

Elderly psychiatric inpatients have more discharge needs than simple outpatient referral. Level of disability, social support, and degree of medical and psychiatric care needs should be evaluated on the first admission day. Caregivers have variable needs: educational, psychiatric, medical, psychosocial, and financial. The inpatient team should assess families' strengths and weaknesses and help them cope while respecting their preferences and autonomy. Bolstering their strengths has the potential to improve quality of life for both patients and caregivers and to delay institutionalization for elderly patients (Schulz et al. 2005). The psychiatric team needs to assess the patient's level of functioning and then link the patient and caregiver dyad to the appropriate services. Following an inpatient geropsychiatric stay, patients may benefit from a partial hospitalization program as an intermediate level of care to ensure further improvement or continued stabiliza-

tion and to prevent rehospitalization (Boyle 1997; Hoe et al. 2005). Alternatively, patients may return home with the appropriate home-based services or, at the other end of the spectrum, be admitted or returned to a long-term-care facility. Cost coverage restrictions imposed by Medicare or other programs, as well as changing eligibility criteria, are ever-present barriers to access to services. The community services network for seniors becomes increasingly complex, and inpatient practitioners must acquire basic information to educate patients, families, and other health professionals about the support services available in each specific community. Cultivating ongoing collaborations between the inpatient psychiatric team and facilities and community programs is crucial to ensuring continuity of care and effective transitions.

Conclusion

Assessment and treatment of geriatric psychiatry inpatients require specially trained multidisciplinary team members skilled in an integrative approach to patient care. Collateral information from families, caregivers, and clinicians and awareness of differential diagnostic issues, including the interplay between medical and psychiatric comorbidities, are essential. The clinician needs to be familiar with acute and continuation geriatric pharmacotherapy and psychotherapy treatment paradigms. Age-appropriate discharge planning with outpatient medical and psychiatric clinicians, family, and caregivers is critical.

References

Abrams RC, Bromberg CE: Personality disorders in the elderly: a flagging field of inquiry. Int J Geriatr Psychiatry 21:1013–1017, 2006

Alexopoulos GS: Clinical and biological findings in late-onset depression, in Psychiatry Update: The American Psychiatric Association Annual Review, Vol 9. Edited by Tasman A, Goldfinger SM, Kaufmann C. Washington, DC, American Psychiatric Press, 1990, pp 249–262

Alexopoulos GS: "The depression-executive dysfunction syndrome of late life": a specific target for D3 agonists? Am J Geriatr Psychiatry 9:22–29, 2001

Alexopoulos GS: Late-life mood disorders, in Comprehensive Textbook of Geriatric Psychiatry, 3rd Edition. Edited by Sadavoy J, Jarvik LF, Grossberg GT, et al. New York, WW Norton, 2004, pp 609–653

Alexopoulos GS, Meyers BS, Young RC, et al: The course of geriatric depression with "reversible dementia": a controlled study. Am J Psychiatry 150:1693–1699, 1993

Alexopoulos GS, Meyers BS, Young RC, et al: Clinically defined vascular depression. Am J Psychiatry 154:562–565, 1997a

Alexopoulos GS, Meyers BS, Young RC, et al: "Vascular depression" hypothesis. Arch Gen Psychiatry 54:915–922, 1997b

Alexopoulos GS, Bruce ML, Hull J, et al: Clinical determinants of suicidal ideation and behavior in geriatric depression. Arch Gen Psychiatry 56:1048–1053, 1999

Alexopoulos GS, Katz IR, Reynolds CF 3rd, et al: The Expert Consensus Guideline series: pharmacotherapy of depressive disorders in older patients. Postgrad Med Spec No Pharmacotherapy:1–86, 2001

Alexopoulos GS, Borson S, Cuthbert BN, et al: Assessment of late life depression. Biol Psychiatry 52:164–174, 2002a

Alexopoulos GS, Kiosses DN, Choi SJ, et al: Frontal white matter microstructure and treatment response of late-life depression: a preliminary study. Am J Psychiatry 159:1929–1932, 2002b

Alexopoulos GS, Kiosses DN, Klimstra S, et al: Clinical presentation of the "depression-executive dysfunction syndrome" of late life. Am J Geriatr Psychiatry 10:98–106, 2002c

Alexopoulos GS, Raue P, Arean P: Problem-solving therapy versus supportive therapy in geriatric major depression with executive dysfunction. Am J Geriatr Psychiatry 11:46–52, 2003

Alexopoulos GS, Streim J, Carpenter D, et al: Expert Consensus Panel for Using Antipsychotic Drugs in Older Patients: using antipsychotic agents in older patients. J Clin Psychiatry 65 (suppl):5–102, 2004

Alexopoulos GS, Jeste DV, Chung H, et al: The Expert Consensus Guideline series: treatment of dementia and its behavioral disturbances. Introduction: methods, commentary, and summary. Postgrad Med Spec No:6–22, 2005a

Alexopoulos GS, Kiosses DN, Heo M, et al: Executive dysfunction and the course of geriatric depression. Biol Psychiatry 58:204–210, 2005b

Almeida OP: The neuropsychology of schizophrenia in late life, in Late Onset Schizophrenia. Edited by Howard R, Rabins PV, Castle DJ. London, Routledge, 1999, pp 181–189

American Psychiatric Association: Practice guideline for the treatment of patients with delirium. Am J Psychiatry 156:1–20, 1999

American Psychiatric Association: Diagnostic and Statistical Manual of Mental Disorders, 4th Edition, Text Revision. Washington, DC, American Psychiatric Association, 2000

American Psychiatric Association: Practice Guideline for the Treatment of Patients With Bipolar Disorder. Washington, DC, American Psychiatric Publishing, 2002

Andreasen NC: I don't believe in late-onset schizophrenia, in Late-Onset Schizophrenia. Edited by Howard R, Rabins PV, Castle DJ. London, Routledge, 1999, pp 111–123

Andreescu C, Mulsant BH, Peasley-Miklus C, et al: Persisting low use of antipsychotics in the treatment of major depressive disorder with psychotic features. Study of Pharmacotherapy of Psychotic Depression (STOP-PD). J Clin Psychiatry 68:194–200, 2007

Arean PA, Cook BL: Psychotherapy and combined psychotherapy/pharmacotherapy for late life depression. Biol Psychiatry 52:293–303, 2002

Arean PA, Perri MG, Nezu AM, et al: Comparative effectiveness of social problem-solving therapy and reminiscence therapy as treatments for depression in older adults. J Consult Clin Psychol 61:1003–1010, 1993

Arias E, Anderson RN, Kung HC, et al: Deaths: final data for 2001. Natl Vital Stat Rep 52:1–115, 2003

Armstrong SC, Cozza KL, Watanabe KS: The misdiagnosis of delirium. Psychosomatics 38:433–439, 1997

Barker SB, Pandurangi AK, Best AM: Effects of animal-assisted therapy on patients' anxiety, fear, and depression before ECT. J ECT 19:38–44, 2003

Bartels SJ, Forester B, Miles KM, et al: Mental health service use by elderly patients with bipolar disorder and unipolar major depression. Am J Geriatr Psychiatry 8:160–166, 2000

Bartels SJ, Blow FC, Brockmann LM, et al: Substance Abuse and Mental Health Among Older Americans: The State of the Knowledge and Future Directions. Rockville, MA, Older American Substance Abuse and Mental Health Technical Assistance Center, 2005

Beier MT: Treatment strategies for the behavioral symptoms of Alzheimer's disease: focus on early pharmacological intervention. Pharmacotherapy 27:399–411, 2007

Blank K, Hixon L, Gruman C, et al: Determinants of geropsychiatric inpatient length of stay. Psychiatr Q 76:195–212, 2005

Blixen CE, McDougall GJ, Suen LJ: Dual diagnosis in elders discharged from a psychiatric hospital. Int J Geriatr Psychiatry 12:307–313, 1997

Borson S, Scanlan JM, Chen P, et al: The Mini-Cog as a screen for dementia: validation in a population-based sample. J Am Geriatr Soc 51:1451–1454, 2003

Borson S, Scanlan JM, Watanabe J, et al: Simplifying detection of cognitive impairment: comparison of the Mini-Cog and Mini-Mental State Examination in a multiethnic sample. J Am Geriatr Soc 53:871–874, 2005

Boyle DP: The effect of geriatric day treatment on a measure of depression. Clinical Gerontology 18:43–63, 1997

Boyle LL, Ismail MS, Porsteinsson AP: The dementia workup, in Principles and Practice of Geriatric Psychiatry. Edited by Agronin ME, Maletta GJ. Philadelphia, PA, Lippincott Williams & Wilkins, 2006, pp 137–152

Brown SL: Variations in utilization and cost of inpatient psychiatric services among adults in Maryland. Psychiatr Serv 52:841–843, 2001

Busch KA, Fawcett J, Jacobs DG: Clinical correlates of inpatient suicide. J Clin Psychiatry 64:14–19, 2003

Casey D, Grant RW: Cognitive therapy with depressed elderly inpatients, in Cognitive therapy With Inpatients: Developing a Cognitive Milieu. Edited by Wright JH, Thase ME, Beck AT, et al. New York, Guilford, 1993, pp 295–314

Cassidy F, Carroll BJ: Vascular risk factors in late onset mania. Psychol Med 32:359–362, 2002

Clauson KA, Marsh WA, Polen HH, et al: Clinical decision support tools: analysis of online drug information databases. BMC Med Inform Decis Mak 7:7, 2007

Cohen-Mansfield JJ: Nonpharmacological interventions for inappropriate behaviors in dementia: a review, summary, and critique. Am J Geriatr Psychiatry 9:361–381, 2001

Colenda CC, Mickus MA, Marcus SC, et al: Comparison of adult and geriatric psychiatric practice patterns: findings from the American Psychiatric Association's Practice Research Network. Am J Geriatr Psychiatry 10:609–617, 2002

Conwell Y, Duberstein PR, Caine ED: Risk factors for suicide in later life. Biol Psychiatry 52:193–204, 2002a

Conwell Y, Duberstein PR, Connor K, et al: Access to firearms and risk for suicide in middle-aged and older adults. Am J Geriatr Psychiatry 10:407–416, 2002b

Cooper AJ, Mendonca JD: A prospective study of patient assaults on nurses in a provincial psychiatric hospital in Canada. Acta Psychiatr Scand 84:163–166, 1991

Covinsky KE, Newcomer R, Fox P, et al: Patient and caregiver characteristics associated with depression in caregivers of patients with dementia. J Gen Intern Med 18:1006–1014, 2003

Cummings JL, Donohue JA, Brooks RL: The relationship between donepezil and behavioral disturbances in patients with Alzheimer's disease. Am J Geriatr Psychiatry 8:134–140, 2000

Cummings JL, Schneider L, Tariot PN, et al: Reduction of behavioral disturbances and caregiver distress by galantamine in patients with Alzheimer's disease. Am J Psychiatry 161:532–538, 2004

de Asis JM, Greenwald BS, Alexopoulos GS, et al: Frontal signal hyperintensities in mania in old age. Am J Geriatr Psychiatry 14:598–604, 2006

de Carle AJ, Kohn R: Risk factors for falling in a psychogeriatric unit. Int J Geriatr Psychiatry 16:762–767, 2001

Depp CA, Jeste DV: Bipolar disorder in older adults: a critical review. Bipolar Disord 6:343–367, 2004

Depp CA, Lindamer LA, Folsom DP, et al: Differences in clinical features and mental health service use in bipolar disorder across the lifespan. Am J Geriatr Psychiatry 13:290–298, 2005

Duman RS, Heninger GR, Nestler EJ: A molecular and cellular theory of depression. Arch Gen Psychiatry 54:597–606, 1997

Elderkin-Thompson V, Kumar A, Bilker WB, et al: Neuropsychological deficits among patients with late-onset minor and major depression. Arch Clin Neuropsychol 18:529–549, 2003

Emery O: Pseudodementia: A Theoretical and Empirical Discussion. Cleveland, OH, Western Reserve Geriatric Education Center, Case Western Reserve University School of Medicine, 1988

Erlangsen A, Zarit SH, Tu X, et al: Suicide among older psychiatric inpatients: an evidence-based study of a high-risk group. Am J Geriatr Psychiatry 14:734–741, 2006

Folks DG, Kinney FC: The medical psychiatry inpatient unit, in Principles and Practice of Geriatric Psychiatry, 2nd Edition. Edited by Copeland JRM, Abou-Saleh MT, Blazer DG. New York, Wiley, 2002, pp 709–712

Folstein MF, Folstein SE, McHugh PR: "Mini-Mental State": a practical method for grading the cognitive state of patients for the clinician. J Psychiatr Res 12:189–198, 1975

Frazer CJ, Christensen H, Griffiths KM: Effectiveness of treatments for depression in older people. Med J Aust 182:627–632, 2005

Gallagher DE, Thompson LW: Treatment of major depressive disorder in older adult outpatients with brief psychotherapies. Psychotherapy: Theory, Research, and Practice 19:482–490, 1982

Gallo JJ, Rabins PV: Depression without sadness: alternative presentations of depression in late life. Am Fam Physician 60:820–826, 1999

Ganzini L, Millar SB, Walsh JR: Drug-induced mania in the elderly. Drugs Aging 3:428–435, 1993

Gerdner LA: Music, art, and recreational therapies in the treatment of behavioral and psychological symptoms of dementia. Int Psychogeriatrics 12:359–366, 2005

Hoe J, Ashaye K, Orrell M: Don't seize the day hospital! Recent research on the effectiveness of day hospitals for older people with mental health problems. Int J Geriatr Psychiatry 20:694–698, 2005

Howard R, Rabins PV: Late paraphrenia revisited. Br J Psychiatry 171:406–408, 1997

Inouye SK, Bogardus ST, Charpentier PA, et al: A multicomponent intervention to prevent delirium in hospitalized older patients. N Engl J Med 340:669–676, 1999

Inventor BR, Henricks J, Rodman L, et al: The impact of medical issues in inpatient geriatric psychiatry. Issues Ment Health Nurs 26:23–46, 2005

Johnson JC, Kerse NM, Gottlieb G, et al: Prospective versus retrospective methods of identifying patients with delirium. J Am Geriatr Soc 40:316–319, 1992

Juby A, Tench S, Baker V: The value of clock drawing in identifying executive cognitive dysfunction in people with a normal Mini-Mental State Examination score. Can Med Assoc J 167:859–864, 2002

Juurlink DN, Mamdani MM, Kopp A, et al: The risk of suicide with selective serotonin reuptake inhibitors in the elderly. Am J Psychiatry 163:813–821, 2006

Kindermann SS, Kalayam B, Brown GG, et al: Executive functions and P300 latency in elderly depressed patients and control subjects. Am J Geriatr Psychiatry 8:57–65, 2000

Kiosses DN: Home-delivered problem solving therapy for depressed, cognitively impaired, disabled elders. Presented at the 20th Annual Meeting of the American Association for Geriatric Psychiatry, New Orleans, LA, March 1–4, 2007

Knopman DS, DeKosky ST, Cummings JL, et al: Practice parameter: diagnosis of dementia (an evidence-based review). Report of the Quality Standards Subcommittee of the American Academy of Neurology. Neurology 56:1143–1153, 2001

Kochanek KD, Sherry L, Murphy BS, et al: Deaths: final data for 2002. Natl Vital Stat Rep 53:1–116, 2004

Krauthammer C, Klerman GL: Secondary mania: manic syndromes associated with antecedent physical illness or drugs. Arch Gen Psychiatry 35:1333–1339, 1978

Krishnan KR, Hays JC, Blazer DG: MRI-defined vascular depression. Am J Psychiatry 154:497–501, 1997

Kunik ME, Mulsant BH, Rifai AH, et al: Diagnostic rate of comorbid personality disorder in elderly psychiatric inpatients. Am J Psychiatry 151:603–605, 1994

Lehmann SW, Rabins PV: Factors related to hospitalization in elderly manic patients with early and late-onset bipolar disorder. Int J Geriatr Psychiatry 21:1060–1064, 2006

Lockwood KA, Alexopoulos GS, van Gorp WG: Executive dysfunction in geriatric depression. Am J Psychiatry 159:1119–1126, 2002

Madhusoodanan S, Shah P, Brenner R, et al: Pharmacological treatment of the psychosis of Alzheimer's disease: what is the best approach? CNS Drugs 21:101–115, 2007

Mancall EL: Neurological assessment of the elderly psychiatric patient, in Principles and Practice of Geriatric Psychiatry. Edited by Agronin ME, Maletta GJ. Philadelphia, PA, Lippincott Williams & Wilkins, 2006, pp 77–91

Mattana J, Charitou M, Mills L, et al: Personal digital assistants: a review of their application in graduate medical education. Am J Med Qual 20:262–267, 2005

McCusker J, Cole M, Abrahamowicz M, et al: Delirium predicts 12-month mortality. Arch Intern Med 162:457–463, 2002

McDonald WM: Epidemiology, etiology, and treatment of geriatric mania. J Clin Psychiatry 61 (suppl):3–11, 2000

Meagher DJ, Norton JW, Trzepacz PT: Delirium in the elderly, in Principles and Practice of Geriatric Psychiatry. Edited by Agronin ME, Maletta GJ. Philadelphia, PA, Lippincott Williams & Wilkins, 2006, pp 332–348

Meltzer HY, Baldessarini RJ: Reducing the risk for suicide in schizophrenia and affective disorders. J Clin Psychiatry 64:1122–1129, 2003

Meltzer HY, Alphs L, Green AI, et al: Clozapine treatment for suicidality in schizophrenia: International Suicide Prevention Trial (InterSePT). Arch Gen Psychiatry 60:82–91, 2003

Meyers BS: Late-life delusional depression: acute and long-term treatment. Int Psychogeriatr 7:113–124, 1995

Meyers BS, Chester JG: Acute management of late-life depression, in Principles and Practice of Geriatric Psychiatry. Edited by Copeland JRM, Abou-Saleh MT, Blazer DG. New York, Wiley, 1994, pp 563–567

Miller MD, Reynolds CF 3rd: Expanding the usefulness of interpersonal psychotherapy (IPT) for depressed elders with co-morbid cognitive impairment. Int J Geriatr Psychiatry 22:101–105, 2007

Miller RJ, Zadolinnyj K, Hafner RJ: Profiles and predictors of assaultiveness for different psychiatric ward populations. Am J Psychiatry 150:1368–1373, 1993

Mulsant BH, Sweet RA, Rosen J, et al: A double-blind randomized comparison of nortriptyline plus perphenazine versus nortriptyline plus placebo in the treatment of psychotic depression in late life. J Clin Psychiatry 62:597–604, 2001

Nadler-Moodie M, Gold J: A geropsychiatric unit without walls. Issues Ment Health Nurs 26:101–114, 2005

Ngoh CT, Lewis ID, Connolly PM: Outcomes of inpatient geropsychiatric treatment: the value of assessment protocols. J Gerontol Nurs 31:12–18, 2005

Owens SJ, Qualls SH: Family involvement during a geropsychiatric hospitalization. J Clin Geropsychology 8:87–99, 2002

Parker SD, Will C, Burke CL: Activities for the Elderly: A Guide to Quality Programming, Vol 1. Ravensdale, WA, Idyll Arbor, 1999

Patel V, Hope RA: Aggressive behaviour in elderly psychiatric inpatients. Acta Psychiatr Scand 85:131–135, 1992

Pollock BG: Psychotropic drugs and the aging patient. Geriatrics 53 (suppl):S20–S24, 1998

Pollock BG, Mulsant BH, Rosen J, et al: Comparison of citalopram, perphenazine, and placebo for the acute treatment of psychosis and behavioral disturbances in hospitalized, demented patients. Am J Psychiatry 159:460–465, 2002

Potter GG, Kittinger JD, Wagner HR, et al: Prefrontal neuropsychological predictors of treatment remission in late-life depression. Neuropsychopharmacology 29:2266–2271, 2004

Rabins P, Blacker D, Bland W, et al: Practice guideline for the treatment of patients with Alzheimer's disease and other dementias of late life. Am J Psychiatry 154:1–39, 1997

Reynolds CF 3rd, Miller MD, Pasternak RE, et al: Treatment of bereavement-related major depressive episodes in later life: a controlled study of acute and continuation treatment with nortriptyline and interpersonal psychotherapy. Am J Psychiatry 156:202–208, 1999

Richards JB, Papaioannou A, Adachi JD, et al: Effect of selective serotonin reuptake inhibitors on the risk of fracture. Arch Intern Med 167:188–194, 2007

Rothschild AJ, Winer J, Flint AJ, et al: Missed diagnosis of psychotic depression at four academic medical centers. J Clin Psychiatry Apr 1:e1–e4 [Epub ahead of print], 2008

Rush AJ: STAR*D: what have we learned? Am J Psychiatry 164:201–204, 2007

Sajatovic M, Madhusoodanan S, Coconcea N: Managing bipolar disorder in the elderly: defining the role of the newer agents. Drugs Aging 22:39–54, 2005

Sanderson DR: Practical geriatrics: use of mood stabilizers by hospitalized geriatric patients with bipolar disorder. Psychiatr Serv 49:1145–1147, 1998

Schneider LS, Sloane RB, Staples FR, et al: Pretreatment orthostatic hypotension as a predictor of response to nortriptyline in geriatric depression. J Clin Psychopharmacol 6:172–176, 1986

Schneider LS, Dagerman KS, Insel P: Risk of death with atypical antipsychotic drug treatment for dementia: meta-analysis of randomized placebo-controlled trials. JAMA 294:1934–1943, 2005

Schneider LS, Tariot PN, Dagerman KS, et al: Effectiveness of atypical antipsychotic drugs in patients with Alzheimer's disease. N Engl J Med 355:1525–1538, 2006

Schulz R, Martire LM, Klinger JN: Evidence-based caregiver interventions in geriatric psychiatry. Psychiatr Clin North Am 28:1007–1038, 2005

Seitz DP, Gill SS, van Zyl LT: Antipsychotics in the treatment of delirium: a systematic review. J Clin Psychiatry 68:11–21, 2007

Shulman KI, Tohen M, Satlin A, et al: Mania compared with unipolar depression in old age. Am J Psychiatry 149:341–345, 1992

Simon GE, VonKorff M: Suicide mortality among patients treated for depression in an insured population. Am J Epidemiol 147:155–160, 1998

Sink KM, Holden KF, Yaffe K: Pharmacological treatment of neuropsychiatric symptoms of dementia: a review of the evidence. JAMA 293:596–608, 2005

Smith M, Specht J, Buckwalter KC: Geropsychiatric inpatient care: what is state of the art? Issues Ment Health Nurs 26:11–22, 2005

Staab JP, Evans DL: Efficacy of venlafaxine in geriatric depression. Depress Anxiety 12 (suppl):63–68, 2000

Tariot PN, Farlow MR, Grossberg GT, et al: Memantine treatment in patients with moderate to severe Alzheimer disease already receiving donepezil: a randomized controlled trial. JAMA 291:317–324, 2004

Teri L, Logsdon RG, Peskind E, et al: Treatment of agitation in AD: a randomized, placebo-controlled clinical trial. Neurology 55:1271–1278, 2000; Erratum in: Neurology 56:426, 2001

Tew JD Jr, Mulsant BH, Haskett RF, et al: Acute efficacy of ECT in the treatment of major depression in the old-old. Am J Psychiatry 156:1865–1870, 1999

Thase ME: Effects of venlafaxine on blood pressure: a meta-analysis of original data from 3744 depressed patients. J Clin Psychiatry 59:502–508, 1998

Thompson LW, Coon DW, Gallagher-Thompson D, et al: Comparison of desipramine and cognitive/behavioral therapy in the treatment of elderly outpatients with mild-to-moderate depression. Am J Geriatr Psychiatry 9:225–240, 2001

Thompson LW, Spira AP, Depp CA, et al: The geriatric caregiver, in Principles and Practice of Geriatric Psychiatry. Edited by Agronin ME, Maletta GJ. Philadelphia, PA, Lippincott Williams & Wilkins, 2006, pp 37–49

Thomson PDR: Physicians' Desk Reference. Montvale, NJ, Thomson PDR, 2007

Tinetti ME, Gordon C, Sogolow E, et al: Fall-risk evaluation and management: challenges in adopting geriatric care practices. Gerontologist 46:717–725, 2006

Tondo L, Hennen J, Baldessarini RJ: Lower suicide risk with long-term lithium treatment in major affective illness: a meta-analysis. Acta Psychiatr Scand 104:163–172, 2001

Trinh NH, Hoblyn J, Mohanty S, et al: Efficacy of cholinesterase inhibitors in the treatment of neuropsychiatric symptoms and functional impairment in Alzheimer disease: a meta-analysis. JAMA 289:210–216, 2003

U.S. Food and Drug Administration: FDA public advisory: deaths with antipsychotics in elderly patients with behavioral disturbances. Rockville, MD, U.S. Food and Drug Administration, 2005. Available at: http://www.fda.gov/cder/drug/advisory/antipsychotics.htm. Accessed April 27, 2007.

Van Gerpen MW, Johnson JE, Winstead DK: Mania in the geriatric patient population: a review of the literature. Am J Geriatr Psychiatry 7:188–202, 1999

Vergare MJ, Binder RL, Cook IA, et al: Practice guideline for the psychiatric evaluation of adults, in Practice Guidelines for the Treatment of Psychiatric Disorders: Compendium 2006. Washington, DC, American Psychiatric Association, 2006, pp 1–64

Wang PS, Schneeweiss S, Avorn J, et al: Risk of death in elderly users of conventional vs atypical antipsychotic medications. N Engl J Med 353:2335–2341, 2005

Weiner RD (ed): The Practice of Electroconvulsive Therapy: Recommendations for Treatment, Training, and Privileging, 2nd Edition. A Task Force Report of the American Psychiatric Association. Washington, DC, American Psychiatric Association, 2001

Weintraub D, Mazour I: Clinical and demographic changes over ten years on a psychogeriatric inpatient unit. Ann Clin Psychiatry 12:227–231, 2000

Woo BK, Rice VA, Legendre SA, et al: The clock drawing test as a measure of executive dysfunction in elderly depressed patients. J Geriatr Psychiatry Neurol 17:190–194, 2004

Wystanski MM: Assaultive behaviour in psychiatrically hospitalized elderly: a response to psychosocial stimulation and changes in pharmacotherapy. Int J Geriatr Psychiatry 15:582–585, 2000

Yazgan IC, Greenwald BS, Kremen NJ, et al: Geriatric psychiatry versus general psychiatry inpatient treatment of the elderly. Am J Psychiatry 161:352–355, 2004

Young J, Inouye SK: Delirium in older people. BMJ 334:842–846, 2007

Young RC, Gyulai L, Mulsant BH, et al: Pharmacotherapy of bipolar disorder in old age: review and recommendations. Am J Geriatr Psychiatry 12:342–357, 2004

Zisselman MH, Rovner BW, Shmuely Y, et al: A pet therapy intervention with geriatric psychiatry inpatients. Am J Occup Ther 50:47–51, 1996

Zubenko GS, Marino LJ Jr, Sweet RA, et al: Medical comorbidity in elderly psychiatric inpatients. Biol Psychiatry 41:724–736, 1997

CHAPTER 6

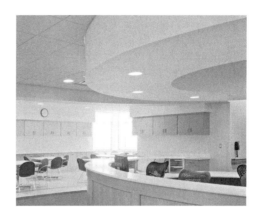

THE EATING DISORDERS UNIT

Harry A. Brandt, M.D.
Katherine A. Halmi, M.D.

The patient with a severe eating disorder poses a substantial challenge to even the highly experienced clinician. The confluence of significant medical compromise, substantial psychological complexity, and serious psychiatric illness comorbidity may necessitate intensive treatment on an inpatient eating disorder unit. Because of the high morbidity and mortality of these illnesses, patients cannot be subjected to randomized controlled studies to assess effectiveness of hospitalization; hence there are no clear evidence-based criteria for either hospitalization or discharge. Instead, on the basis of emerging clinical consensus, established practice guidelines, and several decades of clinical experience from two established eating disorder programs, this chapter provides an overview of inpatient eating disorders treatment and associated issues, as well as the indications for such treatment.

Indications for Hospitalization

Several guidelines have been proposed for determining whether a patient with an eating disorder requires in-

hospital care. The most compelling reasons for hospitalization center on the medical indications listed in Table 6–1. Many patients are hospitalized because of their inability to block the perpetuating core symptoms of their eating disorder, such as marked food restriction, excessive and compulsive exercise, or purging behavior, including self-induced vomiting or laxative abuse. Exacerbation of comorbid psychiatric illness also may be a factor in the decision to recommend intensive in-hospital care. For example, the presence of psychotic depression and/or suicidal ideation or of incapacitating obsessions and compulsions related or unrelated to the eating disorder may necessitate hospitalization. Another common factor in the decision to hospitalize a patient may be the repeated failure of the patient to respond to a well-structured outpatient regimen and/or the need for a highly structured environment to break a cycle of continued destructive symptomatology. Some patients with significant environmental psychosocial stressors coupled with inadequate social support systems may require use of a structured inpatient program to facilitate treatment.

89

TABLE 6–1.   Summary of indications for inpatient eating disorder unit

Significant weight loss—Generally less than 85% of healthy weight for age and height or rapid weight decline secondary to marked food restriction or refusal.

Medical status—

For adults: Heart rate < 40 bpm; blood pressure < 90/60 mm Hg; glucose < 60 mg/dL; potassium < 3mEq/L; electrolyte imbalance; temperature < 97.0°F; dehydration; hepatic, renal, or cardiovascular organ compromise requiring acute treatment; poorly controlled diabetes

For children and adolescents: Heart rate near 40 bpm; orthostatic blood pressure changes (> 20 bpm increase in heart rate or > 10–20 mm Hg drop); blood pressure < 80/50 mm Hg; hypokalemia; hypophosphatemia; or hypomagnesemia

Suicidality—Specific plan with high lethality or intent; admission may be indicated in patient with suicidal ideas or after a suicide attempt, depending on presence or absence of other factors modulating suicidal risk

Motivation—Very poor to poor motivation; patient preoccupied with intrusive repetitive thoughts; patient uncooperative with treatment or cooperative only in highly structured environment

Comorbidity—Any coexisting psychiatric disorder that would require hospitalization

Purging behavior (including laxatives and diuretics)—Needs supervision during and after all meals and in bathrooms; unable to control multiple daily episodes of purging that are severe, persistent, or disabling despite appropriate trials of outpatient care, even if routine laboratory test results reveal no obvious metabolic abnormalities

Environmental stress—Severe family conflict or problems or absence of family so patient is unable to receive structured treatment in home; patient lives alone without support system

Source.   American Psychiatric Association 2006.

Eating Disorder Subtypes and Comorbidity

The majority of eating disorder patients requiring inpatient hospitalization have anorexia nervosa. Those with the restricting type of anorexia nervosa usually have medical complications of dehydration, emaciation, and severe bradycardia. Their overall psychiatric comorbidity is considerably less than that of the binge-purge type of anorexia nervosa patient. Those with a restricting subtype may have a major depressive disorder, and about 15% will have an obsessive-compulsive disorder unrelated to eating behavior, with an additional 30% meeting criteria for a Cluster C anxious personality disorder (Braun et al. 1994). The binge-purge subtype of anorexia nervosa patient and those meeting bulimia nervosa will have a greater prevalence of major depressive disorder (up to 80% of patients), with 30%–50% meeting criteria for alcohol or substance abuse disorder and 30% having a diagnosis of a Cluster B impulsive-type personality disorder. The most prevalent diagnosis in the latter group is borderline personality disorder. For those patients who are bingeing and purging, regardless of whether they have anorexia nervosa or bulimia nervosa, there is the med-

ical problem of hypokalemic alkalosis (described later). Most bulimia nervosa patients can be handled in outpatient or day programs. They are hospitalized only when medical complications are present due to their purging behavior or when they are seriously depressed and suicidal. Patients with binge-eating disorder (BED) are rarely hospitalized because they do not have the medical complications associated with purging. BED patients are usually hospitalized if they are seriously depressed; they may also be hospitalized for a very brief period for the purpose of stopping the bingeing behavior in a highly restricted, controlled environment.

Financing the Cost of Hospitalization

In recent decades there have been major changes in the financing of health care. Previously, eating disorder hospitalizations were primarily covered by private insurance or unrestricted Medicaid. Today, health maintenance organizations and managed care companies overseeing private insurance and public funding have predominately replaced private insurance as the primary source of payment. Eating disorders are unique among psychiatric illnesses because they encompass both serious physical and psychological problems. Managed care companies often opt to treat the physical problems in general hospitals, which cannot cope with the psychological issues that interfere with the physical management. Refeeding severely emaciated anorexia nervosa patients can be time consuming and medically complicated, thus requiring expert and experienced medical and psychiatric staff for effective treatment.

There are serious problems concerning insurance coverage for eating disorder patients. For patients who are admitted at a very low body weight, the mental health inpatient benefit often is only 30 days (or fewer if the patient has used the benefit previously in a year). Studies have found that anorexia nervosa patients who left the hospital while still markedly underweight had a poor outcome and a high rate of relapse (Baran et al. 1995; Commerford et al. 1997; Halmi and Licinio 1989; Howard et al. 1999). Few managed care companies have staff who are knowledgeable about the intricacies of treating eating disorders, and thus they fail to approve ample lengths of stay to provide proper care (Kaye et al. 1996). For example, if anorectic patients are at 75% of ideal body weight or greater, they may be denied coverage even though they might have extreme anxiety about eating and be unable to ingest adequate calories outside of a structured supportive environment. Coverage may also be denied if patients are not suicidal, if they are not given medication, or if medications are not modified. Some insurance companies require intensive on-site family work and will not accept telephone sessions for those families in which distance and scheduling are serious legitimate problems. Bulimia nervosa patients who are incapacitated with bingeing and vomiting and need a period of response prevention in a structured setting are denied coverage either if they are not actively bingeing and purging on the unit or the minute their laboratory tests are within normal limits.

One study comparing eating disorder admissions to an inpatient unit in the 1980s with admissions in the 1990s found that the average length of stay decreased from 120 days to 23 days. During that time, the number of readmissions changed from less than 1% to close to 35% (Wiseman et al. 2001). Overall, this "frequent flyer" model of eating disorder treatment is unlikely to benefit either the patients or the economy.

General Principles

A cognitive-behavioral framework is useful for the overall ward milieu. Exposure and response prevention techniques can be used to prevent patients from purging and exercising. Patients may receive regular feedback about their weight every morning and deal with interpersonal conflicts in a group therapy format.

Group therapy can occur at frequent intervals in the hospital setting and cover a variety of topics. It is a useful format for psychoeducation in which the patients are informed about nutrition and medical complications as well as relapse prevention, assertiveness training, self-control strategies, maturing and autonomy issues, and limit-setting problems. Patients may be given homework assignments of cost–benefit analysis and self-monitoring. For example, the patients could keep a daily diary that includes all foods eaten; symptoms they have had before, during, and after meals; and other distressful symptoms. In a group format, patients can discuss their symptoms and have an increased awareness of their eating behavior, symptom triggers, and coping strategies.

Medical Management and Nutritional Rehabilitation

The medical management and nutritional rehabilitation of eating disorder patients are best accomplished in a specialized inpatient eating disorder setting that provides a team of individuals highly skilled in the multidisciplinary management of these patients. Medical management usually involves weight restoration, nutritional rehabilitation, rehydration, and correction of serum electrolytes. This requires daily monitoring of weight, food and calorie intake, and urine output, and in the patient who is vomiting, frequent assessment of serum electrolytes. Patients must be closely monitored for attempts to purge. Pediatricians and internists are often necessary to supervise the medical management of severely emaciated anorexia nervosa patients or eating disorder patients with specific medical problems. Careful nutritional rehabilitation with the prevention of purging can effectively initiate the correction of most medical problems.

Common Specific Medical Problems in Hospitalized Eating Disorder Patients

Severe Emaciation

When a patient is below 75% of the ideal body weight or has a body mass index (BMI) of 15 or less, that patient is usually regarded as severely emaciated. There are likely to be problems of bradycardia, hypotension, dehydration, and extreme weakness. Rapid, effective nutritional rehabilitation is the essential component of early treatment. Some programs have successfully utilized a strategy based on the primary use of a liquid formula in six equal feedings throughout the day. A liquid formula is efficiently digested and provides necessary fluid, electrolytes, and calories for the patient. Usually additional juices in the amount of one-half of the total daily amount of calories should be added. The total number of calories in these low-weight patients should begin with an intake of 30–40 kcal/kg/day and can be increased very gradually if there is no evidence of peripheral edema or heart failure. Most liquid formulas contain the necessary amounts of vitamins and minerals. One randomly assigned controlled treatment study in a Japanese inpatient setting (Okamoto et al. 2002) showed that a liquid formula given only in the early stages of hospitalization with activity restriction was more effective compared with a general food program with regard to both the amount and rate of increase in BMI measured at the end of hospitalization and 6 months after discharge. Other programs have alternatively advocated providing patients with actual food as early as possible, although some patients will require significant caloric intake to gain weight and will often need to use supplements as part of that intake. There is not clear consensus as to what constitutes "normal" eating, with variability in approaches to vegetarianism and red-meat avoidance. Serum hypophosphatemia may develop during refeeding, requiring phosphate supplements. Bed rest may be necessary, with escorted assisted walks and special observation for development of bedsores.

Cardiovascular and Peripheral Vascular Problems

Most anorexia nervosa patients have bradycardia, which slowly improves with nutritional rehabilitation. An electrocardiogram may reveal ST-T wave abnormalities or QT_c prolongation. Medications known to prolong QT_c intervals should be avoided and electrolyte abnormalities corrected.

Central Nervous System Problems

Anorexia nervosa patients severely ill enough to be hospitalized often have cognitive impairments and are perseverative over issues of food, body weight, and exercising. They are unable to concentrate and are irritable. This will improve with gradual nutritional rehabilitation.

Endocrine/Metabolic Abnormalities

Patients who are admitted because of uncontrolled purging will usually have hypokalemia, hypomagnesemia, hypophosphatemia, and occasionally hypoglycemia. These electrolyte abnormalities may require intravenous correction if severe; otherwise, they will revert to normal with liquid formula feedings. Thyroid and cortisol abnormalities will revert to normal with gradual nutritional rehabilitation. Some patients may have vitamin deficiencies, with low levels of folate, B_{12}, niacin, and thiamine. The liquid nutritional formula may contain sufficient vitamin amounts so that additional supplements may not be necessary.

Gastrointestinal Problems

Patients may complain of feeling bloated after ingesting a small amount. This may due to delayed gastric emptying and usually remits with gradual nutritional rehabilitation. Liver enzymes may be elevated during refeeding and serum amylase levels elevated in purging patients. Constipation is a common problem and may require stool softeners.

Hematological Abnormalities

Leukopenia with relative lymphocytosis is common in emaciated anorectic patients. This will improve with nutritional rehabilitation.

Nutritional Rehabilitation

As mentioned earlier, severely emaciated patients enter a nutritional rehabilitation phase with gradual increases in caloric intake. Nutritional rehabilitation should begin with an intake of 30–40 kcal/kg/day (approximately 1,000–1,600 kcal/day) and increase to a high of 70–100 kcal/kg/day after it is determined that the patient is tolerating the calorie load well. Adding vitamin and mineral supplements when the patients are on food is particularly useful to prevent serum hypophosphatemia and to facilitate adequate nutritional rehabilitation. After the initial nutritional rehabilitation phase, devising individual food plans with food served on trays for each patient is helpful in allowing the patient to have a cognitive recognition of the amount of food she or he is eating and the rate of weight gain. During nutritional rehabilitation, ideally there should be ongoing counseling and education provided by an experienced dietitian. These sessions focus on normalization of eating behavior, reduction of irrational fears about food, and provision of accurate nutritional information. Research has found that nutritional counseling has resulted in marked improvement in eating disorder symptoms and general psychopathology (Laessle et al. 1991).

Patients may eat together as a group around tables but must be supervised carefully by staff to be certain they are not hiding or discarding food. It is desirable for each patient to receive individual nutritional counseling as well as nutritional education in the form of group therapy. Before discharge from the inpatient unit, the patient should be given the opportunity to choose his or her own foods and practice at determining an intake program that will promote either the necessary continued weight gain or weight maintenance. Patients should receive nutritional counseling with devising meal plans to practice after they are discharged from the hospital. If a patient is discharged from the hospital unit with a BMI of 19 or greater, the chances of relapse are significantly less compared with those discharged with a BMI less than 19 (Commerford et al. 1997; Howard et al. 1999).

Physical Structure of an Eating Disorder Unit

To the extent possible, the design of the eating disorder unit should take into consideration the essential importance of sustained behavioral control and blockade of core eating disorder behaviors, including food restriction, compulsive exercise, and purging. Specific attention needs to be given to the dining room space plan such that patients can be directly monitored during meals, reducing opportunities for patients to hide food and avoid caloric intake. Additionally, day room areas should be planned to facilitate ongoing line-of-sight monitoring of patients by nursing staff. Some programs have successfully implemented use of closed-circuit television monitoring of patients to reduce the potential for surreptitious exercise. This strategy requires the informed consent and permission of the patient. The bathrooms on the eating disorder unit need to be locked to ensure patients cannot surreptitiously engage in purging behaviors. One program has successfully utilized electronic key-controlled flush switch on toilets so that patients may have privacy when in the bathroom but must wait for the nurse to check the content of the toilet before it is flushed. This allows for privacy and dignity while preventing destructive behavior.

Therapeutic Approaches During Refeeding and Blocking of Eating Disorder Behaviors

During essential refeeding and/or blockade of compulsive exercise, purging, and/or other core symptomatic behaviors, patients with eating disorders often describe profound psychic stress and anxiety. A number of therapeutic interventions, both pharmacological and psychotherapeutic, may be utilized on the eating disorder unit to provide support, reduce resistance, and facilitate mutative change.

Pharmacological Treatment

Medications may be useful adjuncts in the inpatient treatment of eating disorders. Cyproheptadine in high dosages (up to 24 mg/day) can facilitate weight gain in anorectic restrictors and also provide a mild antidepressant effect (Halmi et al. 1986). Although chlorpromazine was the first drug to treat anorexia nervosa, no double-blind, controlled studies are available to show the efficacy of this drug for inducing weight gain and reducing anxiety in anorectic patients. In open-trial observations, chlorpromazine seemed to be helpful in the severely obsessive-compulsive, agitated anorectic patient. It may be necessary to start at a low dosage of 10 mg three times a day and gradually increase the dosage while monitoring blood pressure. New-generation antipsychotics such as olanzapine have been shown in pilot studies to be useful for severely obsessive-compulsive and agitated anorectic patients (Powers et al. 2002). Tricyclic antidepressants and serotonin reuptake inhibitors are not effective and have undesirable side effects for emaciated anorectic patients (Kaye et al. 2001).

For bulimia nervosa patients who have been admitted due to out-of-control bingeing and purging, the medication approved by the U.S. Food and Drug Administration for treatment of bulimia nervosa is fluoxetine (Romano et al. 2002). The only other selective serotonin reuptake inhibitor studied in a randomized controlled trial and shown to be effective is sertraline (Milano et al. 2004). In patients who do not respond to these agents, topiramate may be helpful (Hoopes et al. 2003). However, because weight loss is a side effect of topiramate, it should be used only in patients at a high normal or overweight weight range. It is necessary to begin topiramate in very low dosages of 25 mg/day, gradually increasing the dosage to avoid adverse side effects such as paresthesias and cognitive word-finding difficulties.

Family Therapy

A clinical family analysis should be conducted on all adolescent patients who are living with their families. On the basis of this analysis, it can be decided what type of family therapy or counseling is advisable. Family therapy and counseling are definitely necessary for all children younger than 18 years (Eisler et al. 1997). The family counseling can begin during the hospitalization phase and continue through partial hospitalization and outpatient treatment. In some cases where family therapy is not possible, issues of family relationships can be addressed in individual therapy or in brief counseling sessions with immediate family members. Teleconferences are an available option for families outside the region. Family therapy often focuses on family psychoeducation, relapse prevention, and improvement of family dynamics. In addition, some programs have utilized multifamily psychoeducational support group meetings.

The randomized controlled studies of family therapy have been conducted with outpatients, usually after a hospitalization phase. At present, there are few empirical data to indicate which type of family therapy is best for a given family dealing with an eating disorder. The family therapy approach developed at the Maudsley Hospital for adolescents tasks parents with the responsibility for overseeing refeeding (Eisler et al. 2000). These authors found that counseling the parents separately from the child was more effective compared with conjoint family therapy in families in which the mother had high expressed emotion. Future family studies are needed to compare family therapies that do not have a parental-control-of-eating component with the Maudsley approach.

Inpatient Cognitive-Behavioral Therapy—Group and Individual

Cognitive-behavioral therapy (CBT) is a well-researched and proven method for the treatment of bulimia nervosa (Fairburn 2006). Although research on the effectiveness of CBT for the treatment of anorexia nervosa is much more limited, clinical evidence and data in support of its utility are emerging (Cooper and Fairburn 1984; Hall and Crisp 1987; Pike et al. 2003). Essentially, the cognitive-behavioral model for the treatment of eating disorders emphasizes the important role of both the cognitive (e.g., attitudes regarding the importance of weight, shape, and their control) and behavioral (e.g., dietary restriction, binge eating) factors that maintain the eating disorder and associated pathology. The treatment is presented in additive stages, with an initial emphasis on stabilization of symptoms and behavioral change. As treatment progresses, the behavioral coping strategies are supplemented with cognitive restructuring techniques, including work on interpersonal issues, body image, and affect regulation. The final stage of CBT concentrates on relapse prevention and maintenance planning.

Although the CBT treatment model was designed as an outpatient intervention, the treatment has been utilized in a variety of settings, including inpatient and partial hospital programs. In this regard, given the high level of symptom severity for patients entering an inpatient program, CBT stands out as one treatment model that is particularly well suited for this population (Bowers 1993). Thus, CBT emphasizes early behavior change in a structured and systematic way. Additionally, once the patient begins to stabilize and becomes more receptive to any form of psychotherapy (American Psychiatric Association 2006), the CBT focus shifts to address salient cognitive and emotional concerns while maintaining symptom control.

It is recommended that hospitalized patients receive intensive CBT in the milieu, in groups, and during individual psychotherapy. Therapists with highly specific training provide a variety of CBT-based group therapies including standard CBT for eating disorders, body image, skills training, self-esteem, and motivation to change. These groups are based on salient elements of the standard CBT treatment protocols (e.g., Fairburn et al. 1993). Each of these important elements of treatment is expanded (and modified for adolescents as compared with adults), creating separate and independent group therapies. The overall effect is that patients receive all elements of CBT, as supported in the literature, but in a more intensive dose. Additionally, other more specialized groups, such as CBT-based trauma groups, can be offered as appropriate.

Hospitalized patients also may benefit from intensive individual CBT in which they can focus in a more specific way on their particular problems and conflicts. In this regard, it is recommended that all patients work individually on stabilization of symptoms through coping skills training, problem solving, and cognitive restructuring around eating disorder beliefs and assumptions. For some patients, however, it may be necessary to expand beyond the standard CBT protocol to address, in a more intensive way, specific areas of concern such as body image, self-esteem, perfectionism, interpersonal difficulties, and emotion regulation (Fairburn 2006). Typically, the individual therapist will concentrate on one or two of these particular areas. The goal is to provide effective, focused, and individually specific therapy.

Examples of Other Eating Disorder Unit Group Approaches

Nutritional Education

Most inpatient units have utilized various nutritional group approaches to impinge on irrational core beliefs common to the eating disorder syndromes. Early in treatment, many patients have little sense of what constitutes "normal" eating and have common misunderstandings that limit food choice. These misunderstandings result in a dietary regimen that is unappealing but makes the patient feel "safe."

Patients often profess to have extensive understanding of human nutrition. However, this knowledge may be highly selective, derived from questionable sources such as popular magazines, and it is often extreme and/or incorrect (Abraham et al. 1981). Inpatient units generally utilize a variety of group nutritional approaches to provide meal planning, basic nutritional education, and family education. Some programs have implemented "therapeutic group meals" later in the course of treatment to provide patients an opportunity to assume greater responsibility for meal selection and consumption in a less structured setting.

Expressive Arts Therapies

Expressive arts therapies may be used as a clinical adjunct to traditional verbal therapies in some eating disorder programs to assist the patient's nutritional goals while he or she is learning appropriate means of tolerating and expressing feelings and reducing anxiety. The appropriate management of anxiety plays a significant role in aiding the patient during refeeding and blockade of eating disorder behavior. Art expression can improve the patient's regulation of body tension. Instead of relying on restricting, bingeing, purging, or other means of self-injury to cope with stress, the patient creates artwork as an alternative, channeling destructive impulses. Cognitive-behavioral principles in art therapy may be utilized to assist patients in both recognizing and challenging the presence of a body image distortion.

Movement Therapies

Some programs have utilized various forms of "movement therapy" groups to improve body tolerance through anxiety reduction and breathing techniques. Patients learn to identify emotions held in their body and to express these emotions through gentle movement. Patients also have the opportunity to learn the differences between obsessive movements for exercise and essential movement for daily activities during movement education groups. Anorexic patients on a rehabilitation protocol learn the direct impact of their high activity levels and frenetic movements on their bodies and body image. The movement therapist can assist these patients toward wellness using a holistic approach to body awareness.

Specific Complexities in Treating Hospitalized Eating Disorder Patients

Involuntary Admission

Involuntary admission may be necessary to manage a life-threatening emergency or a serious medical deterioration when the patient is unwilling to take any steps to cooperate in treatment. Nasal gastric tube feeding may be necessary for involuntary feeding and should be administered by experienced staff. Core goals should be set for the involuntary portion of the treatment, and the involuntary status should be terminated as soon as these goals are met. Both patients and families need to understand that involuntary admission represents management of a life-threatening emergency rather than treatment that would be provided as an ongoing eating disorder treatment program.

Only in extremely rare severe medical situations is total parenteral nutrition (TPN) a necessity. Such severe medical conditions may be severe congestive heart failure or renal failure. TPN is a very complicated procedure associated with infections and metabolic abnormalities and requires an experienced, competent staff with monitoring for the complications of refeeding. Follow-up studies have shown that involuntary admission and feeding do not have a detrimental influence on outcome (Russell 2001).

Core Eating Disorder Psychopathology

The major problem in treating anorexia nervosa patients is their resistance to treatment. These patients have little desire to give up their disorder. The disorder becomes ego-syntonic with strong psychological and most likely physiological reinforcement. The anorexia nervosa becomes a defense mechanism by which the patient can avoid dealing with environmental problems, usually of an interpersonal and developmental nature. To give up this routinized behavior is terrifying to most patients. For patients younger than 18 years, the parents can insist that they stay in a hospital treatment program for an adequate period of time. However, patients ages 18 years and older have the legal right to leave whenever they wish. This forces the treatment staff to proceed with commitment, which usually is not effective unless the patient is dangerously medically ill or suicidal.

Associated Psychiatric Comorbidities

Those patients who are bingeing and purging and require hospitalization often have a comorbid diagnosis of borderline personality disorder and are frequently engaging in substance and/or alcohol abuse. Addiction withdrawal is often better accomplished on a specialized unit with transfer to an eating disorder unit at a later date unless the medical complications of the eating disorder require concurrent management. A structured inpatient setting is usually an effective stabilizing environment for the borderline personality disorder. Dialectical behavior therapy groups are useful for managing emotional dysregulation in borderline bingeing and purging patients.

Discharge Planning From the Inpatient Treatment

The timing of discharge from an inpatient unit is a poorly researched area. However, there is some indication that patients who have reached a BMI of 19 are less likely to relapse (Howard et al. 1999). Currently the transition from a hospital setting to residential treatment, day hospital, or outpatient treatment often depends on available funding and insurance coverage. For patients who require a highly structured environment and 24-hour support but do not require medical intervention or frequent laboratory tests, a stepdown to residential treatment may be beneficial. Partial hospitalization or a day program may be a useful stepdown for patients who need supervision of some meals and a structured day program but are able to live with their families in a less structured environment. Intensive outpatient therapy such as three or four psychotherapy sessions a week may be more effective for patients who have a higher motivation to comply and follow through with techniques to prevent relapse.

Conclusion

Eating disorder patients pose a significant clinical challenge as a result of their complex and often deeply entrenched psychopathology and the presence of multiple medical and psychiatric comorbidities. Despite significant advances over the past decades in our understanding of these illnesses, as well as the refinement of treatment strategies, overall morbidity and mortality remain high. Due to unfortunate changes in health care funding and an overemphasis on providing outpatient care, many patients are not receiving adequate length of treatment in a structured, specialized environment. Based in the experience of two established eating disorders programs, we have summarized and provided the rationale for specific elements of treatment for eating disorders that we have found to be effective.

References

Abraham SF, Beumont PJV, Booth A, et al: Nutritional Knowledge Questionnaire, Part Two. Med J Aust 1(4):39, 1981

American Psychiatric Association: Practice Guidelines for the Treatment of Patients With Eating Disorders, 3rd Edition. Washington, DC, American Psychiatric Association, 2006

Baran S, Weltzin T, Kaye W: Low discharge weight and outcome in anorexia nervosa. Am J Psychiatry 152:1070–1072, 1995

Bowers WA: Cognitive therapy for eating disorders, in Cognitive Therapy With Inpatients: Developing a Cognitive Milieu. Edited by Wright JH, Thase ME, Beck AT, et al. New York, Guilford, 1993, pp 337–356

Braun DL, Sunday SR, Halmi KA: Psychiatric comorbidity in patients with eating disorders. Psychol Med 24:859–867, 1994

Commerford MC, Licinio J, Halmi KA: Guidelines for discharging eating disorder patients. Eat Disord 5:69–74, 1997

Cooper P, Fairburn C: Cognitive-behavioral treatment for anorexia nervosa: preliminary findings. J Psychosom Res 28:493–499, 1984

Eisler I, Dare C, Russell GFM, et al: Family and individual therapy in anorexia nervosa: a 5-year follow-up. Arch Gen Psychiatry 54:1025–1032, 1997

Eisler I, Dare C, Hodes M, et al: Family therapy for adolescent anorexia nervosa: the results of a controlled comparison of two family interventions. J Child Psychol Psychiatry 41:727–732, 2000

Fairburn C: Treatment of bulimia nervosa, in Annual Review of Eating Disorders, Part 2. Edited by Wonderlich S, Mitchell JE, de Zwaan M, et al. Oxford, England, Radcliffe, 2006, pp 144–156

Fairburn C, Marcus M, Wilson G: Cognitive-behavioral therapy for binge-eating and bulimia nervosa: a comprehensive treatment manual, in Binge-Eating: Nature, Assessment, and Treatment. Edited by Fairburn CG, Wilson GT. New York, Guilford, 1993, pp 361–404

Halmi K, Licinio E: Outcome: hospital program for eating disorders. CME Syllabus and Proceeding Summary, 142nd Annual Meeting of the American Psychiatric Association, Washington, DC, May 1989

Halmi KA, Eckert E, Ladu T, et al: Anorexia nervosa: treatment efficacy of cyproheptadine and amitriptyline. Arch Gen Psychiatry 43:177–181, 1986

Hall A, Crisp A: Brief psychotherapy in the treatment of anorexia nervosa: outcome at one year. Br J Psychiatry 151:185–191, 1987

Hoopes SP, Reinherr FW, Hedges DW, et al: Treatment of bulimia nervosa with topiramate in a randomized, double-blind, placebo-controlled trial. J Clin Psychiatry 64:1335–1341, 2003

Howard W, Evans K, Quintero-Howard C, et al: Predictors of success or failure of transition to day hospital treatment for inpatients with anorexia nervosa. Am J Psychiatry 1156:1697–1702, 1999

Kaye W, Kaplan A, Zucker M: Treating eating disorder patients in a managed care environment. Psychiatr Clin North Am 19:793–810, 1996

Kaye W, Nagata T, Weltzin T, et al: Double-blind placebo controlled administration of fluoxetine in restricting and restricting-purging type anorexia nervosa. Biol Psychiatry 49:644–652, 2001

Laessle RG, Beumont PJV, Butow P, et al: A comparison of nutritional management and stress management in the treatment of bulimia nervosa. Br J Psychiatry 159:250–261, 1991

Milano W, Petrella C, Sabatino C, et al: Treatment of bulimia nervosa with sertraline: a randomized controlled trial. Adv Ther 21:232–237, 2004

Okamoto A, Yamashita T, Nagoshi Y: A behavior therapy program combined with liquid nutrition designed for anorexia nervosa. Psychiatry Clin Neurosci 56:515–522, 2002

Pike KM, Walsh BT, Vitousek K, et al: Cognitive behavior therapy in the posthospitalization treatment of anorexia nervosa. Am J Psychiatry 160:2046–2049, 2003

Powers PS, Santana CA, Bannon YS: Olanzapine in the treatment of anorexia nervosa: an open label trial. Int J Eat Disord 32:146–154, 2002

Romano SJ, Halmi KA, Sarkar NP, et al: A placebo controlled study of fluoxetine in continued treatment of bulimia nervosa after successful acute fluoxetine treatment. Am J Psychiatry 159:96–102, 2002

Russell GFM: Involuntary treatment in anorexia nervosa. Psychiatr Clin North Am 24:337–349, 2001

Wiseman CV, Sunday SR, Klapper F, et al: Changing patterns of hospitalization in eating disorder patients. Int J Eat Disord 30:69–74, 2001

APPENDIX 1

Example of an Eating Disorder Unit Milieu Manual for Patients

Introduction to the Unit

The patients are informed that because their eating disorder has rendered them seriously psychiatrically and medically ill, the unit is highly structured and patients are closely monitored 24 hours a day. The main goals of treatment are 1) medical stabilization, 2) weight gain for underweight patients, and 3) interruption of eating disorder thoughts and behaviors for anorectic and bulimic patients. Length of treatment is determined on an individual basis according to a patient's needs. All personnel have had extensive experience in treating eating disorder patients and provide a very intensive treatment program. Family therapy sessions are necessary weekly for all adolescent patients, and when appropriate, spouses and families of adult patients also may have weekly family therapy sessions. All families participate in a weekly supportive family group therapy.

Eating Disorder Rules

On admission your doctor will decide what diet will be ordered for you. If you are severely underweight, you will be given a dietary supplement in the form of a liquid formula. You will be given this supplement six times a day along with juice until your doctor determines you are medically stable. Part of your medical workup will include evaluation of electrolytes and complete blood count weekly, or more often if needed. Once you are medically stable, your doctor will discuss progressing to solid food. Our nutritionist will meet with you to devise a food plan that is in agreement with your medical needs or religious preferences. We cannot accommodate vegan diets, but we will implement vegetarian diets.

The dining room is open for meals at the following times: 8:00–8:30 A.M. for breakfast, 12 noon–12:30 P.M. for lunch, 5:00–5:30 P.M. for dinner, and 8:00–8:30 P.M. for snacks. Supplemental snack times are 10:00–10:30 A.M., 2:30–3:00 P.M., and 8:00–8:30 P.M.

No food is allowed out of the dining room, and no food may be brought onto the unit by patients and visitors. After meals, patients may sit in the den area for 1 hour under staff supervision.

Bathroom Regulations

For medical reasons some patients may require closer observation when going to the bathroom. All efforts will be made to ensure privacy. Bathroom protocol is as follows:

- Supervised bathroom—staff monitors and records all output. The patient is given a commode in which to void to accurately measure urine output.
- Open bathroom—the patient may go to the bathroom without staff supervision. Bathroom times are posted on the unit. Bathrooms are locked after meals. Patients may use the bathroom if there is an urgent need by asking nursing staff.

For medical reasons patients may require closer supervision when showering. Shower protocol is as follows:

- Supervised showers—staff members of same sex observe patients showering.
- Unsupervised showers—patients shower unsupervised.

Weights

All patients are weighed every morning after voiding and before showering. Patients are weighed in a hospital gown. No jewelry is to be worn.

Purging

Purging is not tolerated on the unit. If vomit is found on the unit, a community meeting will be held to discuss the matter. The nursing staff also will meet privately with the individual involved.

Exercise

Exercising is not permitted on the unit. Staff monitor all patient areas and rooms at various intervals to monitor for this behavior.

Room Searches

Patients' rooms may be searched at staff discretion at any time. Regular searches take place to maintain unit safety for all patients. Patients will be informed prior to room search and may be present.

Groups

All patients are expected to attend and participate in all groups prescribed. The unit schedule for groups is posted on the unit bulletin board.

Schooling

Parents are expected to collaborate with the assigned social worker to arrange for supplemental education for adolescents on the unit. Individual tutoring is also available through creative tutoring.

Off-Unit Therapeutic Activities

Off-unit therapeutic activities may be requested through the treatment team.

Requests

Requests for privileges should be discussed with your therapist. Each morning, in rounds, changes in privilege are considered. Your therapist will inform you of the decision of the treatment team regarding your request at the conclusion of morning rounds. Rounds take place 9:00–10:30 A.M., Monday through Friday.

Smoking

This is a no-smoking hospital. Patients with medical clearance and courtyard privileges will be taken out to smoke four times daily. Patients are permitted one cigarette per smoke break and will receive a total of four cigarettes daily. Patients require medical clearance prior to smoking. Patients must be 18 years or older to smoke.

Bedrooms

Patients may not enter another's bedroom. No paper cups, paper towels, or napkins should be kept in rooms. All rooms must be kept tidy, and staff members will check each room daily.

Curfews

Adolescents 17 and under must be in bed by 10:00 P.M. Sunday through Thursday and by 11:00 P.M. Friday through Saturday. Adults must be in bed by 11:00 P.M. Sunday through Thursday and by 12 midnight Friday and Saturday.

Dress

Patients should be appropriately dressed. No tight clothing, sleeveless shirts, shorts, or short skirts. Leggings are to be worn with long shirts. No borrowing or lending of clothes. Undergarments, shoes, and socks must be worn at all times. No bare feet.

Visiting Hours

Visiting hours are Monday through Friday, 4:00–4:45 P.M. and 7:00–8:00 P.M.; and Saturday, Sunday, and holidays, 2:30–4:45 P.M. and 7:00–8:00 P.M. Visiting hours may be restricted for some patients. Visiting hours for each patient will be discussed with the patient by the therapist. All visitors must sign the visitors' book upon arrival. Each family may visit once a day for a maximum of 1 hour. Families may visit for a maximum of 2 hours on weekends. We highly recommend that families limit their visiting to two times per week.

Guidelines for Family Visits

Family visits are important to patients. However, because this in an acute care unit, visits must be closely monitored. Therefore please help us by adhering to the following guidelines:

- We ask that there be no more than two visitors per patient at any given time during visiting hours.
- We ask that no food, beverages, gum, laxatives, or medication be brought to patients.
- Please be aware that bathroom facilities and unit telephones are for patient use only.
- We ask that visitors refrain from bringing personal food or beverages onto the unit.
- Please help us by not entering the nurses' station.
- We will remind visitors that inappropriate personal physical conduct is not part of hospital protocol.
- Please do not include other patients or families in your visit.
- Visitors who give patients contraband items may be restricted from further visits.
- The staff might interrupt the visit if the visit appears disruptive.
- Visitors must leave the immediate area when there is a psychiatric emergency.

Family Group Meetings

The family group meets weekly on Thursday evening from 5:00 to 6:00 P.M. The purposes of the group are

- To provide a forum for parents and spouses to talk together and offer support and understanding to one another and to discuss similarities and differences in their individual and family experiences with an eating disorder.
- To understand family members' questions about psychological medical aspects of anorexia nervosa and bulimia nervosa as well as to provide education about the nature and treatment of psychiatric illness.
- To increase family members' awareness and understanding of their feelings and reactions to the patient's illness as well as the nature of the patient's experience in living with an eating disorder.
- To provide support to family members and to reduce feelings of isolation and discouragement that

they may have in struggling to cope with the patient's illness and its impact on the family.

Group attendance is highly recommended for all families. Participants must respect the confidentiality of patients and families by refraining from informing the patient and their own family of comments made by parents or spouses of other patients.

General Dining Room Rules

1. Everyone must stay in the dining room for 30 minutes for breakfast, lunch, and dinner.
   a. The radio can be on at all times, playing light, soothing music at a low volume.
   b. Patients must clean up after themselves.
   c. There are to be no comments made about food, calories, weight, or body image.
   d. All patients must record their intake with a staff member.
   e. At 30 minutes, all patients, whether finished or not, have to stop and record.
2. Patients on liquid formula sit at one table.
   a. Full glass of liquid formula must be poured.
   b. No switching or passing of liquid formula between patients.
   c. No putting of fingers inside supplement containers.
3. Patients on food trays sit at one table.
   a. Nothing is to be thrown away from the tray.
   b. When finished (and intake recorded), put tray on special shelf.
   c. Extra fluids: 1 cup of either coffee, water, cocoa, or juice once all liquids and half of each food item on the tray are completed.
4. Free foods
   a. Patients eat at one table and serve themselves.
5. After meals everyone must sit in the den area for 1 hour.
   a. Discussions about food and calories are prohibited in the dining room.

APPENDIX II

Example of an Eating Disorder Unit Schedule and Daily Activities

6:00–7:00 A.M.: Patients escorted to the bathroom and weights obtained

7:30–8:00 A.M.: Vital signs measured on all patients

8:00–8:30 A.M.: Breakfast

8:30–9:30 A.M.: Time in the den room, and some group therapies

9:30–10:00 A.M.: Bathroom escorts and courtyard privileges

10:00–10:30 A.M.: Snack time

10:30 A.M.–12 noon: Patients meet with a treatment team member. On some days between 11:00 and 11:45 A.M., there are yoga classes or crafts, and on Monday there is a community meeting. On other days there is an Alcoholics Anonymous meeting and a poetry writing workshop.

11:45 A.M.–12:30 P.M.: Bathroom escorts and lunch

12:45–1:30 P.M.: Cognitive-behavioral group therapy focused on processing issues related to eating behavior and typical eating disorder obsessions and rituals. On some days there are other groups, such as a dialectical behavior therapy group, a news and views group, and a creative arts group.

1:30–2:00 P.M.: Courtyard privileges

2:00–2:30 P.M.: Various groups, including assertiveness and nutritional education groups

2:30–3:00 P.M.: Snack time

3:00–3:45 P.M.: Group therapy, including task groups, leisure planning and stress management groups, and body image group

4:00–4:45 P.M.: Bathroom escorts and visiting hours

5:00–5:30 P.M.: Dinner

5:30–6:30 P.M.: Supervised individual time

7:00–8:00 P.M.: Visiting hours, followed by snack periods and then supervised individual time

CHAPTER 7

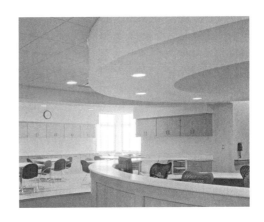

THE TRAUMA DISORDERS UNIT

Richard J. Loewenstein, M.D.
Susan B. Wait, M.D.

Inpatient psychiatric units specializing in treating patients with a history of psychological trauma generally are organized to serve one of two populations: predominantly male active-duty soldiers or veterans with combat-related trauma or predominantly female civilians with trauma related to severe childhood maltreatment (Busuttil 2006). Despite the evidence that posttraumatic stress disorder (PTSD) and dissociative disorders are common in the general population (Kessler 2000; Waller and Ross 1997) and a history of childhood trauma is common in general inpatient psychiatric patients (Loewenstein and Putnam 2004), only a handful of specialized trauma units exist nationwide. Successful inpatient hospital treatment models exist that can help these patients sustain substantial recovery. Hopefully, knowledge from the trauma disorders unit (TDU) can be made more generally available so that these patients receive more appropriate and helpful treatment in all inpatient settings.

This chapter describes the characteristics of an inpatient TDU, specifically the TDU at Sheppard Pratt Health System in Baltimore, Maryland. Sheppard Pratt opened its "Dissociative Disorders Unit" in 1992 to specialize in the inpatient treatment of severe dissociative disorders, primarily dissociative identity disorder (DID) and related severe posttraumatic dissociative psychopathologies. In 1997, the program was renamed the "Trauma Disorders Program" to reflect the clinical reality that we were serving a broader spectrum of patients and to reflect our understanding of the dissociative disorders as part of a broader spectrum of trauma-related disorders (Davidson and Foa 1993; Loewenstein and Putnam 2004).

Excluding patients ultimately diagnosed with non–trauma spectrum disorders (e.g., psychotic disorders, factitious disorders), virtually all TDU patients fit criteria for complex PTSD (Courtois 2004; van der Kolk et al. 1996). Complex PTSD includes a range of disrupted functions beyond the core symptoms of PTSD and is found in survivors of repeated, sustained traumatic experiences occurring over long periods of time and/or multiple developmental periods (Courtois 2004; Putnam 1997). Complex PTSD symptoms include difficulties regulating mood, anxiety, and anger, resulting in severe affective dysregulation; problems regulating state stability and consciousness; difficulties with sense of self and body image, resulting in identity problems, eating disorders, lack of attention to medical needs, and somatization; difficulties in forming stable relationships, with intense mistrust coexisting with vulnerability to victimization and exploitation; deformations in self-attribution and systems of meaning, with the world seen as dangerous and traumatizing and the self seen as damaged, shameful, defective, and responsible for traumatization; and a significant propensity for self-destructiveness, including suicide attempts, substance abuse, self-injury, and risk-taking behaviors (Arnow 2004).

Admission Criteria

Admissions to the TDU must be referred by a treating mental health professional. The admissions coordinator reviews an extensive questionnaire submitted by the referring clinician and discusses the prospective patient with the clinician. Then all potential admissions are reviewed with an attending psychiatrist for suitability for TDU admission, including medical necessity criteria for inpatient level of care. Currently, the TDU accepts both male and female patients, ages 18–65, with a history of psychological trauma. Male patients are screened carefully for their ability to manage in, and not be disruptive to, a mostly female hospital milieu. Given the realities of modern hospital reimbursement, most admissions must meet inpatient "medical necessity" criteria: imminent dangerousness to self or others and/or catastrophic inability to function due to disabling posttraumatic and/or dissociative symptoms.

Because patients must be motivated to participate actively in a demanding treatment program, we generally do not accept involuntary patients or patients referred for court-ordered treatment. Trauma patients with extensive histories of perpetrating childhood abuse, violence toward others, or sexual assaults or with significant antisocial personality features usually are excluded due to their potential negative impact on the TDU milieu and the difficulty in treating these problems in a milieu focused on recovery for abuse survivors. Not uncommonly, however, previously unknown histories of perpetrating child abuse or violence are revealed during TDU hospitalization.

Patients admitted to the TDU must be medically stable. Psychotic and/or manic patients are excluded because of potential disruption to the TDU milieu and difficulty participating in the treatment program. It has been our experience that patients with severe sub-stance and/or alcohol abuse or dependence usually do not respond to the treatment milieu of the TDU until they have achieved sobriety and are motivated to maintain recovery. This is the case even if the substance dependence appears to be "treating" the patient's trauma disorder symptoms. Less severe forms of substance abuse, relapse by a trauma patient in active recovery, and/or recent increase in substance use to medicate trauma symptom exacerbations or distress due to acute life stress may be more treatable in a specialized trauma milieu. Similarly, because we do not have the resources to provide intensive specialized eating disorders treatment during a TDU stay, trauma patients with histories of eating disorders can be admitted only when sufficiently stabilized to manage their eating disorder symptoms.

Diagnostic Workup

TDU patients often present with complex diagnostic issues. Commonly, these include questions about the presence of a dissociative disorder, an intercurrent psychotic process, depression, bipolar disorder, comorbid cognitive disorder, factitious disorder, or personality disorder and the extent to which the clinical picture is influenced by these possible concurrent diagnoses. We also assess psychological factors that affect the patient's ability to undertake psychotherapy for severe trauma-related disorders, such as the ability to form a therapeutic alliance despite severe posttraumatic mistrust and specific transference themes that may occur in therapy. Differential diagnosis is important; DID patients average 6–12 years of psychiatric treatment before correct diagnosis (Loewenstein and Putnam 2004).

On admission, all patients undergo a complete psychiatric history, social and family history, trauma history (to the extent that the patient can tolerate disclosing it on initial interview), physical examination, and basic laboratory evaluation (complete blood count, comprehensive metabolic panel, and thyroid function tests; screenings for drugs of abuse and alcohol, syphilis, and therapeutic drug levels are obtained when indicated). Patients are routinely screened using the office mental status examination for complex dissociative symptoms, which includes assessment of dissociative, mood, somatoform, and PTSD symptoms (Loewenstein 1991).

Specific diagnostic assessment measures that we routinely use for the assessment of dissociative disorders include the Dissociative Experiences Scale (Bernstein and Putnam 1986), the Multiaxial Inventory of Dissociation (Dell 2006), and the Structured Clinical Interview for DSM-IV Dissociative Disorders (Briere et al. 1995; Steinberg 1994). For assessment of PTSD and more general trauma-related issues, we commonly administer the Trauma Symptom Inventory (Briere et al. 1995). More specific diagnostic instruments for PTSD rarely are required because most patients present with obvious PTSD symptoms on clinical evaluation.

More complete psychological assessment, by psychologists familiar with dissociation and trauma, may be needed to fully assess complex differential diagnostic questions. This may include the Wechsler Adult Intelligence Scale, the Minnesota Multiphasic Personality Inventory, the Thematic Apperception Test, neuropsychology screening, and the Rorschach.

Reliability of Traumatic Memories

There is a debate about the reliability of memories of trauma, especially those that reportedly have been subject to lack of recall at some point in the patient's history. This is a complex topic, and the reader is referred to definitive reviews such as those of Brown et al. (1998) and Dalenberg (2006). In short, the current evidence supports the position that recall of trauma memory, like that of all autobiographical memory, is reconstructive, not photographic. Delayed recall for traumatic experiences has not been shown to produce memories that are any more or any less accurate than "continuous" memories. Either kind may be essentially accurate, a mixture of accuracy and confabulation, or entirely confabulated (Dalenberg 2006). Patients are also informed that memories recalled under hypnotic conditions should not be deemed any more or less accurate than memories recalled in their usual behavioral state (Cardena et al. 2000).

In general, TDU staff do not endorse belief or disbelief in any particular uncorroborated memory reported by a patient. Patients and, when indicated, families are educated about the complexity of human memory and the controversies in the field about trauma memory. Patients who report severe childhood trauma sometimes are ambivalent about their own recall, often believing themselves at some times and not at others. It is far more important for the clinician to identify conflicts the patient has about his or her own recall than to validate or discount a patient's memories. We tell patients that rather than offering belief or disbelief, we will do our best to help them begin the process of understanding and integrating memory material. The goal is to allow the patient him- or herself

to resolve questions about what did or did not occur as fully as possible over the course of long-term trauma treatment.

Therapies

Psychotherapy

A variety of studies have shown efficacy of psychotherapy for PTSD and DID (Foa et al. 2000; Loewenstein and Putnam 2004). Evidence-based models support the use of psychodynamic, cognitive-behavioral, hypnotherapeutic, and progressive exposure therapies, among others. Studies of inpatient TDU treatment for DID generally have shown robust improvement using a trauma-/dissociation-focused treatment paradigm (Eliason and Ross 1997).

STAGE-ORIENTED TREATMENT

Expert consensus, buttressed by a variety of evidence-based treatment models, strongly supports the notion of a phasic treatment structure for trauma patients (Brown et al. 1998; Foa et al. 2000). Although a number of models have been proposed, most authorities support the utility of a three-phase treatment structure (American Psychiatric Association 2004; International Society for the Study of Dissociation 2005). In the first phase, the patient works toward basic safety and stability. In the second, the focus is on the detailed and emotionally intense recollection and processing of trauma memories. In the third phase, the therapeutic work is directed toward "reintegration" and living well in the present. In this phase, traumas are relegated more and more to the status of "bad memories" rather than being "relived" as flashbacks, behavioral reexperiencing phenomena, or intense posttraumatic reactivity to current situations. For the DID patient, a major focus in the third phase may be fusion/integration of self states. Finally, the entirety of trauma treatment is directed toward the patient developing a better adaptation to current life.

Contemporary trauma programs generally opt for an inpatient TDU stay focused on developing safety and stability to permit better engagement in outpatient treatment. However, some patients are so mistrustful and demoralized that it may take several weeks for them to develop even a beginning sense of confidence that the TDU can help them. Sadly, at this point, these patients may become just "safe enough" to be discharged due to managed care limitations. This can result in the patient leaving the hospital before having internalized a sense of safety in treatment. Along with ongoing outside stress, this situation may precipitate repeated brief admissions that undermine definitive stabilization even more. Many patients referred to our program are so demoralized, and have such limited ability to manage their symptoms, that hospitalizations of 1–3 months are optimal to help them definitively stabilize and return to productive outpatient treatment.

TRAUMA FOCUS

Our treatment approach begins with a trauma focus toward the patient's difficulties. This involves a mixture of psychodynamic and cognitive therapy models. We attempt to understand the patient's problems as logically related to posttraumatic reactivity; trauma-based cognitive distortions, projections, and projective identifications; and traumatic transference to the staff, other patients, and the hospital environment (Loewenstein 1993). The patient is invited to understand his or her reactions as potentially "triggered" by posttraumatic reminders that set off intense reactivity, often in the form of "unconscious flashbacks" or "emotional flashbacks" (Blank 1985; Loewenstein 2006). This reactivity often leads to self-destructive behavior, maladaptive interactions with others, and emotional dysregulation, usually accompanied by marked cognitive distortions about what is occurring. Remarkably, through powerful projective identifications, others may be drawn into interactions with the patient that seemingly replay reported traumatic situations from the past—"walking into the flashback together," as one patient put it.

Elucidating the traumatic scenario that is being replayed allows the patient to begin to "separate past from present." The patient examines the extent to which current problems, maladaptive behaviors, troubled relationships, inexplicably intense emotional reactivity, and/or self-destructive behaviors result from unconscious "reliving" of past trauma scenarios or attempts at self-protection from anticipated traumas and betrayals based on past traumatic relationships. This task is fundamental to beginning successful treatment for this population. Remarkably, in many of these patients, this approach can ameliorate seemingly intractable problems and maladaptations relatively quickly (Loewenstein 2006). Patients are relieved to understand that behaviors experienced only as "crazy" or "bad" are logically related to past events. Unit staff feel more effective both by understanding better why patients act as they do and by helping to develop specific interventions based on this understanding.

SAFETY FOCUS

Within the overarching trauma framework, establishing safety is usually the central task for the inpatient TDU patient. TDU patients commonly are deeply involved in a plethora of suicidal, parasuicidal, or high-risk behaviors, some of which only become apparent with sequential observation and intensive history taking. Many of these behaviors will be reported to have begun in childhood or adolescence. Frequently, admission has been precipitated by escalation in suicidal or parasuicidal behaviors. Also, these patients may make suicide attempts in the hospital by any means that they find available, commonly strangulation, ingestions, and severe self-cutting.

In addition, most of these patients engage in self-injury that is not suicidal in intent, such as cutting, scratching, and burning, often over extensive parts of the body, including the genital area. Other common self-damaging behaviors include head banging; hitting objects, resulting in orthopedic injuries to the extremities; and nonlethal overdosing, among others. Because patients commonly use these behaviors in an attempt to manage their symptoms, treating these behaviors is one of the central tasks of treatment during hospitalization so that the patients can return to a less restrictive level of care.

Our primary approach to suicidal and self-harming behaviors is to reframe them as attempts at self-regulation and/or management of trauma experiences and related affects and cognitions. Attempts at controlling these behaviors without reframing them in this way are almost invariably doomed to failure, because they reinforce the patient's negative self-assessments. For example, among the manifold cognitive distortions that may drive self-injury is the idea that "I'm going to get hurt anyway, so if I control the timing and intensity of harm, it's less bad. If they [the perpetrators] see that I hurt myself, maybe they won't hurt me as much." These ideas can be reframed as an attempt to survive the helplessness and unpredictability of repeated maltreatment. They also underscore a core belief of many complex PTSD patients: that maltreatment is inevitable, and all one can hope to control is the timing and intensity of it. The therapeutic goal then becomes to exchange this "survival skill" for a "recovery skill" by developing adult non-trauma-based strategies for assessing one's current life situation and level of external danger; gaining a repertoire of skills to keep oneself safe from self and others; and creating overall safety and self-protection in one's current life.

Despite our prescreening, some patients have significant current difficulties with aggression and/or violent dyscontrol (e.g., throwing furniture, threatening staff or patients). These behaviors may also have traumatic antecedents and may involve the patient being in a dissociative state, leading to disorientation to current circumstances. To the extent that this is the case, reframing and understanding the posttraumatic underpinnings of these behaviors may be critical in resolving them. Some violent behavior involves identification/introjection of the aggressor/perpetrator. Working with the patient on these dynamics may be helpful in reframing these behaviors as related logically to trauma dynamics and in helping the patient stop them.

A crucial milieu dynamic is maintaining the TDU as a "safe place" (or safe *enough* place, because no hospital unit is absolutely "safe"). Accordingly, milieu treatment interventions commonly are used to bring social pressure on actively self-destructive and/or violent patients to contain their behavior. Patients who have acted unsafely are required to process the behaviors through writing, discussions with nursing staff, and/or intensive evaluation in individual therapy and attending rounds. Patients also may process the behavior and their commitment to safe alternatives in therapy groups with other patients.

Safety crises and treatment stalemates sometimes result from the patient having been recently victimized in a relationship, or actually *currently* being exploited or victimized in a contemporary relationship. It is important to have a high index of suspicion for this because patients are often profoundly ashamed about these situations and actively conceal them. These destructive relationships can include current interpersonal violence, incestuous involvement with family members into adulthood, and exploitation by psychotherapists and/or medical professionals. Patients may experience contemporary betrayals as even more devastating than their childhood traumas ("I'm grown up. I'm supposed to know better now"). In addition, these situations bring up complex medicolegal issues for staff, as well as excruciating dilemmas for the patients who, just as in childhood, often are attached to those who hurt them. Milieu management may be made more complicated when these patients wish to continue contact in the hospital with individuals who have, or are currently, reportedly exploiting them.

With respect to abuse by current or prior treating therapists, most often patients will report relationships that involve boundary violations and role reversals. Unfortunately, in all too many instances, patients report sexual involvement with a current or former treating clinician. In these cases, for additional perspective on how to proceed, we generally seek consultation from forensic consultants familiar with trauma disorders and issues of professional misconduct.

Patients who threaten harm against others (frequently against reported perpetrators) are assessed with regard to the need to warn intended victims and inform police of their threats, as required by state law. The need to keep *everyone* safe from violence, even those who reportedly have harmed the patient, becomes an important treatment issue.

Finally, patients may report or be suspected of abuse or neglect of their own children. We evaluate these cases carefully, acquiring as much collateral information as possible to assess whether mandated reporting is required. It is optimal if patients collaborate with us in reporting themselves to social services. Mandated reporting may also be required if the patient reveals information about suspected abuse or neglect of children by current or former partners or reported childhood perpetrators who currently have access to minor children.

PSYCHOTHERAPY MODALITIES

In the TDU, each patient has a psychotherapist, a social worker, and an attending psychiatrist. Patients are usually seen in 45- to 50-minute individual psychotherapy sessions three times per week. Individual psychotherapy is psychodynamically informed, emphasizing concepts such as transference, defense, resistance, projective identification, and therapeutic alliance, with optimal treatment drawing from a number of different psychotherapy models.

Patients have daily psychiatric attending rounds that necessarily focus on medication and medical issues as well as administrative issues such as observation levels and privileges. However, TDU attending physicians also carry out brief, focused psychotherapeutic interventions that facilitate goals of the overall treatment. These may include cognitive, psychodynamic, symptom management, and/or educational interventions (S.B. Wait, "Attending Rounds, or How to Establish a Therapeutic Relationship in 15 Minutes a Day," presented at Scientific Day, Sheppard and Enoch Pratt Hospital, Towson, Maryland, June 11, 2000).

Patients attend groups for 3 to 5 hours per day. Some groups are didactic or educational, whereas others focus more on psychotherapy issues and group process. In addition, patients participate in expressive therapy groups, including specialized art therapy and creative writing, as well as trauma-oriented occupational therapy groups.

Psychoeducation. Complex PTSD and dissociative disorder patients require extensive, ongoing psychoeducation. Psychoeducation goes on in all of the unit psychotherapies. Education about treatment risks and benefits primarily is carried out in individual therapy and in rounds.

First, patients are educated about the symptoms of PTSD, complex PTSD, and/or dissociative disorders. Clarification of how dissociative disorders and PTSD are diagnosed and how their symptoms may mimic or overlap those of other disorders is especially helpful to patients who have carried many and varied diagnoses. In addition, patients are educated about the current views of phasic trauma treatment and the risks, benefits, and controversies about current trauma treatment models, including pharmacotherapy. This includes discussing the nature of traumatic memory, delayed recall for trauma (if this is reported), and current controversies about these issues.

Patients who receive a dissociative disorder diagnosis also are educated regarding current controversies about diagnosis and treatment of dissociative disorders, particularly DID. Dissociative patients may have difficulty recalling educational and informed consent information. They may need frequent repetition of information, either because they have amnesia for the discussion or because alternate self states emerge who claim not to have "been present" when the information was originally imparted. The notion that informed consent is best viewed as an ongoing process is amply demonstrated in this population.

Patients are educated about conditioned fear responses and how these relate to PTSD reminders, PTSD reactivity, and intrusive PTSD symptoms. DID patients are educated that all self states make up a single human being and are not "separate people" and that all self states will be held responsible for the behavior of any other, regardless of whether the behavior is recalled and experienced as occurring under voluntary control. They are educated that all self states are adaptations to life circumstances and that there are no "good" or "bad" self states. The self states' harmful, abusive, violent behavior to self or others is not condoned but rather understood and reframed in its adaptive context, generally developed during childhood maltreatment. The clinician explores with the patient what problem the troubling behavior may originally have been intended to solve and what beliefs the self state may have about how the behavior solves the problem. Then more adaptive alternatives are explored.

Psychoeducation also involves discussing the importance of safety and bodily integrity; the nature of relationship boundaries; appropriate behaviors for adults and children; the nature of emotions such as anger, shame, sadness, and grief; the need for medical care; and many other aspects of life that most nontraumatized individuals take for granted. Severely traumatized patients may not believe that they can say "no" when someone wants something from them. Lacking full understanding of some of the most basic aspects of human relationships and of human safety and human dignity, they may be at greater risk for revictimization and exploitation.

Cognitive-behavioral psychotherapy. Cognitive therapy is an essential facet of psychotherapy in addressing the manifold and profound cognitive distortions found in this population (Fine 1990). Cognitive therapy interventions occur in psychotherapy as well as in the milieu and in groups. Most patients attend a weekly cognitive therapy group to help identify and challenge their cognitive distortions.

Basic cognitive distortions may include notions such as "anger is violence"; "self-harm is safety"; "sex is love"; "I made my abuser bad"; "sex is all I'm good for"; "if something good happens, it will just get taken away, so I should destroy it first"; and so on. In the trauma population, the apparent fixity of cognitive distortions may conceal significant trauma memory material that seemingly is held at bay by the cognitive distortion.

Cognitive distortions also interconnect with profound shame scripts that dominate these patients' cognitive/affective universe. One should never underestimate the importance of shame in the psychotherapeutic approach to these patients. Recognition of, systematic psychotherapeutic attention to, and education of the patient about shame-based cognitions and behaviors best described by Nathanson's "compass of shame"—attack self, attack other, avoidance, and withdrawal—may lead to significant clinical leverage (Nathanson 1992). Attack-self scripts typically take forms such as "I'm a loser"; "I'm disgusting"; "I'm hideous and loathsome"; or "I wish I could disappear off the face of the earth." In attack-other mode, patients may wish vengeance to get back at reported perpetrators for the humiliations caused by childhood abuse, but they commonly turn this back on themselves (Lewis 1990).

Dialectical behavior therapy. Dialectical behavior therapy (DBT) was developed by Marsha Linehan (1993a) primarily for outpatient treatment of patients diagnosed with borderline personality disorder. It is a staged treatment that focuses first on modifying life-threatening behaviors; second, on modifying behaviors that interfere with therapy; and then on modifying a defined hierarchy of problematic behaviors. In its establishment of priorities, it has much in common with the stages of treatment for complex PTSD and similarly advocates deferring intensive treatment of traumatic memories until initial safety issues are well controlled. In Linehan's model of treatment, the DBT skills group is only one component of the treatment. However, in our program, it is the one most adaptable to an inpatient setting with a constantly changing patient group. In our program, the DBT skills group meets twice a week for 45 minutes, and each group focuses on one of the four basic skills: mindfulness, distress tolerance, emotion regulation, or interpersonal effectiveness.

Group sessions start with a 2-minute mindfulness practice, followed by group leaders discussing one of the skills. We use handouts from Linehan's DBT manual (Linehan 1993b). Patients read sections aloud and give examples from their own experience of situations where they might find the skills useful. The group leaders are active and positively reinforce patients' participation in group discussions and use of the skills being taught. Patients have homework assignments to practice the skills and to discuss in individual therapy how they are using them.

Symptom management skills training. "Grounding" is the most basic skill taught to TDU patients. This relates to patients frequently experiencing themselves as depersonalized, detached, spaced out, out of their bodies, not oriented to current circumstance, "lost" in memories or internal experiences, rapidly switching among alternate self states, and so on. Grounding techniques are methods to counter these experiences, often by attempting to accomplish simple orienting tasks using all the senses. These may include helping the patient to keep his or her eyes open, to become aware of his or her feet touching the floor or arms touching the chair, and to look around the room, identifying where he or she is and with whom he or she is speaking. Patients with marked difficulties maintaining orientation to current circumstances, for example, continuously going into spontaneous self-hypnotic states, can be given a "15-Minute Check-In" sheet. Here, the patient fills out a rating scale every 15–30

minutes to assess feelings, behaviors, and degree of orientation. Severely dissociative patients may be so ungrounded as to forget to do the task as often as mandated. Nonetheless, patients can find this helpful in "staying present" and gradually becoming more grounded in reality.

DID patients have the highest hypnotizability of any clinical group on standardized assessment measures (Frischholz et al. 1992). Many non-DID PTSD and complex PTSD patients are also highly hypnotizable. Accordingly, hypnotherapeutic imagery and relaxation interventions may be particularly useful for symptom management in the acute management of TDU patients (Brown et al. 1998; Kluft and Loewenstein 2007).[1] Hypnosis represents a set of adjunctive therapeutic techniques that vary widely and may be used for many different clinical problems (Spiegel and Spiegel 2004). Formal hypnotherapeutic interventions must only be performed by those with specific training in hypnosis and additional training in hypnosis for traumatized/dissociative patients.

Patients may be taught to use images in formal hypnosis. TDU patients also can be taught self-hypnosis for a variety of symptom containment purposes. Induction of self-hypnosis may increase the potency of imagery for this population and allow a greater depth of relaxation and symptom control. Patients with DID and dissociative disorder not otherwise specified in particular may be able to use imagery to reduce the intensity of traumatic intrusions without formal induction of hypnosis. Typically, patients are taught to visualize themselves in a "safe place" where they experience a reduction in panic, flashbacks, and hyperarousal. Patients may learn to visualize "containment" of traumatic memory material in imagined vaults or boxes in outer space or at the bottom of the sea, for example. Some patients visualize a "remote control" that can take away intrusive trauma images and superimpose benign images. Patients can be taught to imagine a volume control to "dial down" intense affects and intrusive symptoms.

SAFETY AGREEMENTS

Agreements to maintain safety are frequently used with TDU patients by the therapist, attending physician, and nursing staff. These agreements have *no* le-

---

[1] We do not have space to review the controversies over use of hypnotic techniques in this population. See Brown et al. (1998) and International Society for the Study of Dissociation (2005). See also guidelines of the American Society of Clinical Hypnosis Committee on Hypnosis and Memory (1995). However, in general, in the TDU patient population these techniques are used to *attenuate* and *contain* intrusive traumatic memories, not explore them.

gal force and should *never* be substituted for the judgment of the clinician or nursing staff about the actual state of the patient's safety (International Society for the Study of Dissociation 2005; Loewenstein and Putnam 2004). However, they have considerable therapeutic utility. It is best to conceptualize these as *delaying* agreements rather than as safety agreements per se. These agreements emphasize the patient's ambivalence about self-harm or suicide, greater awareness of the impact these behaviors have on the patient and others around him or her, and development of honesty about the state of one's safety.

These agreements are most effective when paired with a "safety plan"—a repertoire of alternatives to acting unsafely. Alternatives to unsafe behavior include grounding, not isolating from others, using imagery or self-hypnosis, or going to staff and asking for help with psychotherapeutic interventions or as-needed medication. Some patients find it frightening to verbalize a need for help, based on past traumatic experiences in which they attempted to do so and were rejected, disbelieved, or additionally mistreated. We provide a "help chair" where patients can sit to nonverbally indicate their need for staff assistance. Some patients write their need for help on index cards if they are posttraumatically terrified of speaking but are less "triggered" by conveying their needs in writing.

Pharmacotherapy

Here we give a brief overview of pharmacotherapy for the TDU patient. The reader is referred to reviews of neurobiology and pharmacotherapy of PTSD and dissociative disorders (Friedman 2000; Loewenstein 2005). Complex PTSD may involve extreme fear states, terror, profound existential despair, grief, guilt, self-loathing, and shame, among other extreme emotions, none of which may be clear-cut targets of current psychopharmacology.

Psychopharmacological treatments for PTSD for the most part have excluded complex PTSD and DID patients in their protocols. In addition, studies suggest that the more trauma exposure, and the more long-standing the PTSD, the less robust the pharmacological response (Loewenstein 2005). Nonetheless, double-blind studies in male combat veterans support the specific efficacy in PTSD of the selective serotonin reuptake inhibitors (SSRIs) sertraline, paroxetine, and fluoxetine (there also was a successful fluoxetine trial in childhood trauma patients); the tricyclic antidepressants (TCAs) amitriptyline and imipramine; and the monoamine oxidase inhibitor (MAOI) phenelzine (Friedman 2000) Also, in controlled studies, the anti-

hypertensive prazosin has been found to reduce PTSD nightmares in combat veterans (Loewenstein 2005). Our clinical experience supports this indication in TDU patients with severe, recurrent nightmares who can tolerate the hypotensive effects of the medication.

Clinical experience by TDU psychiatrists suggests that other SSRIs and serotonin–norepinephrine reuptake inhibitors (SNRIs) such as venlafaxine and duloxetine, TCAs, and MAOIs are equally as effective as those that have been studied in double-blind trials, although the U.S. Food and Drug Administration (FDA) has approved only sertraline and paroxetine for use in PTSD. Other medications represent off-label uses. In particular, a subgroup of these patients presents with significant obsessive-compulsive symptoms and may respond preferentially to clomipramine or fluvoxamine (Loewenstein 2005).

Open-label studies using anticonvulsant mood stabilizers (carbamazepine, valproate, topiramate, and gabapentin) primarily in male combat veterans suggest these agents may alleviate PTSD symptoms (Friedman 2000). In addition, one small double-blind study supported efficacy for lamotrigine in PTSD (Friedman 2000). In several double-blind studies, the benzodiazepines have not been shown to have specific effects for PTSD, although they improved sleep and general anxiety responses. However, many TDU patients report significant symptom relief with benzodiazepines.

The benzodiazepines are safe and effective anxiolytic agents that have generated significant concern about their use, overuse, and misuse in psychiatric practice in general and in the treatment of patients with trauma-related disorders specifically. Their safety and efficacy are flawed by their potential for dependence and tolerance. It is important to caution patients about this and warn them against stopping these agents suddenly or without the advice of a physician. Not all patients develop tolerance, however, and many can use benzodiazepines successfully at the same dosage for long periods of time (Soumerai et al. 2003). The risk of tolerance may be higher in patients with histories of alcohol abuse or dependence and with family histories of alcoholism.

Clonazepam and lorazepam are the most commonly used benzodiazepines on the TDU; they are both relatively long acting and as such are preferable to alprazolam, which can cause rebound anxiety between doses and life-threatening withdrawal symptoms due to its short half-life. Diazepam is occasionally used as well; it is often less expensive than other benzodiazepines in its generic formulation, which may be a consideration. In addition to decreasing anxiety, the benzodiazepines are sedating and cause skeletal muscle relaxation. Patients sometimes associate the skeletal muscle relaxation with the antianxiety effect and seem to experience it as an indicator that the medication is "working."

Benzodiazepines may be given as scheduled medications, as needed, or both. Patients often have difficulty asking for as-needed medications and wait until their anxiety is extreme to do so, which makes the medications less likely to help. A twice-daily dosing regimen with as-needed doses available seems to help keep anxiety at a more manageable level. A rule of thumb for clonazepam and lorazepam is to limit the total daily dosage to 4–8 mg. If a patient requires more than this, especially if there are repeated requests for dosage increases, it is likely that tolerance is developing, and other classes of medications should be considered, including neuroleptics and agents that decrease sympathetic response, such as propranolol or clonidine.

One study of a small group of complex PTSD patients treated with risperidone showed this medication was helpful in reducing intrusive symptoms of PTSD (Reich et al. 2004). Again, clinical experience in the TDU shows that subgroups of patients respond to each of the atypical antipsychotics, and a smaller subgroup responds preferentially to some of the older typical antipsychotic tranquilizers, primarily for reduction of thought disorganization caused by repeated intrusive PTSD and dissociative symptoms; reduction in repetitive, severe flashbacks and behavioral reexperiencing episodes; and severely disrupted sleep. TDU patients with true comorbid psychotic symptoms (as opposed to dissociative pseudopsychotic symptoms), subtle thought disorder, pervasive lack of reality testing, or particularly bizarre PTSD or dissociative symptoms, especially with lack of robust response to other antipsychotics, may respond to a trial of clozapine.

Other medications found to be helpful for PTSD symptoms in open-label trials include α_2 agonists such as clonidine, β-blockers such as propranolol (especially for hyperarousal symptoms), and the μ- and δ-opiate receptor antagonist naltrexone, for reduction of compulsive self-injury, particularly when accompanied by a "high" (Friedman 2000). We find each of these agents helpful in subgroups of TDU patients.

PRAGMATICS

It is particularly vital to make the trauma patient a partner in psychopharmacological management. The complex PTSD patient is informed that pharmacolog-

ical treatments are primarily "shock absorbers" in this context and unlikely to be curative. Patients may be more readily able to identify helpful medication treatments in this context: "I don't feel 'good,' but if I wasn't taking this medication and all this stuff was happening to me, I wouldn't be able to get out of bed." In the DID patient, it is important to assess the attitudes toward medications of different self states; some may seek medications in an addictive way, whereas others are medication phobic. Some complex PTSD/DID patients report being drugged as part of abuse, creating even more complex reactivity to medication management. Accordingly, in DID patients, assent of the whole alter self state "system" may be important in adherence to a medication regimen. In DID, symptoms such as depressed mood that are found only in one or a few self states, not across the "whole human being," are less likely to be medication responsive (see Loewenstein 2005 for additional discussion).

Because there are few good studies of psychopharmacology in the complex PTSD/dissociative disorders population, there are no formally developed algorithms for medication management. However, commonsense principles can guide clinical decision making. The most important first step is a careful assessment of the symptom picture to assess the contribution of comorbid affective, PTSD, and dissociative disorders, among others. Next it is vital to take as complete a medication history as possible. It is common in this population that a medication works for a period of time and then appears to become ineffective as the patient is overwhelmed by additional life stress. Reintroduction of the medication at a later time may lead to a response.

A logical first step is to maximize dosages of medications that the patient is already taking. Medication subtraction also can be important, because patients commonly arrive on multiple medications, often stating that they have been put on several medications at the same time, confounding assessment of efficacy and side effects. Next, augmentation strategies may be useful, such as adding bupropion to an SSRI, especially if there is significant motoric retardation; a low-dose TCA to an SSRI (carefully monitoring TCA blood levels); or mirtazapine to an SSRI. Addition of an anticonvulsant mood stabilizer may be indicated if there is significant irritability or agitation as part of the symptom picture. Lamotrigine may be useful due to its preferential effects on depressed mood.

Addition of a neuroleptic, either typical or atypical, usually in low dosages, may be helpful for intrusive symptoms, posttraumatic panic, loss of reality orien-

tation, thought disorganization due to PTSD and repeated dissociation, and sleep. Neuroleptics may also
be given on an as-needed basis, although some, like
risperidone, have a relatively slow onset of action that
may limit use as an as-needed medication.

Pharmacological interventions for sleep may involve
any of a number of medications, including trazodone,
mirtazapine, benzodiazepines, and related sedative hyp-
notics such as zolpidem, sedating antihistamines, low-
dose TCAs, prazosin (for nightmares), and low-dose
neuroleptics (Loewenstein 2005).

Group Therapy

TDU patients attend a large number of groups on a
daily basis. Groups are led by nursing staff, physicians,
psychology postdoctoral fellows, social work staff, rehabilitation therapists, and the consulting pharmacol-
ogist. Groups include those with a more didactic focus:
Containment I (a group that educates patients about
PTSD, dissociation, and symptom management strategies), Medication Education, DBT Skills, Cognitive
Therapy, Health and Stress Management, and Ask
Anything (a group led by the service chief in which the
patients can ask anything), among others. Process
groups that have a more psychodynamic structure include Family Issues, Transitions (related to a variety of
life transitions but especially to discharge issues), and
Containment II (a group focused on patients' processing thoughts and feelings related to issues that brought
them into the hospital, problems with symptom management strategies, and so on).

Patients also attend a daily Goals Group in the
morning to establish goals for themselves for the day
and to discuss living together on the unit. Patients may
process safety problems that have affected the whole
hospital community as well. Evening groups include a
Community Meeting and a smaller group for each team
(half of the patients), primarily directed to identifying
containment skills and safety strategies for evening and
nighttime, usually times of day that childhood trauma
survivors have heightened PTSD reactivity.

Certain groups require a referral by the treatment
team; these include Tension Reduction, an occupational therapy group involving leather work; Journal
Making; Family Issues; and Applied Containment.
The latter is a group in which patients developing
skills using symptom containment strategies discuss
the application of those skills to specific problem areas
in life. In order to be referred to these groups, patients
must demonstrate the ability to manage their safety
and to use containment skills to tolerate discussions
of potentially triggering topics.

Groups provide an opportunity for patients to assist each other in work on common issues and problems. In addition, therapeutic groups represent a potential laboratory for interpersonal skills for trauma
patients. Patients often have difficulty with self-asser-
tion, confusing this with aggression and avoiding it at
all costs. This can be helpfully addressed "in vivo" in
group settings where patients can see that the feared
consequences of assertiveness do not occur. Additionally, patients who are repeatedly harming themselves
may more readily hear about the impact of these behaviors when challenged by their fellow patients
rather than staff.

Not all patients can tolerate groups equally. Very
disorganized, overwhelmed patients or cognitively
limited patients may find process groups destabilizing.
These patients can be frustrating to the patients who
are more insight oriented, and it may be necessary to
remove the former from process groups until they are
more stable and can participate in these groups more
effectively. Nonverbal groups such as art therapy or occupational therapy may be particularly helpful for
these patients.

Family Therapy/Psychoeducation

Family interventions are discussed in treatment team
meetings and are organized around what will benefit
the *patient*. The goal is to help the patient move toward stabilized symptoms and improved ability to use
outpatient therapy. Interventions that seem unlikely
to result in these outcomes are deferred, with recommendations as to when they might be revisited (including "never," with an appropriate explanation of
the rationale for this recommendation).

We eschew "confrontation" by patients in our program with reported intrafamilial perpetrators of abuse.
In general, these are disastrous for patient and family
members alike, no matter in what stage of therapy they
occur. In particular, patients who are so unsafe and
symptomatic as to require inpatient TDU treatment for
stabilization are not in clinical circumstances to work
through the complex psychodynamics that usually underlie a wish to confront reported perpetrators. In general, the patient harbors a fantasy that the reported perpetrator will apologize or acknowledge wrongdoing
when confronted, an event that rarely occurs and that,
even if it does, almost never leads to the immediate positive resolution imagined by the trauma patient. Typically, when the desire to confront arises, we attempt to
educate the patient about the complexity of this issue,
the risks of engaging in a confrontation, and the need to
focus on the goals of stabilization in the hospital while

postponing the question of confrontation until fully worked through in long-term treatment.

Increasing effective family communication is another important goal of the family meeting. Openness, clarity, honesty, and directness are the ideals. The social worker gives feedback about communication styles and helps family members to explore what seems to work and what does not. Family members are encouraged to find their own sources of support for the feelings evoked by the patient's illness rather than making the patient responsible.

Boundaries are often problematic for the patients and their support systems, particularly with respect to the disclosure of details of traumatic experiences. It is hard for patients and families to believe that therapy is the only place these details should be discussed, and then only when significant stability has been achieved. Setting limits on these discussions is an important way of making a patient's support system more supportive. It is important to clarify that the patient is responsible for managing his or her own safety issues, with the help of the therapist, and that this mostly is not a responsibility to be shared with the family.

Expressive and Rehabilitative Therapies

Expressive and rehabilitation therapies may be particularly helpful for complex PTSD/DID patients because these patients often have particular difficulties putting their experiences into words. Observing the patient's creations can provide understanding of traumatic experiences, coping strategies, safety issues, and specific posttraumatic reminders, among others. Art therapy has developed a rigorous system of diagnostic indicators, including an assessment for DID (Cohen et al. 1994). Accordingly, art therapy may be particularly helpful in differential diagnosis of dissociative disorders.

In the TDU, the occupational therapy assessment provides crucial information about the adverse effects of trauma disorders and symptoms on personal hygiene, meal preparation, money management, work, school, leisure, and unstructured time as well as the patient's social life or lack thereof. This may bring vital information into therapy that the patient finds too shameful to discuss and that may contrast with the patient's outward presentation of apparent competence in everyday activities. It can help the patient begin to develop specific strategies to alleviate critical hidden difficulties. For example, a patient who avoids bathing may be reacting to intrusive memories of sexual assaults in the family bathroom. He or she can be helped to develop specific symptom management and past/present separation strategies to allow better hygiene with decreased posttraumatic reactivity. Usually this is accompanied as well by relief of deep shame, not only about experiencing the traumas but also about having had such difficulty with routine personal hygiene.

Journaling

Pennybaker (1993) and others have studied rigorously the clinical utility of therapeutic journaling for the improvement of symptoms in a variety of disorders. Significant benefit in psychological well-being and improvement in stress management, medical symptoms, and even immune function have been shown to occur by using this intervention (Spiegel 1999). Accordingly, journaling tasks may be very helpful in the treatment of complex PTSD/dissociative disorder patients. Benefits can include access to dissociated thoughts and feelings, more coherence of experience, ability to track the relationship between behaviors and consequences, expression of negative affects, and better concentration. In DID, journaling can assist in identification of, and communication and coordination among, self states.

Milieu Management

Management of the therapeutic milieu is critical for functioning of the TDU. As in every true therapeutic milieu, all members of the milieu, staff and patients alike, must participate in ensuring a safe and therapeutic environment.

Staff Management Issues

It is important that the TDU staff be a functional team with mutual respect between individual members and between disciplines. The staff team must be able to model interactions that are different from those experienced by TDU patients in their traumatic relationships—for example, there should be clarity of roles and boundaries between staff members. Staff education is crucial, and we work on it continually. In addition to teaching opportunities in regular team meetings to discuss patient management, we hold weekly hourlong educational meetings for nursing staff, either with the nurse manager or with the attending staff. In addition, more experienced staff members mentor newer staff to help them develop facility at working with symptom management and cope with the stress of the milieu. A weekly hourlong "Service Conference" is designed to foster discussion of milieu issues, management problems regarding specific patients, and staff discussion of their coping with the milieu. At times, a specific weekly meeting has been held, either with one of the TDU psychotherapists or with an outside counselor, to assist staff with discussing group process issues that they might be reluctant to discuss with program leadership.

In addition, we have periodic half-day retreats to work on program development, team building, and problem solving. We also have sponsored daylong didactic training programs with lectures and other learning activities for all program staff. This has been especially important when there has been a critical level of new staff members who need basic overall education.

Many new staff members have limited knowledge and understanding of basic psychological concepts such as transference, countertransference, and defense mechanisms. Staff members working with trauma populations are continuously exposed to traumatic material. Patients often go into flashbacks, lose reality orientation, harm themselves, and describe or reenact horrific trauma scenes. Staff may be pulled between patients' negative transference responses to staff and their direct or indirect entreaties to staff for rescue. New staff members often have difficulty setting limits with patients, at some level believing that the patients are fragile and will be harmed by firm limit setting. In addition, staff members may be fearful of provoking patients' anger or of precipitating a more extreme crisis. It is important to allow staff to talk about their reactions to patients' self-harm and suicidal behaviors and to help staff achieve therapeutic distance from, and insight into, the posttraumatic origins of patients' frequent negative transference reactions to helpers. Staff need help understanding that, fundamentally, limits and boundaries provide safety and protection.

In terms of helping staff work most effectively with patients, use of the trauma frame of reference can be of great assistance. This model tends to help make explicable behavior that otherwise seems incomprehensible, alienating, and exasperating. For example, patients' overreactions to minor medical issues may be enervating for staff. However, the understanding that many TDU patients suffered some form of medical neglect may be helpful in reframing the behavior. In the overreacting patient's history, he or she may report not getting medical attention unless it was a life-or-death matter. Accordingly, the patient, fearing neglect, adopts the strategy of complaining as loudly as possible for any problem, no matter how small. In addition to feeling less blaming, staff members can also let the patient know that he or she is shouting so loudly that no one can hear him or her and that decent medical care will be provided routinely in the TDU.

Patient Management Issues

A functional TDU milieu provides a significant healing component to treatment of trauma patients. Issues that have been enumerated previously in the sections on psychotherapy are applicable to milieu management of trauma patients. The milieu program is focused on making the unit as safe a place as possible for all members to do the serious work of recovery, but this is always a work in progress. The TDU is an open system, with stabilized patients being discharged and new unstable patients being admitted, concerned others visiting and coming for family meetings, fire alarms going off, and so on. A focus on safety includes developing honesty about the state of one's safety, recognizing the impact of one's unsafe behavior on the others in the community, and learning to take real responsibility for one's behavior in the interest of genuine change.

In addition, traumatic transference themes are continuously made explicit in the milieu, with patients helping one another recognize out-of-place and posttraumatic reactions to current situations. Patients are encouraged to follow the "golden rule": to behave toward others as one wishes they would behave toward oneself. Patients can help challenge one another's cognitive distortions, including cognitive distortions regarding safety, such as "If I hurt or kill myself, it's not hurting anyone else; it doesn't involve anyone else."

Community members may play out many core traumatic transference themes. For example, TDU patients, like other survivors of childhood violence, may enact interpersonal themes of "victim-perpetrator-rescuer" (Davies and Frawley 1994) and of victim and uninvolved, uncaring "co-abuser" (Loewenstein 1993). All these attributions may shift between individual patients, patient subgroups, individual staff members, and the staff group as a whole. Frequent group interpretations and confrontations in Goals Group, Community Meeting, and process groups, among others, may be needed to move the community toward a functional milieu.

Behavior that undermines others' treatment must be vigorously challenged and confronted directly as such by staff. This is true of repeated self-harm as well as aggression toward others. For example, "staff bashing" is confronted as verbal aggression toward other patients who may be inhibited by this peer pressure from working with staff for their own recovery. The patient community is invited to look at the possibility that they are re-creating the dynamics of a violent family: the aggressive or self-harming patient may be unconsciously replaying the idea that no one can, or will, take a stand to stop violence that family members perpetrate on one another. Here, as in individual therapy, we emphasize the tasks of separating past from present and discovering safe, non-trauma-based alternatives to problem solving.

When there has been a prolonged or repeated failure of patients to use their ability to control their behavior and a failure to respond to other group and individual interventions, we may "shut down" the community, an intervention that has been used fewer than 10 times in 15 years. It is important that the TDU leadership not overuse this type of intervention and reserve it for only the most serious, prolonged community breakdown. In general, this is a highly successful intervention to restore safety and a renewed focus on treatment goals.

This intervention involves an extended community meeting with *all* patients required to attend and all available staff, including individual therapists, joining the meeting. All other groups and individual therapy sessions are cancelled. Each patient is required to speak. Here, the task is not to rehash old difficulties or engage in mutual recriminations. Each patient is asked to identify problems that are contributing to the current situation in the community, including how he or she is contributing to the difficulties, and to describe practical steps that he or she can take to work toward meaningful change. During this meeting, the leadership maintains a tight focus for the group. This may involve vigorously confronting patients who have been undermining the community's function and redirecting patients who are having difficulty following the group task. The group only ends after all members of the community have spoken. After the group, community members focus on making changes based on goals generated in the meeting.

Management of Patient Boundaries in the Milieu

Boundaries between TDU patients are a continual challenge. This has led to a series of unit rules for behavior between patients and specific rules for DID patients. Some examples are given in the following sections.

TOUCH

Sustained touch such as hugging, hand holding, and so on is forbidden between TDU patients. Although many of our patients hunger for touch and feel "untouchable," they also may react with anxiety, panic, and even physical discomfort when touched. In DID, some self states may seek repeated hugs or touch, but others are phobic of touch, recalling that, in the past, "nice" touches may have progressed to inappropriate touch. Some patients take issue with this rule; they may accuse staff of "being mean" and thwarting what they "know" will help them heal. Discussion in individual and group therapy can help educate the patients about the complex issue of touch in the complex PTSD population. Other patients may be particularly articulate about the complexity of the problem for them and may help their peers understand that if the TDU staff really thought this was a helpful intervention, we would encourage it, not eschew it.

TRIGGERS

Patients are enjoined from a variety of topics that may engender significant PTSD reactivity in their peers, in part due to the nature of the topics and in part due to the natural high hypnotizability and consequent liability to experiencing vivid visualization in the TDU population. Discussing details of one's traumatic experiences is considered potentially damaging to others and, if persistent, is viewed as a form of verbal aggression in the milieu. In TDU patients, increased PTSD intrusive symptoms, dissociative episodes, and/or deterioration in safety are virtually an inevitable outcome of detailed descriptions of trauma experiences by peers.

In general, TDU patients are asked to be sensitive to each other's idiosyncratic PTSD reminders or "triggers." Many everyday, apparently neutral topics may be upsetting to individual milieu members due to increased PTSD reactivity. On the other hand, patients are asked to work on developing resilience in coping with all manner of "triggers" because attempts at restricting life to avoid PTSD triggers usually result in the patient being deeply inhibited from engaging in many quotidian activities. Managing the dialectical tensions involving the problem of "graphic" language is an ongoing task for patients and staff. There is no clear line that shows where graphic discussions or triggers begin and end. Patients and staff must struggle with the "gray" areas that inevitably arise in attempts to work with these issues. These patients commonly struggle with polarized, "all or nothing," "black and white" thinking (Armstrong 1995). Accordingly, as in other aspects of trauma treatment, it is usually a productive endeavor to work on the "gray areas" and the dialectical tension inherent in the recovery.

ADDITIONAL MILIEU RULES FOR PATIENTS WITH DISSOCIATIVE IDENTITY DISORDER

Management of DID patients in an inpatient TDU milieu requires additional guidelines and rules. Patients are required to use *one* name consistently in the milieu, no matter which self state is "out." Also, the patient must be responsive to his or her legal name when this is required for administrative purposes, even if that is not the preferred name for regular usage. The various names of self states may be used in individual interaction with treatment team members, including nursing staff, but not in the milieu.

Management of Acute Behavioral Dyscontrol

TDU staff manage acute episodes of impending or actual dyscontrol and/or dangerousness to self or others with a hierarchy of interventions. First, they attempt psychotherapeutic interventions to discuss precipitants of problems (upsetting phone call, being triggered by something in the milieu) and to talk through the problem to find alternatives to help settle down. Other interventions may include using symptom management techniques such as relaxation, deep breathing, and imagery. Patients may be asked to journal or to use the quiet room to reduce stimulation. Staff may work with DID patients to encourage a safe self state to "come forward" and a dyscontrolled self state to "step back" within the mind.

Staff may then offer as-needed medication such as oral benzodiazepines or neuroleptics. If the patient already has lost control of his or her behavior, or acutely appears to be doing so, staff may administer parenteral medication to reduce anxiety, agitation, and dyscontrol. Commonly used medications for acute dyscontrol are listed in Table 7–1.

If the patient cannot stabilize acute serious danger to self or others with psychotherapeutic or pharmacological methods, or is so acutely agitated and unsafe that he or she refuses or cannot use these interventions, staff is urged to quickly move to physical methods to control the patient to provide optimal safety for all. In most cases, going "hands on," and giving medication, with the patient secluded in the quiet room with an open door, is sufficient to change the patient's state to a safer and more grounded one. However, in some cases, physical restraint may be needed. In many cases, TDU patients rapidly de-escalate and can be safely moved out of the quiet room or restraints quickly. Often, a period of sleep induced by medications allows the patient to become less overwhelmed and/or permits a more grounded and safe alter self state to come forward.

Intensive Observation Levels

Overall, TDU patients are managed at the least restrictive observation level possible. Despite the severity and chronicity of some TDU patients' self-destructive behavior, we attempt to avoid interventions such as constant observation and intensive suicide observation, although we do place acutely, intractably suicidal or severely, acutely, or violently self-injurious patients on these levels. In our experience, the chronicity of many patients' dangerousness to self and many patients' tendency to externalize and look for outside solutions for safety may make it difficult to find an endpoint for these intensive observation levels. Also, other patients may see these patients as receiving more staff time and may attempt to find ways to get staff to observe them more closely as well. Accordingly, we almost never place patients on these levels for parasuicidal behaviors, preferring to move them, as well as less acutely suicidal patients, to areas where staff can observe them more or less continuously but not necessarily on a one-to-one basis. The overarching safety focus on the unit means that staff are skilled in anticipating, evaluating, detecting, managing, and developing longer-term treatment strategies for dangerousness to self or others, often obviating the need for intensive one-on-one observation.

Discharge Planning

Basic discharge planning is the same for the TDU as for other inpatient units, with a few salient differences. Many of our patients come from outside the local region or state. Therefore, the logistics of discharge planning with family and the referring providers may be more complex than for local patients. Family involvement may have been done mostly by phone, and discharge may allow the first face-to-face family psychoeducation meeting.

Patients, especially those who have had a longer-term hospitalization, may need careful preparation to reenter the everyday world. Due to managed care standards for inpatient care, in most cases therapeutic passes are no longer a possibility to help prepare the patient for the impact of stepdown. TDU patients should be carefully counseled that stimuli will increase and that the "speed" of life outside the hospital

TABLE 7–1.   Commonly used medications for acute dyscontrol in patients with complex PTSD or dissociative identity disorder

Benzodiazepines

Lorazepam 0.5–2 mg po or im every 2–4 hours

Clonazepam 0.5–2 mg po every 2–4 hours

Diazepam 5–10 mg po every 6 hours

Neuroleptics

Haloperidol 2–5 mg po or im every 4 hours

Fluphenazine 2–5 mg po or im every 4 hours

Chlorpromazine 25–100 mg po or im every 4 hours

Olanzapine 2–5 mg po, im, or sl every 4 hours

Ziprasidone 5 mg po or im every 4 hours*

Droperidol 5 mg every 1–4 hours (can only be given with electrocardiographic monitoring)

Other

Hydroxyzine 25–50 mg po or im every 4–6 hours

Diphenhydramine 25–50 mg po or im every 4–6 hours

Note.   im = intramuscular; po = by mouth; sl = sublingual; PTSD = posttraumatic stress disorder.

*Requires electrocardiogram to assess QT interval for safety from arrhythmias.

may seem disconcerting. Patients are encouraged to practice their symptom management "skills" sets. The most common cause that patients cite for relapse and rehospitalization is "I stopped using my skills. I stopped communicating with my 'parts'" (in DID patients).

Patients may regard the TDU, notwithstanding their complaints about the staff and the program, as the safest place they have ever known. They feel understood by staff and surrounded by patients who share their difficulties. They may feel "at home" in ways that they never have before. They may live a solitary existence or be enmeshed in chronically problematic, unsatisfactory relationships. They may feel ashamed of deficits in functioning that they can avoid facing while in the hospital. Some patients may attempt to thwart discharge by acting unsafely whenever discharge looms or by insisting that they will commit suicide upon discharge, although they can maintain themselves safely with the support of the hospital setting.

In the past, we were more able to consider transferring patients like these to other units in our hospital or to other hospitals or trauma programs. Discussion of transfer was often sufficient to motivate the patient to

resolve issues seemingly blocking discharge. However, transfer is very difficult to accomplish in the current psychiatric care environment. We discuss directly with patients their inhibitions and fears of discharge and gently confront their anxiety over returning to problematic outpatient situations. More direct confrontation may be needed to focus patients about failure to use skills or failure to be honest about their core safety. Patients may need to be restricted from TDU readmission, and told so, if they do not make good-faith efforts to "work the program" and move toward discharge when this is a reasonable expectation. Discussion of future restrictions from readmission may help galvanize some of these patients toward discharge.

Conclusion

PTSD and dissociative disorders are common in the general population (Kessler 2000; Loewenstein and Putnam 2004). In addition, history of childhood trauma is common in general inpatient psychiatric patients (Carlson et al. 1998). Despite the difficulties presented by these patients, there are inpatient and partial hospital treatment models, as well as outpatient treatment models, that can help them sustain substantial recovery. Hopefully, knowledge from the TDU can be made more generally available, so that these patients receive more appropriate and helpful treatment in all inpatient and day hospital settings.

References

American Psychiatric Association: Practice Guideline for the Treatment of Patients With Acute Stress Disorder and Posttraumatic Stress Disorder. Washington, DC, American Psychiatric Association, 2004

American Society of Clinical Hypnosis Committee on Hypnosis and Memory: Clinical Hypnosis and Memory: Guidelines for Clinicians and for Forensic Hypnosis. Des Plaines, IL, American Society of Clinical Hypnosis Press, 1995

Armstrong JG: Reflections on multiple personality disorder as a developmentally complex adaptation. Psychoanalytic Study of the Child 50:349–364, 1995

Arnow BA: Relationships between childhood maltreatment, adult health and psychiatric outcomes, and medical utilization. J Clin Psychiatry 65 (suppl):10–15, 2004

Bernstein EM, Putnam FW: Development, reliability, and validity of a dissociation scale. J Nerv Ment Dis 174:727–735, 1986

Blank AS: The unconscious flashback to the war in Vietnam veterans: clinical mystery, legal defense, and community problem, in The Trauma of War: Stress and Recovery in Vietnam Veterans. Edited by Sonnenberg SM, Blank AS, Talbott JA. Washington, DC, American Psychiatric Press, 1985, pp 293–308

Briere J, Elliott DM, Harris K, et al: Trauma Symptom Inventory: psychometrics and association with childhood and adult trauma in clinical samples. J Interpers Violence 10:387–340, 1995

Brown D, Scheflin AW, Hammond DC: Memory, Trauma, Treatment, and the Law. New York, WW Norton, 1998

Busuttil W: The development of a 90-day residential program for the treatment of complex posttraumatic stress disorder. Journal of Aggression, Maltreatment, and Trauma 12:29–55, 2006

Cardena E, Maldonado J, van der Hart O, et al: Hypnosis, in Effective Treatments for PTSD: Practice Guidelines from the International Society for Traumatic Stress Studies. Edited by Foa EB, Keane TM, Friedman MJ. New York, Guilford, 2000, pp 247–279

Cohen BM, Mills A, Kijak AK: An introduction to the diagnostic drawing series: a standardized tool for diagnostic and clinical use. Art Therapy 11:111–115, 1994

Courtois CA: Complex trauma, complex reactions: assessment and treatment. Psychotherapy: Theory, Research, Practice, Training 41:412–425, 2004

Dalenberg CJ: Recovered memory and the Daubert criteria: recovered memory as professionally tested, peer reviewed, and accepted in the relevant scientific community. Trauma Violence Abuse 7:274–311, 2006

Davidson JRT, Foa EB: Posttraumatic Stress Disorder: DSM-IV and Beyond. Washington, DC, American Psychiatric Press, 1993

Davies JM, Frawley MG: Treating the Adult Survivor of Childhood Sexual Abuse: A Psychoanalytic Perspective. New York, Basic Books, 1994

Dell PF: A new model of dissociative identity disorder. Psychiatr Clin North Am 29:1–26, 2006

Eliason JW, Ross CA: Two-year follow-up of inpatients with dissociative identity disorder. Am J Psychiatry 154:832–839, 1997

Fine CG: The cognitive sequelae of incest, in Incest-Related Disorders of Adult Psychopathology. Edited by Kluft RP. Washington, DC, American Psychiatric Press, 1990, pp 161–182

Foa EB, Keane TM, Friedman MJ (eds): Effective Treatments for PTSD: Practice Guidelines from the International Society for Traumatic Stress Studies. New York, Guilford, 2000

Friedman MJ: What might the psychobiology of posttraumatic stress disorder teach us about future approaches to pharmacotherapy? J Clin Psychiatry 61 (suppl):44–51, 2000

Frischholz EJ, Lipman LS, Braun BG, et al: Psychopathology, hypnotizability, and dissociation. Am J Psychiatry 149:1521–1525, 1992

International Society for the Study of Dissociation: Guidelines for treating dissociative identity disorder in adults. J Trauma Dissociation 6:69–149, 2005

Kessler RC: Posttraumatic stress disorder: the burden to the individual and to society. J Clin Psychiatry 61 (suppl):4–14, 2000

Kluft RP, Loewenstein RJ: Dissociative disorders and depersonalization, in Gabbard's Treatment of Psychiatric Disorders, 4th Edition (G. O. Gabbard, Editor in Chief). Washington, DC, American Psychiatric Publishing, 2007, pp 547–572

Lewis HB: Shame, repression, field dependence, and psychopathology, in Repression and Dissociation: Implications for Personality Theory, Psychopathology, and Health. Edited by Singer JL. Chicago, IL, University of Chicago Press, 1990, pp 233–257

Linehan MM: Cognitive-Behavioral Treatment of Borderline Personality Disorder. New York, Guilford, 1993a

Linehan MM: Skill Training Manual for Treating Borderline Personality Disorder. New York, Guilford, 1993b

Loewenstein RJ: An office mental status examination for chronic complex dissociative symptoms and multiple personality disorder. Psychiatr Clin North Am 14:567–604, 1991

Loewenstein RJ: Posttraumatic and dissociative aspects of transference and countertransference in the treatment of multiple personality disorder, in Clinical Perspectives on Multiple Personality Disorder. Edited by Kluft RP, Fine CG. Washington, DC, American Psychiatric Press, 1993, pp 51–85

Loewenstein RJ: Psychopharmacological treatments for dissociative identity disorder. Psychiatr Ann 35:666–673, 2005

Loewenstein RJ: DID 101: a hands-on clinical guide to the stabilization phase of dissociative identity disorder treatment. Psychiatr Clin North Am 29:305–332, 2006

Loewenstein RJ, Putnam FW: The dissociative disorders, in Comprehensive Textbook of Psychiatry, 8th Edition. Edited by Sadock BJ, Sadock VA. Baltimore, MD, Williams & Wilkins, 2004, pp 1844–1901

Nathanson DL: Shame and Pride: Affect, Sex, and the Birth of the Self. New York, WW Norton, 1992

Pennybaker JW: Putting stress into words: health, linguistic therapeutic implications. Behav Res Ther 31:539–548, 1993

Putnam FW: Dissociation in Children and Adolescents: A Developmental Model. New York, Guilford, 1997

Reich DB, Winternitz S, Hennen J, et al: A preliminary study of risperidone in the treatment of posttraumatic stress disorder related to childhood abuse in women. J Clin Psychiatry 65:1601–1606, 2004

Soumerai SB, Simoni-Wastila L, Singer C, et al: Lack of relationship between long-term use of benzodiazepines and escalation to high dosages. Psychiatr Serv 54:1006–1011, 2003

Spiegel D: Healing words: emotional expression and disease outcome. JAMA 281:1328–1329, 1999

Spiegel H, Spiegel D: Trance and Treatment. Washington, DC, American Psychiatric Publishing, 2004

Steinberg M: The Structured Clinical Interview for DSM-IV Dissociative Disorders–Revised (SCID-D-R). Washington, DC, American Psychiatric Press, 1994

van der Kolk B, Pelcovitz D, Roth S, et al: Dissociation, somatization, and affect dysregulation: the complexity of adaptation to trauma. Am J Psychiatry 153 (suppl):83–93, 1996

Waller NG, Ross CA: The prevalence and biometric structure of pathological dissociation in the general population: taxonometric and behavioral genetic findings. J Abnorm Psychol 106:499–510, 1997

CHAPTER 8

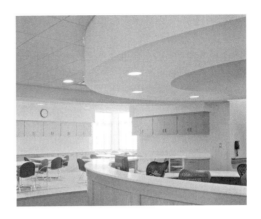

THE PSYCHOTIC DISORDERS UNIT

John J. Boronow, M.D.

Psychosis is a ubiquitous phenomenon in general psychiatry. No inpatient setting can avoid treating psychotic patients. Why then should we consider a specialty program targeting this all-too-common syndrome? The mission of a specialized psychotic disorders unit is to serve the needs of patients with severe and persistent mental illness whose psychosis is likely to be chronic and whose resulting disability is both widespread and profound.

The history of American inpatient psychiatry is very much bound up in the story of caring for these patients. Ever since the Pennsylvania Hospital volunteered to care for "the sick-poor and the insane who were wandering the streets of Philadelphia" in 1751 (University of Pennsylvania Health System 2007), there has been a recognition in American society that there is a population of severely disturbed people whose illness is both chronic and refractory to treatment. The asylum movement was begun in the nineteenth century to provide humane care, if not cure, for these unfortunate people. By the end of the twentieth century, this national enterprise, implemented on a state-by-state basis as the state hospital system, was largely dismantled under the rubric of deinstitutional-

ization. This historic change was fueled by advances in treatment, especially the promulgation of antipsychotic medication; by social concerns about the rights of patients to live unsegregated in society in the least restrictive manner; by documented abuses of patients within the confines of total institutions; and by powerful economic pressures to reduce the cost of care. Deinstitutionalization coalesced with managed care in recent decades, yet the challenge of how to best provide services for the chronically psychotic patient at all levels of care has not been resolved. Many, if not most, such patients receive so-called crisis stabilization for their acute psychotic relapses on general inpatient units within local community hospitals. The restrictions on length of stay placed by commercial managed care organizations, using severely curtailed and often arbitrary criteria for hospital care, can result in patients being discharged prematurely, with consequent readmissions and the evolution of the all-too-familiar "revolving door" scenario. In addition, the mixing of severely psychotic chronic patients with younger, higher-functioning patients and/or with older, more fragile geriatric patients leads to a predictable additional pressure within the milieu to extrude patients with illnesses characterized by disruptive behavior by discharging them early.

The mission, then, of a specialized psychotic disorders inpatient unit is to implement state-of-the-art diagnostic and therapeutic techniques, coupled with a sophisticated appreciation of the patients' illness in its community context, for the treatment of some of the most ill patients with the most treatment-resistant disorders. That community context includes social (family, friends, care providers, and all manner of outpatient treatment team members), historical (onset of illness, precipitators of relapse or noncompliance, motivators of positive change, response to past treatments), economic (available therapeutics of all sorts, from medications to assertive community treatment teams and cognitive-behavioral therapy–competent therapists), and even legal (restraining orders, criminal charges, mandated treatment orders) considerations. The vision of such a unit is to accurately diagnose the acutely ill or relapsed patient in the broadest DSM-IV-TR (American Psychiatric Association 2000) multiaxial biopsychosocial framework (Engel 1977), implement the optimal therapeutics that can be realistically expected to be followed up within the patient's community setting, control inpatient behavioral problems with the greatest efficiency for the patient and the least adverse impact on other patient groups, and coordinate the handoff of treatment to the next level on the continuum of care with minimal disruption to the flow of treatment.

Admission Criteria

The admission criteria for such a program can be formulated both diagnostically and functionally. Diagnostically, the core target population would include patients with schizophrenia, including schizoaffective disorder and psychotic disorder not otherwise specified; bipolar disorder, when the course of the illness resembles persistent schizophrenia and enduring psychotic features remain a central treatment focus; developmental disorders, including mental retardation and pervasive developmental disorders in which there is a significant psychotic component; neuropsychiatric disorders with psychotic features, including psychoses due to epilepsy, head injury, or Wilson's disease; and personality change due to these kinds of medical etiologies, especially paranoid, aggressive, and disinhibited types. Some geriatric patients with dementia and behavioral dyscontrol may at times be more successfully treated in a psychotic disorders milieu as well.

Functionally, diagnosis notwithstanding, the hallmark of a patient treated in an inpatient psychosis program is the patient's cognitive dysfunction, including other negative symptoms, and its attendant disability. Nursing staff view such patients as requiring "hands on" nursing, compared with higher-functioning patients on general units where verbal interaction is a much more important medium of therapeutics. By hands-on, we mean the need to guide such patients through many, if not all, of their activities of daily living; prompt them continuously to attend to the milieu schedule; set limits (often physically) around boundaries and socially inappropriate behavior; and restore order and good hygiene on the unit if there is destruction of property or soiling of linen, clothing, or the unit environment.

Patients with schizophreniform disorders present a special challenge. Ideally, this population would be best served with its own specialized program. However, the point prevalence of these cases, even in a metropolitan region as large as the Baltimore Metropolitan Statistical Area (2.6 million), is too low to support such a unit, at least within the current commercial managed care health insurance paradigm. Moreover, the diagnostic stability of schizophreniform disorder is notoriously low (Addington et al. 2006), and although it is likely that true schizophreniform patients will go on to develop unambiguous schizophrenia within 5 years, there are certainly some patients in the schizophreniform mix who will ultimately turn out to have bipolar disorder or a substance-induced psychosis. There is legitimate concern that these latter patients may not be well served by programming that emphasizes the rehabilitation needs of the chronically ill at the expense of more appropriately focused therapeutics aimed at their affective and/or chemical dependency illnesses. In addition, even the truly schizophreniform patient (and the patient's family) may be frightened by a milieu composed of older, more persistently ill and often dilapidated peers. In our experience, the decision of where to admit young first-episode patients is often made on an initial best approximation, based on prognostic features and level of functioning. It is not uncommon for the young first-episode person to start off on a general short-term unit, only to be transferred to the psychosis program because of failure to improve within the short-term milieu.

Special Populations

One specific population that bears mentioning is the mentally retarded. The management of psychotic disorders in the context of mental retardation can often be considerably problematic. Mentally retarded patients may have an *organic personality* (a term used in the *International Classification of Diseases,* Ninth Revision [ICD-9; World Health Organization 1977]), referred to in DSM-IV-TR as *personality change due to a general medical condition.* The general medical disorder in this case is characterized by mental retardation, or what more recently is termed *intellectual disability.* They may also have personality disorders, like anyone else. The impact on treatment, and on the rest of the milieu, of an organic personality can be huge, depending on the subtype (DSM-IV-TR specifies labile, disinhibited, aggressive, apathetic, paranoid, combined, other, and unspecified). Such a patient not only may present with hallucinations, delusions, a formal thought disorder, negative symptoms, and a mood syndrome but also may be impulsive, perseverative, attention seeking, histrionic, childish, and grossly primitive, superimposed on the cognitive limitations, which makes communication, learning, and participation in higher-functioning groups difficult. Add to that the not-uncommon associated physical disabilities, ranging from frequent expressive language and speech disorders to more disabling problems such as ataxia or spasticity, and the need to assist the patient with most activities of daily living, from toileting to feeding, and one begins to appreciate why this population is often shunned at the time of admission. Such patients often are unable to take advantage of the programming designed for the rest of the psychotically ill peers in the milieu; the services of a behavioral psychologist are often very helpful, but they are rarely available. Access to the outpatient behavioral treatment plan, often forgotten by psychiatrists unfamiliar with this population, can be enlightening, especially in framing the patient's baseline behaviors before the psychotic disorder episode developed, but it can be practically very difficult to implement such a plan in an inpatient milieu, where the staffing and training simply are incongruent with the context of the outpatient behavioral plan.

Aggressive patients constitute another challenging population. Although aggression is common in the untreated psychotic population (Krakowski et al. 1999; Steinert et al. 1999), the psychosis program must not allow itself to become the de facto intensive care unit for the whole hospital, where every violent adolescent patient or sociopathic patient is sent to keep the other units safe. There tends to be a dynamic of the "state hospital ward" even within a single hospital. It is important that clinical staff throughout the hospital have the skills to successfully manage nonpsychotic aggressive patients without triaging them to a psychosis program. Similarly, a psychosis unit is not

(necessarily) a forensic unit. Unless there are additional specialized resources available for the safe management of potentially violent forensic patients, it is necessary to screen out such patients at the point of admission. Screening criteria that we have found useful include determination of the most serious violence up to that point; whether there is a criminal history; whether a weapon was used; whether the violence was self-limited or sustained; whether it was in the context of a clear and avoidable precipitant, such as substance intoxication or the presence of specific conflict with another person; whether the referral is coming from an unreliable source; what the patient's behavior in the emergency department was subsequently; and so on. Even with such screening, both internally and externally, it is unfortunately to be expected that a psychosis unit will experience a significant amount of violence, and management of this violence is discussed later in the chapter.

Dual Diagnosis

The patient with co-occurring substance abuse presents a clinical challenge. Although comprehensive programming for chemical dependency may exist on other specialty units, the psychotic patient may not be able to take advantage of it, at least during the first part of the hospitalization. There is also a concern that such patients may be victimized by the more sociopathic patients who are sometimes present in the chemical dependency unit. Even when they are stabilized, there is well-documented evidence that patients with co-occurring severe and persistent mental illness and substance use disorders can have trouble accessing traditional therapeutics for chemical dependency because of such obstacles as residual paranoia and thought disorder, which make participation in verbal 12-Step groups highly problematic (Green et al. 2007). As with the first-episode psychotic patient, the decision of where to admit the dually diagnosed psychotic patient is often a difficult one, and the flexibility to transfer the patient (in either direction) should be anticipated after determining how the patient does in one or the other setting for a few days.

Dissociative Identity Disorder and Posttraumatic Stress Disorder

The psychotic patient with dissociative symptoms and a history of physical abuse is another unique challenge. There are both differential diagnostic aspects (Is the patient truly dissociative? Is what appears to be posttraumatic stress disorder essentially a complicating factor in an otherwise clear-cut case of schizophrenia?) as well as practical considerations (If the patient has dissociative identity disorder, is the thought disorder so severe that the patient would not be appropriate on a trauma disorder specialty unit, because he or she would not be able to make use of the higher-order cognitive/behavioral therapies employed on such a unit?). The triaging of such patients is further complicated by the common occurrence that the dissociative or psychotic elements are only uncovered subsequent to the admission, so a certain amount of collegial reassessment and cross-consultation between programs is required.

Other Considerations

Finally, certain nonmedical considerations such as insurance and placement resources cannot be dismissed from a complete understanding of why some patients are not admitted. A specialty psychosis unit has a very specific set of skills and objectives to bring to the care of patients with some of the most disabling illnesses in psychiatry. Depending on the setting, it may have an intermediate or long-term average length of stay. State hospitals, Department of Veterans Affairs hospitals, and forensic settings may all have programs explicitly designed for a length of stay measured in months. Our program, located in the context of a private freestanding psychiatric hospital, has an average length of stay of 2–3 weeks and a range of 3 days to 6 months. Our entire program is designed around what can typically be accomplished in a month, and this directly affects admission criteria. For example, if a patient has only 5 days left of insurance, has no insurance coupled with a state mandate to admit regardless, or has a managed care company that is unlikely to authorize a hospital length of stay to carry out comprehensive patient care, it is probably better to triage the patient to a conventional short-term crisis unit where the entire program is focused on finding an immediate disposition and where crisis psychopharmacology is the order of the day. Likewise, specialty units will understandably at times receive referrals of the most ill patients in the state, if not the country, and yet the patients will not have the portfolio of resources needed to support any kind of adequate treatment planning. Such are the fiscal realities of psychiatry today.

Diagnostic Workup

The differential diagnostic evaluation of the psychotic patient can be extensive (Sheitman et al. 1997), particularly when considering all the rare but possible neuropsychiatric manifestations of a host of medical and neurological disorders. However, as a practical matter in the contemporary American urban health care system, a great deal of screening is done prior to the referral of a patient to a psychotic disorders unit. One cannot stress enough the importance and value of the two most basic evaluation tools: a good history and a neurological examination. These alone, when combined with basic laboratory tests (comprehensive metabolic profile, complete blood count, urinalysis, toxicology screen, and syphilis serology), will identify the vast majority of "organic" psychoses that warrant medical-surgical, rather than psychiatric, triage. The addition of computed tomography scanning or magnetic resonance imaging, often now routinely done in urban emergency rooms for any mental status changes, further improves such screening, although these tests can sometimes be ordered by the busy emergency physician in lieu of a good history and neurological examination. A lumbar puncture is warranted for the catatonic or deliriously psychotic patient, again usually done in the emergency department prior to admission. The only other routine test not usually available in the emergency setting is the electroencephalogram, and here history is usually able to at least identify epilepsy as a diagnosis needing further assessment. In addition, electroencephalograms are usually readily available on the psychiatric inpatient service. Copper and other heavy metal assays, urine porphobilinogens, chromosome testing for Huntington's disease or specific mental retardation diagnoses, antinuclear antibody, and other more obscure testing can be obtained on the inpatient psychiatric unit as needed, once the clinical presentation and history are clarified after admission. Brain metabolic studies such as positron emission tomography, single photon emission computed tomography, and functional magnetic resonance imaging, as well as brain electrical activity mapping, remain primarily research investigations.

Psychological testing is a much neglected evaluation tool, possibly related to the influence of managed care in recent decades. Psychological testing, when done properly by skilled doctoral-level psychologists in sufficient depth (unhampered by clinically arbitrary managed limits on units of testing), can shed important light on matters of diagnosis, prognosis, and rehabilitation. Projective testing can document the severity of otherwise "sealed over" paranoia, the extent of formal thought disorder and its impact on functioning, and the otherwise hidden delusional themes that motivate the patient. The Continuous Performance

Test (Beck et al. 1956) and the Wisconsin Card Sorting Test (Berg 1948) can document the degree of attentional and frontal deficit in the medicated patient as a guide to appropriate discharge and rehabilitation planning. IQ testing and even simple proxies for IQ, such as the Wide Range Achievement Test–Reading subtest (Jastak et al. 1993), give a snapshot of both overall cognitive functioning and the degree to which that functioning has declined over the course of the illness. More specific neuropsychological testing, such as tests of memory and praxis, can further clarify the specific domains of cognitive deficit, which in turn have immediate bearing on disposition planning and rehabilitation.

As in the emergency department, taking a good history is important on the inpatient unit. The focus here is not to rule out the occasional outlier with a neuropsychiatric illness but rather to deepen the understanding of the course of illness, once confirmed as primarily psychiatric in nature. The timeline, first championed by Kraepelin (Kraepelin and Quen 1990) and later expanded upon by Adolf Meyer (Meyer and Winters 1950), is a very helpful tool in this regard. One draws a line from birth to the present and identifies key historical dates, such as developmental milestones (e.g., preschool problems, school problems, highest level of education, marriage/divorce/loss of a parent), as well as psychiatric history (first contact with any mental health provider, first treatment with medications, first hospitalization, any legal problems). Below the line one documents treatments, including names and dosages of medications as available, episodes of psychotherapy, residential placements, and so on. Inspection of the timeline makes it clear what necessary data are still lacking (e.g., Why was the patient at the state hospital for 5 years? What did the state hospital do to be able to discharge the patient eventually?). It also reveals trends, such as the increase in treatment failures (six hospitalizations in the past 8 months compared with two in the previous 5 years). The timeline also can reveal episodes of wellness, an especially important datum in the clinical history (e.g., Why was the patient stable between 1999 and 2004? Was there a certain medication, or certain psychosocial support, that enabled stability during that time?).

The timeline usually results in the need to request old records from previous treatments in order to answer some of these questions, because it is virtually impossible to do so directly with this patient population, owing to the fundamental brain deficits that afflict them in the first place. Our treatment algorithms are all predicated on knowledge of historical facts regarding prior response to treatment, and the lack of such knowledge severely constricts the likely accuracy of any cross-sectional treatment decisions. Patients being transferred to a specialty unit from another inpatient setting should always have their medication record sent along. One can immediately understand what exactly was being tried, and what exactly the patient actually received, without having to wait for a discharge summary to be dictated. The central premise here is that the inpatient hospitalization is not a self-contained island but rather a point along a temporal continuum of care for a chronic condition. It must address itself to what happened before, and what will happen after, the hospitalization, if it is to be successful.

The genogram is another underutilized tool that is useful for understanding the chronically mentally ill patient as well as most other psychiatric populations. The genogram quickly enables the clinician to understand the social reality of the patient in terms of family and other intimate relationships as well as living arrangements, which are often paramount in undertaking discharge planning and understanding relapses. Knowing who the players are in the patient's family nexus, including the sad possibility that there are none, as well as what their attitudes toward the patient and treatment are, is an indispensable part of evaluating the patient in the broader psychosocial context, and it is usually necessary in order to develop a realistic aftercare plan.

Therapies

Medication Treatments, Including Drug–Drug Interactions

A comprehensive discussion of antipsychotic therapeutics is well beyond the scope of this chapter, so let us focus instead on certain core principles of treatment. The most important single point to make about psychopharmacology with this population is not about the pharmacology itself. It is simply that no amount of pharmacology will be helpful if the patient does not take the medication reliably. The problem of nonadherence is the single biggest obstacle to outpatient success in this population (Lacro et al. 2002). The challenge on the inpatient unit is to assess the reasons for nonadherence and develop a treatment plan that can optimally address them. Concerns about side effects certainly rise to the top of patients' expressed reasons for nonadherence and should be actively elicited and responded to by the inpatient psychiatrist. Complaints about weight gain, sedation, and extrapyramidal symptoms can all be responded to in a rational way with alternative medications, although helping the patient appreciate nuances may be difficult if paranoia causes the patient to disparage all medications with a broad brush. First and foremost, however, the psychiatrist and medication nurse should present patients with the clearest possible message that they can exercise choice over the medications and that their opinion about side effects is sincerely respected and responded to. Equally difficult may be sorting out whether prior failures on certain medications were due to true medication failures (as described as common in the Clinical Antipsychotic Trials in Intervention Effectiveness studies [Lieberman et al. 2005]) or to nonadherence. Successful treatment with clozapine, for example, can be sustained by discharging to a supervised residential setting that ensures adherence, but it may be unnecessary if one knows for a fact that a previous clozapine trial was a failure.

Identification of nonadherence early in the admission process should alert the psychiatrist to considering depot neuroleptics as a pharmacological strategy. This technology, although more than 40 years old (Kurland and Richardson 1966), is still much underutilized in the United States compared with Western Europe (Glazer and Kane 1992). The inpatient setting is often a good place to initiate such treatment. The hospitalization often brings with it a certain impetus for change from the patient, the family, or the outpatient treatment team. The patient's resistance to recommendations for depot treatment in a 15-minute clinic "medication check" visit may change over a period of several days, with daily psychoeducation from doctor, nurses, and activity therapists with access to videos and pamphlets and with input from family and outpatient treatment team members. (Bringing to bear such a "full-court press" to motivate a recalcitrant patient about an important treatment decision is another unique advantage of the specialized psychotic disorders unit.) If the patient does indeed cooperate with initiating depot neuroleptics, careful consideration needs to be given to the details of treatment in terms of initial dosing; choice of drug, including payment limitations; and the handoff to the next level of care. Choosing a drug that cannot be delivered after discharge is a serious but avoidable error.

If depot neuroleptics are not indicated or agreed to, the inpatient team must still ensure that oral medications are being swallowed during the hospitalization.

Some nonadherent patients will appear to take their medications but will not, in fact, do so, which may require administration of the medications in liquid form for a period of time. Mouth checks may be needed for some patients at the time of medication administration, or patients may need to be kept in view of staff for an hour or so. Administering the medication just once a day may be helpful, as well as writing an order to re-offer all refused doses of medications for the next three medication times within the next 24-hour medication cycle before documenting that day's medications as refused. This latter tactic has proved extremely helpful over the years. Many acutely relapsed patients are so disorganized that medication refusal is not really a rational decision. Offering the same medication that was refused at 9 A.M. again at 1 P.M., at 6 P.M., and at bedtime often results in successful administration as the patient's mood or suspiciousness fluctuates during the course of the day and with ongoing interaction with the other therapeutic aspects of the milieu, including one-to-one talks, peer conversations, illness educational classes, and family visits.

The second most important psychopharmacological principle is to find out what has or has not worked previously. Patients who are known to have done well on a certain regimen and who are agreeable to continuing should not be subjected to trials of newer medications unless there is a persuasive (preferably evidence-based) rationale for making a change.

Dosing is occasionally an issue with successful antipsychotic treatment. There is good evidence that first-episode patients may respond to lower-than-average dosages of neuroleptics (Lieberman et al. 2003; McEvoy et al. 1991). However, a common problem in patients with persistent mental illness is that they receive dosages of medication that are too low and therefore insufficiently effective. Tobacco dependence may exacerbate this problem in some patients whose liver enzymes are induced by the effects of tar in the smoke, resulting in increased metabolism and clearance of neuroleptics. There is also a less well-documented but nevertheless strongly held clinical observation that many patients with persistent mental illness have developed a tolerance to neuroleptics, resulting in a remarkable persistence of symptoms and lack of side effects in the face of objectively monitored robust dosing. Why this should be so is a matter of some speculation (Sramek et al. 1990). One strategy worth considering with such a scenario is to obtain neuroleptic serum levels. Such levels are not routinely available for the atypical antipsychotics and many of the typical agents, and even if available, they are not easily interpretable unless the result is zero or very high, given the lack of studies of clinical correlation. The one drug for which levels are reliably interpretable is haloperidol, which is fortunately a widely used product. Obtaining a steady-state haloperidol level of 2 ng/mL in a patient on 40 mg/day of elixir in a well-supervised inpatient setting, for example, suggests that rapid metabolism may indeed play a role in nonresponse. Such a finding might well lead to a decision to pursue an ultra-high-dosage strategy or switch to a product or a route (e.g., depot) that is more likely to achieve a therapeutic level. This problem can be further compounded by the artificially imposed vicissitudes of cigarette availability. In the contemporary environment, cigarette smoking is being eliminated altogether from many hospital campuses. The lack of access to cigarettes, coupled with the relatively longer length of stay with this population, may result in deinduction of liver enzyme metabolism during the course of inpatient treatment, with subsequent lowering of neuroleptic dosages. However, the patient may then relapse within a week of discharge because he or she returns to smoking two packs a day or more, and the liver enzymes are reinduced as a result.

Duration of treatment with neuroleptics cannot be emphasized enough in the assessment of response to treatment. Managed care has artificially distorted what has otherwise been extremely well documented since the 1960s (Casey et al. 1960)—namely, that neuroleptics take time to work. Even if rapid response to initial treatment results in quick behavioral improvement in some critical target behaviors, such as violence, the overall response to neuroleptic treatment can take up to 3 months to optimize and even as long as 6 months for clozapine (Conley et al. 1997). No amount of dosage increase will speed up this process once the dosage has reached the therapeutic threshold for a particular patient. Finding each patient's threshold has become a bit more difficult with the atypical antipsychotics, because there are often no side effects to document bioavailability of the dosing (another reason why old records become so important!). Nevertheless, once an optimal dosage has been settled on, there is much value in waiting for the neuroleptic to show benefit before making changes (e.g., at the behest of the managed care company), although the waiting may often be done at a lower level of care.

Because the illness of patients in the chronic population is by definition so characteristically treatment refractory, a structured, rational, and evidence-based approach to psychopharmacology is necessary. Between the complexity of the clinical presentation and

the host of medications available, there is a very real danger of these patients winding up on all sorts of irrational polypharmacy regimens prescribed by well-intentioned but time-stressed psychiatrists or other physicians. It is quite common for patients to be admitted to the psychosis unit while taking two neuroleptics, and those taking three or even four can even be seen. Partly owing to the increased tolerability of the atypical antipsychotics, to the fact that antipsychotic medications are still frequently carved out from otherwise managed formularies, and also perhaps to the aggressive marketing of products, psychiatrists are often adding multiple neuroleptics for patients who continue to display refractory symptoms. It has been our experience that regimens of three and four neuroleptics are almost never necessary and that even combinations of typical and atypical antipsychotics beg the question, If the patient improved only after adding a full dose of a typical antipsychotic to an atypical one, what is the added value of continuing the atypical agent? The Texas Implementation of Medication Algorithms (TIMA) has provided a readily accessible Web-based resource for guiding clinicians in the evidence-based sequential treatment of patients with refractory psychosis (Texas Department of State Health Services 2007). One may quibble with a detail here or there, but overall it is vastly superior to the ad hoc and idiosyncratic treatment combinations that arrive at our doorstop on admission. TIMA also has built into it the same fundamental assumptions about adequate length of treatment trials described earlier.

Because the severely and persistently mentally ill population has illnesses that are so often treatment refractory, there is always a certain risk of unwarranted complacency with suboptimal outcomes. This is only further bolstered by the medical necessity standards of some commercial managed care companies, which appear to be structured to contain long-term risk with their psychotic patients, because such patients often transfer from the commercial policy risk pool to the public-sector risk pool (either Medicare, Medicaid, or local state hospital). We have often seen commercial managed care companies deny continued inpatient care for the sickest of young psychotic patients, not because they were not sick enough but because they were not making progress and thus were categorized as "custodial" and not meeting the contractual definition of "acute care."

Nevertheless, one should not succumb to economic pressures or despair. Rather, when faced with a failure in treatment, one must continue to take care of the patient, and the first medical consideration should always be a reevaluation of the diagnosis. The major differential diagnosis to consider when otherwise appropriate treatment for psychosis fails is a mood disorder. Kraepelin (1921) himself continued to reevaluate the validity of his famous dichotomy between dementia praecox and manic depression even at the end of his career, and mood disorders remain today the most common confounding syndromes in assessing persistently psychotic patients. Aggressive treatment for atypical mania, atypical depression, and coexisting anxiety disorders (including obsessional states and panic disorders) should always be considered in refractory cases. Other potential but harder-to-treat complications that may thwart forward progress in inpatient treatment include co-occurring personality disorders, personality changes due to other neurological disorders, dissociative disorders, and even malingering. Finally, one should not lightly dismiss the somewhat vague but all-too-real problem of demoralization (Clarke and Kissane 2002). The ravages of chronic psychosis, which extend across the biopsychosocial continuum from cognitive decline at the biological level to the crushing of self-esteem and hope at the psychological level and to loss of friends, family, vocation/role, and income at the social level, can so converge and impact the patient that he or she is left with virtually no reason or motivation to get out of bed every day and face the bleakness of current life circumstances. Such patients are extremely difficult to engage in any setting and represent the greatest collective fear we all experience when we hear that someone we love has schizophrenia.

When confronted with this specter, it is easy to understand how clozapine has achieved a unique place in the therapeutic armamentarium. Although not the "magic bullet" it was originally touted to be (Wallis and Willwerth 1992), clozapine remains the gold standard for the treatment of refractory psychosis. The difficulty of using the drug is not to be minimized, however, because the problems with agranulocytosis are only the tip of the iceberg. Sedation, hypotension, tachycardia, constipation, drooling, enuresis, hyperthermia, myoclonic jerking, and generalized seizures are also common side effects, as are the more recently documented complications of weight gain, diabetes, acute myocarditis, and chronic cardiomyopathy. However difficult this drug can be to tolerate, many patients do so, and some patients have indeed been saved by it, remaining out of the hospital and living independently. It therefore remains an important therapeutic tool to offer the patient with a treatment-refractory illness, and the inpatient setting is often the best place to initiate therapy, due to the host of potential complications described earlier.

Finally, electroconvulsive therapy (ECT) must be considered in the treatment of difficult schizophrenia spectrum cases. Mood symptoms in schizophrenia will respond to ECT, as in any other mood disorder, and the same criteria should apply in both instances: severity of symptoms, urgency of lifesaving treatment, and failure of pharmacological treatment. It should be remembered, however, that unlike bipolar I disorder, schizophrenia spectrum disorders will have enduring psychotic symptoms that persist even as the acute mood disorder remits with ECT. It is particularly important not to unduly continue ECT after the mood disorder symptoms have improved nor to inappropriately target the residual schizophrenic positive and negative symptoms, which are unlikely to respond in any fundamental way to ECT. On the other hand, catatonic symptoms, especially frank stupor, whether seen in a pure mood disorder or in schizoaffective disorder or catatonic schizophrenia, usually respond well to ECT (Taylor and Fink 2003). Catatonic excitement is also a legitimate target for ECT. Some patients with schizophrenia or schizoaffective disorder who are unresponsive to psychopharmacology may also benefit from ECT (Fink and Sackeim 1996), including maintenance ambulatory ECT (Chanpattana and Andrade 2006).

One final point to add is the powerful role that cigarette smoking has had in the treatment of patients with chronic psychoses. The powerful attraction to nicotine observed in many patients with chronic illnesses has led to some fascinating research on the possible role of nicotinic receptors in the pathogenesis of psychotic symptoms (Simosky et al. 2002). The nursing management challenges associated with smoking are daunting and include problems such as theft, contraband, patient conflicts and assaults, and a never-ending barrage of smoking-related demands that can literally consume whatever precious time staff have to actually relate to patients. Our recent experience in becoming a smoke-free hospital, although I initially opposed it, proved to be a complete success, particularly in terms of the reduction in countertherapeutic staff-related interactions with patients. We have made all forms of nicotine replacement available (e.g., patch, lozenge, gum, and inhaler). Patients often like the inhaler, and it is interesting to find that they frequently forget to "recharge" it with a new nicotine cartridge. Our recent experience with the new nicotine agonist varenicline is also quite promising. Together, such interventions can significantly reduce the hostility and demandingness of the occasional patients for whom the smoke-free hospital is truly an additional stress compounding their already exacerbated illness.

Psychotherapies

The inpatient unit is designed to bring specialized care to the treatment of very sick patients, but it must not be forgotten that the setting is quite intentionally designed within a larger continuum of care. The criteria for inpatient treatment nowadays are extremely narrow and focused on the most acute and disturbed behaviors that threaten life and safety of the patient and/or others. Patients in such a state are, for the most part, densely psychotic, and their capacity to engage in psychotherapy is consequently gravely diminished. By the time they are stabilized adequately to be able to engage in psychotherapy, they are usually considered ready for treatment at a lower level of care, such as partial hospitalization coupled with supervised residential care. In addition, the demands of contemporary inpatient medical practice, which place tremendous time and productivity pressures on psychiatrists in the context of high volumes of service, extensive documentation requirements, managed care reviews, and collateral meetings with team members and families, leave little time in the day for psychotherapy. Until recently, this constraint did not seem to represent a problem, because the landmark Chestnut Lodge study (McGlashan 1986) on schizophrenia outcomes concluded that high-quality psychodynamic intensive inpatient psychotherapeutic treatment did not significantly alter the course of the disorder.

Newer, interesting, and evidence-based cognitive-behavioral psychotherapies have been utilized as components of treatment for patients with schizophrenia in Great Britain and Europe in recent years (Dickerson 2000); however, such modalities are simply not appropriate for the short-term crisis-oriented inpatient setting as it presently exists in the United States. The most helpful thing the inpatient team can do is to educate the patient and family about the existence of these therapies and steer them toward outpatient resources as part of comprehensive discharge planning.

Patient and Family Education

If individual psychotherapy is not practicable for the acute inpatient setting, one can nevertheless attempt to educate patients and families about the core issues surrounding a diagnosis of schizophrenia or other severe and persistent mental illnesses. There has been significant progress in this domain over the past generation. As documented by Miller and Mason (2002),

it was not so long ago that psychiatrists would actually teach residents not to tell their patients and families the correct diagnosis if it was schizophrenia because of the devastating impact the "S word" would have on them. It is now commonly held, in our present era of patient empowerment and the widespread availability of patient information materials on the Internet, that patients and families need truthful, accurate information. To be sure, the impact of such information can be traumatic, and in the spirit of *primum non nocere* the clinician must skillfully deliver the message with hope and a promise to try and help the patient regardless of the prognosis. A variety of tools are now available for illness education, including pamphlets, books, videos, and Internet sites. Referral of patients and their families to their local chapter of the National Alliance on Mental Illness and its excellent Web site is an equally important intervention in this regard. Personal support from other families afflicted with the pain of schizophrenia can be sustaining in an hour of despair.

Rehabilitation and Recreational Therapies

With the ever-decreasing lengths of stay in contemporary American managed care inpatient settings, the role of rehabilitation and recreational therapies has diminished to a huge degree. As with the psychotherapies discussed earlier, true rehabilitation of the chronically psychotic patient needs to be conducted in the context of community living for patients whose positive symptoms are not acute and distracting, and where consistent and content-specific instruction, repetition, practicing, reinforcement, and peer support can all combine to achieve slow but meaningful learning of specific interpersonal, survival, and vocational skills. The acuity of the inpatient milieu, coupled with the relatively short length of stay, during only part of which any given patient is likely to be well enough to actually be able to process rehabilitation groups effectively, severely limits what can be accomplished during an admission.

The primary content focus of our rehabilitation groups is on illness and medication education. Patients leaving inpatient status should at least have a rudimentary grasp of what their illness is all about and the integral role of medication in their lifelong self-management of the illness. Because of these patients' cognitive deficits and psychotic symptoms (both positive and negative), achieving such "psychoeducation" effectively is no small task and requires a good deal of flexibility and creativity on the part of the group leader. In addition to traditional group and didactic modalities, group leaders may rely on the same kind of multimodal sensory learning used in the education of children with attention-deficit/hyperactivity disorder, including rapid rotation from one modality to another; use of video, interactive educational games, and writing exercises; and so on to communicate a few essential teaching objectives. More ambitious goals, such as vocational assessment, social skills training, and life skills associated with successful independent living, must wait for lower levels of outpatient care in the continuum. The rehabilitation group leader is in an excellent position to provide the treatment team with valuable data about the patient's cognitive level, degree of disorganization, motivation, and negative symptoms, all of which can guide disposition planning to the extent that a continuum of different outpatient programming is actually available in the patient's geographical location.

Purely recreational groups, on the other hand, can be tremendously important in "keeping the lid on" an otherwise chaotic milieu comprised of 20 or more acutely psychotic human beings. Particularly with the advent of the smoke-free hospital campuses across the United States, patients need other opportunities besides smoking to channel their energy, contain their anxiety, and experience a modicum of pleasure. Limitations on groups may be imposed by the overarching need to maintain safety, including control over elopement or impulsive self-injury. Contemporary psychiatric hospital design can provide secure, enclosed, but very attractive outdoor courtyard space that can offer patients "fresh air" and an opportunity to walk and experience the outdoor weather as well as offer quiet private space on a bench in the sun, away from the "madding crowd" of the unit. Within the confines of the indoor unit, gross motor therapeutic activities associated with music and group participation, such as exercise and dance groups, can decrease tension and lead to a sense of community. The long hallways in hospitals lend themselves to a variety of bowling and pitching games with soft, quiet equipment. Arts and crafts activities are often nonthreatening and appealing to psychotic patients when they can experience mastery and pleasure and pride at creating something attractive that they can even proudly wear and call their own. In our setting, the television is usually not a primary focus of patient attention or interest. Likewise, reading is seldom the preferred activity of choice for most patients, usually due to significant impairment of attention and concentration. Music can be particularly

soothing, and judicious use of relaxation CDs with natural sounds of waterfalls or rain or beach sounds can be very effective in quieting a milieu that has become overstimulated. The most common inappropriate "recreation" that staff need to constantly work with patients on is, of course, sleeping. Now that cigarettes are gone from the unit, the easiest way to recognize that one is on a unit for the chronically mentally ill is to notice that many, if not most, of the patients are in their rooms, in bed, in the middle of the day. This withdrawal, so common that it is measured in some detail in the Positive and Negative Syndrome Scale (Kay et al. 1987), can be addressed by offering the kinds of activities described earlier as well as assertive and motivated nursing staff who literally go to rooms to draw patients out and into the milieu. At times, locking the bedroom areas during activities can be a last (but effective) resort if presented in a therapeutic way to the patient. It should never be done punitively and should be abandoned immediately if it has the adverse consequence of heightening the patient's antagonism.

Other Modalities

The psychotic disorders unit is often the venue for treating patients with highly treatment-refractory conditions, often of considerable complexity. The ability to work with such patients in a safe, coherent, and controlled inpatient setting with an experienced multidisciplinary team over a period of weeks is truly a luxury compared with the fragmented and chaotic everyday outpatient world of the chronically mentally ill. The inpatient stay in such a setting can be viewed as a unique opportunity, like the eye of a storm, to pause and reflect thoughtfully on the case and, if possible, breathe new life into the treatment. For this to happen, of course, a certain vision must be established and maintained under the leadership of the psychiatrist as team leader. This vision is based on a deep commitment to empiricism as embodied in DSM-IV-TR and evidence-based diagnosis as well as evidence-based treatment. Time is spent in team meetings revisiting preliminary assessments of the patient during the course of the current treatment. On such units it is still possible for patients to remain in a single admission for several months, and procedures usually reserved for research settings can become very helpful, including the use of actual rating scales. The goal of such a comprehensive and synthesizing approach is to provide the patient, the family, and the outpatient team with a new perspective on the nature of the problem(s), the treatment, and the prognosis. At its best, such an inpatient stay serves as an extended consultation for the ongoing treatment of the patient, which, if well documented in an in-depth discharge summary that is proactively distributed to all the relevant members of the patient's treatment team, can provide an ongoing guidepost to future clinicians as they wrestle with an illness that is notoriously chronic and confusing.

Milieu Management

The art of managing a unit composed of psychotic people requires close collaboration between the psychiatric and the nursing staff as well as a modicum of understanding from the hospital administration. The most common complication in running such a program is the oversaturation of the milieu with agitated, disorganized, needy, attention-seeking, and aggressive patients, which can result in a contemporary state of "bedlam." Despite progress in psychopharmacology in the past 50 years, effective inpatient management cannot be reduced to just aggressive medication practices (Coffman et al. 1987), and no amount of oral and intramuscular medication will consistently allow all 20 or more psychotic patients to remain perfectly calm at all times.

This patient population lends itself to a more highly structured milieu, and ideally, with a sufficiently long length of stay, a fully implemented token economy can be extremely therapeutic. As first described by Ayllon and Azrin (1965) and later refined and demonstrated effective by Paul and Lentz (1977), the token economy offers a comprehensive approach to milieu management that includes a systematic approach not only to the manifold behavioral challenges presented by a group of actively psychotic patients but also to the education and training of the nursing staff. The modified token economy, based on a point card and real-time reports of both patient and staff behaviors, has been demonstrated to improve long-term outcomes after discharge (Dickerson et al. 2005). In an environment where patient behaviors can be wildly unpredictable and bizarre, disorienting even experienced staff, there is something very reassuring and steadying in an approach that calls for close attention to the specifics of patient and staff behaviors, reasoned analysis, and problem-oriented interventions.

The shortened lengths of stay in recent years, coupled with the pressure to reduce hospital labor costs, have made the fully featured model of a token economy untenable in all but a few exceptional settings nowadays. However, modifications of the original model are still useful in organizing a psychotic disorders program. Although principles of a more generic "milieu therapy" may apply fruitfully in any inpatient setting, a specifically behavioral focus for a psychotic disorders program remains helpful. General principles include 1) defining the patient and the target psychopathology using a robust behavioral perspective, with specific behavioral descriptors of the precipitants, reinforcers, and contingencies surrounding the target behaviors; 2) paying close attention to the degree of expressed emotion (Wearden et al. 2000) used by staff and making continuous efforts to minimize and re-express that emotion in more neutral ways; 3) minimizing reliance on complex higher-order verbal interpersonal interactions (such as might occur in confrontational or interactive community meetings) in favor of a simpler, more concrete problem-oriented review of the day's events and requirements; 4) avoiding any purposeful, although artificial, therapeutic "neutrality" in favor of a more globally affirming and continuously positive stance toward the patient; and 5) focusing on core activities of daily living that are typically disrupted in the course of an acute psychotic episode and that can often be taken for granted in higher-functioning nonpsychotic patient populations.

One tool that we have found to be useful is the incorporation of structured behavioral observations into the daily charting of the staff. Certain frequent and clinically urgent target behaviors are routinely queried and documented on every shift and include nighttime sleep, use of as-needed medication (and for which specific behaviors and contexts), incontinence, vomiting, and the use of any limit-setting interventions such as time-out in the bedroom or quiet room or use of seclusion or restraint. In addition, a dictionary of patient-specific target behaviors is used for any staff to spontaneously add to ongoing tracking of specific patients, including such things as yelling, cursing, threats, sexual self-stimulation, inappropriate touching of others, intrusive attention seeking, failure to get out of bed, or medication refusal. Such documentation can be readily reviewed, can provide insight into whether treatment interventions (be they medical or behavioral) are helpful, and can guide ongoing treatment planning.

The management of such a milieu can be configured in a variety of ways, each with its own strengths and weaknesses. In an ideal world, even without a true token economy, there is plenty of work for a doctoral-level clinical psychologist to do as a behavioral consultant, both to the milieu in general and to specific problem patients in particular. If such a clinician is not available, a physician with interest and experience in behavioral psychology can fill a similar role, or a psychology consultant can be requested on a case-by-case basis as needed. For behavioral interventions to work best, however, a certain amount of ongoing training and education of staff is necessary, particularly if there is a high degree of turnover in the staff and the pool of new mental health worker recruits is inexperienced. A nurse manager who has had experience with behavioral therapy can be invaluable in enhancing the effectiveness of the model in terms of technical expertise, but perhaps even more importantly as a role model for the rest of the staff to "think behaviorally." One final caveat, however: at times, even the most comprehensive and technically well-executed behavioral program will fail if the patient's underlying psychopathology is so extreme, and so poorly controlled, as to make it virtually impossible for the patient to interact successfully with a behavioral learning paradigm. Examples of this include florid mania, paranoid states of panic, and dementia, all of which can overwhelm the patient's ability to engage with and learn from an otherwise commendable behavioral treatment plan.

Management of Suicidal and Aggressive Behaviors

The psychotic patient presents certain unique challenges in terms of suicidal and aggressive behaviors. The suicidal impulses of an acutely psychotic person with schizophrenia can be particularly powerful, in part due to the compelling force of auditory and other hallucinations, which bring a whole new level of "reality" to the already depressed and/or frightened patient. Patients with schizophrenia may hurt themselves in a panic of violence in order to appease the command of "God" or the "Devil," or to escape the (mis)perceived threat from the paranoid "other," in which case death itself is viewed as a better outcome than the horror of being trapped by the other. The power of such delusions, coupled with tremendously real affective and often religious energy, can result in such acts as throwing oneself through a window, cutting (not scratching) clear through tendons and arteries, shooting one's head with a shotgun, putting a knife into one's heart, setting oneself on fire, jumping in front of a subway train, or castrating oneself or removing one's eyes ("cast off the offending organ"). Simple overdosing is often not the schizophrenic way of suicide (Hunt et al. 2006).

Similarly, aggression directed toward others can be extreme and quite dangerous. In general it is fair to say

that violence comes with the territory when running a psychotic disorders inpatient program. Persecutory delusions, ideas of reference, and thought broadcasting can all create a state of panic or hostility in patients that makes them a potential risk to themselves, peers, visitors, and staff. Although scrupulously careful and appropriate psychopharmacology can certainly mitigate such violence, it is not a panacea, especially for the acutely admitted patient. First-episode patients, substance-intoxicated patients, patients who have suffered abuse, manic patients, head-injured patients, mentally retarded patients, antisocial patients, and patients with treatment-refractory illnesses all can present an increased risk of violence.

The psychopharmacological approach to violence is straightforward and evidence based and has been well described repeatedly in the literature (Petit 2005). Besides such psychopharmacological interventions, it is imperative for the staff to have training and confidence in behavioral approaches to the agitated patient. Principles of effective management of the potentially violent patient include 1) transparency and clarity in explaining the rules of the milieu and the patient's legal rights; 2) a neutral but respectful attitude toward the patient at all times, even when the patient is menacing or grossly out of control; 3) avoidance of any threats, coupled with clear limits on what is and is not tolerated in the milieu; 4) recognition of the countertransference fear of the patient or the projective identification of rage toward the patient, either of which can contaminate the therapeutic relationship and poison any treatment alliance; and 5) availability of sufficient power (i.e., expertly trained staff) to implement any limit setting in as humane and safe and efficient a way as possible. Perhaps the single most important rule to follow, but not always the easiest, is the prompt and effective confrontation of threatening behavior when it first occurs. The failure to intervene immediately, with a clear expression to the patient of the nature and reason for the limit, the possible consequences, and the need to accept additional therapeutics from the staff, almost invariably leads to "escalation" of the aggressive behavior until it reaches a crisis that may, by that point, unavoidably result in someone being injured. The choices of additional therapeutics that should be presented to the out-of-control patient are diverse and include providing as-needed medication, adding a new medication, changing to a different medication, taking a time-out, making restitution to a peer, or removing oneself from the milieu in general or from a specific peer or staff member. Teaching staff to be facile with any and all of these options, either singly or in combination, can greatly enhance the therapeutic leverage of the team and is certainly more helpful than merely relying on as-needed medications, which unfortunately can become the final common pathway of least effort in an underresourced and overly stressed hospital with high acuity.

Seclusion and restraint in particular are often considered when dealing with the acutely psychotic patient. This can begin before the hospitalization, if the police need to subdue a violent patient emergently or if the emergency department staff need to seclude or restrain the patient. To be sure, seclusion and restraint are, and should always be, the last resort in responding to the potential for violence in psychotic patients. Iatrogenic worsening of an already bad situation can occur if the paranoid patient is kept in a locked room with a camera and one-way mirror. Restraints can at times exacerbate fear because of the total helplessness and consequent vulnerability the patient experiences, coupled with the psychotic distortions that convince the patient that the people in control are lying and wish to kill him or her. Every effort should be made to avoid using seclusion and restraint or, if not possible, to minimize their duration and address any iatrogenic morbidity that they may introduce. Nevertheless, it must be said that in our experience, complete renunciation of seclusion and restraint with the psychotic population has never been possible, and seclusion and restraint remain a necessary option in the safe management of psychotically aggressive patients.

Discharge Planning

Involvement of Community Providers, Resources, and Significant Others

The effective treatment of the persistently psychotic patient must always be considered within the broader context of the patient's ongoing outpatient treatment and rehabilitation/housing situation. It is incumbent upon the inpatient program to reach out to the outpatient treatment team, including family and significant others, if it is to do more than merely put yet another pharmacological bandage on what is, in fact, a complicated biopsychosocial system in crisis. Remarkably, despite the ravages of managed care, the inpatient team usually still has more resources at its disposal than the beleaguered outpatient team and can create a kind of therapeutic shelter or interlude during which the relevant parties can afford to (briefly) pause and reassess

the entire treatment system, determining what may need to be changed. We routinely arrange team conferences with family, outpatient case managers, housing care providers, and service coordinators from other agencies such as developmental disabilities, social services, protective services, vocational services, educational services, and mobile treatment (or assertive community treatment) teams. We also find the modern speakerphone and conference calling technologies to be an invaluable way to engage concerned outpatient parties who cannot physically attend such conferences and yet keep the discussion totally transparent to the patient, if the patient is clinically well enough to attend. It is often the outpatient psychiatrist who is least able to participate in such conferences due to huge caseloads and clinical assignments spread over a variety of geographical locations. In fact, just reaching the outpatient psychiatrist when he or she has the patient's chart available to review is often impossible in a 1-week length of stay when the outpatient psychiatrist is only in that particular office once a week. We have found that most agencies are cooperative, with appropriate consents, to fax copies of the psychiatrist's medication log and recent progress notes, which can often shed important light on the precipitants to the admission.

Families are always relevant in helping the chronically mentally ill. We always begin with the view of the family as an ally, until proven otherwise. We try to join with them, form a shared therapeutic alliance, and learn from them as much as we can: What motivates the patient? To whom is the patient closest? To whom will he or she listen? Why does the patient feel this way or that? Sometimes, the family itself becomes a secondary patient, when we identify their unmet needs in response to the patient's illness. If supporting the patient in the home of 80-year-old parents has become too much, we try to facilitate disengagement and transition to a new developmental level. If the patient's risk of violence has become too great, we provide specific warning and legal advice. Although one must of course obtain the patient's consent to collaborate with the family in this way, such collaboration is critical to long-term success. When families are actively caring for their relative with persistent mental illness, the old-fashioned "individual therapy" patient-centric model may be completely inappropriate and even hurtful and should be utilized on a case-by-case basis when there are specific clinical reasons for following such a model (Glynn et al. 2006).

Transition to Next Level of Care

Mobilizing psychotic patients who have begun to "seal over" the acute psychosis that precipitated inpatient admission requires careful clinical assessment and comprehensive planning. Despite the economic pressures to discharge patients as soon as they cease being aggressive or self-destructive, the clinical fact remains that psychotic patients remain fragile for some time even after the more florid symptoms remit. Putting patients back into stressful environments before they are able to cope with them can merely result in an exacerbation of symptoms and rehospitalization.

Finding appropriate transitional levels of care, however, can be quite challenging. In our uniquely American health insurance paradigm, so-called acute treatment (i.e., short-term hospital care) is paid for by most commercial insurances, but "chronic" or "rehabilitation" or "custodial" services are viewed as uncovered and hence the responsibility of the public sector, the family if they have resources, or no one at all in many instances. Criterion B for schizophrenia in DSM-IV-TR is the classic Kraepelinean failure to ever fully recover *(restitutio ad integrum)* from what Adolf Meyer (Meyer and Winters 1950) later called "the life break," which in contemporary America is usually translated operationally into chronic disability and poverty. Disabled patients may become eligible for Social Security Disability Insurance (which comes with Medicare) or Supplemental Security Income (which comes with Medicaid), but getting these entitlements is no small task, the difficulty of which literally varies from administration (the Reagan administration raised the bar) to administration (the Clinton administration lowered it). Without these entitlements, paying for long-term ancillary services in the community can be impossible. It is not uncommon, for example, for the newly psychotic child of middle-class parents with good commercial insurance to be unable to access the local psychiatric rehabilitation program because it is not possible to get Medicaid and neither the commercial insurer nor Medicare will pay for it. Likewise, paying for housing can be a tremendous obstacle to successful community adjustment for the person with persistent mental illness. Although some states may have dedicated funding lines to provide supervised residential care for the mentally ill, access often requires years of being on waiting lists. In urban areas of many states, a literal cottage industry has evolved in the past 30 years in which local homeowners will rent out rooms and provide meals and sometimes medication supervision ("board and care"). In our setting, the existence of, and collaboration with, such providers is absolutely essential to the overall successful management of this chronically mentally ill population. Although there are certainly occasional, potentially lethal drawbacks of using essentially unlicensed and untrained laypersons (Barnhardt 2002), the alternative of literally "dumping" patients on the streets, as has been reported in Los Angeles (Winton and DiMassa 2005), is simply unacceptable. The other alternative final common pathway for homeless mentally ill—jails and prisons—can result in unspeakable horror, such as the recent death by dehydration of a bipolar man kept in restraints in a Michigan jail (Pelley 2007).

Specialty Day Hospital

Because the transitional period can be a vulnerable one for patients recovering from an acute psychosis, there is a role for a day hospital model that delivers programming specifically tailored to the persistently ill patient. General partial hospital programs, which are run out of a psychiatric unit embedded in a general hospital, are typically geared for higher-functioning patients, with programming that emphasizes recovery and return to work and family. Such a milieu may be even less tolerant than the inpatient unit of the deviant, deficit behavior characteristic of the persistently ill patient, precisely because the high-functioning patients are themselves no longer so symptomatic and wish to focus on higher-level problem solving. We have found that with the economies of scale inherent in a large freestanding psychiatric hospital, we can easily fill a special day hospital that services the chronic patient. Such a model is a natural extension of the longer-length-of-stay inpatient model of 30 years ago, only now delivered in a partial setting. Whereas patients on the inpatient unit are not there long enough when they are stable to benefit from social skills groups such as a cooking group, for example, they can definitely take advantage of such occupational therapy programming in a partial setting. Coordinating such a day hospital with the inpatient unit allows for continuity of physician coverage as the patient is stepped down to a lower level of care and higher level of psychosocial stress and performance demands. This can be invaluable when medications need to then subsequently be adjusted. A registered nurse can coordinate closely with the care provider, and a social worker can do family work now that the patient is back at home. We have been able to, in effect, provide a 2- to 3-month length of treatment, if not length of stay, in such a continuum and as a result see fragile patients successfully stabilized in the community and then handed off to the next level of care, namely a psychiatric rehabilitation program and office practice.

Conclusion

In summary, the treatment of the psychotic patient is in a state of flux and has been so since deinstitutionalization got under way in the 1960s. Although length of stay in the hospital has been greatly shortened, the severity of illness and psychosocial needs of this very vulnerable population have not decreased. Creative programming that targets these patients with specialized services can result in relatively better outcomes, occasionally dramatically so. Such programming speaks well of the progress that the mental health professions together have made over the years in bringing rational, caring, and effective therapeutics to the sickest patients we treat. This is work we can all be proud of, even as we wait for the breakthroughs in neuroscience that we expect to come in the future.

References

Addington J, Chaves A, Addington D: Diagnostic stability over one year in first-episode psychosis. Schizophr Res 86:71–75, 2006

American Psychiatric Association: Diagnostic and Statistical Manual of Mental Disorders, 4th Edition, Text Revision. Washington, DC, American Psychiatric Association, 2000

Ayllon T, Azrin NH: The measurement and reinforcement of behavior of psychotics. J Exp Anal Behav 8:357–383, 1965

Barnhardt L: Owings Mills woman killed in apartment. Baltimore Sun, July 11, 2002, p B1

Beck LH, Bransome ED Jr, Mirsky AF, et al: A continuous performance test of brain damage. J Consult Psychol 20:343–350, 1956

Berg EA: A simple objective test for measuring flexibility in thinking. J Gen Psychol 39:15–22, 1948

Casey JF, Bennett IF, Lindley CJ, et al: Drug therapy in schizophrenia: a controlled study of the relative effectiveness of chlorpromazine, promazine, phenobarbital, and placebo. Arch Gen Psychiatry 2:210–220, 1960

Chanpattana W, Andrade C: ECT for treatment-resistant schizophrenia: a response from the Far East to the UK. NICE report. J ECT 22:4–12, 2006

Clarke DM, Kissane DW: Demoralization: its phenomenology and importance. Aust N Z J Psychiatry 36:733–742, 2002

Coffman JA, Nasrallah HA, Lyskowski J, et al: Clinical effectiveness of oral and parenteral rapid neuroleptization. J Clin Psychiatry 48:20–24, 1987

Conley RR, Carpenter WT Jr, Tamminga CA: Time to clozapine response in a standardized trial. Am J Psychiatry 154:1243–1247, 1997

Dickerson FB: Cognitive behavioral psychotherapy for schizophrenia: a review of recent empirical studies. Schizophr Res 43:71–90, 2000

Dickerson FB, Tenhula WN, Green-Paden LD: The token economy for schizophrenia: review of the literature and recommendations for future research. Schizophr Res 75:405–416, 2005

Engel GL: The need for a new medical model: a challenge for biomedicine. Science 196:129–136, 1977

Fink M, Sackeim HA: Convulsive therapy in schizophrenia? Schizophr Bull 22:27–39, 1996

Glazer WM, Kane JM: Depot neuroleptic therapy: an underutilized treatment option. J Clin Psychiatry 53:426–433, 1992

Glynn SM, Cohen AN, Dixon LB, et al: The potential impact of the recovery movement on family interventions for schizophrenia: opportunities and obstacles. Schizophr Bull 32:451–463, 2006

Green AI, Drake RE, Brunette MF, et al: Schizophrenia and co-occurring substance use disorder. Am J Psychiatry 164:402–408, 2007

Hunt IM, Kapur N, Windfuhr K, et al: Suicide in schizophrenia: findings from a national clinical survey. J Psychiatr Pract 12:139–147, 2006

Jastak JF, Jastak SR, Wilkinson GS: The Wide Range Achievement Test, Revised 2. Wilmington, DE, Guidance Associates of Delaware, 1993

Kay SR, Fiszbein A, Opler LA: The positive and negative syndrome scale (PANSS) for schizophrenia. Schizophr Bull 13:261–276, 1987

Kraepelin E: Manic-Depressive Insanity and Paranoia. Edinburgh, Scotland, Churchill Livingstone, 1921

Kraepelin E, Quen JM: Psychiatry: A Textbook for Students and Physicians. Canton, MA, Science History Publications, 1990

Krakowski M, Czobor P, Chou JC: Course of violence in patients with schizophrenia: relationship to clinical symptoms. Schizophr Bull 25:505–517, 1999

Kurland AA, Richardson JH: A comparative study of two long acting phenothiazine preparations, fluphenazine-enanthate and fluphenazine-decanoate. Psychopharmacologia 9:320–327, 1966

Lacro JP, Dunn LB, Dolder CR, et al: Prevalence of and risk factors for medication nonadherence in patients with schizophrenia: a comprehensive review of recent literature. J Clin Psychiatry 63:892–909, 2002

Lieberman JA, Tollefson G, Tohen M, et al: Comparative efficacy and safety of atypical and conventional antipsychotic drugs in first-episode psychosis: a randomized, double-blind trial of olanzapine versus haloperidol. Am J Psychiatry 160:1396–1404, 2003

Lieberman JA, Stroup TS, McEvoy JP, et al: Effectiveness of antipsychotic drugs in patients with chronic schizophrenia. N Engl J Med 353:1209–1223, 2005

McEvoy JP, Hogarty GE, Steingard S: Optimal dose of neuroleptic in acute schizophrenia: a controlled study of the neuroleptic threshold and higher haloperidol dose. Arch Gen Psychiatry 48:739–745, 1991

McGlashan TH: The Chestnut Lodge follow-up study, III: long-term outcome of borderline personalities. Arch Gen Psychiatry 43:20–30, 1986

Meyer A, Winters EE: The Collected Papers of Adolf Meyer. Baltimore, MD, Johns Hopkins University Press, 1950

Miller R, Mason SE: Diagnosis: Schizophrenia. New York, Columbia University Press, 2002

Paul GL, Lentz RJ: Psychosocial Treatment of Chronic Mental Patients: Milieu Versus Social-Learning Programs. Cambridge, MA, Harvard University Press, 1977

Pelley S: The Death of Timothy Souders. 60 Minutes, February 11, 2007. Available at: http://www.cbsnews.com/stories/2007/02/08/60minutes/main2448074.shtml. Accessed April 21, 2007.

Petit JR: Management of the acutely violent patient. Psychiatr Clin North Am 28:701–711, 2005

Sheitman BB, Lee H, Strous R, et al: The evaluation and treatment of first-episode psychosis. Schizophr Bull 23:653–661, 1997

Simosky JK, Stevens KE, Freedman R: Nicotinic agonists and psychosis. Curr Drug Targets CNS Neurol Disord 1:149–162, 2002

Sramek JJ, Gaurano V, Herrera JM, et al: Patterns of neuroleptic usage in continuously hospitalized chronic schizophrenic patients: evidence for development of drug tolerance. DICP 24:7–10, 1990

Steinert T, Wiebe C, Gebhardt RP: Aggressive behavior against self and others among first-admission patients with schizophrenia. Psychiatr Serv 50:85–90, 1999

Taylor MA, Fink M: Catatonia in psychiatric classification: a home of its own. Am J Psychiatry 160:1233–1241, 2003

Texas Department of State Health Services: Texas Implementation of Medication Algorithms. Austin, Texas Department of State Health Services, 2007. Available at: http://www.dshs.state.tx.us/mhprograms/TIMA.shtm. Accessed April 21, 2007.

University of Pennsylvania Health System: In the Beginning: The Story of the Creation of the Nation's First Hospital. Philadelphia, University of Pennsylvania Health System, 2007. Available at: http://www.uphs.upenn.edu/paharc/features/creation.html. Accessed April 15, 2007.

Wallis C, Willwerth J: Awakenings: schizophrenia—a new drug brings patients back to life. Time, July 6, 1992, p 57

Wearden AJ, Tarrier N, Barrowclough C, et al: A review of expressed emotion research in health care. Clin Psychol Rev 20:633–666, 2000

Winton R, DiMassa CM: L.A. county makes plans to end patient "dumping." Los Angeles Times, November 30, 2005, p B6

World Health Organization: International Classification of Diseases, 9th Revision. Geneva, Switzerland, World Health Organization, 1977

CHAPTER 9

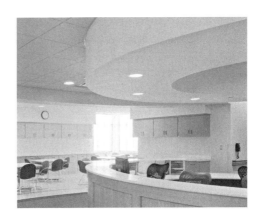

THE CO-OCCURRING (SUBSTANCE ABUSE/MENTAL ILLNESS) DISORDERS UNIT

Patricia R. Recupero, J.D., M.D.
Michael C. Fiori, M.D.
Mary Ella Dubreuil, R.N., L.C.D.P.

Admission Criteria

The goal of the co-occurring disorders (CODs) unit is to provide safe and effective psychiatric care to patients with co-occurring mental illness and substance abuse. In the literature, patients with CODs may also be referred to as dual-diagnosis patients or mentally ill chemical abusers, among other terms. In this chapter, "patients with CODs" refers to all patients with at least one primary psychiatric disorder *and* at least one substance use disorder (SUD). True CODs units are specifically designed to meet the needs of patients with both significant active psychiatric illnesses and significant active substance dependence issues. Such units may be rare. Far more prevalent are units whose primary orientation and expertise are in the treatment of either chemical dependence or primary psychiatric

disorders. In reality, however, all units at various levels of care and expertise are faced with caring for patients with clinically significant CODs. Ideally, patients are evaluated for admission to a continuum of care, their needs in all realms are assessed, and a treatment plan is devised and implemented in the most effective, least restrictive, safest level of care possible.

The American Society of Addiction Medicine (ASAM; 2001) placement criteria have been devised in an attempt to address how to *safely and efficiently* match patient assessment to modality of treatment and treatment setting. The placement criteria are a set of guidelines for placement, care planning, and discharge of patients with SUDs. *Safety* must be the clinician's top priority in assessing whether a patient meets criteria for admission to a CODs unit.

The American Association of Community Psychiatrists has also produced a software system to assist in patient placement decisions. The system, Level of Care Utilization System for Psychiatric and Addiction Services (LOCUS), helps to determine psychiatric and/or substance use treatment level-of-care needs (Sowers et al. 2003) using criteria similar to ASAM. LOCUS is somewhat more sensitive to psychiatric domains. The patient's acute and chronic issues determine where treatment should be delivered. From a psychiatric perspective, there are three main safety concerns shaping level-of-care decisions:

1. Presence and intensity of suicidal, self-harming, homicidal, or violent/aggressive ideation or behavior;
2. Severity of a patient's depression, psychosis, or personality dysfunction; and
3. The patient's acute or chronic cognitive dysfunction.

From a medical perspective, additional safety concerns relate to medical risks associated with the patient's substance abuse, health status, and risks associated with different treatment options. For example, patients with a history of delirium tremens (DTs) and/or seizures are most at risk for those to occur during detoxification; patients with tachycardia and hypertension, despite the presence of intoxication, are at higher medical risk. Risks posed by level of intoxication, withdrawal history, the current episode's amount and frequency of intake, and what psychosocial supports a patient possesses all interrelate to indicate whether a patient meets criteria for treatment on a CODs unit.

The ASAM placement criteria function best when patients are assessed in each dimension independently and also in the interactions across dimensions. For example, a patient may meet criteria for admission to a CODs unit, but a high level of psychosocial support might mitigate against the need for inpatient treatment. However, clinicians must be careful not to minimize the importance of any one dimension by simply *averaging* patients' scores across domains. Although consideration of the interactions across dimensions is an important aspect of sophisticated patient evaluation, if a patient requires admission to a CODs unit as evidenced by severity of ratings in substance dependence or psychiatric illness, then strength in other dimensions does not generally alter the clinical necessity for admission.

Diagnostic Workup

The mainstay of the initial assessment is the taking of an adequate history. The type of assessment should be tailored to the setting of the evaluation; an initial outpatient office evaluation of a patient complaining of depression and fatigue is different from the patient who comes to a hospital emergency department and self-identifies as having depression and addiction.

The diagnostic workup must include a multiaxial assessment, including evaluation for psychiatric disorders, SUDs, medical disorders, general functioning, and personality and psychosocial issues that relate to the patient's presentation or treatment. The evaluation must also address the relationship between these issues. Are the psychiatric problems relatively distinct from the substance dependence issues? Does the substance abuse simply exacerbate and complicate the psychiatric illness, or does it cause the psychiatric problems? Does the substance abuse arise from the psychiatric illness, perhaps as a maladaptive attempt at self-treatment? A careful gathering of the history from the patient and, ideally, from significant others is the most instructive procedure at the clinician's disposal. Examples of pertinent information include

1. To the extent a working hypothesis can be established, which came first, the psychiatric problem or the substance abuse disorder?
2. What is the effect of the substance usage on the psychiatric symptoms and on the treatment of the psychiatric illnesses?
3. Is there a family history of psychiatric illness or substance dependence?
4. What is the severity of the patient's psychiatric symptoms during periods of sobriety?

Laboratory testing can be a helpful adjunct to the history in the diagnostic assessment and can aid in monitoring and motivating patients with CODs. All diagnostic and treatment-monitoring laboratory testing described in other chapters of this book apply to patients with CODs. However, some laboratory services more specifically apply to the treatment of patients with known or suspected SUDs.

Virtually any body fluid or tissue can be assayed for drugs of abuse, but most testing is performed on urine and blood samples. Urine is the primary fluid collected when testing for the presence of drugs of abuse because it is easily and noninvasively collected, and drugs are often present in high concentrations. In the acute care setting, laboratory testing for substance abuse can help to identify specific drugs of abuse, history of use, and amounts or levels of substances in the body, which can help to guide treatment decisions. This chapter provides a brief overview of some of the laboratory tests available; more detailed information may be found in textbooks of substance abuse treatment, such as *The American Psychiatric Press Textbook of Substance Abuse Treatment* (Galanter and Kleber 2008) and Lowinson et al.'s (2005) *Substance Abuse: A Comprehensive Textbook.*

Immunoassays of urine samples for drugs of abuse can cross-react with endogenous metabolites or prescribed medications, thus causing false positive results. Gas chromatography with mass spectroscopy is more expensive, sensitive, and specific for confirming positive immunoassays. Negative tests will be reported if the concentration in the urine is below the cutoff for the drug or its metabolite. The amount and duration of usage, coupled with the timing of the last dosage, all affect urine screen results.

Codeine and heroin are metabolized to morphine, which is the target of urine assays for opioids. Poppy seeds famously can cause false positives at the 300-ng/mL cutoff level for 48 hours after ingestion. Commonly used immunoassays are less sensitive for oxycodone and hydrocodone, resulting in unexpected false negatives. Methadone, propoxyphene, and buprenorphine require specific assays, because standard assays often yield negative results.

The interpretation of benzodiazepine immunoassays is complicated by the diverse number of compounds and their metabolites that may show poor cross-reactivity. Different screening assays will result in false negatives depending on the benzodiazepine type and concentration. Therefore, a positive finding will affect treatment decisions, but a negative finding should not override a history or a clinical concern. Similarly, a positive finding of a long-acting, fat-soluble benzodiazepine should not be taken as a sign of recent usage.

The major cannabinoid metabolites in marijuana are present and detected for 1–2 days after a single episode of smoking, whereas long-term usage will result in positive assays for as long as 2 months and can be positive even in abstinent individuals after a negative urine, where the concentration may be fluctuating around the cutoff level. False-positive urine screenings for marijuana due to passive inhalation are rare.

Assays for the short-acting barbiturates are positive for 1–4 days after last usage.

Phencyclidine, if tested for, is positive for about 7 days after a single usage.

Cocaine usage is detected by the presence of its primary metabolite, benzoylecgonine, in urine immunoassays; there are few false positives.

Urine tests for *d*-amphetamine and *d*-methamphetamine are widely available and commonly used, but medications such as decongestants and appetite suppressants frequently cause false positives. Commonly used assays often miss the hallucinogenic amphetamines, methylenedioxyamphetamine, and methylenedioxymethamphetamine ("ecstasy") unless they are present in high concentration.

Acute usage of alcohol can be estimated by the blood alcohol level (BAL), which can be noninvasively obtained by having the patient exhale a deeply drawn breath into a measuring device. Longer-term usage of alcohol can be estimated by blood tests. For tests reflecting the function of the liver, the γ-glutamyl transferase (GGT) is the most sensitive marker of alcohol abuse. The aspartate aminotransferase (AST) and the alanine aminotransferase (ALT) are also elevated in alcohol dependence (AST greater than ALT) and are commonly drawn on admission to CODs units, but the transaminases are not as sensitive as the GGT. Increased red blood cell mean corpuscular volume is also associated with alcohol dependence and is commonly obtained; it takes 3 months for this level to normalize after initiating abstinence. Although the carbohydrate deficient transferrin, which normalizes after roughly a month of abstinence, may be informative on admission, it may be more helpful in an abstinent, long-term care setting.

In addition to screening for the usage of drugs of abuse, laboratory testing can be useful in other ways, including blood tests for ammonia levels, which are correlated with cognitive dysfunction in alcoholics and may be significantly elevated in the presence of mild or even nonexistent transaminase elevation.

Treatment Planning and Therapeutic Programming

Challenges in Treating Patients With Co-Occurring Disorders

The successful treatment of patients with CODs requires coordinated and integrated care for each of the patient's psychiatric disorders and SUDs. The focus of the COD inpatient program is to provide safety, assessment, education, and assistance in the development of follow-up and relapse prevention plans. An inpatient stay is also an opportunity to work with the patient toward enhancing motivation for ongoing treatment. Patients can be introduced to information that will help guide ongoing efforts toward recovery.

It is important for both the treatment team and the patient to understand the unique relationship between the psychiatric disorder and the pattern of substance use. It is not uncommon for one disorder to trigger the other or for one to interfere with recovery from the other. Psychosocial factors common among patients with CODs (e.g., financial hardship, homelessness, unemployment, legal difficulties, isolation, poor social support, and interpersonal conflict) may complicate treatment and recovery (Laudet et al. 2000). The difficulty in formulating a treatment plan is further compounded by the lack of published studies in this area as well as problems with countertransference and burnout among clinical staff.

Difficulties may also vary by the specific diagnoses, further complicating the treatment plan and emphasizing the need for treatment plans to be individualized. Substance-abusing patients with posttraumatic stress disorder (PTSD) have greater numbers of hospitalizations for inpatient substance abuse treatment than those without PTSD (Brown et al. 1995). For these PTSD patients, therapy focusing on trauma and recovering from trauma may be helpful (Ford and Russo 2006). Patients with severe trauma and CODs may come to be known as "difficult" patients, and monitoring and controlling countertransference may be particularly challenging for coworkers. These patients may have found substance abuse effective in relieving psychic distress because they lack healthy coping skills (Cramer 2002). Thus, patients may not be motivated to cease abusing substances until they can learn healthy and adaptive coping strategies. In patients with eating disorders, those with bingeing and purging behaviors seem to be correlated with a higher rate of substance misuse than patients with purely restricting eating disorders (i.e., patients with nonpurging anorexia nervosa). Impulse control may be a problem for addictions treatment in these patients (Corcos et al. 2001). Substance abuse in patients with schizophrenia is associated with increased rates of homelessness, more severe psychosis, lack of medication adherence, violent behavior, and poor clinical outcomes (Soyka 2000). Finally, comorbid personality disorders and SUDs may present challenges not only for acute care but also for long-term treatment planning and discharge placement.

Staff Selection, Education, Training, and Supervision

Creating a therapeutic milieu begins with people. Selecting staff with a commitment to the population, patience, self-awareness, and an understanding of the process of change is important in creating an environment where patients can feel safe to learn and grow. Patients often enter treatment with shame and guilt.

They may not possess the information necessary to truly understand the illnesses they are struggling with or why they continue to behave in ways that are detrimental to themselves and others. They frequently enter treatment vulnerable and defensive. Clinical staff must care for patients with CODs in a way that does not reinforce patients' negative self-image, so that patients can gradually let down their defenses. The optimal treatment team consists of people who have experience working with both addictions and other psychiatric disorders. Biases in either direction can be problematic in the overall care of the patient. Important relationships between the two illnesses can be missed, unrealistic expectations might be set, and relapse management and prevention plans may not meet the needs created by both diagnoses.

Staff should be oriented to the treatment philosophy of the program, program goals, and expectations. Ongoing performance feedback should be given. Core competencies should be clearly established and reflected in the annual performance evaluation so that staff may plan appropriate professional growth initiatives. Ongoing education for staff on the CODs unit may take advantage of training interventions currently being developed (Hunter et al. 2005), and unit supervisors may wish to provide clinical staff with copies of the American Psychiatric Association's practice guidelines and other resource documents, such as the Substance Abuse and Mental Health Services Administration's Treatment Improvement Protocol (TIP), "Substance Abuse Treatment for Persons With Co-Occurring Disorders" (Center for Substance Abuse Treatment 2005). Ongoing clinical supervision, which allows for continued learning, support, and self-evaluation, is a critical ingredient in the delivery of compassionate care.

Staff members need to be able to provide a safe environment, crisis management, and group and individual therapies. They must be able to function as a team to continuously assess the patient and to develop and work with individualized treatment plans. Staff members also need a venue to process countertransference they may experience in response to the behavior of patients with complicated, chronic, relapsing, and sometimes treatment-resistant conditions. Clinical supervision should provide staff with a safe place to discuss attitudes and judgments that might arise toward patients in their day-to-day interactions.

Stages of Change and Readiness for Change

Two major factors in formulating and carrying out a successful intervention include the patient's readiness to change (or stage of change) and the ability of the unit's staff and structure to match treatment to the patient's individual needs and capabilities.

Prochaska et al.'s (1992) five-step transtheoretical model of change is especially applicable to the treatment of individuals with addictions and those with co-occurring mental illness. In this model, individuals go through five stages before finally achieving change. The first stage is that of *precontemplation*, during which the individual is not seriously contemplating change. During the second stage, *contemplation*, one recognizes the problem and thinks about change. The third stage, *preparation*, involves taking steps to prepare oneself for the action that will effect change. Fourth, one *engages in action*—that is, takes direct steps—such as chewing nicotine gum instead of smoking cigarettes. Finally, during the fifth stage, *maintenance*, one's goal is to maintain the change. Individuals undergoing behavioral changes frequently go through several cycles of the five steps before achieving permanent change; relapse is a normal phase in this process (DiClemente et al. 2004). A patient with CODs may be at different and potentially conflicting stages of change for each disorder. Relapse or decompensation in one area may impact change status in other areas. The Center for Mental Health Services recommends the use of the stages-of-change model for identifying and serving patients' needs in the treatment of individuals with CODs (Center for Mental Health Services Managed Care Initiative 1997).

DiClemente et al. (2004) noted that readiness to change is distinct from readiness for treatment: "Individuals can come to treatment and be open to participating in treatment without being ready to abstain from alcohol and drugs" (p. 105). For many individuals with CODs, substance misuse has become a trusted coping mechanism despite its undesirable consequences. Therefore, abstinence may be implausible for patients who have not yet developed alternative coping skills and who have not yet worked through the trauma or symptoms that trigger maladaptive coping behaviors. Brunette and Mueser (2006) offered a helpful review of treatment components and treatment plans at each stage of change, emphasizing the importance of fully integrated and flexible treatment for patients with CODs.

Integrated Treatment and Individualized Treatment Plans

There is insufficient evidence (due to a dearth of studies on CODs) to recommend one type of treatment plan over another for all patients with severe mental illness and comorbid substance misuse (Jeffery et al. 2000). New treatment models are continually emerging (Bellack et al. 2006), making large-scale comprehensive reviews unlikely. However, integrated programs emphasizing core elements, such as active engagement and smaller case loads, have produced noticeable improvements in patient outcomes (Jerrell and Ridgely 1999).

Although patients with CODs are known to have lower treatment success rates, most persons with CODs do not receive adequate, integrated treatment for both disorders (Watkins et al. 2001). This is a significant and unfortunate unmet need, because epidemiological data suggest that CODs are the norm rather than the exception in substance-using populations (Minkoff 2001). Furthermore, integrated treatment has been shown to improve clinical outcomes. When substance-abusing patients were provided with additional services for their comorbid depression, the course and outcomes of their treatment were similar to those of substance-abusing patients who did not have comorbid depression (Charney et al. 2001). For many patients with CODs, successfully treating the affective or anxiety disorder may remove the patient's need to "self-medicate." Treatment must also address the SUD in order to establish insight into the maladaptive substance use and to develop relapse prevention strategies. In a study comparing integrated versus standard treatment for dually diagnosed homeless adults, the group receiving integrated treatment "had fewer institutional days and more days in stable housing, made more progress toward recovery from substance abuse, and showed greater improvement of alcohol use disorders than the standard treatment group" (Drake et al. 1997, p. 298). In a study of patients with schizophrenia and substance abuse, the integration of motivational interviewing, cognitive-behavior therapy, and family sessions produced improvements in general functioning and abstinence from substance abuse as well as reductions in positive schizophrenia symptoms (Barrowclough et al. 2001).

The Center for Mental Health Services Managed Care Initiative (1997) called for increased availability of integrated treatment for patients with CODs as well as programs that can adapt to the needs and readiness of individual patients. The Institute of Medicine also called for integrated treatment for persons with CODs, highlighting the value of collaboration and coordination of care (Institute of Medicine Committee on Crossing the Quality Chasm 2006). The committee recommended routine sharing of information about the patient's problems and treatment (with the patient's consent), increased screening and monitoring for CODs, and policies and incentives to encourage collaboration. Better outcomes with integrated treatment appear to be related to overall administrative or system changes that facilitate collaborative programming and enhanced support to direct-care clinical staff (Minkoff 2001).

Smoking Cessation

The decision whether (or how) to include treatments for smoking cessation is a critical aspect of treatment planning on the CODs unit. The integration of smoking cessation strategies is especially recommended for facilities with smoking bans, because such bans have little to no effect on long-term smoking cessation (el-Guebaly et al. 2002) but may affect patients' comfort and agitation related to nicotine withdrawal. Cigarette smoking is highly prevalent in individuals with CODs and accounts for substantial morbidity and mortality in these patients; smoking may even impede successful pharmacological treatment of underlying psychiatric or addictive disorders by affecting the metabolism of other drugs (Williams and Ziedonis 2004). Among people discharged from inpatient treatment for addictions, more die from tobacco-related disease than from alcohol-related disease (Hurt et al. 1996). Additionally, there appears to be a link between current cigarette smoking and suicide, even after controlling for potentially confounding factors (Tanskanen et al. 1998).

There are conflicting schools of thought on treating nicotine addiction in early recovery. Few deny the negative consequences of nicotine addiction. However, it has long been felt that pushing smoking cessation concurrently with other addictions treatment puts the person at greater risk for relapse to alcohol and other drugs. Such beliefs do not appear to be supported by empirical research, which has shown that smoking cessation does not impair sobriety. On the contrary, data suggest that continued cigarette smoking may make abstinence from other substances more difficult for patients (Gulliver et al. 2006). Cigarette smokers are thought to be in a nearly constant state of withdrawal, and agitation from nicotine withdrawal may impair an individual's ability to resist cravings and impulses to relapse on other substance abuse. In one study, smoking cessation during intervention for other substance abuse resulted in a 25% increased likelihood of long-term (at least 6 months) sobriety from alcohol or other drugs (Prochaska et al. 2004). In another study, continued cigarette smoking was found to impair recovery from alcoholism in measures of neurocognitive performance, such as reasoning, problem solving, and short-term memory (Durazzo et al. 2007).

It is also sometimes assumed that people with psychiatric illnesses and/or addictions would not want to stop smoking. This thinking has led to numerous programs not addressing the issue of nicotine addiction at a time when the opportunity to at least educate and increase motivation is present. Although it is true that many patients arrive at the CODs unit ready to address psychological issues or other SUDs but still in the precontemplation stage for changing their nicotine addiction, therapeutic programming on the unit may provide the support and resources a patient needs to become motivated or even to begin to effect change. Even if the philosophy of the inpatient COD program does not include the recommendation of concurrent smoking cessation, it should at least provide education for all patients, motivational enhancement efforts, and treatment for those who decide to engage in smoking cessation during treatment.

Therapies

Medication Treatments

Skillful usage of medications helps to engage patients in treatment. Generally speaking, medications may be utilized to treat states of intoxication, treat withdrawal syndromes, prevent relapse, and treat co-occurring psychiatric conditions.

LIFE-THREATENING INTOXICATION STATES

States of intoxication can be dangerous to patients, and associated belligerence can be dangerous to staff and other patients and may undermine treatment before it has even begun. Life-threatening intoxication states are generally treated by specialists in emergency medicine, but clinicians involved in the treatment of patients with CODs should be able to recognize potentially dangerous states in order to make appropriately rapid referrals and initiate treatment. Two of the best-studied medications are the opioid antagonist naloxone and the benzodiazepine antagonist flumazenil, which are used for the treatment of opiate, benzodiazepine, and polydrug overdose.

Naloxone is parenterally active and binds with high affinity to all three subtypes of opioid receptors but is without intrinsic activity at the receptors. Thus, in opiate-dependent patients, intravenous doses of 0.05–0.4 mg may be given to patients with central nervous system (CNS) depression and may be repeated every 3 minutes until that depression is completely reversed. For patients with respiratory depression, 2 mg intravenously is given, up to 10 mg. The half-life of naloxone at the level of the brain is much shorter than that of opioid agonists, so close monitoring of the patient and repeated administration of naloxone may be necessary. Supportive treatment for the induced state of opiate withdrawal should be provided as clinically indicated.

Flumazenil is a competitive antagonist at the central synaptic γ-aminobutyric acid (GABA) receptor, which briefly antagonizes in a dose-dependent fashion both benzodiazepine and nonbenzodiapine agonists at the GABA receptor (American Psychiatric Association 2007). Flumazenil must be administered cautiously to benzodiazepine- and polydrug-dependent patients, with the knowledge that withdrawal seizures may be precipitated with GABA blockade. Patients who become obtunded or exhibit respiratory suppression may require it as an emergency lifesaving intervention. The effects and bioavailability of benzodiazepines usually outlast flumazenil, requiring multiple administrations of flumazenil to prevent relapsing into an intoxicated state. Patients should be managed without flumazenil whenever possible (American Psychiatric Association 2007).

Special precautions are necessary when treating patients who are showing signs and symptoms of both intoxication and withdrawal simultaneously. For example, patients with a blood alcohol level above 200 mg/dL (0.2) who show tachycardia, hypertension, and tremulousness are at greater risk for withdrawal seizures and DTs. Furthermore, patients with polysubstance dependence can be intoxicated from one substance while in withdrawal from another, necessitating caution and careful monitoring to safely begin detoxification.

DETOXIFICATION AND WITHDRAWAL

What is detoxification? Volumes of scholarly articles have been written on this subject, but detoxification can be defined as "intervention that manages an individual safely through the process of acute withdrawal" (McCorry et al. 2000, p. 9). Detoxification of a patient on a CODs unit should include ongoing evaluation and refining of the psychiatric diagnoses. Detoxification is a necessary acute intervention in the treatment of many SUDs; to be clinically useful, it must be integrated into the continuum of treatments. Connecting safe and humane detoxification to long-term psychiatric and substance abuse treatment helps to save money and prevents needless further suffering.

Alcohol. The prediction of need for detoxification and risk for severe withdrawal syndrome rests on the patient's reported history and knowledge of the alcohol withdrawal syndrome. Mild to moderate withdrawal includes anxiety, irritability, tremulousness, anorexia, insomnia, and mild cognitive and perceptual changes. More severe withdrawal may include complications such as autonomic instability with tachycardia, hypertension, frank delirium, psychosis, and seizures. Alcohol abuse may lead to dehydration, and mild changes in vital signs can often be correlated with excessive alcohol consumption. Restoring adequate fluid intake may normalize all vital signs for such patients. However, fever greater than 100.5°F should not be simply attributed to the alcohol withdrawal syndrome. A complete medical assessment may be warranted in order to rule out underlying disorders such as urinary tract infections.

Traditional detoxification protocols may involve a "loading and taper" methodology. A standardized 4-day protocol for alcohol withdrawal treatment might call for the administration of 50–100 mg of chlordiazepoxide four times daily (or every 6 hours) on day 1; 50–100 mg three times (or every 8 hours) on day 2; twice (or every 12 hours) on day 3; and once at bedtime on day 4. A flexible 4-day protocol might call for 50–100 mg of chlordiazepoxide every 4–6 hours as needed (e.g., if pulse exceeds 90 beats per minute, if diastolic blood pressure exceeds 90 mm Hg, or if the patient exhibits signs of withdrawal) on day 1; 50–100 mg every 6–8 hours as needed on day 2; every 12 hours as needed on day 3; and at bedtime as needed on day 4. Another alternative is a front-loading protocol. A front-loading protocol for treating alcohol withdrawal with chlordiazepoxide might call for 50–100 mg of chlordiazepoxide as often as every 2–4 hours until signs of withdrawal are controlled, then 50–100 mg every 4–6 hours as needed on day 1, and 50–100 mg every 4–6 hours as needed on days 2 and 3. No doses may be needed on days 2 and 3, because the long half-life of chlordiazepoxide allows it to self-taper while withdrawal symptoms are controlled. (These withdrawal treatment protocols are drawn from Prater et al. 1999 and Burant 1990.)

A substantial body of evidence supports benzodiazepines as the drugs of choice for ameliorating the symptoms of alcohol withdrawal. There are advantages and disadvantages to the long- and short-acting benzodiazepines. Various protocols for the use of long-acting benzodiazepines, including using loading doses and monitoring the patient as the long-acting benzodiazepine self-tapers, are well documented. Many studies have shown the utility of long-acting benzodiazepines such as diazepam and chlordiazepoxide, but their erratic absorption intramuscularly and their association with sedation and cognitive impairment both in patients with hepatic dysfunction and in the elderly have led to the use of other benzodiazepines for alcohol detoxification. Lorazepam and oxazepam, with their lack of active metabolites, moderate half-lives, more predictable intramuscular absorption, and pharmacokinetics less affected by age and liver disease, have become popular with some clinicians. However, there are concerns that short-acting benzodiazepines may require more frequent dosing and longer periods of monitoring. These shorter-acting benzodiazepines may be preferred for patients with compromised hepatic functioning, whereas longer-acting benzodiazepines may be preferred for DTs and seizure prophylaxis in most other patients. Further research is needed to clarify the relative risks and benefits of the various types of benzodiazepines.

Benzodiazepines are essential to providing humane detoxification from alcohol, and a primary goal of their usage is the prevention of seizures and delirium tremens. Although it is hoped and often thought that adequate dosages of benzodiazepines given early enough in the alcohol detoxification process will prevent DTs (Center for Substance Abuse Treatment 2006), the data to support this contention are lacking. Furthermore, once DTs are established, high doses of benzodiazepines do not abort the syndrome rapidly but nonetheless remain vitally important in the safe management of patients. Patients with DTs require trained clinical observation for withdrawal or excess sedation. Severe DTs, with autonomic instability, fever, and inability to maintain adequate oral nutrition, is beyond the capabilities of most CODs units and may require intensive care unit monitoring and treatment.

Although benzodiazepines are central to the attenuation of moderate to severe alcohol withdrawal syndrome, other medications may be employed. For severe withdrawal with psychosis, the use of high-potency antipsychotics can decrease the need for very-high-dose benzodiazepines, which can result in paradoxical disinhibition, falls, and toxic confusion and delirium perhaps caused by the benzodiazepines themselves (Center for Substance Abuse Treatment 2006). Anticonvulsants have been utilized especially in Europe for the treatment of alcohol withdrawal, with carbamazepine and valproic acid the best studied (Malcolm et al. 2001; Reoux et al. 2001). Dilantin has not been shown to be effective in preventing alcohol withdrawal seizures (Chance 1991; Hilbon and Hjelm-

Jager 1984; Rathlev et al. 1994). The use of β-blockers, clonidine, and other antihypertensives has been shown to be useful in the treatment of tachycardia and hypertension not well controlled by adequate doses of benzodiazepines, but these do not prevent seizures nor delirium (Center for Substance Abuse Treatment 2006). Additionally, their use can mask withdrawal, potentially leading to underdosing of necessary benzodiazepines.

All patients suspected of alcohol abuse should be started on a multivitamin with minerals as well as 100 mg daily of supplemental thiamine. Some clinicians recommend parenteral or even intravenous thiamine administration as well as additional thiamine supplementation, particularly in the presence of Wernicke's encephalopathy. However, experimental data are limited, and at the time of this writing, data are insufficient to guide decisions about dosage, frequency, route of administration, or duration of thiamine replacement therapy for the treatment or prevention of Wernicke's encephalopathy or Wernicke-Korsakoff syndrome in patients with alcohol abuse (Day et al. 2004). Some clinicians favor folate supplementation as well, but data supporting this practice are limited. If folate is given, the failure of the mean corpuscular volume to normalize should arouse suspicion of a vitamin B_{12} deficiency. Additional mineral supplementation may also be important in malnourished alcoholic patients.

Sedative-hypnotics. The issues involved in sedative-hypnotic intoxication, dependence, and detoxification are similar in many respects to those discussed in the treatment of alcohol dependence. However, extreme alcohol intoxication can be life threatening, whereas overdose on benzodiazepines alone is rarely fatal. The combination of high-dose benzodiazepines with other CNS depressants such as alcohol or opiates must be managed aggressively to prevent mortality.

When possible, gradual detoxification by tapering dosages from benzodiazepines is the ideal. However, many patients who take benzodiazepines have anxiety disorders, and even very slow detoxification will result in flares of anxiety symptomatology; it is very difficult to ascertain whether these symptoms are due to the withdrawal process or represent the patient's underlying anxiety. This clinical conundrum makes it very difficult to detoxify benzodiazepine-dependent patients on an outpatient basis, and the patients may do best on an inpatient unit. However, the length of stay on inpatient units is usually quite brief, and it is generally not safe to rapidly taper benzodiazepine-dependent patients (Ashton 2005; Center for Substance

Abuse Treatment 2006). Anticonvulsants such as carbamazepine, valproate (Dickinson et al. 2003; Rickels et al. 1999), and gabapentin have proven quite helpful. The anticonvulsants may be initiated and raised more rapidly in benzodiazepine-dependent patients while the patient is simultaneously stabilized and then tapered off the benzodiazepines.

To safely taper patients off CNS depressants such as benzodiazepines and alcohol, symptom-triggered administration of benzodiazepines has proven effective and safe. The Clinical Institute Withdrawal Assessment of Alcohol Scale—Revised (Sullivan et al. 1989) is commonly utilized. Symptom-triggered medication administration allows treatment to be tailored to the individual patient's needs, and when properly done, it avoids the under- and overmedicating of patients that can occur when medications are given according to standardized protocols.

Opiates. Although symptom-triggered medication administration is quite effective for alcohol- and benzodiazepine-dependent patients, this may be problematic with opioid-dependent patients. The signs of opioid withdrawal include anxiety, irritability, agitation, mydriasis, diarrhea, vomiting, piloerection, yawning, rhinorrhea, lacrimation, and anorexia. Seizures and delirium do not occur. However, before the physical signs and symptoms become evident, there is an emergence of dysphoria, anxiety, irritability, and agitation; thus, symptom-triggered medication administration, which relies on vital signs and objective criteria, will leave the patient in great subjective distress. The dissatisfaction the patient feels with the detoxification process can decrease patient retention in treatment and may impair the therapeutic alliance between patient and staff. Psychotherapeutic interventions and improved staff education, as discussed elsewhere in this chapter, may have a special role for improving the therapeutic alliance with patients undergoing opioid detoxification. Additionally, protocols are available for the use of clonidine and clonidine–naltrexone for the treatment of patients undergoing opioid detoxification (Kleber 1999). A sample clonidine-aided opioid detoxification protocol for patients with short-acting opioid dependence might call for 0.1–0.2 mg of clonidine three times a day (or every 4 hours), up to 1 mg, on day 1; 0.1–0.2 mg three times a day (or every 4 hours), up to 1.2 mg, on days 2 through 4; and a specified taper protocol (e.g., reduce dosage by half each day) from day 5 until detoxification is completed (Kleber 1996). Clonidine may also be used to aid in the detoxification of methadone-maintained patients, but detoxification may take longer and may require additional modifica-

tion of tapers and monitoring to minimize withdrawal symptoms. Buprenorphine and methadone may also be useful, but special caution may be warranted to minimize the risk of respiratory suppression. A thorough discussion of pharmacotherapy for opioid detoxification is beyond the scope of this chapter; clinicians are urged to consult addictions treatment textbooks and other clinical resources that deal with this subject in more detail.

The half-life of the abused opiate determines the peak of the opiate withdrawal symptomatology. Heroin withdrawal peaks at 36–72 hours, whereas oxycodone and methadone peak at 72–96 hours (Kosten and O'Connor 2003). Even after the symptoms of acute withdrawal have subsided, persistent fatigue, insomnia, and dysphoria may last for weeks to months, and Goldstein and Volkow (2002) have shown significant changes in brain functioning persisting for a year post abstinence. This delayed abstinence syndrome may contribute to the high rate of relapse seen in patients who are detoxified but not engaged in either long-term rehabilitation or maintenance treatment. For many patients, long-term maintenance on methadone or buprenorphine may be appropriate.

Stimulants. Although detoxification from CNS depressants such as alcohol and benzodiazepines may result in life-threatening physiological problems, the detoxification from CNS stimulants does not usually involve severe physiological morbidity. However, abrupt discontinuation of stimulants can lead to depression and a sense of hopelessness that puts patients at risk for suicide even in the protected environment of the hospital (Coffey et al. 2000; Cottler et al. 1993). Although this state of intense dysphoria can be persistent, it often improves after a few days (Coffey et al. 2000). Although there is a growing body of literature both on the lasting CNS effects of stimulant dependence and possible medication treatments of stimulant dependence, no agents have shown reliable efficacy in ameliorating the symptoms of withdrawal (Kosten and O'Connor 2003).

Nicotine. Nicotine dependence is very common in patients with psychiatric and other substance abuse issues and is associated with significant morbidity and mortality. Pharmacological treatments include forms of nicotine replacement and bupropion. For an excellent review of the treatment of nicotine dependence, the reader is referred to the American Psychiatric Association's (2007) revised "Practice Guideline for the Treatment of Patients With Substance Use Disorders." Varenicline, which functions as a partial agonist at the nicotine receptor, shows some promise for the treatment of nicotine dependence (Oncken et al. 2006), but data are insufficient to endorse its use in the acute hospital setting at this stage. The U.S. Food and Drug Administration has recently raised concerns about potential serious neuropsychiatric side effects of the drug.

Cannabis. Contrary to the view of some clinicians and patients, marijuana (cannabis) has been associated with complicating the course and treatment of co-occurring psychiatric disorders. In vulnerable individuals, cannabis abuse is associated with new-onset psychosis and earlier onset of psychosis as well as increased risk of other substance abuse (American Psychiatric Association 2007). The genetics underlying the vulnerability for cannabis-related psychosis are being investigated (D'Souza 2007). Withdrawal symptoms include significant anxiety, dysphoria, insomnia, and nightmares. No specific pharmacotherapies have been proven efficacious in treating cannabis withdrawal, nor in preventing relapse, at this time.

Further reading. Withdrawal syndromes are discussed in more detail in substance abuse treatment textbooks (see, for example, Galanter and Kleber 2008; Lowinson et al. 2005), which typically include detoxification protocols as well.

POSTDETOXIFICATION PSYCHOPHARMACOLOGICAL TREATMENT

One of the central challenges of the CODs unit is the initiation of medications for maintaining sobriety. Postdetoxification medications are utilized both in the treatment of substance dependence and in the treatment of CODs. There is no evidence to suggest that duration of treatment of psychiatric disorders is different in patients with co-occurring SUDs, but the timing of the initiation of treatment is controversial. For example, there are abundant data showing that clinically significant depression and anxiety commonly coexist with opiate and alcohol dependence disorders; there are also data suggesting that with weeks to months of sobriety, a significant proportion of these patients improve. Clinicians must consider many factors, including the following (American Psychiatric Association 2007):

1. Whether the psychiatric disorder(s) predates the onset of substance dependence
2. The status of the psychiatric disorder during periods of sobriety
3. Family history of psychiatric illness

4. Whether the psychiatric symptoms are commonly seen in the postacute withdrawal state.

Although the recommendations for psychopharmacological treatment of patients with and without CODs are largely identical, there is controversy regarding the usage of psychotropic medications with a known abuse potential, such as sedative-hypnotics, stimulants, and opiates. These medications may be utilized successfully if carefully monitored. Education of the patient and other caregivers, coupled with monitoring of the quantity prescribed and refill dates, can help to lessen the risks these medicines may pose to patients with CODs.

Psychopharmacological treatment in the postwithdrawal period of the SUD per se may be initiated on the CODs unit. Emphasis on informed consent ensures that thoughtful caution will be exercised. For example, disulfiram should be avoided in a patient who for neuropsychiatric reasons cannot appreciate the risks of alcohol ingestion on this medication.

Appropriate treatment of comorbid mental illness has been shown to improve outcomes for patients with SUDs, although research on maintenance pharmacology for patients with CODs is currently lacking (Cornelius et al. 2003). Successful treatment of psychiatric symptoms has been found to lower rates of comorbid substance abuse in patients with schizophrenia (Green et al. 2007; Scheller-Gilkey et al. 2003). Patients with comorbid anxiety disorders and SUDs may find anxiolytics such as buspirone helpful in lessening reliance on substances of abuse (Cornelius et al. 2003; Pettinati et al. 2003). Patients with comorbid PTSD and alcohol dependence had both improved PTSD symptoms and decreased alcohol consumption following treatment with sertraline (Brady et al. 1995). Patients with comorbid alcoholism and major depression may find selective serotonin reuptake inhibitors and tricyclic antidepressants helpful (Cornelius et al. 2003).

However, some questions remain. Antidepressants appear to reduce drinking in depressed alcohol-abusing men but not depressed alcohol-abusing women (Graham and Massak 2007). Furthermore, data are mixed concerning the use of antidepressants for the treatment of severe SUDs; selective serotonin reuptake inhibitors appear less effective for patients with more severe alcoholism and more severe depressive symptoms, for example (Pettinati et al. 2003). It is unclear what role, if any, anticonvulsants and mood stabilizers might play in the long-term pharmacotherapy of patients with CODs. Lithium has not yet been studied for comorbid bipolar affective disorder and

SUDs, but it has been studied for alcoholic patients with depression and those with no affective disorder, and in both cases it was not associated with increased abstinence from alcohol (Cornelius et al. 2003).

DRUG–DRUG INTERACTIONS

Patients admitted to a CODs unit will not only have both classic psychiatric disorders *and* SUDs, but many will also have medical complications of these illnesses; thus, multiple medications are often utilized in their treatment and detoxification. The potential for clinically significant drug–drug interactions is ever present. Even top physicians cannot know every potential drug–drug interaction; it appears that the best practice is to have a system in place to alert the medical doctor to the probability and severity of potential pharmacological interactions. Pharmacy software programs now routinely alert the nursing and physician staff to potential problems; if properly implemented, they may improve patient safety.

Computer-assisted monitoring of known potential drug–drug interactions is ideally suited to supplement but not supplant physician knowledge of pharmacology and careful monitoring of patients' response to the medications introduced. In addition to the very specific knowledge of whether a medicine induces or inhibits a particular cytochrome system and how this will affect the next medication's efficacy and toxicity, the more general clinical evaluation of the patient's global condition must be considered. For example, because a small number of patients in France had lethal respiratory depression when intravenous buprenorphine was combined with intravenous high-potency benzodiazepines, many computer programs and pharmacological review papers will caution about the combination of oral benzodiazepines with sublingual buprenorphine; in fact, there are very few clinical problems reported with this commonly used combination. However, the patient's overall clinical status must be carefully considered. The combination of benzodiazepines and buprenorphine in patients taking methadone is particularly dangerous. Patients who are grossly sedated from other causes, such as alcohol intoxication, should be administered benzodiazepines and buprenorphine with caution.

Many Web sites are available where medical staff may access data regarding drug–drug interactions. Two Web sites popular at the time of this writing are http://www.uptodate.com and http://www.epocrates.org.

Psychotherapies

Relationships formed with treatment staff can be among the most powerful experiences the patient has in treatment, because they provide an opportunity for patients to learn to share uncomfortable thoughts and emotions and to build deeper relationships. A strong therapeutic relationship can also assist in the management of the unit milieu by building trust and promoting a feeling of safety. Patients are often uncomfortable and even irritable when they enter treatment and will better respond to someone with whom they have a positive relationship. There may be some concern over staffing constraints, but individual sessions can be brief and still yield positive results.

COGNITIVE-BEHAVIORAL THERAPY

Cognitive-behavioral therapy (CBT) has been shown to be effective in the treatment of many disorders, including addiction, depression, and anxiety. The basic premise of CBT is that our thoughts result in emotional responses that, in turn, motivate behavior. If thoughts are negative or irrational, then the result will be negative emotions and problematic behavior. CBT, offered in individual sessions or in groups, can help patients to identify situations that trigger irrational thinking and negative emotions. Once the antecedents to the behavior have been identified by the patient, the work will focus on assisting the patient in cognitive restructuring. Beck's cognitive therapy, although it focuses more on changing thoughts rather than behaviors, is a similar model (National Institute on Drug Abuse 1998).

Analyzing the consequences of the problem behavior is also an important part of the process. Patients often have a difficult time understanding why they continue to behave in ways that cause problems. Teaching patients to identify the consequences of their behavior reinforces why they continue to engage in behaviors that have negative consequences for them. It also allows them to begin to think about finding healthier ways to produce similar positive results. Finally, identifying negative consequences of the behavior serves as a way to motivate change; however, one of the main goals of CBT is to facilitate the patient's access to positive alternatives.

CBT for CODs may involve helping patients to relearn new responses to cues for substance abuse and may include coping skills training, because substance abuse is often indicative of poor coping skills (Kadden 2003). In the Matching Alcoholism Treatments to Client Heterogeneity ("Project MATCH") study, outpatients preferred CBT over motivational enhancement and 12-Step therapies (Donovan et al. 2002). Dual-focus schema therapy (24-week manual-guided CBT model with integrated relapse prevention and targeted intervention) shows promise for treating individuals with co-occurring substance abuse and personality disorders (Ball 1998). A CBT training manual is available from the Project MATCH study (Kadden et al. 1992).

MOTIVATIONAL INTERVIEWING OR MOTIVATIONAL ENHANCEMENT THERAPY

Motivational interviewing and motivational enhancement therapy (MET) have also been used to treat patients with CODs. Essentially, motivational interviewing is meeting the client where he or she is in terms of readiness to change, and working with the person to resolve any ambivalence. One might use a "pros and cons" list, for example. MET, a time-limited, adapted form of motivational interviewing, can also be integrated into group therapies. A group designed to enhance motivation might look at positive consequences of remaining sober compared with the negative consequences of substance abuse. Either approach can be used in conjunction with CBT, for example, in a phased approach, using motivational interviewing first, until the patient is sufficiently motivated for the work of CBT (National Institute on Drug Abuse 1998). In a study with psychiatric and dually diagnosed inpatients, those from both groups who received motivational interviewing in addition to standard treatment were more likely to attend their first outpatient appointment (Swanson et al. 1999). This approach involves better and more frequent measurement of readiness to change and stages of change in addictions treatment. It may therefore be helpful in matching treatment plans to individual patient needs (DiClemente et al. 2004). MET enjoyed high patient satisfaction rates in the Project MATCH study (Donovan et al. 2002), and as with CBT, training manuals are available (Miller et al. 1992).

CONTINGENCY MANAGEMENT

Contingency management can also be added as an adjunct to standard treatment, and it has been shown to improve abstinence rates (Prendergast et al. 2006). This approach involves providing incentives or vouchers to the patient for success; incentives may include cash, prizes, privileges, and other rewards for meeting treatment goals. Contingency management seeks to identify specific goals for achievement, such as group attendance, drug abstinence, continuing to take medicines, and other clinically significant progress. Use of contingency management or its addition to standard treatment may be helpful for patients with a wide range of psychiatric conditions (Weinstock et al. 2007)

as well as those for whom other therapies have failed (Petry et al. 2001).

RELAPSE PREVENTION THERAPY

Relapse prevention therapy (RPT; Weiss et al. 1999) is a type of psychotherapy focused specifically on relapse prevention; it combines several different elements, overlaps with skills-training methods (Kadden 2003), and is distinct from relapse prevention, an important component of any treatment plan. Research has shown mixed results for RPT as a psychosocial treatment for substance abuse. It appears to be better than no treatment, but there is less evidence to suggest that it is any *better* than other treatments for long-term results (Schmitz et al. 2004). Most studies, however, support the use of RPT for smoking cessation (Carroll 1996). If RPT is used, it may be most helpful as an adjunct to standard treatment.

DIALECTICAL BEHAVIOR THERAPY

Dialectical behavior therapy's (DBT) ability to address affect dysregulation may have significant potential for helping patients with CODs, such as individuals with PTSD and comorbid substance abuse. Research in this area has been scant. However, DBT has been shown to be more effective than treatment as usual for patients with drug dependence and borderline personality disorder, as evidenced by greater reductions in drug abuse, improvement in treatment retention, and greater gains in global and social adjustment at follow-ups (Linehan et al. 1999). For heroin-dependent women with borderline personality disorder, DBT appears to be effective in reducing opioid abuse, maintaining reductions in use, and improving the accuracy of self-reported substance abuse (Linehan et al. 2002).

SUPPORTIVE PSYCHOTHERAPY

Supportive psychotherapy, which typically follows a strengths-based perspective, is often useful for establishing a strong therapeutic alliance, which can be difficult in patients with CODs. It may be helpful for beginning to build healthy coping skills even in resistant patients (Winston et al. 2004). Supportive psychotherapy can be integrated with other therapeutic methods, such as motivational interviewing, MET, or RPT.

OTHER THERAPIES AND CONCLUDING POINTS

Interpersonal psychotherapy follows an exploratory approach, aiming to connect substance use to deficits in interpersonal functioning. In this approach, substance abuse is a symptom of other problems, so therapy may not address SUDs as directly as other therapies (National Institute on Drug Abuse 1998). Interpersonal therapy has been reviewed positively for the treatment of psychiatric illnesses and has been adapted for use in groups, but it is not well studied for treating CODs or substance abuse (DiClemente et al. 2003).

Similarly, psychodynamic therapy and rational emotive therapy have received mixed results in substance abusing populations and are not currently recommended for the treatment of SUDs (DiClemente et al. 2003).

Marital and family therapy, however, shows significant promise in the treatment of substance abuse and CODs. Behavioral couples therapy has been shown to be effective for treating SUDs, reducing the cost of treatment and improving clinical outcomes as well as psychosocial consequences of problematic substance use (Fals-Stewart et al. 1997). Because therapeutic approaches may vary and different therapies may be used in marital and family therapy, additional research is needed to determine which models are most effective for patients with CODs.

Researchers in the Project MATCH study found that patient satisfaction with the mode of therapy is associated with higher levels of attendance, greater reductions in problematic substance abuse, and improved outcomes at the conclusion of treatment (Donovan et al. 2002). Echoing the concerns of the Center for Mental Health Services and the Institute of Medicine, research suggests that successful treatment requires well-integrated therapeutic programming that addresses a patient's stages of change and readiness to change as well as the relationship between SUDs and other psychiatric disorders. Individualized treatment plans, highly skilled staff, and flexible clinical resources may improve clinical response to psychotherapies for patients with CODs.

Group Programming

SKILLS-BUILDING GROUPS

Patients with CODs have a variety of skills deficits, including social skills, leisure and vocational skills, and occasionally even the skills necessary to engage in the activities of daily living. Daily skills-building groups might include assertiveness training, giving and receiving compliments, dealing with anger, time management, goal setting, leisure skills, and developing healthy alternatives. Group and individual time should also focus on assisting patients to become more proficient in activities of daily living.

ACTIVITY GROUPS

Weaving in a variety of activities for patients is helpful in several ways. It provides a model for practicing healthy alternatives, serves as a way for patients to be exposed to social situations, fosters group cohesiveness, and allows for stress reduction. Some examples of group activities might include meditation, yoga, art therapy, recovery games, and various exercise groups.

SPIRITUALITY GROUPS

Dealing with spiritual issues is an important aspect of recovery. The limited research available on religion and spirituality in addictions treatment supports the widely accepted notion that spirituality and religious involvement are strong protective factors against substance abuse and dependence and that addressing spirituality in substance abuse treatment may improve outcomes for many patients (Miller 1998). Spirituality may also successfully reach some of the most challenging clients in substance abuse treatment; inner-city drug users, for example, found a Buddhist-based, spirituality-focused therapy helpful for increasing motivation (Beitel et al. 2007).

Spiritual needs of people with CODs vary depending on the diagnoses. People with SUDs often benefit from talking about relationships, core values, and hopes for the future. Most have witnessed themselves behaving in ways that do not match what they truly believe is right. Many patients describe guilt and shame related to this or related to their behaviors or to their illness in general. However, needs may differ significantly among different diagnoses. People with schizophrenia, for example, may be less focused on relationship building and more focused on being part of a safe, accepting, and compassionate environment.

12-STEP GROUPS

12-Step groups, such as Alcoholics Anonymous (AA) and Narcotics Anonymous (NA) enjoy a well-deserved reputation for their effectiveness in reducing substance abuse (Humphreys 2003). Inpatient settings, such as the CODs unit, offer a valuable opportunity to introduce patients to these groups as well as to support continued involvement with the groups following a relapse. 12-Step groups enjoyed high patient satisfaction ratings in the Project MATCH study (Donovan et al. 2002), and manuals for staff training are readily available (Nowinski et al. 1992). Attendance at self-help meetings is a critical component of membership in 12-Step groups, and these communities can form a supportive social network for patients to support continued abstinence following discharge.

Critics of 12-Step groups have identified some conflict between what patients learn about their behaviors in the groups and what they learn in CBT (National Institute on Drug Abuse 1998). In the 12-Step model, addiction is a disease over which the individual is powerless, whereas CBT teaches patients that addiction is a learned behavior that can be unlearned. Nonetheless, CBT and AA can be integrated into an effective relapse prevention plan by focusing on individual needs and goals. Patients should be aware that they may hear conflicting information regarding the use of psychotropic medication, because some individuals in recovery groups advocate complete and total abstinence from all psychotropic substances based on the assumption that total abstinence will alleviate psychological symptoms. This is rarely true for individuals with CODs, so patients should be fully informed about the nature of their illnesses prior to discharge. Despite limitations to 12-Step groups and other self-help models, many patients credit them with improved abstinence from relapse.

EDUCATION GROUPS

Education groups should include illness education for the CODs, medication education, nutrition education, and information about available community supports. Providing education can result in increased understanding and awareness, can assist patients in feeling more control around managing their illness, and may decrease shame and guilt. Techniques to enhance motivation and awareness are particularly useful.

OTHER GROUPS

Other groups that may be included in the therapeutic programming of a CODs unit include CBT groups, family education and support groups, relapse management and prevention groups, and discharge preparedness groups. Aspects of these groups are addressed elsewhere in this book.

Risk Management and Safety

There are many safety issues that arise on a CODs unit, including suicidal behavior, use of illicit drugs, unstable psychiatric symptoms, and aggressive behavior. It is important to have procedures in place to monitor patient activity and status. An observation status reflecting the patient's level of functioning and potential risk should be ordered by the physician and monitored by staff. The observation status should be reviewed at least daily and changed when there is a significant change in risk factors. There should be a plan in place for dealing with patients found in possession of illicit drugs. Discharge is sometimes an option but may not be possible if the patient has an unstable COD. The Web site for the Substance Abuse and Mental Health Services Administration's Center for Excellence in the treatment of CODs (www.coce.samhsa.gov) has numerous resources to assist unit administrators in implementing sound risk management practices on the CODs unit.

Suicide

The risk of patient suicide is a serious concern for clinicians on the CODs unit. Suicide risk assessments are a requirement for accreditation by the Joint Commission (2008). Individuals with CODs often have numerous markers for suicide risk, and these risk factors may compound one another, particularly in interactions between certain psychiatric diagnoses and specific types of substance abuse. Knowing the risk factors may improve the accuracy of a risk assessment, allowing clinicians to identify and monitor those patients most at risk and to select interventions that address patients' needs, thereby minimizing the risk of suicide as well as reducing the need for seclusion or restraint.

Affective disorders carry a 15% lifetime risk of suicide and compose 50%–70% of completed suicides; the high-risk profile includes anxiety or panic symptoms or moderate alcohol abuse (Jacobs et al. 1999). Schizophrenia carries a 10% lifetime risk of suicide and accounts for 10%–15% of completed suicides; the high-risk profile is a formerly high-functioning person or the presence of depressive symptoms (Jacobs et al. 1999). SUDs carry a 2%–3% lifetime risk of suicide and account for 15%–25% of completed suicides; the high-risk profile includes interpersonal loss or comorbid depression (Jacobs et al. 1999). Additionally, "[s]ubstance abuse is associated with greater frequency and repetitiveness of suicide attempts, more medically lethal attempts, more serious suicidal intent, and higher levels of suicidal ideation" (Moscicki 1999, p. 47). Cocaine abuse is a contributor to completed suicide and a risk factor for attempted suicide (Moscicki 1999).

Alcohol abuse increases the risk of suicide in both alcoholic and nonalcoholic persons. Up to 50% of individuals who commit suicide were drinking at or near the time of death, and 89% of alcoholic persons who commit suicide were drinking at the time of their suicide (Jacobs et al. 1999). In suicides where multiple substance abuse is involved, alcohol is the substance most frequently found (Moscicki 1999). Alcohol misuse is a well-known risk factor for suicide for all age groups, including the elderly (Waern 2003) and youth (Moscicki 1999). Adverse consequences of alcohol misuse on the life course of a patient are common during the last months of life in alcoholic persons who complete suicide (Pirkola et al. 2000). Future suicide attempts in alcohol-dependent patients are more common when the patient has the following risk factors (Preuss et al. 2003):

- Prior suicide attempts
- Younger age
- Separated or divorced
- Other drug dependence
- Substance-induced psychiatric disorders
- Indicators of a more severe course of alcoholism

Regarding the effect of alcohol abuse on suicide risk, Brady (2006) wrote:

> There is evidence to suggest alcohol misuse predisposes to suicidal behavior through its depressogenic effects and promotion of adverse life events, and both behaviors may share a common genetic predisposition. Acute alcohol use can also precipitate suicidal behaviors through induction of negative affect and impairment of problem-solving skills, as well as aggravation of impulsive personality traits, possibly through effects on serotonergic neurotransmission. (p. 473)

Comorbid factors increase risk level and can potentially interact to compound risk. Comorbid mood disorders and SUDs are associated with an increased lethality risk (Moscicki 1999). Furthermore, research has uncovered strong evidence suggesting a possible genetic link to suicide attempts among persons with alcohol dependence (Hesselbrock et al. 2004), recurrent early onset depression (Zubenko et al. 2004), and bipolar disorder (Willour et al. 2007), underscoring the importance of obtaining a thorough family history during the evaluation and risk assessment.

General risk factors for suicide, such as family history of completed suicide, still apply equally to patients with CODs. It is therefore important for clinicians to follow general risk-management guidelines for suicidal patients, taking into consideration the additional risk factors specific to the patient's particular diagnoses and individual situation. One should also consider the risk of suicide postdischarge, inquire about availability of lethal means (such as firearms), provide psychoeducation to patients and family members about the increased risk of suicidality if the patient relapses, and provide phone numbers to call in the event of a relapse or other warning signs.

Successful treatment of SUDs and comorbid psychiatric illness reduces the risk of suicidal behavior, in part by reducing two of the major risk factors for suicide. Unit supervisors and other clinicians seeking to improve the management of suicidal patients will find the American Psychiatric Association's practice guidelines and the Center for Substance Abuse Treatment's TIPs especially helpful. TIP 42 includes a section devoted especially to management of suicidality in patients with CODs. The CODs unit staff must be aware of the increased suicide risk among patients with CODs and must implement a correspondingly higher level of safeguards on the inpatient unit than is found in residential facilities or social-setting detoxification. Such safeguards might include quality improvement efforts targeting environment-of-care issues, lower staff-to-patient ratios, and 24-hour coverage by registered nurses, among others.

Violence

The treatment and prevention of violence is of utmost importance in the care of patients with CODs. Active CODs increase the risk of violence (Scott et al. 1998), so risk assessments and measures to manage potentially violent patients should be firmly in place on any unit treating patients with SUDs. Generally speaking, the greater the number of comorbid diagnoses, the greater the risk of violence. A comorbid SUD was found in three-quarters of mentally ill homicide offenders, and the presence of a "triple diagnosis" (involving antisocial personality disorder, psychotic mental illness, and SUD) was found in roughly half of all homicide offenders with a psychotic illness (Putkonen et al. 2004).

Beyond the "triple diagnosis" red flag, clinicians should learn to recognize additional risk factors that may increase the risk of violence in patients on the CODs unit. These other risk factors may include higher drinking levels, younger age, minority status, and the interaction of alcohol and cocaine (Chermack and Blow 2002) as well as DTs, phencyclidine intoxication, cocaine-induced paranoia, amphetamine abuse, flunitrazepam (Rohypnol) intoxication, psychosis, and agitation. Alcohol abuse is associated with increased severity in violence and resulting injuries (Martin and Bachman 1997) and is frequently involved in family violence and child abuse (Yudko et al. 1997). Among early onset drinkers (i.e., problematic drinking before age 20 years), "low plasma levels of tryptophan—a precursor of 5-HT—were associated with high levels of depression and aggression" (Pettinati et al. 2003, p. 254). Patients with both cocaine and alcohol abuse have higher rates of criminal behavior, including violent aggression (Denison et al. 1997), and among patients in substance abuse treatment, violence perpetration is associated with alcohol and cocaine abuse (Chermack and Blow 2002). The abuse of flunitrazepam, especially when used in conjunction with other substance abuse, such as alcohol, amphetamines, or cannabis, is associated with a marked risk for severely violent criminal behavior as well as impaired reasoning and empathy (Dåderman et al. 2002).

Among persons with severe mental illness, three variables were found to have a cumulative association with the risk of violent behavior: previous victimization by violence, the presence of violence in the surrounding environment, and substance abuse (Swanson et al. 2002). Mental illness per se is not a reliable predictor of violent behavior (Corrigan and Watson 2005), but substance abuse is associated with an increased rate of violence in both mentally ill and non–mentally ill persons (Steadman et al. 1998). Such violence is most frequently targeted at family members and friends and occurs most often at home (Steadman et al. 1998).

Given these troubling facts, clinicians must also consider the risk of violence postdischarge and should incorporate a risk assessment and reduction plan in the discharge planning if a risk of violence is present. Additional caution is warranted if a patient is known to have been violent in the past or on the unit, or if he or she has shown warning signs for violent behavior. Violent behavior in the previous year significantly predicted suicide, independent of alcohol misuse history (Conner et al. 2001). Violence prevention may also perform a dual function, also reducing the risk of suicide. Clinicians must remain conscious of the legal duty to warn or to protect known intended victims of potentially violent patients. This duty is articulated in the oft-cited case of *Tarasoff v. Regents of the University of California* (1976), in which a troubled young man had expressed to his therapist his intention to kill a young woman; he subsequently followed through on these threats, and the girl's family sued numerous parties involved in the case.

Discharge planning and risk assessments should take into account not only the potential for violence perpetration but also the patient's prior history and current risk of violence victimization. Trauma and victimization are risk factors for substance abuse and relapse, and rates of violence victimization are likely to be high among patients treated on a CODs unit. Patients with CODs experience higher rates of violence victimization than individuals with only a psychiatric

or only a substance use diagnosis (Sells et al. 2003). Women with co-occurring schizophrenia and SUDs, for example, are at increased risk for violent victimization and HIV (Gearon and Bellack 1999). Intimate partner violence is highly prevalent and frequently bidirectional among suicidal psychiatric inpatients, many of whom have CODs such as depression and alcohol abuse (Heru et al. 2006). As noted elsewhere in this chapter, patients with CODs often misuse substances due to a lack of healthy coping skills. Poor conflict resolution and poor anger management, combined with maladaptive substance use (likely leading to disinhibition), often contribute to the escalation of conflict and aggression in relationships of persons with CODs, which can further complicate the recovery process. The inpatient stay can be an ideal time to introduce patients and, possibly, their families, to conflict management skills and proper anger management. Standardized, manual-guided group treatment resources are available from numerous sources.

Evidence suggests that successful clinical treatment substantially reduces the risk of violence in substance-abusing patients, possibly by decreasing patient agitation and escalation. Integrating a contingency management model (token economy) for dually diagnosed patients within an acute inpatient psychiatric ward was found to result in decreased violence and increased patient participation in group activities (Franco et al. 1995). Treatment for alcohol dependence has been found to result in significantly decreased levels of intimate partner violence perpetrated both by individuals in treatment and by their partners (Stuart et al. 2003). For patients with CODs and a history of trauma, not only integrating treatments for psychiatric diagnosis and substance abuse diagnosis but also addressing trauma issues may improve clinical outcomes (Morrissey et al. 2005).

Seclusion and restraint should be used only as a remedy of last resort, when attempts to de-escalate a patient through other clinical means have failed or when there is imminent risk of physical harm to the patient or to others on the unit. To minimize the risk of violence, as well as reduce the use of seclusion and restraint, clinicians should carefully monitor the patient's treatment to ensure that clinical needs are met before agitation escalates.

Discharge Against Medical Advice

Discharge against medical advice is a frequent problem in the treatment of patients with co-occurring SUDs and psychiatric illness. Criteria for holding a patient with CODs should match that of the general psychiatric inpatient population. If the patient presents an acute risk to self or to others, involuntary commitment for safety should be considered. The patient (and his or her family, if possible) should be fully informed of the risks associated with a discharge against medical advice. If involuntary commitment is not an option, a 24-hour observation period is usually reasonable for patients with CODs; however, state law varies by jurisdiction, and unit supervisors should be aware of the governing law and legal rights of psychiatric patients. In the event that a patient discharges him- or herself against medical advice, clinicians should record in the patient's chart the reasons for the patient's release and the rationale for recommending against discharge.

Discharge Planning

The goal of discharge planning is to secure for the patient ongoing integrated treatment, supported by diagnosis-specific interventions. Effective treatment for dually diagnosed patients requires "a comprehensive, long-term, staged approach to recovery; assertive outreach; motivational interventions; provision of help to clients in acquiring skills and supports to manage both illnesses and to pursue functional goals; and cultural sensitivity and competence" (Drake et al. 2001, p. 469). Once the psychiatric condition is stable, partial hospital and individual outpatient provider levels of care can be useful as a stepdown option for people with COD, because they provide opportunities to practice healthy coping skills in the context of the person's own environment. The experience of having the support of a treatment program while working on recovery in a natural environment can help decrease denial about the challenges of the recovery process, increase awareness of trigger situations, improve self-confidence, and offer an opportunity for people to discuss alternatives that are working as well as those they may need to change. Medications can be monitored closely and adjusted as needed for both the SUD and any psychiatric disorder.

When planning outpatient follow-up care, there are several things to consider. Most often there will be a need for both an outpatient psychiatrist and a therapist or case manager. It is helpful to establish patient preference as to location, type of therapy and gender of the therapist. Transportation problems and any financial restrictions that might interfere with follow-through should be resolved prior to making a referral. If the patient already has an outpatient clinician, it is important to make contact when the patient arrives in the program in order to gather assessment information, and, at discharge, to review the course of treatment and outstanding issues to be addressed by the outpatient therapist.

Follow-up planning and patient placement can become a challenge when working with people who have CODs, especially if they require long-term residential placement. Most residential programs are set up to work with either addictions patients or psychiatric patients, but rarely both. Addictions facilities may not have staff members trained to work with CODs or may not be able to cope with the multiple problems that can arise out of an exacerbation of the psychiatric condition. Medication management sometimes becomes an issue as well. In some cases, addressing the patient's CODs conflicts with the treatment philosophy of the program itself. On the other hand, facilities working with patients with psychiatric illnesses may not feel comfortable accepting addictions patients for fear of relapse and the impact of potential substance use on the premises.

For patients with hostility and more severe dimensional psychiatric symptoms, retention in long-term treatment programs is difficult because they are at higher risk for dropping out. For these patients, on-site mental health services in long-term residential programs seem to improve retention rates (Broome et al. 1999). Fortunately, there appears to be growing support for progressive models such as Assertive Community Treatment, which can be useful for delivering integrated treatment (Essock et al. 2006), and the Community Reinforcement Approach (Meyers and Miller 2001). The latter may be a component of outpatient discharge planning and sometimes includes contingency management approaches as well as a variety of counseling services, including vocational counseling, drug refusal training, and behavioral skills (National Institute on Drug Abuse 1998).

For individuals with CODs, sustained employment is often viewed as a benchmark of successful treatment. Moreover, working has been correlated with long-term improvements in self-esteem, self-confidence, and feelings about life in general among adults with severe mental illness (Salyers et al. 2004). In a study of veterans with severe SUDs in a partial hospitalization program, Kerrigan et al. (2000) found that returning to work was correlated with completion of an alcohol or drug treatment program, placement in supported sober housing, and participation in work therapy. Individual placement and support has shown some promise for improving employment and housing outcomes for homeless veterans with psychiatric or substance use disorders (Rosenheck and Mares 2007). Because financial difficulties and unstructured time are known risk factors for individuals with CODs, helping patients to obtain and retain gainful employment is an important goal of treatment. Incorporating referrals to vocational rehabilitation or supported employment into the discharge plan may help to sustain treatment gains achieved during the inpatient stay. For placement to be effective, however, it must be tailored to the individual patient's needs and preferences (Becker et al. 2005).

Leaving the hospital can be a frightening event for patients. Length of stay is typically short and focused on crisis stabilization. Patients may be entering unfamiliar facilities after discharge or may face severe psychosocial difficulties, such as family dysfunction or homelessness. In addition to presenting options for follow-up, groups or clinical discussions about the patient's discharge preparedness should include discussion regarding the emotional aspects of leaving the safety of the hospital, what it might be like to enter a new treatment environment, and fear of relapsing to the addiction and/or other illness.

Relapse Management and Prevention

During inpatient treatment the patient should be assisted in developing an individualized relapse prevention plan. For each high-risk situation, ideally the patient should have a corresponding plan of action. Teaching patients to anticipate high-risk situations and to problem-solve ways to deal with them can decrease the risk of impulsive responses and falling back on dysfunctional coping mechanisms. Education should be provided about the various community self-help programs, such as AA, NA, Double Trouble, and Gamblers Anonymous, so these groups may be incorporated into the overall relapse prevention plan.

Although it would be wonderful if prevention were the only issue related to relapse, clinicians must acknowledge the reality that people often do slip back into old patterns before making a successful change. The symptoms of psychiatric illnesses can return through no fault of the patient, and a relapse management plan coupled with an ongoing treatment program can make the difference in the opportunity for early intervention. Among substance abusers, individuals with earlier onset of substance abuse and those with comorbid psychiatric disorders (particularly major depression) are more likely to relapse (Landheim et al. 2006). It is important to help people understand the importance of taking positive action in the event of

a slip or exacerbation of illness. Helping patients to recognize the difficulty of change can help remove some of the irrational thoughts, guilt, and shame that occur after relapse. People are often self-critical after relapse, and such thinking may actually reinforce the relapse rather than prompt help-seeking behaviors.

Relapse prevention discussions should focus on helping the patient to recognize early warning signs of relapse and to develop an action plan should they occur. For example, staff may educate patients about depression and how it can recur; early recognition and treatment of depressive symptoms may help the patient to avert a relapse to substance abuse. It is useful to talk about the difficulty of change and the importance of building a support network, especially in early recovery. Relapse management and prevention can be dealt with successfully in the group setting when resources and time are limited, as is often the case on the acute inpatient unit.

When possible, family members should be included in the relapse prevention plan. Family members should be aware of triggers and symptoms in order to assist the patient in relapse prevention, and families should agree on how to respond to warning signs of an impending relapse. The patient and family members also need to reach an agreement as to what the family should do if a relapse does occur. Discussing and reaching an agreement beforehand can help family members to feel less conflicted if, for example, they need to call a treatment provider following a relapse.

Patient and Family Education

Although it is difficult enough for someone to come to terms with having a chronic illness of any kind, having CODs comes with an additional challenge. Although much has improved through the years, there still remains a certain stigma attached to both SUDs and other psychiatric disorders. These misconceptions, biases, and judgments may be held by community members, family, staff, and even the patient him- or herself. Community and family support is important in the recovery process for both addictions and psychiatric disorders. Families can be of great help to the patient, and most would like to be. They may not always know exactly how to help and may, in fact, react in ways that have the opposite result they intended. For patients experiencing family conflict, clinicians should consider the possibility that intimate partner or other family violence may be occurring. The link between substance abuse and such violence is well established, but families may need help to recognize the importance of addressing family conflict and the fact that treatment for substance abuse and mental illness can also help to reduce violence within the family. Illness education and a support system for the family can make a big difference in the ability of the family to provide support to the person in recovery and to participate effectively in a relapse prevention plan.

It has been shown that including families in treatment produces positive outcomes in the treatment of addictions. It is not always possible to meet individually with every family in a short-term acute inpatient setting. Family education and support groups offer an excellent opportunity for families to come together and receive information and to network with other families. Meeting families who are experiencing similar challenges can be very healing. Families of patients with psychiatric illnesses often feel different and can become isolated from others. Introduction to community supports, such as the National Alliance on Mental Illness, AA, Al-Anon, and other groups for both patients and family members can be reviewed in a group setting.

Patient and family education is a critical component of discharge planning. Families can be very helpful in recognizing a patient's triggers and symptoms of relapse, and they can also help to reinforce adherence to a treatment plan. When a patient shows signs of relapse or noncompliance, families can notify treatment teams and arrange for crisis intervention when necessary. Beyond merely *educating* patients and families, experts also call for the *involvement* of patients and families in designing and overseeing service delivery to patients with CODs, including activities such as serving on quality improvement teams (Center for Mental Health Services Managed Care Initiative 1997).

Conclusion

The successful CODs unit assists patients undergoing a very difficult process of change for both psychiatric and substance-use disorders. Most units provide detoxification services as well as some psychotherapy and group activities. Treatment plans should be individualized and should address the patient's substance misuse, psychiatric illness, and the relationship between the CODs. Psychopharmacology for patients with CODs can be particularly challenging, as there are numerous risk factors to consider. Electronic tools and evidence-based treatment protocols help to reduce the risk of adverse events. It is important for clinical staff on the CODs unit to act cohesively as a team to identify early warning signs and to mitigate risks re-

lated to suicide, violence, and discharge against medical advice.

An inpatient stay on a CODs unit is a crucial event in the life of a patient with both psychiatric illness and substance abuse and can be conceptualized as a transition point in the recovery process. Treatment teams on CODs units work together to enable patients to progress toward the next level of care while minimizing the risk of relapse. During hospitalization, patients begin to build the skills, knowledge, and motivation to abstain from substance misuse and to maintain gains achieved toward better psychiatric outcomes. The goals of treatment in a CODs unit are twofold: simultaneous resolution of medical and psychological crises, so that patients may progress toward lasting, stable change.

References

American Psychiatric Association: Practice guideline for the assessment and treatment of patients with suicidal behaviors. Am J Psychiatry 160 (suppl):1–60, 2003

American Psychiatric Association: Practice guideline for the treatment of patients with substance use disorders. Am J Psychiatry 164 (suppl):1–124, 2007

American Society of Addiction Medicine: Patient Placement Criteria for the Treatment of Substance-Related Disorders, 2nd Edition, Revised. Chevy Chase, MD, American Society of Addiction Medicine, 2001

Ashton H: The diagnosis and management of benzodiazepine dependence. Curr Opin Psychiatry 18:249–255, 2005

Ball SA: Manualized treatment for substance abusers with personality disorders: dual focus schema therapy. Addict Behav 23:883–891, 1998

Barrowclough C, Haddock G, Tarrier N, et al: Randomized controlled trial of motivational interviewing, cognitive behavior therapy, and family intervention for patients with comorbid schizophrenia and substance use disorders. Am J Psychiatry 158:1706–1713, 2001

Becker DR, Drake RE, Naughton WJ Jr: Supported employment for people with co-occurring disorders. Psychiatr Rehabil J 28:332–338, 2005

Beitel M, Genova M, Schuman-Olivier Z, et al: Reflections by inner-city drug users on a Buddhist-based spirituality-focused therapy: a qualitative study. Am J Orthopsychiatry 77:1–9, 2007

Bellack AS, Bennett ME, Gearon JS, et al: A randomized clinical trial of a new behavioral treatment for drug abuse in people with severe and persistent mental illness. Arch Gen Psychiatry 63:426–432, 2006

Brady J: The association between alcohol misuse and suicidal behavior. Alcohol Alcohol 41:473–478, 2006

Brady KT, Sonne SC, Roberts JM: Sertraline treatment of comorbid posttraumatic stress disorder and alcohol dependence. J Clin Psychiatry 56:502–505, 1995

Broome KM, Flynn PM, Simpson DD: Psychiatric comorbidity measures as predictors of retention in drug abuse treatment programs. Health Serv Res 34:791–806, 1999

Brown PJ, Recupero PR, Stout R: PTSD substance abuse comorbidity and treatment utilization. Addict Behav 20:251–254, 1995

Brunette MF, Mueser KT: Psychosocial interventions for the long-term management of patients with severe mental illness and co-occurring substance use disorder. J Clin Psychiatry 67 (suppl):10–17, 2006

Burant D: Management of withdrawal, in Review Course Syllabus. Edited by Wilford BB. New York, American Society of Addiction Medicine, 1990, pp 173–194

Carroll KM: Relapse prevention as a psychosocial treatment: a review of controlled clinical trials. Exp Clin Psychopharmacol 4:46–54, 1996

Center for Mental Health Services Managed Care Initiative: Co-Occurring Psychiatric and Substance Disorders in Managed Care Systems: Standards of Care, Practice Guidelines, Workforce Competencies, and Training Curricula. Rockville, MD, Center for Mental Health Services, 1997

Center for Substance Abuse Treatment: Substance Abuse Treatment for Persons With Co-Occurring Disorders. Treatment Improvement Protocol (TIP) Series 42. DHHS Publication No. (SMA) 05-3992. Rockville, MD, Substance Abuse and Mental Health Services Administration, 2005

Center for Substance Abuse Treatment: Detoxification and Substance Abuse Treatment. Treatment Improvement Protocol (TIP) Series 45. DHHS Publication No. (SMA) 06-4131. Rockville, MD, Substance Abuse and Mental Health Services Administration, 2006

Chance JF: Emergency department treatment of alcohol withdrawal seizures with phenytoin. Ann Emerg Med 20:520–522, 1991

Charney DA, Paraherakis AM, Gill KJ: Integrated treatment of comorbid depression and substance use disorders. J Clin Psychiatry 62:672–677, 2001

Chermack ST, Blow FC: Violence among individuals in substance abuse treatment: the role of alcohol and cocaine consumption. Drug Alcohol Depend 66:29–37, 2002

Coffey SF, Dansky SB, Carrigan MH, et al: Acute and protracted cocaine abstinence in an outpatient population: a prospective study of mood, sleep and withdrawal symptoms. Drug Alcohol Depend 59:277–286, 2000

Conner KR, Cox C, Duberstein PR, et al: Violence, alcohol, and completed suicide: a case-control study. Am J Psychiatry 158:1701–1705, 2001

Corcos M, Nezelof S, Speranza M, et al: Psychoactive substance consumption in eating disorders. Eat Behav 2:27–38, 2001

Cornelius JR, Bukstein O, Salloum I, et al: Alcohol and psychiatric comorbidity, in Recent Developments in Alcoholism, Vol 16: Research on Alcoholism Treatment. Edited by Galanter M. New York, Kluwer Academic/Plenum, 2003, pp 362–374

Corrigan PW, Watson AC: Findings from the national comorbidity survey on the frequency of violent behavior in individuals with psychiatric disorders. Psychiatry Res 136:153–162, 2005

Cottler LB, Shillington AM, Compton WM III, et al: Subjective reports of withdrawal among cocaine users: recommendations for DSM-IV. Drug Alcohol Depend 33:97–104, 1993

Cramer MA: Under the influence of unconscious process: countertransference in the treatment of PTSD and substance abuse in women. Am J Psychother 56:194–210, 2002

D'Souza DC: Cannabinoids and psychosis. Int Rev Neurobiol 78:289–326, 2007

Dåderman AM, Fredriksson B, Kristiansson M, et al: Violent behavior, impulsive decision-making, and anterograde amnesia while intoxicated with flunitrazepam and alcohol or other drugs: a case study in forensic psychiatric patients. J Am Acad Psychiatry Law 30:238–251, 2002

Day E, Bentham P, Callaghan R, et al: Thiamine for Wernicke-Korsakoff syndrome in people at risk from alcohol abuse. Cochrane Database Syst Rev 1:CD004033, 2004

Denison ME, Pardes A, Booth JB: Alcohol and cocaine interactions and aggressive behaviors, in Recent Developments in Alcoholism, Vol 13: Alcohol and Violence. Edited by Galanter M. New York, Kluwer Academic/Plenum, 1997, pp 283–303

Dickinson WE, Mayo-Smith MF, Eickelberg SJ: Management of sedative-hypnotic intoxication and withdrawal, in Principles of Addiction Medicine, 3rd Edition. Edited by Graham AW, Schultz TK, Mayo-Smith MF, et al. Chevy Chase, MD, American Society of Addiction Medicine, 2003, pp 633–649

DiClemente CC, Haug N, Bellino L, et al: Psychotherapy and motivational enhancement, in Recent Developments in Alcoholism, Vol 16: Research on Alcoholism Treatment. Edited by Galanter M. New York, Kluwer Academic/Plenum, 2003, pp 115–132

DiClemente CC, Schlundt D, Gemmell L: Readiness and stages of change in addiction treatment. Am J Addict 13:103–119, 2004

Donovan DM, Kadden RM, DiClemente CC, et al: Client satisfaction with three therapies in the treatment of alcohol dependence: results from Project MATCH. Am J Addict 11:291–307, 2002

Drake RE, Yovetich NA, Bebout RR, et al: Integrated treatment for dually diagnosed homeless adults. J Nerv Ment Dis 185:298–305, 1997

Drake RE, Essock SM, Shaner A, et al: Implementing dual diagnosis services for clients with severe mental illness. Psychiatr Serv 52:469–476, 2001

Durazzo TC, Rothlind JC, Gazdzinski S, et al: Chronic smoking is associated with differential neurocognitive recovery in abstinent alcoholic patients: a preliminary investigation. Alcohol Clin Exp Res 31:1114–1127, 2007

el-Guebaly N, Cathcart J, Currie S, et al: Public health and therapeutic aspects of smoking bans in mental health and addiction settings. Psychiatr Serv 53:1617–1622, 2002

Essock SM, Mueser KT, Drake RE, et al: Comparison of ACT and standard case management for delivering integrated treatment for co-occurring disorders. Psychiatr Serv 57:185–196, 2006

Fals-Stewart W, O'Farrell TJ, Birchler GR: Behavioral couples therapy for male substance-abusing patients: a cost outcomes analysis. J Consult Clin Psychol 65:789–802, 1997

Ford JD, Russo E: Trauma-focused, present-centered, emotional self-regulation approach to integrated treatment for posttraumatic stress and addiction: Trauma Adaptive Recovery Group Education and Therapy (TARGET). Am J Psychother 60:335–355, 2006

Franco H, Galanter M, Castañeda R, et al: Comorbid behavioral and self-help approaches in the inpatient management of dually diagnosed patients. J Subst Abuse Treat 12:227–232, 1995

Galanter M, Kleber HD (eds): The American Psychiatric Press Textbook of Substance Abuse Treatment, 4th Edition. Washington, DC, American Psychiatric Press, 2008

Gearon JS, Bellack AS: Women with schizophrenia and co-occurring substance use disorders: an increased risk for violent victimization and HIV. Community Ment Health J 35:401–419, 1999

Goldstein RZ, Volkow ND: Drug addiction and its underlying neurobiological basis: neuroimaging evidence for the involvement of the frontal cortex. Am J Psychiatry 159:1642–1652, 2002

Graham K, Massak A: Alcohol consumption and the use of antidepressants. Can Med Assoc J 176:633–637, 2007

Green AI, Drake RE, Brunette MF, et al. Schizophrenia and co-occurring substance use disorder. Am J Psychiatry 164:402–408, 2007

Gulliver SB, Kamholz BW, Helstrom AW: Smoking cessation and alcohol abstinence: what do the data tell us? Alcohol Res Health 29:208–212, 2006

Heru AM, Stuart GL, Rainey S, et al: Prevalence and severity of intimate partner violence and associations with family functioning and alcohol abuse in psychiatric inpatients with suicidal intent. J Clin Psychiatry 67:23–29, 2006

Hesselbrock V, Dick D, Hesselbrock M, et al: The search for genetic risk factors associated with suicidal behavior. Alcohol Clin Exp Res 28 (suppl):70S–76S, 2004

Hilbon ME, Hjelm-Jager M: Should alcohol withdrawal seizures be treated with anti-epileptic drugs? Acta Neurol Scand 69:39–42, 1984

Humphreys K: Alcoholics Anonymous and 12-step alcoholism treatment programs, in Recent Developments in Alcoholism, Vol 16: Research on Alcoholism Treatment. Edited by Galanter M. New York, Kluwer Academic/Plenum, 2003, pp 149–164

Hunter SB, Watkins KE, Wenzel S, et al: Training substance abuse treatment staff to care for co-occurring disorders. J Subst Abuse Treat 28:239–245, 2005

Hurt RD, Offord KP, Croghan IT, et al: Mortality following inpatient addictions treatment: role of tobacco use in a community-based cohort. JAMA 275:1097–1103, 1996

Institute of Medicine Committee on Crossing the Quality Chasm: Adaptation to Mental Health and Addictive Disorders: Improving the Quality of Health Care for Mental and Substance-Use Conditions. Washington, DC, National Academies Press, 2006

Jacobs DG, Brewer M, Klein-Benheim M: Suicide assessment: an overview and recommended protocol, in The Harvard Medical School Guide to Suicide Assessment and Intervention. Edited by Jacobs DG. San Francisco, CA, Jossey-Bass, 1999, pp 3–39

Jeffery DP, Ley A, McLaren S, et al: Psychosocial treatment programmes for people with both severe mental illness and substance misuse. Cochrane Database Syst Rev 2:CD001088, 2000

Jerrell JM, Ridgely MS: Impact of robustness of program implementation on outcomes of clients in dual diagnosis programs. Psychiatr Serv 50:109–112, 1999

Joint Commission: 2008 National Patient Safety Goals: Behavioral Health Care Program. Available at: http://www.jointcommission.org/PatientSafety/NationalPatientSafetyGoals/08_bhc_npsgs.htm. Accessed April 2008.

Kadden RM: Behavioral and cognitive-behavioral treatments for alcoholism: research opportunities, in Recent Developments in Alcoholism, Vol 16: Research on Alcoholism Treatment. Edited by Galanter M. New York, Kluwer Academic/Plenum, 2003, pp 165–182

Kadden RM, Carrol KM, Donovan DM, et al: Cognitive Behavioral Coping Skills Therapy Manual: A Clinical Research Guide for Therapists Treating Individuals With Alcohol Abuse and Dependence (Project MATCH Monograph Series, Vol 3). Rockville, MD, National Institute on Alcohol Abuse and Alcoholism, 1992

Kerrigan AJ, Kaough JE, Wilson BL, et al: Vocational rehabilitation outcomes of veterans with substance use disorders in a partial hospitalization program. Psychiatr Serv 51:1570–1572, 2000

Kleber HD: Outpatient detoxification from opiates. Prim Psychiatry 1:42–52, 1996

Kleber HD: Opioids: detoxification, in The American Psychiatric Press Textbook of Substance Abuse Treatment, 2nd Edition. Edited by Galanter M, Kleber HD. Washington, DC, American Psychiatric Press, 1999, pp 251–270

Kosten TR, O'Connor PG: Management of drug and alcohol withdrawal. N Engl J Med 348:1786–1795, 2003

Landheim AS, Bakken K, Vaglum P: Impact of comorbid psychiatric disorders on the outcome of substance abusers: a six year prospective follow-up in two Norwegian counties. BMC Psychiatry 6:44, 2006

Laudet AB, Magura S, Vogel HS: Recovery challenges among dually diagnosed individuals. J Subst Abuse Treat 18:321–329, 2000

Linehan MM, Schmidt III H, Dimeff LA, et al: Dialectical behavior therapy for patients with borderline personality disorder and drug-dependence. Am J Addict 8:279–292, 1999

Linehan MM, Dimeff LA, Reynolds SK, et al: Dialectical behavior therapy versus comprehensive validation therapy plus 12-step for the treatment of opioid dependent women meeting criteria for borderline personality disorder. Drug Alcohol Depend 67:13–26, 2002

Lowinson JH, Ruiz P, Millman RB, et al. (eds): Substance Abuse: A Comprehensive Textbook, 4th Edition. Philadelphia, PA, Lippincott Williams & Wilkins, 2005

Malcolm R, Myrick H, Brady KT, et al: Update on anticonvulsants for the treatment of alcohol withdrawal. Am J Addict 10 (suppl):16–23, 2001

Martin SE, Bachman R: The relationship of alcohol to injury in assault cases, in Recent Developments in Alcoholism, Vol 13: Alcohol and Violence. Edited by Galanter M. New York, Kluwer Academic/Plenum, 1997, pp 41–56

McCorry F, Garnick DW, Bartlett J, et al: Developing performance measures for alcohol and other drug services. Washington Circle Group. Jt Comm J Qual Improv 26:633–643, 2000

Meyers WR, Miller WR (eds): A Community Reinforcement Approach to Addiction Treatment. Cambridge, UK, Cambridge University Press, 2001

Miller WR: Researching the spiritual dimensions of alcohol and other drug problems. Addiction 93:979–990, 1998

Miller WR, Zweben A, DiClemente CC, et al: Motivational Enhancement Therapy Manual: A Clinical Research Guide for Therapists Treating Individuals With Alcohol Abuse and Dependence (Project MATCH Monograph Series, Vol. 2). Rockville, MD, National Institute on Alcohol Abuse and Alcoholism, 1992

Minkoff K: Developing standards of care for individuals with co-occurring psychiatric and substance use disorders. Psychiatr Serv 52:597–599, 2001

Moscicki EK: Epidemiology of suicide, in The Harvard Medical School Guide to Suicide Assessment and Intervention. Edited by Jacobs DG. San Francisco, CA, Jossey-Bass, 1999, pp 40–51

Morrissey JP, Jackson EW, Ellis AR, et al: Twelve-month outcomes of trauma-informed interventions for women with co-occurring disorders. Psychiatr Serv 56:1213–1222, 2005

National Institute on Drug Abuse: A Cognitive-Behavioral Approach: Treating Cocaine Addiction. Therapy Manuals for Drug Addiction, Vol 1 (NIH Publication No 98-4308). Rockville, MD, U.S. Department of Health and Human Services, 1998

Nowinski J, Baker S, Carroll K: Twelve-Step Facilitation Therapy Manual: A Clinical Research Guide for Therapists Treating Individuals With Alcohol Abuse and Dependence (Project MATCH Monograph Series, Vol 1). Rockville, MD, National Institute on Alcohol Abuse and Alcoholism, 1992

Oncken C, Gonzales D, Nides M, et al: Efficacy and safety of the novel selective nicotinic acetylcholine receptor partial agonist varenicline for smoking cessation. Arch Intern Med 166:1571–1577, 2006

Petry NM, Petrakis I, Trevisan L, et al: Contingency management interventions: from research to practice. Am J Psychiatry 158:694–702, 2001

Pettinati HM, Kranzler HR, Madaras J: The status of serotonin-selective pharmacotherapy in the treatment of alcohol dependence, in Recent Developments in Alcoholism, Vol 16: Research on Alcoholism Treatment. Edited by Galanter M. New York, Kluwer Academic/Plenum, 2003, pp 247–262

Pirkola SP, Isometsa ET, Heikkinen MT, et al: Suicides of alcohol misusers and non-misusers in a nationwide population. Alcohol Alcohol 35:70–75, 2000

Prater CD, Miller KE, Zylstra RG: Outpatient detoxification of the addicted or alcoholic patient. Am Fam Physician 60:1175–1183, 1999

Prendergast M, Podus D, Finney J, et al: Contingency management for treatment of substance use disorders: a meta-analysis. Addiction 101:1546–1560, 2006

Preuss UW, Schuckit MA, Smith TL, et al: Predictors and correlates of suicide attempts over 5 years in 1,237 alcohol-dependent men and women. Am J Psychiatry 160:56–63, 2003

Prochaska JJ, Delucchi K, Hall SM: A meta-analysis of smoking cessation interventions with individuals in substance abuse treatment or recovery. J Consult Clin Psychol 72:1144–1156, 2004

Prochaska JO, DiClemente CC, Norcross JC: In search of how people change: applications to addictive behaviors. Am Psychol 47:1102–1114, 1992

Putkonen A, Kotilainen I, Joyal CC, et al: Comorbid personality disorders and substance use disorders of mentally ill homicide offenders: a structured clinical study on dual and triple diagnoses. Schizophr Bull 30:59–72, 2004

Rathlev NK, D'Onofrio G, Fish SS, et al: The lack of efficacy of phenytoin in the prevention of recurrent alcohol-related seizures. Ann Emerg Med 23:513–518, 1994

Reoux JP, Saxon AJ, Malte CA, et al: Divalproex sodium in alcohol withdrawal: a randomized double-blind placebo-controlled clinical trial. Alcohol Clin Exp Res 25:1324–1329, 2001

Rickels K, DeMartinis N, Rynn M, et al: Pharmacological strategies for discontinuing benzodiazepine treatment. J Clin Psychopharmacol 19 (suppl):12S–16S, 1999

Rosenheck RA, Mares AS: Implementation of supported employment for homeless veterans with psychiatric or addiction disorders: two-year outcomes. Psychiatr Serv 58:325–333, 2007

Salyers MP, Becker DR, Drake RE, et al: A ten-year follow-up of a supported employment program. Psychiatr Serv 55:302–308, 2004

Scheller-Gilkey G, Woolwine BJ, Cooper I, et al: Relationship of clinical symptoms and substance use in schizophrenia patients on conventional versus atypical antipsychotics. Am J Drug Alcohol Abuse 29:553–566, 2003

Schmitz JM, Stotts AL, Sayre SL, et al: Treatment of cocaine-alcohol dependence with naltrexone and relapse prevention therapy. Am J Addict 13:1333–1341, 2004

Scott H, Johnson S, Menezes P, et al: Substance misuse and risk of aggression and offending among the severely mentally ill. Br J Psychiatry 172:345–350, 1998

Sells DJ, Rowe M, Fisk D, et al: Violent victimization of persons with co-occurring psychiatric and substance use disorders. Psychiatr Serv 54:1253–1257, 2003

Sowers W, Pumariega A, Huffine C, et al: Level-of-care decision making in behavioral health services: the LOCUS and the CALOCUS. Psychiatr Serv 54:1461–1463, 2003

Soyka M: Substance misuse, psychiatric disorder and violent and disturbed behavior. Br J Psychiatry 176:345–350, 2000

Steadman HJ, Mulvey EP, Monahan J, et al: Violence by people discharged from acute psychiatric inpatient facilities and by others in the same neighborhoods. Arch Gen Psychiatry 55:393–401, 1998

Stuart GL, Ramsey SE, Moore TM, et al: Reductions in marital violence following treatment for alcohol dependence. J Interpers Violence 18:1113–1131, 2003

Sullivan JT, Sykora K, Schneiderman J, et al: Assessment of alcohol withdrawal: the revised Clinical Institute Withdrawal Assessment for Alcohol scale (CIWA-Ar). Br J Addict 84:1353–1357, 1989

Swanson AJ, Pantalon MV, Cohen KR: Motivational interviewing and treatment adherence among psychiatric and dually diagnosed patients. J Nerv Ment Dis 187:630–635, 1999

Swanson JW, Swartz MS, Essock SM, et al: The social-environmental context of violent behavior in persons treated for severe mental illness. Am J Public Health 92:1523–1531, 2002

Tanskanen A, Viinamäki H, Hintikka J, et al: Smoking and suicidality among psychiatric patients. Am J Psychiatry 155:129–130, 1998

Tarasoff v. Regents of the University of California, 551 P2d 334 (Cal 1976)

Waern M: Alcohol dependence and misuse in elderly suicides. Alcohol Alcohol 38:249–254, 2003

Watkins KE, Burnam A, Kung FY, et al: A national survey of care for persons with co-occurring mental and substance use disorders. Psychiatr Serv 52:1062–1068, 2001

Weinstock J, Alessi SM, Petry NM: Regardless of psychiatric severity the addition of contingency management to standard treatment improves retention and drug use outcomes. Drug Alcohol Depend 87:288–296, 2007

Weiss RD, Najavits LM, Greenfield SF: A relapse prevention group for patients with bipolar and substance use disorders. J Subst Abuse Treat 16:47–54, 1999

Williams JM, Ziedonis D: Addressing tobacco among individuals with a mental illness or an addiction. Addict Behav 29:1067–1083, 2004

Willour VL, Zandi PP, Badner JA, et al: Attempted suicide in bipolar disorder pedigrees: evidence for linkage to 2p12. Biol Psychiatry 61:725–727, 2007

Winston A, Rosenthal RN, Pinsker H: Introduction to Supportive Psychotherapy (Core Competencies in Psychotherapy series). Washington, DC, American Psychiatric Publishing, 2004

Yudko E, Blanchard DC, Henrie JA, et al: Emerging themes in preclinical research on alcohol and aggression, in Recent Developments in Alcoholism, Vol 13: Alcohol and Violence. Edited by Galanter M. New York, Kluwer Academic/Plenum, 1997, pp 123–138

Zubenko GS, Maher BS, Hughes III HB, et al: Genome-wide linkage survey for genetic loci that affect the risk of suicide attempts in families with recurrent, early onset, major depression. Am J Med Genet B Neuropsychiatr Genet 129:47–54, 2004

CHAPTER 10

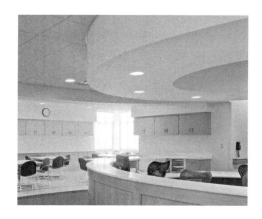

THE ADOLESCENT NEUROPSYCHIATRIC UNIT

Developmental Disabilities and Mental Illness

Margaret E. Hertzig, M.D.

Pediatric neuropsychiatry is a rapidly evolving clinical discipline concerned with the diagnosis and treatment of behavioral and emotional symptoms in children and adolescents with disturbances of brain function. As such, it is not a new discipline, but in recent years the growth of interest in and attention to the neurological underpinnings of behavioral and emotional impairment has been greatly enhanced by advances in neuroscience, neuroimaging, and neuropharmacology. Increasingly, conceptualizations of neuropsychiatry are redefining the mind–brain dichotomy so that clinicians as well as investigators have come to accept without question that "the brain is the organ of the mind." Thus, the scope of pediatric neuropsychiatry has broadened to encompass consideration of the neuropsychiatric underpinnings of the entire panoply of psychiatric and behavioral disorders as they occur during the developmental years (Coffey and Brumback 2006). Despite this expansion of focus, traditionally organized psychiatric services are generally well able to meet the needs of children and adolescents whose behavioral and/or emotional disorders are not additionally complicated by significant cognitive impairment. It is when behavioral and emotional disturbance is comorbid with mental retardation that specialized services specifically dedicated to the needs of this subgroup of psychiatrically disturbed children and adolescents may be required.

Mental retardation is defined by significantly subaverage intellectual and adaptive functioning, with onset before 18 years of age. Commonly used synonyms include *intellectual disability, learning disability,* and *developmental disability*. The presence of mental retardation has been recorded on Axis II of DSM since 1980, with the publication of DSM-III (American Psychiatric Association 1980), and continues to be so located in all subsequent revisions. The DSM-IV-TR (American Psychiatric Association 2000) definition establishes an IQ of approximately 70 as obtained on an independently administered test of intelligence coupled with impairment in adaptive functioning in at least two of the following skill areas: communication, self-care, home living, social/interpersonal skills, use of community resources, self-direction, functional academic skills, work, leisure, health, and safety. The measurement of both IQ and adaptive functioning may be affected by a range of factors, including the individual's sociocultural background, native language, and associated communicative, motor, and sensory handicaps as well as education, motivation, personality characteristics, social and vocational opportunities, and comorbid psychiatric and general medical conditions (American Psychiatric Association 2000).

Mental retardation is a heterogeneous condition. Individuals meeting criteria for a diagnosis of mental retardation display a broad spectrum of abilities and disabilities, liabilities and strengths. The prevalence of mental retardation is estimated at about 1% of the population. Approximately 85% of persons with mental retardation are classified as mildly retarded (IQ level 50–70), 10% as moderately retarded (IQ level 35–55) 3%–4% as severely retarded (IQ level 20–40) and 1%–2% profoundly retarded (IQ level below 20) (American Psychiatric Association 2000). Advances in medicine and most particularly in molecular genetics have led to the identification of more than 500 genetic causes of intellectual disability alone (Harris 1995) that account for some 35% of individuals with mental retardation. Some 95 mental retardation syndromes have been linked to the X chromosome, with the fragile X syndrome accounting for some 40% of all X-linked retardation (Feldman 1996). In less than 10%, retardation may be the consequence of a malformation syndrome of as yet unknown origin. External, prenatal, perinatal, or postnatal factors including infections, trauma, toxins, perinatal complications, and prematurity account for about one-third of cases, with etiology unknown in the remainder. The prevalence of mental retardation caused by a number of specific medical conditions including congenital syphilis, Rh hemolytic disease of the newborn, measles, *Haemophilus influenzae* type B meningitis, congenital hypothyroidism, phenylketonuria, and congenital rubella has decreased sharply over the past 50 years. However, the incidence of each

of these conditions is relatively low. Combined, they represented, at most, 16.5% of the total number of cases of mental retardation in 1950. Consequently, although improved medical interventions have prevented thousands of cases of mental retardation, the contribution to the overall prevalence of mental retardation is relatively small (Brosco et al. 2006).

The increased prevalence of psychiatric disorder among individuals with mental retardation is well established, although reported rates vary significantly from study to study—ranging from a low of 10% to upward of 60% (State et al. 1997). Differences in prevalence rates are the consequence of differences in diagnostic criteria employed, whether the sample was drawn from the community or from institutions, the level of mental retardation, and the ages and gender of the study sample (Dosen and Day 2001). The risk of psychopathology in children and adolescents with mental retardation is most significantly increased with moderate cognitive impairment as compared with those with either mild or severe/profound intellectual disability (Holden and Gitlesen 2004; Koskentausta et al. 2007). The term *dual diagnosis* is frequently used to describe mental retardation complicated by mental illness, although this use may be confusing to some because this term is also used to refer to the comorbidity of mental illness and substance abuse (American Academy of Child and Adolescent Psychiatry 1999; Bongiorno 1996).

Higher prevalence rates of psychiatric disorder among those with mental retardation are associated with a range of neurological, social, psychological, and personality risk factors including impaired cognition, organic brain damage, communication problems, physical disabilities, family psychopathology, and psychosocial factors. Singly or in combination, these factors increase the vulnerability of persons with mental retardation to psychiatric or behavioral disturbance (Dosen and Day 2001; Wallander et al. 2006). Currently it is recognized that children and adolescents with mental retardation can have the full range of psychopathology experienced by children of normal intelligence. Anxiety disorders, depression, bipolar affective disorders, attention-deficit/hyperactivity disorder (ADHD), schizophrenia, and psychotic disorders have all been described in young people with significant cognitive impairments. The types of psychopathological disorders in children with mild mental retardation are more likely to resemble those found in the general population. The more severe the level of cognitive impairment, the more difficult it becomes for clinicians to apply existing diagnostic criteria with confidence.

Additionally, specific chromosomal/genetic abnormalities may also be associated with the emergence of constellations of behavioral and emotional symptoms that do not fit neatly into conventional diagnostic categories. Behavioral phenotypes—the increased likelihood that persons with a given syndrome will display certain behavioral and developmental characteristics when compared to those without the syndrome—have been described in children with genetic abnormalities associated with fragile X, Williams, Prader-Willi, Smith-Magenis, Down, and 5p syndromes. The maladaptive vulnerabilities of affected children include problems relating to others as well as difficulties regulating attention, arousal, and activity levels in fragile X syndrome; indiscriminate relatedness and social disinhibition in Williams syndrome; hyperphagia, food preoccupations, non-food-related obsessions, temper tantrums, and skin picking in Prader-Willi syndrome; inattention, hyperactivity, aggression, self-injury, stereotypies, and self-hugging in Smith-Magenis syndrome; noncompliance, stubbornness, inattention, withdrawn behavior, and depression in Down syndrome; and infantile, high-pitched, cat-like crying, hyperactivity, inattention, stereotypies, and self-injury in 5p (cri du chat) syndrome (Dykens 2000). A pattern of self-injurious and aggressive behavior has also been described in Lesch-Nyhan disease—an X-linked disorder of purine metabolism caused by a near absence of the enzyme hypoxanthine–guanine phosphoribosyltransferase (Schretlen et al. 2005).

The co-occurrence of autism and other pervasive developmental disorders (PDDs) and mental retardation is well established. Despite differences in instrumentation and the bands of intellectual level reported, the results of 19 recently conducted studies have noted that about 30% of children with PDD scored in the normal range of intelligence, about 30% scored in the mild-to-moderate mental retardation range, and about 40% scored in the serious-to-profound mental retardation range (Fombonne 2005). An overall increase in the prevalence of autism and the other PDDs has also been reported over the past 15 years. Although surveys conducted during the 1960s and 1970s estimated that four children per 10,100 had autism, recent estimates have conservatively estimated the prevalence of autism to be 13 per 10,000, and of all PDDs to be about 60 per 10,000. This increased prevalence has been attributed to a broadening of the concept and diagnostic criteria as well as to increased awareness and improved detection of the PDDs at all ages and at all levels of intellectual ability. These higher prevalence rates have been confirmed in a new survey utilizing an identical

methodology that was applied in the same community some 4 years earlier (Chakrabarti and Fombonne 2005). Prevalence data deriving from special education sources have suggested a rising administrative prevalence of autism and a falling administrative prevalence of mental retardation. However, because schools do not necessarily use standard DSM-IV-TR criteria for assigning a label of autism to children in special education, and Special Education Child Count data report only counts of primary classification without noting the presence of comorbid conditions, such data cannot be considered to accurately reflect the epidemiology either of autism and the other PDDs or of mental retardation (Shattuck 2006).

Throughout the nineteenth and well into the twentieth century, care for persons with mental retardation—regardless of whether they had comorbid psychiatric illness and/or displayed significant patterns of maladaptive or "challenging" behaviors—was provided in large public institutions. The phasing out and subsequent closure of these large facilities for people with mental retardation, beginning in the late 1960s, served to highlight the special needs of those with psychiatric problems. Initially it was hoped that the level of behavioral and psychiatric disturbance found in individuals with mental retardation might have been over exaggerated—a consequence of institutionalization—and would therefore substantially diminish with the introduction of large-scale community care programs. However, as it became increasingly apparent that this was not the case, proponents of the "normalization" movement argued that the behavioral and emotional difficulties of individuals with comorbid mental retardation should be treated within ordinary mental health services as part of a general policy of integration (Moss et al. 1997). It was opined that specialized services would lead to increased stigmatization, labeling, and negative professional attitudes (Day 1994). With the passage of time, it has become possible to examine the impact of this approach in practice. Day (1994, 2001) cogently summarized the evidence demonstrating that generic mental health services, whether provided by default or design, cannot satisfactorily meet the treatment and care needs of persons with mental retardation and comorbid psychiatric and behavioral problems.

Day (2001) included the following in making the case for specialized services for this population:

1. The accurate diagnosis and treatment of psychiatric disorder in persons with mental retardation require special expertise and experience in the face of

atypical presentation, communication difficulties, and the frequent absence of subjective complaints.

2. Special regimens and careful monitoring of drug treatment are necessary because side effects and unusual responses occur frequently among those with mental retardation.

3. Highly specialized assessment and treatment techniques are required to effectively manage disruptive, self-abusive, and aggressive behaviors, many of which are unique to this population, accounting for approximately half of the presenting problems.

4. Underlying dependency levels and coexisting physical disabilities, including epilepsy, have to be taken into account in treatment, rehabilitation, and aftercare.

5. Persons with mental retardation are disadvantaged and vulnerable in generic treatment settings. They do not on the whole integrate easily with other mentally disordered patients, the pace of ward life is usually too fast for them, and it is difficult for staff to tailor therapeutic interventions to their specific needs, resulting in the prolongation of treatment and rehabilitation.

6. Specialist services increase staff competence and skills, permit the application of knowledge gained from cumulative experience, and increase ownership of the task at hand, therefore increasing the probability of successful treatment.

7. Specialist services facilitate the establishment of a cadre of experts to carry out teaching and research (Day 1994, 2001).

Although these conclusions have face validity, the database underlying them derives from a limited number of studies of adults with comorbid cognitive impairment and psychiatric disorder. In reviewing available evidence, Chaplin (2004) concluded that further evaluation of differing patterns of service delivery is needed to provide robust evidence as to which services are to be preferred.

Admission Criteria

Acute neuropsychiatric inpatient units are the most common form of hospital-based care for adolescents in whom behavioral and emotional disturbance is comorbid with significant cognitive impairment. The inpatient unit is an important component of a continuum of care that addresses the provision of ongoing psychiatric treatment in the least restrictive environment while also providing for the educational, voca-

tional, residential, and recreational requirements (including respite care) of patients and their families. Many, if not most, dually diagnosed persons with mental retardation can be treated as outpatients provided that there are no significant unresolved diagnostic problems, the illness can safely be managed in the community, there are no anticipated difficulties in implementing the treatment program, and family and other caregivers are adequately supported (Day and Dosen 2001). However, services to meet the needs of this population are few and far between, and adolescents are frequently referred from agency to agency because they fall between the cracks of many human-service systems (McGee et al. 1984). Consequently, patients may present for admission with an array of symptoms and challenging behaviors that are more severe than they would have been if appropriate treatment had been available at an earlier point in time.

The overall goals of inpatient treatment are assessment, stabilization, disposition planning, and transition to less restrictive settings. Little information is available that specifically addresses the factors leading to the hospitalization of dually diagnosed adolescents. Nonetheless, admission criteria can be extrapolated from the results of a review by Smith and Berney (2006) of the reasons for admission of 96 patients between the ages of 6 and 19 years (two-thirds of whom were males) accepted for treatment in specialized psychiatric inpatient units. Cognitive impairment was described as borderline to mild in 41%, moderate in 31%, and severe in 26% of this study sample. Primary reasons for admission included 1) admission was necessary to provide an independent assessment of environmental contributions to escalating disruptive behavior (23%); 2) required treatment was too complex or hazardous to be undertaken on an outpatient basis (16%); 3) there was an acute risk of harm to the patient or to others (14%); 4) the patient required protection from abuse (4%); 5) the environment was unable to cope with severely disruptive or destructive behavior (27%); 6) previous treatment plans had failed (1%); and caregivers were unable to implement the current treatment plan (15%).

Admission to adolescent neuropsychiatric units should be available to individuals between the ages of 13 and 21 years of age—the upper age limit being selected to coincide with the termination of educational entitlements for children and adolescents with disabilities under Public Law 94–142, the federal legislation that establishes the basis for the provision of appropriate educational services for all handicapped children from birth to age 21 years. Admission should be provided for those whose cognitive impairments preclude admission to mainstream adolescent units. Consideration for admission most often arises in the context of increasing concern on the part of usual caretakers about their ability to maintain safety of either the patient or staff because of escalating aggressive, destructive, suicidal, or other self-abusive behavior. Additionally, patients whose behavior falls short of acute dangerousness may benefit from an admission directed toward clarifying diagnosis and/or refining pharmacological treatment. Admission may also be appropriate in circumstances when the patient's current living, educational, or working environment is a major precipitating or aggravating factor in the illness, or community resources have identified a need to review and revise current treatment plans. While unnecessary hospitalizations should, of course, be avoided, it also should be recognized that hospital admission should not be "avoided at all costs" or delayed unnecessarily for ideological reasons. Such attitudes may well have detrimental consequences for family, other caregivers, and subsequent management of the patient in the community. Hospitalization can be a positive therapeutic intervention because it provides an opportunity to assess the possible aggravating effects of environmental factors, and it provides a setting in which required changes in ongoing treatment plans can be initiated (Day and Dosen 2001).

Diagnostic Workup

The evaluation of behavioral and emotional difficulties in persons with mental retardation should follow the general rules of psychiatric assessment. In principle, the manifestations of mental illness in people with mild and borderline retardation are similar to those in the general population, although special skills may be required to elicit symptoms in the face of communication difficulties and a paucity of subjective complaints. Mental disorders in patients with mental retardation are often underdiagnosed—perhaps because clinicians may restrict their focus only to the symptomatic treatment of disruptive behaviors. "Diagnostic overshadowing," the assumption that symptoms can be fully accounted for by retardation, may further impede diagnostic accuracy (Jopp and Keys 2001). It is generally agreed that it is difficult to establish a diagnosis of mental illness with confidence in the severely retarded (American Academy of Child and Adolescent Psychiatry 1999; Dosen and Day 2001). Nevertheless, having a formal diagnosis rather than a

nonspecific description of "challenging behavior" is important for the following reasons: 1) the comprehensive evaluation and resulting diagnosis may indicate a specific treatment and 2) the patient's difficulties can be reframed for staff and other caregivers as manifestations of illness as contrasted with "bad behavior." Mental retardation itself usually has been fully assessed prior to presentation for admission to an inpatient neuropsychiatric unit. However, for some patients a critical review of this aspect of the clinical picture may be indicated, most particularly because certain behavioral patterns may suggest "behavioral phenotypes" that had not yet been identified at the time of initial presentation (State et al. 1997).

Accurate diagnosis begins with a full and detailed history. Persons with mental retardation, even those who are only mildly impaired, may have considerable difficulty in reliably describing their own behavior and symptoms. They are usually dependent on multiple service providers and supportive services. Therefore the history must incorporate information derived from multiple informants. Moreover, maladaptive behaviors may be situation specific—disruptive behavior may occur only in the relatively unstructured home setting but not at school where more support and supervision is available.

Components of a comprehensive history should include a clear description of the presenting concerns, including behavioral descriptions of symptoms in various settings and situations and their evolution over time, antecedent events, and the effectiveness of already applied management strategies. Possible predisposing or precipitating factors should be thoroughly explored, and the results of previous assessments should be reviewed. Information about current strengths and impairments in adaptive skills including communication, self-care, social/interpersonal, community integration, self-direction, academic, work, leisure, health, and safety should be specified. Behavioral changes with respect to sleep, appetite, and weight loss, as well as loss of interest in usual pursuits, deterioration of social skills, bizarre behavior, and other deviations from well-established behavioral patterns should be specified. Information should be sought regarding premorbid personality and functioning, together with full details about any previous psychiatric illnesses and treatment experienced by the patient and other family members. The attitudes of parents and other caregivers toward the patient and their understanding of his or her disability should be assessed. Information regarding medication and possible medication side effects should be carefully explored. A developmental and medical history, including inquiry about past etiological assessments as well as past and/or current general medical disorders and their treatments, should be obtained.

The standard approach to interviewing adolescent patients will require modifications appropriate to the patient's level of cognitive functioning. Ample time should be allocated or several briefer interviews may be required to complete a full mental status assessment. An effort should be made to assess mental status in the context of conversation. It is desirable to begin the interview with a discussion of the patient's strengths and interests rather than problems. Only later can the focus shift to clarifying the patient's understanding of problems, disability, limitations, and reasons for hospitalization. An effort should be made to avoid leading questions or questions requiring yes or no answers. Of necessity, the general paucity of subjective complaints requires that the examiner be attentive to objective data, including the patient's appearance, degree of relatedness, expressions of affect, impulse control, activity level, attention span, distractibility, and the presence of unusual behaviors or seizures. Evidence of hallucinations may be inferred by behaviors that suggest the patient is talking to him- or herself or responding to internal stimuli.

Rating scales for the assessment of psychopathology in individuals with comorbid mental retardation can provide guides to further inform history taking and the direct examination of the patient. Although not designed to provide a clinical diagnosis, measures such as the Aberrant Behavior Checklist (Aman et al. 1996; Rojahn et al. 2003) or the Behavior Problem Inventory (Rojahn et al. 2001) can be used to track symptom change during the course of treatment. Although the Autism Diagnostic Inventory may well be too lengthy and cumbersome to use in its entirety, it is a useful guide to obtaining information about both early development and current functioning in adolescents with PDD (Lord et al. 1994). Elements of the Autism Diagnostic Observation Schedule (Lord et al. 2000) can augment the clinical interview of adolescents with PDD. In addition, the Children's Yale-Brown Obsessive-Compulsive Scale has been modified for use in children and adolescents with PDD (Scahill et al. 2006), as has the Children's Global Assessment Scale (Wagner et al. 2007). Additionally, it may be appropriate to update previously conducted assessments of IQ and adaptive functioning.

Consultation with pediatricians and pediatric neurologists should be readily available. Physical illness can be easily missed in individuals with significant communication deficits. Undiagnosed medical conditions may result in or contribute to an exacerbation of behavioral symptoms. Ryan and Sunada (1997) found that 75% of adults with mental retardation referred for psychiatric assessment had one or more undiagnosed or undertreated medical problems. In 6.5% of the patients studied, psychiatric symptomatology remitted after effective treatment of the primary medical condition. In addition, many individuals with mental retardation have co-occurring motor and sensory impairments or seizure disorders (American Academy of Child and Adolescent Psychiatry 1999; Dosen and Day 2001). The incidence of epilepsy, often in a medically intractable form, is higher among patients with mental retardation than in the general population, and its incidence increases with the severity of cognitive impairment. However, the diagnosis of epilepsy in this population is often challenging, both over- and underdiagnosis is frequent, and pharmacological control of seizures may be difficult to obtain, resulting in a high level of polypharmacy (Smith 2006). Pediatric neurological consultation can assist in clarifying these and other complex issues at the interface between neurology and psychiatry.

Although traditional nosological classifications are not entirely adequate to accommodate the phenomenology of emotional and/or behavioral disturbance in individuals with mental retardation, an effort should be made to clearly establish a DSM-IV-TR Axis I diagnosis. A patient's verbal productions provide the basis for a full assessment of many DSM-IV-TR criteria. Nevertheless, the nomenclature does make some provision for situations in which the patient's language is insufficient to describe symptoms. For example, the criteria for major depressive episode include "observations made by others" (American Psychiatric Association 2000, p. 356). For nonverbal patients, "not otherwise specified" designations may have to be used. Commonly occurring comorbid conditions include autism and other PDDs, psychoses and major mood disorders, anxiety disorders (including posttraumatic stress disorder and obsessive-compulsive disorder), tic disorders, ADHD, and stereotypic movement disorders. With this population, care should be taken to summarize the basis for diagnosis in individual cases (American Academy of Child and Adolescent Psychiatry 1999).

The diagnostic formulation should interpret clinical data in the context of the individual patient's developmental level, communicative abilities, and possible associated motor and/or sensory handicaps as well as life experiences, education, and familial and sociocultural factors. Although caregivers may seek to distinguish between behaviors that are thought to be deliberate attempts to gain attention or avoid disliked activities and those that are viewed as more genuine symptoms of psychiatric illness, such efforts are overly simplistic and misguided. Persistent overtly disturbed behavior is the observable result of a complex interplay of biological, psychological, and social factors and comprises elements that are learned, conditioned by environmental factors, and under voluntary control (American Academy of Child and Adolescent Psychiatry 1999). Nevertheless, persons with mental retardation frequently exhibit an array of "challenging" behaviors including frequent temper tantrums, aggression, stereotypes, physical disruption, rituals, hyperactivity, and self-injurious behaviors that cut across diagnostic lines but are a necessary and appropriate focus of treatment (Murphy et al. 2005; Pilling et al. 2007; Schroeder et al. 2001).

Therapies

The diagnostic assessment provides the basis for the development of a comprehensive individualized treatment plan. Although most of the therapeutic methods used for the treatment of psychiatric disorder in the nonretarded are applicable, with little or no modification, to individuals who are mildly retarded, treatment of those with moderate and severe retardation must take into account lower intelligence, often greatly impaired communication skills, and associated neurological disorders as well as specific behavioral syndromes. Each individualized treatment plan reflects the integration of biological and psychosocial interventions, including specifically targeted behavioral treatments, family education and therapy, and habilitative, educational, and recreational therapies. Although it should go without saying that comprehensive treatment must include both biological and psychosocial interventions, too often these two primary modalities are conceptualized as antithetical. Through the development of a comprehensive, multidisciplinary treatment plan, the inpatient unit plays an important role in educating family and other caretakers about the potential for mutual reinforcement that the judicious use of both interventions offers patients with intellectual disabilities (Dosen 2007).

Medication

Medications are the principal biological interventions employed in the treatment of psychiatric disorder in

individuals with comorbid mental retardation. As a general rule, medications should be prescribed only for the treatment of specific mental disorders as part of a comprehensive treatment plan. Because medication effects are generally not different from those expected in the absence of mental retardation, the rules governing usual pharmacological practice may be applied without major modification. Nevertheless, response rates tend to be poorer and side effects more frequent (Handen and Gilchrist 2006). Individuals with compromised central nervous system function can be especially vulnerable to the anticholinergic effects of low-potency neuroleptics (Madrid et al. 2000). Other side effects that may occur with increased frequency in this population include disinhibition in response to sedative-hypnotics; irritability and hyponatremia with carbamazepine; cognitive dulling and an increased likelihood of toxicity as a consequence of erratic fluid intake with lithium; social withdrawal and motor tics with methylphenidate; tardive and other dyskinesia, withdrawal, irritability, self-injury, and akathisia with neuroleptics; and pancreatitis and hepatotoxicity with valproate (American Academy of Child and Adolescent Psychiatry 1999).

Antochi et al. (2003) observed that although the number of studies devoted to the use of psychotropic medications in persons with dual diagnosis of psychiatric disorders and developmental disabilities is small, there is adequate evidence to suggest that a range of antidepressants, mood stabilizers, anxiolytics, antipsychotics, and stimulants can be efficacious, with selective serotonin reuptake inhibitors, newer anticonvulsants, and atypical neuroleptics being preferred medication choices. Persons with intellectual disabilities are more vulnerable to side effects, with potentially catastrophic results, including fatalities. Consequently, the risk–benefit ratio of a proposed pharmacological regimen must be carefully examined and thoroughly reviewed with parents or other legal guardians who must provide informed consent before pharmacological treatment can be undertaken. Initial dosages should be low, increases introduced slowly, and the emergence of possible side effects carefully monitored. Efforts should be made to limit polypharmacy by ensuring the clear documentation of specific indications for each medication prescribed (American Academy of Child and Adolescent Psychiatry 1999). Caution should be exercised with regard to the prescription of as-needed medications, and their use should be carefully monitored. A retrospective chart review has revealed that as-needed medications were more commonly prescribed for hospitalized children and adolescents with comorbid mental retardation or PDD as compared with nonretarded patients housed on the same integrated 12-bed acute-care unit. In this unit, as-needed medications were also used more frequently in patients receiving other psychotropic treatments, raising the risk of drug interactions or other adverse effects (Dean et al. 2006).

Although it is highly desirable that the prescription of psychotropic medication follows diagnosis, it is sometimes difficult to entirely avoid using medications to target specific symptoms in the absence of a clearly established clinical diagnosis. Sometimes this is the result of gaps in our current nomenclature. For example, DSM-IV-TR does not allow a diagnosis of separation anxiety disorder, generalized anxiety disorder, social phobia, or ADHD in individuals with PDD, yet symptoms of anxiety, rigidity, inflexibility, repetitive behaviors, inattention, easy distractibility, and impulsivity often associated with the diagnosis of PDD may well be appropriate targets for treatment (Leyfer et al. 2006). Among the most frequent reasons for the use of psychotropic medication in persons with mental retardation are various forms of disruptive behavior including self-injurious behaviors, stereotyped behaviors, and aggression. These behaviors are often grouped together as disorders of impulse control, although the pathogenesis may be quite different, and there is no uniform response to pharmacological agents (American Academy of Child and Adolescent Psychiatry 1999).

The use of medications to address target symptoms has been perhaps best studied in autism and other PDDs. When administered at relatively low dosages, antipsychotics, most particularly risperidone, have been shown to reduce repetitive behaviors, stereotypies, and social withdrawal as well as hyperactivity, aggression, self-abusive behavior, temper tantrums, lability of mood, and irritability. Adverse effects in the PDD population include increased appetite, weight gain, drooling, hyperprolactinemia, and risk of drug-related dyskinesias. Although less well studied, available evidence suggests that selective serotonin reuptake inhibitors may be effective in reducing repetitive behaviors and expanding the range of interest of children and adolescents with PDD. Restlessness, agitation, and insomnia are commonly reported side effects. Stimulant medications have been shown to reduce hyperactivity and improve focus, but they may result in increases in disruptive behavior, weight loss, and increased stereotypic behavior (Malone et al. 2005). Second-generation antipsychotics, most particularly risperidone, have been found to be efficacious in controlling hyperactivity, irritability, and aggressive, self-injurious, and other

repetitive behaviors in individuals with mental retardation. Side effects include serious ongoing weight gain, predisposing to the metabolic syndrome, and the emergence of type 2 diabetes. Although data regarding efficacy are limited, aripiprazole's weight neutrality may make it a good treatment alternative (Handen and Gilchrist 2006).

Electroconvulsive Therapy

There is a paucity of empirical data regarding the efficacy of electroconvulsive therapy (ECT) in patients with mental retardation and psychiatric disorders. Specific difficulties in using ECT in this patient population have included diagnostic dilemmas, difficulties with measurement of outcome, and monitoring of side effects as well as professional reluctance and difficulties in obtaining informed consent. Nevertheless, although the number of treated cases is small, the responses of adults with mental retardation and severe or refractory psychotic symptoms or treatment-resistant mood disorders are encouraging (Aziz et al. 2001; Cutajar and Wilson 1999; Reinblatt et al. 2004). In addition, four cases of catatonic stupor in adolescents with autism, all of whom have been successfully treated with ECT, have been reported (Bailine and Petraviciute 2007; Ghaziuddin et al. 2005; Zaw et al. 1999). Thus, albeit limited, the available evidence suggests that ECT certainly should be considered as a treatment option for adolescents with mental retardation and psychiatric disorders for which ECT is otherwise warranted.

Psychosocial Interventions

Psychosocial interventions for psychiatrically ill adolescents with developmental disabilities include specifically targeted behavioral treatment, family education and treatment, and habilitative, educational, and recreational therapies provided in an environment structured to address challenging behaviors safely and effectively while reducing symptomatology to a level that will allow the patient to return to appropriate community-based services.

INDIVIDUALIZED BEHAVIORAL TREATMENT

Behavior therapy represents the mainstay of psychologically based treatment of persons with moderate to severe retardation. Behavioral techniques provide a consistent and structured framework for teaching appropriate behavioral patterns and adaptive life skills. Although it is beyond the scope of this chapter to provide details of specific behavioral treatment techniques, it should be noted that behavioral interventions should be individualized based on data derived from a comprehensive contextual analysis that identifies to the greatest extent possible the external and internal conditions that influence the occurrence and persistence of problem behaviors. Care should be taken to distinguish description from explanation in clarifying events that precede the targeted behavior, consequences of the behavior, and patient characteristics that increase vulnerability to adverse events (Gardiner et al. 2001). The behavioral treatment of persistent inappropriate behaviors should utilize techniques of ignoring, redirection, and positive reinforcement. All three steps may be employed simultaneously; for example, when a request for action on the part of staff results in screaming behavior, the screams can be ignored while the caretaker assists the patient in executing the task by providing hand-over-hand guidance. This approach does not mean that maladaptive behavior is completely ignored. Rather, the focus is shifted to the acquisition of appropriate skills and interactions so that the patient gradually learns that he or she will gain attention for appropriate behaviors and interactions and, conversely, will regularly be ignored when behaving inappropriately (McGee et al. 1984). Aversive behavioral techniques, including electric shocks, food deprivation, noxious tastes, the delivery of white noise through ear phones, and limitation of movement when used as a punishing consequence, are clearly outside of the mainstream of current psychiatric practice and have no place in the therapeutic armamentarium of an adolescent neuropsychiatric unit.

FAMILY EDUCATION AND TREATMENT

It has long been recognized that parents of children with mental retardation, most particularly those with comorbid behavioral and emotional problems, report more parenting stress and mental health problems than parents of children without disabilities. Parental stress may occur in response to episodic life events that may impact on any family, such as marital breakdown or bereavement, as well as from family life-cycle transitions that may be especially pertinent to families of children with disabilities. Relevant transition points include early childhood events such as initial diagnosis and starting school. The adolescent years may bring additional challenges as families begin to learn how to cope with the difficulties that physical maturation may impose on previously well-established routines (Hastings and Beck 2004; Schneider et al. 2006). Although the adolescent years usually herald increased independence and autonomy for typically developing children, those with intellectual dis-

abilities continue to require close supervision, and their increasing size may render them harder to control and discipline. A survey of parents of children and adolescents with intellectual disability and comorbid behavioral and emotional problems identified numerous unmet support needs, including "a friendly ear" with whom to share worries and concerns; respite care and other practical and material help; mental health care for themselves and their children; and information about additional services and recreational and leisure time activities (Douma et al. 2006). Although work with families of adolescents admitted to an acute care unit must of course be individualized, providers should be alert to the emergence of common themes. Admission can stimulate recall of the experience of initial diagnosis, and parents and other family members may benefit from an opportunity to process these experiences anew from the expanded perspective gained in the course of the passage of time. At the time of initial diagnosis, parents often experience considerable anxiety in the face of uncertainty about the future. During adolescence, as future expectations are increasingly clarified, parents must begin to address questions about the provision of lifetime care. Work with families provides an opportunity to examine the impact of the patient's disability on other family members, most particularly siblings (Lobato and Kao 2002), and to explore each family member's need for ongoing mental health treatment. Parents also should be actively involved in planning the hospital treatment as well as provisions for aftercare. Even if the patient is to be admitted to, or returned to, an out-of-home placement, the role of the family should be carefully examined because available evidence stresses the importance of sustaining ongoing relationships with parents for the adjustment of institutionalized patients (Ruedrich and Menolascino 1984). Additional referrals to either professionally led groups or to a group organized and run by other parents to provide a source of ongoing support can be considered (Hastings and Beck 2004).

MILIEU MANAGEMENT AND EDUCATIONAL AND RECREATIONAL THERAPIES

An adolescent neuropsychiatric acute care unit requires a multidisciplinary staff and a higher staff-to-patient ratio than would be found on a traditional psychiatric unit. Typically, overall staffing is 2–3:1, with the availability of 1:1 staffing on an as-needed basis. The staff should have experience and training in the developmental disabilities and include a child and adolescent psychiatrist with training and experience in the psychiatric aspects of developmental disabilities and mental retardation, including pharmacological interventions; psychiatric nurses; social workers; special education teachers; recreational therapists; and behaviorally trained direct-care workers. Additionally, the services of speech and language and occupational therapists should be available on an as-needed basis, and consultation with pediatricians and pediatric neurologists should be similarly accessible. The milieu should be organized to provide patients with a closely scheduled, active, and developmentally appropriate treatment day. The execution of activities of daily living must be closely supervised and guided to facilitate the assumption of increasing responsibility for personal care. A typical daily schedule may include school attendance and sessions with the occupational therapist and speech and language therapist as indicated by each patient's individualized educational plan. Organized recreational groups and supplementary therapeutic groups designed to provide social skills and anger management training, as well as individual behavioral therapy and individual and family therapy as prescribed by each patient's individualized treatment plan, complete the day (McGee et al. 1984). All staff should be familiar with the content of each patient's individual behavioral plan, which at a minimum should be implemented during all scheduled activities throughout the day.

Maintenance of Safety

Because a large proportion of patients on an acute care adolescent neuropsychiatry unit are admitted because they exhibit a high intensity and/or frequency of maladaptive behaviors that render them unsafe either to themselves or others, the maintenance of unit safety is clearly of paramount importance. Currently, standard practice in psychiatric hospitals accredited by the Joint Commission (http://www.jointcommission.org) and regulated by the Centers for Medicare and Medicaid Services (http://www.cms.hhs.gov) requires that the use of restraint and seclusion be limited to emergencies in which there is an imminent risk of patients harming themselves or others, including staff. Because regulations regarding seclusion and restraint are revised frequently, practitioners should review these organizations' Web sites at frequent intervals.

The practice parameters prepared by the American Academy of Child and Adolescent Psychiatry (2001) note that approaches to the use of restrictive interventions with developmentally disabled children and ado-

lescents are generally the same as for children without disabilities, although actual procedures may vary according to state law, regulations, statutes, and mandates. Because seclusion and restraint have the potential to produce serious consequences, including physical and psychological harm, loss of dignity, violation of an individual's rights, and even death (Mohr et al. 2003; Nunno et al. 2006; Petti et al. 2001), in recent years unit administrators have actively embarked on programs directed toward reducing the use of these practices in children and adolescent inpatient settings (Delaney 2006; LeBel et al. 2004; Miller et al. 2006; Schreiner et al. 2004). Strategies directed toward the prevention of aggression and self-aggression are at the core of a program to maintain unit safety. Prevention begins at intake and continues through the admission process as a history of aggressive behavior including triggers, warning signs, repetitive behaviors, responses to previous treatments, and prior episodes of seclusion and restraint is obtained. Additionally, cognitive limitations and neurological deficits should be identified as well as medical conditions that might require modification of usual seclusion and restraint practices. Treatment planning should include the development of individualized strategies to minimize aggressive behavior, de-escalate behavior before safety is significantly jeopardized, and specify treatment for underlying psychopathology. Furthermore, it is essential that staff receive extensive training in the management of aggressive behavior and documentation requirements (American Academy of Child and Adolescent Psychiatry 2001).

Every unit should have its own program directed toward the de-escalation of potentially threatening and dangerous behavior. Such a program can be conceptualized as consisting of three levels:

- *Level 1:* Nonrestrictive interventions designed to increase the patient's behavioral self-control while preserving safety of patient, others, and property. Examples of Level 1 interventions include verbal prompting; reward programs, including token economies; and short periods (less than 30 minutes) of timeout.
- *Level 2:* Restrictive interventions are employed when concern for safety of patient, others, and property is greater and use contingencies that are directed to supporting adaptive behavior without reinforcing maladaptive behaviors. Optimally, Level 2 interventions require advance planning and may include ignoring behavior (extinction), time-outs lasting more than 30 minutes, and room restriction.

- *Level 3:* These most restrictive interventions should only be used when clinical judgment indicates that they are necessary to ensure safety of patient, others, and property and after documented failure of less restrictive interventions. Examples include seclusion, mechanical restraint, and medication (American Academy of Child and Adolescent Psychiatry 2001).

The practices and procedures at all three levels require the availability of one-to-one staffing. These procedures should never be used for the purpose of punishment. Moreover, the use of seclusion and/or restraint should be followed by a debriefing session that allows the patient to process and understand the episode to the extent that cognitive limitations may permit.

Although there has been increasing scrutiny of seclusion and restraint use in recent years, research on the use of these practices with children and adolescents is limited. Available evidence suggests that rates of seclusion and restraint are highest for hospitalized children and adolescents with diagnoses of mental retardation, developmental disability, and neurological impairments (Fryer et al. 2004). Additionally, youths restrained during an acute inpatient hospitalization are more likely to be male, to have been previously hospitalized, to be enrolled in special education, to be in foster care, or to have a history of voicing suicidal ideation and attempting suicide (Delaney and Fogg 2005).

In reviewing physical restraint procedures for managing the challenging behaviors of adults and children with mental retardation, Harris (1996) distinguished between contingent and noncontingent restraint. Although contingent restraint is initiated to ensure safety in the face of escalating aggressive behavior, noncontingent restraints are used to suppress self-injurious behaviors. Examples include mechanical devices employed to limit movement or specially adapted clothing to attenuate the self-injurious consequences of a person's actions, including helmets, masks, and mittens. Self-injurious behavior, which may occur in between 4% and 14% of people with intellectual disabilities, is often persistent and difficult to treat, and when untreated, it can have serious consequences, including permanent tissue damage and secondary problems such as infection, sensory and neurological impairment, and even death (Jones et al. 2007). Although noncontingent restraint can be effective in reducing self-injury, mechanical restraint can also have a number of detrimental side effects, which may include reinforcement of target behaviors; muscular atrophy; demineralization of bones or shortening

of tendons as a consequence of long-term restriction; disruption or prevention of opportunities to engage in activities associated with daily living, education, and leisure; and reduced levels of interaction with caregivers (Jones et al. 2007). Nevertheless, the use of mechanical devices to limit self-injury may be appropriate in selected cases. The most recent (January 2008) iteration of the *Comprehensive Accreditation Manual for Hospitals*, the official handbook of the Joint Commission, provides for this possibility in an exception to the applicability of the behavioral health care restraint and seclusion standards by allowing

> [t]he use of restraint with patients who receive treatment through formal behavior management programs (to which the behavior management standard in this manual applies—standard PC13.70). Such patients exhibit intractable behavior which is severely self-injurious or injurious to others, have not responded to traditional interventions and are unable to contract with staff for safety (for example, understand the concept of or act on criteria for discontinuing restraint or seclusion). (Joint Commission 2008)

Discharge Planning

When the lives of persons with developmental disabilities are complicated by comorbid psychiatric disorder, successful integration into community life becomes additionally problematic. Acute psychiatric inpatient services are but one point on the continuum of care required to meet both the residential and programmatic needs of this population over time. Residential services can be conceptualized as extending from long-term institutional care at one end of the continuum, through specialized group homes in the community, group homes offering less intensive supervision, and family-based care as provided by biological families or specialized foster home settings at the other end. Programmatic provision may include day hospital settings, special educational placements, sheltered workshops, group and/or individual counseling, case management, and preventive services (McGee et al. 1984).

It is to be expected that most adolescents admitted to an acute inpatient unit for adolescents will return to the residential and programmatic settings from which they were admitted. Relatively few individuals will be in need of ongoing institutional care, but this may be necessary in those instances when behavioral and pharmacological interventions have not been successful in controlling severely aggressive and/or self-abusive behavior to levels that can be safely managed in less restrictive settings. All discharge plans must be closely coordinated with receiving service providers to ensure continuity of care and that treatment goals can be sustained following discharge. Existing services may require expansion to include arrangements for ongoing pharmacological treatment, referral for individual/family therapy, or case management services. Prior to discharge, caregivers should receive training in the implementation of behavioral interventions. If possible, home and school visits should be provided to allow for generalization of behavioral expectations to other settings. If patients are to return home, referral to ongoing case management services should be considered to provide a means by which the various components of ongoing care—including outpatient psychiatric services, educational/vocational placements, and recreational activities—can be coordinated. Arrangements for ongoing care should also include provision for working with families to address issues surrounding planning for long-term out-of-home placement.

Access to appropriately experienced professionals should not be limited to inpatient settings. Persons with developmental disabilities and severe behavioral and emotional problems can be served in the community if an appropriate range of educational, vocational, and residential services is available to meet their needs. Both inpatient and outpatient services must be responsive to the needs of individual patients. Unfortunately, services are too often defined as being appropriate for only the mentally ill *or* only those with developmental disabilities. Individuals who are dually diagnosed are the losers in this either/or diagnostic game (Fleisher et al. 2001). A unit dedicated to the treatment of those who are both developmentally disabled *and* mentally ill goes a considerable distance toward remedying this historical crack in the continuum of care available to some of society's most vulnerable members.

Conclusion

The overall goals of inpatient treatment for adolescents with mental retardation and psychiatric disorder include diagnostic assessment, stabilization, disposition planning and transition to less restrictive settings. While it is often difficult to establish a diagnosis of mental illness with confidence in the severely retarded, efforts should be made to obtain a complete history using multiple informants. The full assessment of mental status may require multiple developmentally appropriate interviews. Neurological and pediatric consultation should be readily available as

physical illness can be easily missed in individuals with significant communication deficits. A diagnostic formulation, interpreting clinical data in the context of the individual patient's developmental level, communicative abilities, life experiences, education and familial and sociocultural factors provides the foundation for the development of a comprehensive individualized treatment plan integrating both pharmacological and psychosocial interventions. Ideally, medication should be prescribed for the treatment of specific mental disorders, but the use of pharmacological agents to target specific symptoms in the absence of a clearly established clinical diagnosis may be required. As response rates tend to be poorer and side effects more frequent in individuals with compromised central nervous system function, the risk–benefit ratio of psychopharmacological regimens must be carefully assessed and reviewed with legal guardians who must provide informed consent. Psychosocial interventions including specifically targeted behavioral treatments, family education and therapy, and habilitative educational and recreational therapies should be provided in a milieu which permits challenging behaviors to be safely and effectively addressed, while also facilitating the reduction of symptomatology to a level that will allow the patient to return to appropriate community based services. An acute care unit for adolescent neuropsychiatric patients requires a multidisciplinary staff and a staff-to-patient ratio sufficient to insure the provision of 1:1 staffing on an as needed basis. Every unit should have its own program directed toward the de-escalation of potentially threatening and dangerous behaviors consistent with standard practice in psychiatric hospitals accredited by the Joint Commission and regulated by the Centers for Medicaid and Medicare Services. Acute psychiatric inpatient services are but one point on the continuum of care required to meet both the residential and programmatic needs of persons with developmental disability complicated by comorbid psychiatric disorder. Most adolescents admitted to an acute inpatient unit will return to the settings from which they were admitted. Nevertheless, discharge plans must be closely coordinated with receiving facilities to insure that treatment goals are sustained following discharge.

References

Aman MG, Tasse MJ, Rojahn J, et al: The Nisonger CBRF: a child behavior rating form for children with developmental disabilities. Res Dev Disabil 17:41–57, 1996

American Academy of Child and Adolescent Psychiatry: Practice parameters for the assessment and treatment of children, adolescents and adults with mental retardation and comorbid mental disorders. J Am Acad Child Adolescent Psychiatry 38 (suppl):5S–31S, 1999

American Academy of Child and Adolescent Psychiatry: Practice parameter for the prevention and management of aggressive behavior in child and adolescent psychiatric institutions, with special reference to seclusion and restraint. J Am Acad Child Adolesc Psychiatry 41 (suppl):4S–25S, 2001

American Psychiatric Association: Diagnostic and Statistical Manual of Mental Disorders, 3rd Edition. Washington, DC, American Psychiatric Association, 1980

American Psychiatric Association: Diagnostic and Statistical Manual of Mental Disorders, 4th Edition, Text Revision. Washington, DC, American Psychiatric Association, 2000

Antochi R, Stavrakaki C, Emery PC: Psychopharmacological treatments in persons with dual diagnosis of psychiatric disorders and developmental disabilities. Postgrad Med J 79:139–146, 2003

Aziz M, Maixner DF, DeQuardo J, et al: ECT and mental retardation: a review and case reports. J ECT 17:149–152, 2001

Bailine SH, Petraviciute S: Catatonia in autistic twins: role of electroconvulsive therapy. J ECT 23:21–22, 2007

Bongiorno FP: Dual diagnosis: developmental disability complicated by mental illness. South Med J 89:1142–1146, 1996

Brosco JP, Mattingly M, Sanders LM: Impact of specific medical interventions on reducing the prevalence of mental retardation. Arch Pediatr Adolesc Med 160:302–309, 2006

Chakrabarti S, Fombonne E: Pervasive developmental disorders in preschool children: confirmation of high prevalence. Am J Psychiatry 162:1133–1141, 2005

Chaplin R: General psychiatric services for adults with intellectual disability and mental illness. J Intellect Disabil Res 48:1–10, 2004

Coffey CE, Brumback RA: Pediatric Neuropsychiatry. Philadelphia, PA, Lippincott Williams & Wilkins, 2006, pp ix–x

Cutajar P, Wilson D: The use of ECT in intellectual disability. J Intellect Disabil Res 43:421–427, 1999

Day K: Psychiatric services in mental retardation: generic or specialized provision? in Mental Health in Mental Retardation. Edited by Bouras N. Cambridge, UK, Cambridge University Press, 1994, pp 275–292

Day K: Service provision and staff training: an overview, in Treating Mental Illness and Behavior Disorders in Children and Adults With Mental Retardation. Edited by Doson A, Day K. Washington, DC, American Psychiatric Publishing, 2001, pp 469–492

Day K, Dosen A: Treatment: an integrative approach, in Treating Mental Illness and Behavior Disorders in Children and Adults With Mental Retardation. Edited by Doson A, Day K. Washington, DC, American Psychiatric Publishing, 2001, pp 519–528

Dean AJ, McDermott BM, Marshall RT: PRN sedation: patterns of prescribing and administration in a child and adolescent mental health inpatient service. Eur Child Adolesc Psychiatry 15:277–281, 2006

Delaney KR: Evidence base for practice: reduction of restraint and seclusion use during child and adolescent inpatient treatment. Worldviews Evid Based Nurs 3:19–30, 2006

Delaney KR, Fogg L: Patient characteristics and setting variables related to the use of restraint on four inpatient psychiatric units for youths. Psychiatr Serv 56:186–192, 2005

Dosen A: Integrative treatment in persons with intellectual disability and mental health problems. J Intellect Disabil Res 51:66–74, 2007

Dosen A, Day K: Epidemiology, etiology, and presentation of mental illness and behavior disorders in persons with mental retardation, in Treating Mental Illness and Behavior Disorders in Children and Adults With Mental Retardation. Edited by Dosen A, Day K. Washington, DC, American Psychiatric Publishing, 2001, pp 3–24

Douma JCH, Dekker MC, Koot HM: Supporting parents of youths with intellectual disabilities and psychopathology. J Intellect Disabil Res 50:570–581, 2006

Dykens EM: Annotation: psychopathology in children with intellectual disability. J Child Psychol Psychiatry 41:407–417, 2000

Feldman EK: The recognition and investigation X-linked learning disability syndromes. J Intellect Disabil Res 40:400–411, 1996

Fleisher M, Faulkner EH, Schalock RL, et al: A model for inpatient services for persons with mental retardation and mental illness, in Treating Mental Illness and Behavior Disorders in Children and Adults With Mental Retardation. Edited by Dosen A, Day K. Washington, DC, American Psychiatric Publishing, 2001, pp 503–518

Fombonne E: Epidemiology of autistic disorder and other pervasive developmental disorders. J Clin Psychiatry 66 (suppl):3–8, 2005

Fryer MA, Beech M, Byrne GJA: Seclusion use with children and adolescents: an Australian experience. Aust NZ J Psychiatry 38:26–33, 2004

Gardiner WI, Graeber-Whalen JL, Ford DR: Behavioral therapies: individualizing interventions through treatment formulations, in Treating Mental Illness and Behavior Disorders in Children and Adults With Mental Retardation. Edited by Dosen A, Day K: Washington, DC, American Psychiatric Publishing, 2001, pp 69–100

Ghaziuddin M, Quinlan P, Ghaziuddin N: Catonia in autism: a distinct subtype? J Intellect Disabil Res 49:102–105, 2005

Handen BL, Gilchrist R: Practitioner review: psychopharmacology in children and adolescents with mental retardation. J Child Psychol Psychiatry 47:871–882, 2006

Harris J: Developmental Neuropsychiatry, Vol 2. Oxford, England, Oxford University Press, 1995

Harris J: Physical restraint procedures for managing challenging behaviors presented by mentally retarded adults and children. Res Dev Disabil 17:99–134, 1996

Hastings RP, Beck A: Practitioner review: stress intervention for parents of children with intellectual disabilities. J Child Psychol Psychiatry 45:1338–1349, 2004

Holden B, Gitlesen JP: The association between severity of intellectual disability and psychiatric symptomatology. J Intellect Disabil Res 48:556–562, 2004

Jones E, Allen D, Moore K, et al: Restraint and self-injury in people with intellectual disabilities: a review. J Intellect Disabil 11:105–118, 2007

Joint Commission: Restraint and Seclusion, in Comprehensive Accreditation Manual for Behavioral Health Care (CAMBHe). Oakbrook Terrace, IL, Joint Commission, 2008, PC–50

Jopp DA, Keys CB: Diagnostic overshadowing reviewed and reconsidered. Am J Ment Retard 106:416–433, 2001

Koskentausta T, Livanainen M, Almqvist F: Risk factors for psychiatric disturbance in children with intellectual disability. J Intellect Disabil Res 51:43–53, 2007

LeBel J, Stromberg N, Duckworth K, et al: Child and adolescent inpatient restraint reduction: a state initiative to promote strength-based care. J Am Acad Child Adolesc Psychiatry 43:37–45, 2004

Leyfer OT, Folstein SE, Bacalman S, et al: Comorbid psychiatric disorders in children with autism: interview development and rates of disorders. J Autism Dev Disord 36:849–861, 2006

Lobato DJ, Kao BT: Integrated sibling-parent group intervention to improve sibling knowledge and adjustment to chronic illness and disability. J Pediatr Psychol 27:711–716, 2002

Lord C, Rutter M, Le Couteur A: Autism Diagnostic Interview–Revised: a revised version of a diagnostic interview for caregivers of individuals with possible pervasive developmental disorders. J Autism Dev Disord 24:659–685, 1994

Lord C, Risi S, Lambrecht L, et al: The Autism Diagnostic Observation Schedule-Generic: a standard measure of social and communication deficits associated with the spectrum of autism. J Autism Dev Disord 30:205–223, 2000

Madrid AL, State MW, King BH: Pharmacological management of psychiatric and behavioral symptoms in mental retardation. Child Adolesc Psychiatr Clin N Am 9:225–243, 2000

Malone RP, Gratz SS, Delaney MA, et al: Advances in drug treatments for children and adolescents with autism and other pervasive developmental disorders. CNS Drugs 19:923–934, 2005

McGee JJ, Folk L, Swanson DA, et al: A model inpatient psychiatric program: its relationship to a continuum of care for the mentally retarded-mentally ill, in Handbook of Mental Illness in the Mentally Retarded. Edited by Menolascino FJ, Stark JA. London, Plenum, 1984, pp 249–272

Miller JA, Hunt DP, Georges MA: Reduction of physical restraints in residential treatment facilities. Journal of Disability Policy Studies 16:202–208, 2006

Mohr WK, Petti TA, Mohr BD: Adverse effects associated with physical restraint. Can J Psychiatry 48:330–337, 2003

Moss D, Emerson E, Bouras N, et al: Mental disorders and problematic behaviours in people with intellectual disability: future directions for research. J Intellect Disabil Res 41:440–447, 1997

Murphy GH, Beadle-Brown J, Wing L, et al: Chronicity of challenging behaviours in people with severe intellectual disabilities and/or autism: a total population sample. J Autism Dev Disord 35:405–418, 2005

Nunno MA, Holden MJ, Tollar A: Learning from tragedy: a survey of child and adolescent restraint fatalities. Child Abuse Negl 30:1333–1342, 2006

Petti TA, Mohr WK, Somers JW, et al: Perceptions of seclusion and restraint by patients and staff in an intermediate-term care facility. J Child Adolesc Psychiatr Nurs 14:115–127, 2001

Pilling N, McGill P, Cooper V: Characteristics and experiences of children and young people with severe intellectual disabilities and challenging behaviours attending 52-week residential special schools. J Intellect Disabil Res 51:184–196, 2007

Reinblatt SP, Rifkin A, Freeman J: The efficacy of ECT in adults with mental retardation experiencing psychiatric disorders. J ECT 20:208–212, 2004

Rojahn J, Matson JL, Lott D, et al: The Behavior Problems Inventory: an instrument for the assessment of self-injury, stereotyped behavior, and aggression/destruction in individuals with developmental disabilities. J Autism Dev Disord 13:577–588, 2001

Rojahn J, Aman MG, Matson JF, et al: The aberrant behavior checklist and the behavior problems inventory: convergent and divergent validity. Res Dev Disabil 24:391–404, 2003

Ruedrich S, Menolascino FJ: Dual diagnosis of mental retardation and mental illness: an overview, in Handbook of Mental Illness in the Mentally Retarded. Edited by Menolascino FJ, Stark JA. London, Plenum, 1984, pp 45–82

Ryan R, Sunada K: Medical evaluation of persons with mental retardation referred for psychiatric assessment. Gen Hosp Psychiatry 19:274–280, 1997

Scahill L, McDougle CJ, Williams S, et al: Children's Yale-Brown Obsessive Compulsive Scale modified for pervasive developmental disorders. J Am Acad Child Adolesc Psychiatry 45:1114–1123, 2006

Schneider J, Wedgewood N, Llewellyn G, et al: Families challenged by and accommodating to the adolescent years. J Intellect Disabil Res 50:926–936, 2006

Schreiner GM, Crafton CG, Sevin JA: Decreasing the use of mechanical restraints and locked seclusion. Adm Policy Ment Health 31:449–463, 2004

Schretlen DJ, Ward J, Meyer SM, et al: Behavioral aspects of Lesch-Nyhan disease and its variants. Dev Med Child Neurol 47:673–677, 2005

Schroeder SR, Oster-Granite ML, Berkson G, et al: Self-injurious behavior: gene-brain-behavior relationships. Ment Retard Dev Disabil Res Rev 7:3–12, 2001

Shattuck PT: The contribution of diagnostic substitution to the growing administrative prevalence of autism in US special education. Pediatrics 117:1028–1037, 2006

Smith MC: Optimizing therapy of seizures in children and adolescents with developmental disabilities. Neurology 67:S52–S55, 2006

Smith P, Berney TP: Psychiatric inpatient units for children and adolescents with intellectual disability. J Intellect Disabil Res 50:608–614, 2006

State MW, King BH, Dykens E: A review of the past 10 years (mental retardation, part 1). J Am Acad Child Adolesc Psychiatry 36:1664–1668, 1997

Wagner A, Lecavalier L, Arnold LE, et al: Developmental disabilities modification of the children's global assessment scale. Biol Psychiatry 61:504–511, 2007

Wallander JL, Dekker MC, Koot HM: Risk factor for psychopathology in children with intellectual disability: a prospective longitudinal population-based study. J Intellect Disabil Res 50:259–268, 2006

Zaw FKM, Bates GDL, Murali V, et al: Catatonia, autism and ECT. Dev Med Child Neurol 41:843–845, 1999

CHAPTER 11

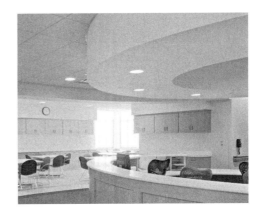

THE ETHNIC/MINORITY PSYCHIATRIC INPATIENT UNIT

Francis G. Lu, M.D.

Since the late 1990s, national attention has focused increasingly on the importance of reducing health care disparities by increasing the cultural competence and workforce diversity in the delivery of health care to meet the needs of an ever more culturally diverse patient population (Agency for Healthcare Research and Quality 2007; U.S. Department of Health and Human Services Office of Minority Health 2000). During this time, there has been a parallel development in these areas for mental health care. After first reviewing the issues relevant to the mental health care of culturally diverse patients, this chapter will describe one example of a psychiatric inpatient service that has focused on cultural competence and reducing mental health disparities: the Ethnic/Minority Psychiatric Inpatient Programs at San Francisco General Hospital (SFGH), which began its journey toward cultural competence in 1980 to provide services for underserved populations.

Mental Health Care Disparities and Cultural Competence

In August 2001, the Surgeon General issued a supplement to the 1999 *Mental Health: A Report of the Surgeon General* entitled *Mental Health: Culture, Race, and Ethnicity* (U.S. Surgeon General 2001). This landmark report for the first time documented comprehensively striking disparities in mental health care for racial and ethnic minorities involving access, appropriateness, quality, and outcomes. Minorities were documented to be woefully underrepresented in research studies. Taken as a whole, these disparities imposed a greater disability burden on racial and ethnic minorities. The following are some examples from the four chapters on the four major racial and ethnic groups:

- Disproportionate numbers of African Americans are represented in the most vulnerable segments of the population—people who are homeless, incarcerated, in the child welfare system, or victims of trauma—all populations with increased risks for mental disorders.
- As many as 40% of Hispanic Americans report limited English-language proficiency. Because few mental health care providers identify themselves as Spanish-speaking, most Hispanic Americans have limited access to ethnically or linguistically similar providers.
- The suicide rate among American Indians/Alaska Natives is 50% higher than the national rate; rates of co-occurring mental illness and substance abuse (especially alcohol) are also higher among native youth and adults. Because few data have been collected, the full nature, extent, and sources of these disparities remain a matter of conjecture.
- Asian Americans/Pacific Islanders who seek care for a mental illness often present with more severe illnesses than do other racial or ethnic groups. This, in part, suggests that stigma and shame are critical deterrents to service utilization. It is also possible that mental illnesses may be undiagnosed or treated later in their course because they are expressed in symptoms of a physical nature.

The report concluded with a chapter titled "A Vision for the Future" in which recommendations were grouped in several areas. The first recommendation area was to "continue to expand the science base." Within this recommendation the report noted that

> clinicians' awareness of their own cultural orientation, their knowledge of the client's background, and their skills with different cultural groups may be essential to improving access, utilization, and quality of mental health services for minority populations. While no rigorous, systematic studies have been conducted to test these hypotheses, evidence suggests that culturally oriented interventions are more effective than usual care at reducing dropout rates for ethnic minority mental health clients. While the efficacy of most ethnic-specific or culturally responsive services is yet to be determined, models already shown to be useful through research could be targeted for further efficacy research and, ultimately, dissemination to mental health providers. (U.S. Surgeon General 2001, p. 161)

The inclusion of a "Glossary of Culture-Bound Syndromes" and the "Outline for Cultural Formulation" within DSM-IV (American Psychiatric Association 1994) was a significant step forward in recognizing the impact of culture, race, and ethnicity on mental health. The report also noted that

> A few studies have examined racial and ethnic differences in the metabolism of clinically important drugs to treat mental illnesses. As the evidence base grows, improved treatment guidelines will help clinicians be aware that differences in metabolic response, as well as differences in age, gender, family history, lifestyle, and co-occurring illnesses, can alter a drug's safety and efficacy. For example, clinicians are becoming sensitized to the possibility that a significant proportion of racial and minority patients will respond to some common medications at lower-than-usual dosages. (U.S. Surgeon General 2001, p. 161)

The second recommendation made was to "improve access to treatment." The report noted the importance of improving geographic access for those living in rural and other medically underserved areas as well as ensuring language access: "A major barrier to effective mental health treatment arises when provider and patient do not speak the same language" (U.S. Surgeon General 2001, p. 163). In 2000, nearly 47 million people—18% of the U.S. population—spoke a language other than English at home. The 2000 census documented that more than 28% of all Spanish speakers, 22.5% of Asian and Pacific Island language speakers, and 13% of Indo-European language speakers spoke English "not well" or "not at all." Limited English proficiency affects the person's ability to access and receive health and mental health care.

The third recommendation, to "reduce barriers to treatment," is related to the subsequent President's New Freedom Commission on Mental Health (2003) report *Achieving the Promise: Transforming Mental Health Care in America*, which was issued in July 2003. Within the New Freedom Commission report, the primary goal for culturally diverse populations was that "disparities in mental health services are eliminated." By way of background, this report noted that racial and ethic minorities face additional barriers to accessing and receiving quality care such as mistrust and fear of treatment; different cultural ideas about illnesses and health; differences in help-seeking behaviors, language, and communication patterns; racism; varying rates of being uninsured; and discrimination by individuals and institutions.

The fourth recommendation area in the surgeon general's report was to "improve quality of care." As stated in the report,

Culture and language affect the perception, utilization, and, potentially, the outcomes of mental health services. Therefore, the provision of culturally and linguistically appropriate mental health services is a key ingredient for any programming designed to meet the needs of diverse racial and ethnic populations. The programming should include: 1) language access for persons with limited English proficiency; 2) services provided in a manner that is congruent, rather than conflicting, with cultural norms; and 3) the capacity of the provider to convey understanding and respect for the client's worldview and experiences. (U.S. Surgeon General 2001, p. 166)

A fifth recommendation was to "support capacity development." Here, the importance of continuing education for mental health staff was noted: "…many providers and researchers of all backgrounds are not fully aware of the impact of culture on mental health, mental illness, and mental health services. All mental health professionals are encouraged to develop their understanding of the roles of age, gender, race, ethnicity, and culture in research and treatment" (U.S. Surgeon General 2001, p. 167). Lu and Primm (2006) provided specific analysis and recommendations for how the field of psychiatry can play an important role in increasing cultural competence and reducing disparities in medical student education consistent with LCME accreditation standards. The President's New Freedom Commission on Mental Health (2003) report also highlighted that "culturally competent services are essential to improve the mental health system" (p. 52). The following definition of cultural competence was given:

Culturally competent services [italics in text] are "the delivery of services that are responsive to the cultural concerns of racial and ethnic minority groups, including their language, histories, traditions, beliefs, and values (U.S. Surgeon General 2001)." Cultural competence in mental health is a general approach to delivering services that recognizes, incorporates, practices, and values cultural diversity. Its basic objectives are to ensure quality services for culturally diverse populations, including culturally appropriate prevention, outreach, service location, engagement, assessment, and intervention. (President's New Freedom Commission on Mental Health 2003, p. 52)

As also noted in the report, "Despite widespread use of the concept of cultural competence, research on putting the concept into practice and measuring its effectiveness is lacking" (President's New Freedom Commission on Mental Health 2003, p. 52).

Case Example: The Ethnic/Minority Psychiatric Inpatient Programs at San Francisco General Hospital

History and Overview

The Ethnic/Minority Psychiatric Inpatient Programs that began in 1980 on one inpatient unit at the University of California San Francisco (UCSF) Department of Psychiatry at SFGH strive to provide the highest quality of care to individuals with severe mental illnesses who largely depend on public sector services due to Medicare or Medi-Cal insurance or lack of health insurance. From 1985 to 2008, the inpatient programs were on five inpatient units with a total of 97 beds. As of July 2008, the inpatient programs consist of four acute diagnostic and treatment units with a total of 75 beds. Each inpatient unit has developed a single or dual focus reflecting the cultural diversity of both San Francisco and the patients served by the SFGH, the only acute public hospital in San Francisco funded by the Department of Public Health of the City and County of San Francisco. The U.S. Census Bureau reported that in 2005, 33.3% of the San Francisco population was Asian/Pacific Islander, 7.3% black, 13.7% Hispanic, 0.5% American Indian, 44.1% white (not Hispanic), and 2.3% two or more races (U.S. Census Bureau 2005). In 1987, the American Psychiatric Association awarded a Certificate of Significant Achievement to these programs "in recognition of the innovative model program that provides specialized services for four previously underserved groups, including Asian/Asian American, Latino, African American, and AIDS/HIV patients as well as services geared to the special needs of women." In 1999, the programs were awarded the American College of Psychiatrists Award for Creativity in Psychiatric Education "in official recognition of creativity in addressing significant educational issues and sustained commitment to excellence in psychiatric education that can serve as a model for other programs." Finally, in 2006, the programs were awarded the San Francisco Department of Public Health Award of Excellence for Cultural Competence.

These Ethnic/Minority Psychiatric Inpatient Programs began in March 1980, before the start of the initiatives in cultural competence and reducing mental health disparities described earlier in the chapter, when I initiated the Asian Focus Psychiatric Inpatient Unit, which was the first inpatient psychiatric program in the United States with a focus on the cultural needs of Asians/Asian Americans. It linked with preexisting Asian-focused outpatient/day treatment mental health services in the San Francisco Department of Public Health Community Mental Health Services to provide a comprehensive system of care for the Asian population of San Francisco, then 22% of the city of 685,000 people. The focus service concept was highlighted in the 1978 report of President Carter's Commission on Mental Health, Subpanel on Asian Americans (President's Commission on Mental Health 1978), as a cost-effective way to efficiently utilize scarce human resources of bilingual/bicultural staff to care for this underserved population. The focus service concept brings together multidisciplinary staff, faculty, and trainees to work with patients who could benefit from their cultural and linguistic expertise related to diagnosis, assessment, and treatment. The Asian Focus Program Unit has served as a model for the initiation and development of the other four focus units. Psychiatrists, nursing staff, social workers, occupational therapists, and psychologists comprise the staff. SFGH has been a major teaching hospital at UCSF since the late 1800s. Trainees include UCSF postgraduate year–1 psychiatric residents (23-week rotation on several inpatient units); year-3 and year-4 medical students; psychology fellows; and students of social work, nursing, and occupational therapy. A 1991 article by Zatzick and Lu described the concept of the ethnic/minority focus unit as a training site in transcultural psychiatry, with specific discussion of two patients treated on the Asian Focus Program Unit.

Each inpatient program, led by an attending psychiatrist unit chief and nurse manager, has developed expertise and experience in working with individuals from underserved populations who may have needs best served by the unit. The department is committed to recruiting and retaining a culturally and linguistically diverse staff with this expertise. The focus service concept is not a form of segregation, because we have staff and patients of many ethnicities on all units. Despite their focus on different populations, the programs share a commitment to providing care that is sensitive and responsive to the complex cultural identity and particular needs of every individual patient and family rather than prematurely stereotyped patients. The DSM-IV-TR "Outline for Cultural Formulation" provides a concise clinical tool to help guide clinicians and is incorporated routinely in department case conference presentations (American Psychiatric Association 2000). The Outline was incorporated into the *Practice Guideline for the Psychiatric Evaluation of Adults,* 2nd Edition (American Psychiatric Association 2006) and has been the subject of several impor-

tant recent publications (Group for the Advancement of Psychiatry 2002; Koskoff 2002; Lim 2006). Staff are provided diversity training modeled after the small group experiential work of Elaine Pinderhughes (1988) to explore differences across race, ethnicity, gender, and sexual orientation, especially when these differences intersect with power differentials between staff and patients; staff comfort with such differences is important in working with our culturally diverse patients.

Ethnic/Minority Psychiatric Inpatient Programs: Descriptions and Admission Indications

Almost all patients admitted to Ethnic/Minority Psychiatric Inpatient Programs are first assessed in the Psychiatric Emergency Service. Nearly 100% of patients admitted to the inpatient units are involuntarily committed because of dangerousness to self, dangerousness to others, or grave disability (inability to provide food, clothing, or shelter) due to a mental disorder and because the patient is either unwilling or incapable to accept treatment voluntarily. The department has a procedure for admission indications based on staff expertise and patient needs, which in turn is based on the San Francisco Department of Public Health Policy Number 102 on Cultural and Linguistic Competency. This policy states that health care organizations should ensure that patients/consumers receive from all staff members effective, understandable, and respectful care provided in a manner compatible with the patients' cultural health beliefs and practices and preferred language. The extent to which patients are admitted to the unit that best meets their needs is contingent on many factors such as bed availability and unit acuity.

ASIAN FOCUS PROGRAM

The unit's staff share common linguistic and cultural backgrounds with many of the patients. The staff speak 16 Asian languages and dialects of Chinese (including Cantonese, Mandarin, Toishanese), Tagalog, and Vietnamese. About two-thirds of the staff are Asian; many have migrated from countries outside the United States. Family assessment and dealing with the intense stigma of mental illness are particularly emphasized. The unit operations are more fully described later in the chapter to exemplify how such ethnic/minority focus units provide care (Gee et al. 1999). A key textbook for staff and trainees on this unit was edited by the late Evelyn Lee, Ed.D., M.S.S.A., Clinical

Professor of Psychiatry at UCSF, who worked on the unit from 1982 to 1988 (Lee 1997).

Admission indications for the Asian Focus Program Unit are as follows:

A. Patients who have Asian languages as their primary or preferred language.
B. Patients whose families or significant others have Asian languages as their primary or preferred language.
C. Patients and significant others who are culturally identified as Asians, Asian Americans, or Pacific Islanders.
D. Patients who have clinically significant issues related to culture. Examples include
   1. Immigration stress
   2. Acculturation differences among family members
   3. Victims of racial violence and discrimination
   4. Victims of political oppression, colonization, and war
   5. Cultural expressions or explanations of illness
   6. Use of indigenous healing systems
   7. Cultural supports (e.g., family or religion) or stressors that need assessment
E. Patients who have had prior or ongoing treatment with Asian-focused inpatient or outpatient programs in order to maintain treatment continuity.
F. Patients who state a preference/request for the Asian Focus Program Unit.

Contraindications for admission include the following:

A. Patients who have a history of severe physical assault, strong ideation of assault, or history of verbal abuse/racial harassment, specifically against or by Asians.
B. Patients who actively decline to be admitted to the unit.

LATINO FOCUS PROGRAM

Started in 1982, the Latino Focus Program works with Spanish-speaking patients and families that have limited English proficiency as well as with patients and families that are English-speaking. The patients have national origins from Mexico and Central and South American countries. A key textbook was edited by two former faculty members, Alberto Lopez, M.D., M.P.H., and Ernestina Carrillo, M.S.W., who initiated the Latino Focus Program and worked on the unit from the early 1980s to the early 1990s (Lopez and Carrillo

2001). Herrera and Collazo (1999) described a similar Latino-focused milieu in New York City.

Admission indications for the Latino Focus Program Unit are as follows:

A. Patients who have Spanish as their primary or preferred language.
B. Patients whose families or significant others have Spanish as their primary or preferred language.
C. Patients and significant others who are culturally identified as Latinos or Hispanic.
D. Patients who have clinically significant issues related to culture (such as those noted earlier in the Asian Focus Program indications).
E. Patients who have had prior or ongoing treatment for Latino-focused issues with inpatient or outpatient programs in order to maintain treatment continuity.
F. Patients who state a preference/request for the Latino Focus Program Unit.

Contraindications for admission include the following:

A. Patients who have a history of severe physical assault, strong ideation of assault, or history of verbal abuse/racial harassment specifically against or by Latinos.
B. Patients who actively decline to be admitted to the unit.

WOMEN'S FOCUS PROGRAM

Started in 1982 by Anna Spielvogel, M.D., Ph.D. (now Clinical Professor and Associate Residency Training Director), the Women's Focus Program works with women needing psychiatric assessment and treatment during pregnancy, postpartum, and menopause; women dealing with parenting issues; women experiencing past and present trauma (such as physical and sexual abuse, rape, and domestic violence); and women diagnosed with major psychiatric disorders. This team developed innovative treatment approaches for severely mentally ill women, first focusing on treating psychotic pregnant women and later developing specialized treatment approaches for women who self-mutilate, those doing sex trade work, and women with severe drug and alcohol dependence.

Admission indications for the Women's Focus Program Unit are as follows:

A. Women who have histories of severe trauma, including recent sexual assault, domestic violence, and childhood trauma, and women with dissociative disorders.

B. Women with obstetric/gynecological and reproductive issues, including pregnancy, menopause, and reproductive choice.
C. Women struggling with multiple gender roles.
D. Women with child-rearing issues, including relinquishment.
E. Patients who have had prior or ongoing treatment with Women's Focus inpatient or outpatient programs, in order to maintain treatment continuity.
F. Patients who state a preference/request for the Women's Focus Program Unit.

Contraindications for admission include the following:

A. Patients who have a history of physical/sexual assault against women, strong ideation of assault, stalking, and/or harassing of women or children or who have a history of such acts by women against them.
B. Patients who actively decline to be admitted to the unit.

BLACK FOCUS PROGRAM

Started in 1985, the Black Focus Program has expertise in African American, African Caribbean, and African patient issues. Family assessment, spirituality, and understanding of racism, racial discrimination, and racial identity development are some of the relevant issues seen on this unit (Ridley 2005; Whaley 2004). Michelle O. Clark, M.D., Associate Clinical Professor, who was the Unit Chief from the late 1980s to the late 1990s, described the unit in 1999 (Clark 1999).

Admissions indications for the Black Focus Program Unit are as follows:

A. Patients or significant others who self-identify as black, African American, or African.
B. Patients who have conflicts about racial identity and prefer a black-focused program.
C. Patients who have clinically significant issues related to culture. Examples include
   1. Social stressors of racism/discrimination that affect development or functional ability
   2. Black cultural family issues
   3. Black religious or spiritual supports or conflicts
   4. Cultural expressions or explanations of illness
   5. Use of indigenous healing systems
   6. Patient or family communication in primarily African American vernacular English, African Caribbean, Arabic, or other African language.

D. Patients who have had prior or ongoing treatment with black-focused inpatient or outpatient programs in order to maintain treatment continuity.
E. Patients who have had difficulty linking with white-dominated mental health providers.
F. Patients who state a preference/request for the Black Focus Program Unit.

Contraindications for admission include the following:

A. Patients who have a history of severe physical assault, strong ideation of assault, or history of verbal abuse/racial harassment specifically by or against blacks.
B. Patients who actively decline to be admitted to the unit.

HIV/AIDS FOCUS PROGRAM

Started by Jay Baer, M.D., in 1982, the HIV/AIDS Focus Program has experience in working on this medical/psychiatric interface since the start of the HIV/AIDS epidemic that greatly affected San Francisco. Two articles by Baer (1989; Baer et al. 1987) described the initial history of this program. In July 2008, this program was integrated into the other psychiatric programs.

Admission indications for the HIV/AIDS Focus Program Unit were as follows:

A. Patients with medical complications of HIV/AIDS that could benefit from the close liaison with the AIDS consultation team. Examples include those with new opportunistic infections and new medications to be considered.
B. Patients with psychological or neuropsychiatric complications of HIV/AIDS, such as recent seroconversion leading to depression, depression due to catastrophic losses, and AIDS dementia.
C. Patients with social issues complicated by HIV/AIDS, including complex relationships with significant others and complex dispositions.
D. Patients with prior or ongoing treatment at the HIV/AIDS medical service or HIV/AIDS-focused inpatient or outpatient programs in order to maintain treatment continuity.
E. Patients who state a preference/request for the HIV/AIDS Focus Program Unit.

The only contraindication for this unit was patients who actively declined to be admitted to the unit.

Lesbian/Gay/Bisexual/Transgender Focus Program

Started in 1992, the Lesbian/Gay/Transgender (LGBT) Focus Program has expertise in working with patients with these sexual orientation identities and relevant clinical issues. A key textbook was edited by Robert Cabaj, M.D., Director of the San Francisco Community Behavioral Health Service, on homosexuality and mental health (Cabaj and Stein 1996).

Admission indications for the LGBT Focus Program Unit are as follows:

A. Patients who state a preference/request for the LGBT team, especially those who are identified with these sexual orientations or who are transgendered (pre- or postsurgery).
B. Patients who have clinically significant issues related to sexual orientation/sexual identity and who prefer/request the LGBT team. Examples include

   1. Conflicts about coming out
   2. Alienation from family/friends/religious communities
   3. Complex social relations related to sexual orientation/sexual identity
   4. Victims of homophobic violence or discrimination

C. Patients with prior or ongoing treatment at LGBT-focused inpatient or outpatient programs in order to maintain treatment continuity.

Contraindications for admission include the following:

A. Patients who are clearly homophobic or actively decline to be admitted to the unit.
B. Patients who have been violent or have strong assault ideation toward LGBT persons.
C. Patients who are in an acute homosexual panic.

Forensic Focus Program

This 10-bed inpatient unit provides acute emergency evaluation and treatment for patients in the San Francisco County Jail system. Patients are mostly newly charged and admitted awaiting a pretrial hearing. Unlike the other three inpatient units, only patients with charges are admitted to this unit, and their disposition is return to jail unless their charges are dropped. Staff have developed knowledge and skills to work with patients from the jail system.

Unit Operations: The Example of the Asian Focus Program Unit

Diagnostic Workup

The role of culture and inpatient care infuses many aspects of unit operation, from staff relations to clinical assessment and diagnosis to milieu therapy to family work and treatment planning (Lu 2004). The contribution of the Asian Focus Program Unit to the diagnostic workup relates to the staff's ability to communicate both verbally and nonverbally with the many patients with limited English proficiency who are admitted. Members of the staff are able to speak 16 Asian languages and dialects of Chinese, and the SFGH Interpreters Service has access to interpreters for additional languages. Staff are familiar with working with interpreters (Tribe and Raval 2003). Language access in health care has become an important goal, as demonstrated by the National Health Law Program (2007) Language Access in Health Care Statement of Principles, signed by more than 70 organizations. In addition, the staff members not only are fluent in the various languages but also are trained mental health professionals across multiple disciplines. For example, Cantonese is the predominant Asian language spoken by the patients; we have Cantonese-speaking staff on the unit in the following disciplines: psychology, nursing, social work, occupational therapy, and unit clerk. Such a concentration of Cantonese speakers on the same unit permits true multidisciplinary assessment and treatment planning with both the patient and families. At times, even though the patient speaks English, the families have limited English proficiency. The ability to communicate with the patients and families in their preferred language facilitates rapport and information gathering with patients and families and the conduct of diagnostic tests such as laboratory work, which can sometimes be difficult with more traditionally acculturated Asian patients, who may have divergent explanatory models of illness and treatment pathway preferences.

Secondly, the staff use the DSM-IV-TR "Outline for Cultural Formulation" to facilitate understanding of the sociocultural issues as they affect diagnosis and management. This is especially important for the differential diagnosis as to whether a particular phenomenon represents a cultural norm, an idiom of distress, a culture-bound syndrome, a condition that warrants clinical attention, a sign or symptom of a mental disorder, or some combination of any of these possibilities. Misdiagnosis and resultant mistreatment can be reduced through the use of the outline. The large numbers of multicultural staff who have direct and long-standing experience with patients from diverse Asian cultures greatly helps in the differential diagnosis.

It is also important to note that the cultural assessment involves for all patients not only the primary focus of the unit (Asian in this case) but also any possible issues involving gender (Burt and Hendrick 2005), religion/spirituality (Josephson and Peteet 2004; Koenig 2007), sexual orientation, and socioeconomic status, among others, especially as they intersect the other cultural identity variables (Hays 2007). Finally, family assessment in working with Asian patients has proven to be an essential aspect of the diagnostic workup. As discussed in Evelyn Lee's (1997) book and the classic *Ethnicity and Family Therapy* edited by McGoldrick et al. (2005), the clinician must be sensitive and responsive to the complexities of family dynamics across different Asian ethnic subgroups, generations, genders, and levels of acculturation within the family, which may need to be defined beyond the nuclear family. Family support and stress, as noted in the third part of the "Outline for Cultural Formulation," relates often to the culture of the patient and family.

Therapies

Care is provided through one of two multidisciplinary teams, each led by an attending psychiatrist. Pharmacotherapy strategies take into account the possibility that some Asian patients may require lower dosages of medications to achieve therapeutic improvement and to avoid side effects (Ruiz 2000). It is critically important to understand the patient and families' explanatory model and treatment pathway preferences in order to negotiate differences with the clinicians' model to maximize treatment adherence. Psychotherapy may need modification to accommodate diverse levels of English proficiency and health literacy, cultural identities and worldviews, and explanatory models and treatment pathway preferences. For example, Hays and Iwamasa (2006) demonstrated the important modifications necessary to optimize cognitive-behavioral therapy for culturally diverse populations. Psychoeducational material for patients and families must also take these issues into consideration. Due to the value placed on work and education by traditional Asian families, rehabilitation approaches that promise hope to return to functioning are very important for these patients and families.

Milieu Management

The milieu is designed to provide a multicultural, supportive environment for diagnostic and therapeutic purposes. First, the physical design includes signage in Chinese and Vietnamese languages for patients with limited English proficiency. Patient orientation brochures, description of patients' rights, legal and consent forms, and unit schedules are also translated. The unit decor reflects Asian sensibilities, with appropriate posters, pictures, and paintings. One of the unit televisions is tuned to the Chinese-language station, and newspapers in various Asian languages are present. Rice and tea are available at meals, and an Asian food–cooking group is a popular activity. Consistent with traditional Asian family norms, family members are generally allowed to bring in home-cooked meals for patients.

Group activities include community meetings, occupational therapy groups, small group discussions, medication groups, and patio and recreational activities. The occupational therapy staff include Cantonese-speaking personnel, which allows the conduct of these activities using the predominant Asian language spoken by the patients in addition to English. Activities are scheduled that are popular with the Asian patients; these include the Asian food cooking group, physical exercise group incorporating Asian themes, and a meditation group. Because of the critical mass of patients with limited English and the multicultural and multilingual staff, those patients who might feel isolated on most inpatient units due to their limited English proficiency are able to interact not only with the multidisciplinary staff but also with other patients and family members. This process encourages socialization and group cohesion and support when discussing cultural stressors such as acculturation, refugee and immigrant experiences, and intergenerational stress due to different levels of acculturation within a family.

Management of Suicidal and Aggressive Behaviors

All the ethnic/minority focus units, including the Asian Focus Program Unit, pay particular attention to how culture—broadly speaking—may increase the risk for or protect a particular person from suicidal ideation and acts (Gold 2006; Horton 2006; Wendler and Matthews 2006). Use of the "Outline for Cultural Formulation" can help uncover specific cultural stressors as well as cultural supports that otherwise might be neglected or ignored in the assessment. For example, an individual's religious or spiritual beliefs or practices might not be assessed by the clinician due to personal or professional training issues, yet this might be an important area of either stress or support for the patient. Regarding violent patient behaviors, all of our units have been engaged in a violence reduction project since 2006 to reduce both patient assaults on other patients and staff and the use of seclusion and restraints consistent with national trends.

Discharge Planning

On the Asian Focus Program Unit, as with all the ethnic/minority focus units, the team social worker provides the family/significant other with assessment and disposition planning. The social workers on the Asian Focus Program Unit are both bicultural and bilingual, which facilitates family assessments when there is language concordance with the family. Other staff members with language capability are called on to help with interpretation when needed. Furthermore, the social workers have developed over the years an in-depth knowledge of the cultural resources as well as culturally focused outpatient programs that exist in the San Francisco Community Behavioral Health Services, such as Chinatown/North Beach Clinic, Chinatown Child Development Center, the Richmond Area Multi-Services (Asian and Russian focus), and the South of Market Clinic (Filipino focus) as well as specialized services for battered Asian women and Asian substance abusers. A retrospective study by Mathews et al. (2002) demonstrated that a statistically significantly higher number of patients matched to the appropriate focus unit accepted a referral as compared with patients who were not hospitalized on the appropriate focus unit.

Conclusion

The goal of reducing health care disparities is an important one that has implications for psychiatric hospital treatment. Achieving this goal is facilitated by increasing cultural competence and workforce diversity in the delivery of psychiatric hospital care in order to meet the needs of an increasingly culturally diverse U.S. patient population. The programs described from the SFGH are innovative and may be adapted to other cities and locations with consideration of the cultural diversity in the local population. In addition, some of the treatment principles may be extrapolated to the general inpatient unit when working with individuals

of different ethnic and/or minority status. The specific benefits of providing care on culturally designated units as opposed to units not focused on these groups have not been systematically investigated. More research is needed to address this important issue.

References

Agency for Healthcare Research and Quality: 2007 National Healthcare Disparities Report (AHRQ Publ No. 08-0041). Rockville, MD, Agency for Healthcare Research and Quality, 2007. Available at: http://www.ahrq.gov/qual/qrdr07.htm. Accessed May 27, 2008.

American Psychiatric Association: Diagnostic and Statistical Manual of Mental Disorders, 4th Edition. Washington, DC, American Psychiatric Association, 1994

American Psychiatric Association: Diagnostic and Statistical Manual of Mental Disorders, 4th Edition, Text Revision. Washington, DC, American Psychiatric Association, 2000

American Psychiatric Association: Practice Guideline for the Psychiatric Evaluation of Adults, 2nd Edition. Washington, DC, American Psychiatric Association, 2006

Baer JW: Study of 60 patients with AIDS or AIDS-related complex requiring psychiatric hospitalization. Am J Psychiatry 146:1285–1288, 1989

Baer JW, Hall JM, Holm K, et al: Challenges in developing an inpatient psychiatric program for patients with AIDS and ARC. Hosp Community Psychiatry 38:1299–1303, 1987

Burt V, Hendrick V: Clinical Manual of Women's Mental Health. Washington, DC, American Psychiatric Publishing, 2005

Cabaj RP, Stein TS (eds): Textbook of Homosexuality and Mental Health. Washington, DC, American Psychiatric Press, 1996

Clark M: Development of a client-centered inpatient service for African Americans, in Cross Cultural Psychiatry. Edited by Herrera JM, Lawson WB, Sramek JJ. New York, Wiley, 1999, pp 287–294

Gee K, Du N, Akiyama K, et al: The Asian Focus Unit at UCSF: an 18-year perspective, in Cross Cultural Psychiatry. Edited by Herrera JM, Lawson WB, Sramek JJ. New York, Wiley, 1999, pp 275–286

Gold L: Suicide and gender, in The American Psychiatric Publishing Textbook of Suicide Assessment and Management. Edited by Simon RI, Hales RE. Washington, DC, American Psychiatric Publishing, 2006, pp 77–106

Group for the Advancement of Psychiatry: Cultural Assessment in Clinical Psychiatry. Washington, DC, American Psychiatric Publishing, 2002

Hays PA: Addressing Cultural Complexities in Practice, 2nd Edition. Washington, DC, American Psychological Association, 2007

Hays PA, Iwamasa GY (eds): Culturally Responsive Cognitive-Behavioral Therapy: Assessment, Practice, and Supervision. Washington, DC, American Psychological Association, 2006

Herrera J, Collazo Y: The effectiveness of a culturally sensitive milieu on hospitalized Hispanic patients, in Cross Cultural Psychiatry. Edited by Herrera JM, Lawson WB, Sramek JJ. New York, Wiley, 1999, pp 295–302

Horton L: Social, cultural, and demographic factors in suicide, in The American Psychiatric Publishing Textbook of Suicide Assessment and Management. Edited by Simon RI, Hales RE. Washington, DC, American Psychiatric Publishing, 2006, pp 107–137

Josephson AM, Peteet JR (eds): Handbook of Spirituality and Worldview in Clinical Practice. Washington, DC, American Psychiatric Publishing, 2004

Koenig HG: Spirituality in Patient Care: Why, How, When, and What, 2nd Edition. Philadelphia, PA, Templeton Foundation Press, 2007

Koskoff H: The Culture of Emotions (DVD). Boston, MA, Fanlight Productions, 2002

Lee E (ed): Working With Asian Americans: A Guide for Clinicians. New York, Guilford, 1997

Lim R (ed): The Clinical Manual of Cultural Psychiatry. Washington, DC, American Psychiatric Publishing, 2006

Lopez A, Carrillo E (eds): The Latino Psychiatric Patient: Assessment and Treatment. Washington, DC, American Psychiatric Publishing, 2001

Lu F: Culture and inpatient psychiatry, in Cultural Competence in Clinical Psychiatry. Edited by Tseng W-S, Streltzer J. Washington, DC, American Psychiatric Publishing, 2004

Lu FG, Primm A: Mental health disparities, diversity, and cultural competence in medical student education: how psychiatry can play a role. Acad Psychiatry 30:9–15, 2006

Mathews CA, Glidden D, Murray S, et al: The effect on treatment outcomes of assigning patients to ethnically focused inpatient psychiatric units. Psychiatr Serv 53:830–835, 2002

McGoldrick M, Giordano J, Garcia-Preto (eds): Ethnicity and Family Therapy, 3rd Edition. New York, Guilford, 2005

National Health Law Program: Language Access in Health Care Statement of Principles (June 2007 Update). Washington, DC, National Health Law Program, 2007. Available at: http://www.healthlaw.org/search/item.121215-Language_Access_in_Health_Care_Statement_of_Principles_Explanatory_Guide_Oc?tab=pane_search-results-1. Accessed May 27, 2008.

Pinderhughes E: Understanding Race, Ethnicity and Power. New York, Free Press, 1988

President's Commission on Mental Health: Report to the President. Washington, DC, U.S. Government Printing Office, 1978

President's New Freedom Commission on Mental Health: Achieving the Promise: Transforming Mental Health Care in America. Final Report (DHHS Publ No SMA-03-3832). Rockville, MD, U.S. Department of Health and Human Services, 2003

Ridley C: Overcoming Unintentional Racism in Counseling and Therapy, 2nd Edition. Thousand Oaks, CA, Sage, 2005

Ruiz P (ed): Ethnicity and Psychopharmacology. Washington, DC, American Psychiatric Press, 2000

Tribe R, Raval H: Working With Interpreters in Mental Health. New York, Brunner-Routledge, 2003

U.S. Census Bureau: State and Country QuickFacts. Washington, DC, U.S. Census Bureau, 2005. Available at: http://quickfacts.census.gov/qfd/states/06/06075.html. Accessed May 27, 2008.

U.S. Department of Health and Human Services Office of Minority Health: National Standards on Culturally and Linguistically Appropriate Services (CLAS) in Health Care, 2000. Rockville, MD, U.S. Department of Health and Human Services Office of Minority Health, 2000. Available at: http://www.omhrc.gov/templates/content.aspx?ID=87. Accessed May 27, 2008.

U.S. Surgeon General: Mental Health: Culture, Race, and Ethnicity. A Supplement to Mental Health: A Report of the Surgeon General. Rockville, MD, U.S. Department of Health and Human Services, Public Health Service, Office of the Surgeon General, 2001

Wendler S, Matthews D: Cultural competence in suicide risk assessment, in The American Psychiatric Publishing Textbook of Suicide Assessment and Management. Edited by Simon RI, Hales RE. Washington, DC, American Psychiatric Publishing, 2006, pp 159–176

Whaley AL: Paranoia in African American men receiving inpatient psychiatric treatment. J Am Acad Psychiatry Law 32:282–290, 2004

Zatzick DF, Lu F: The ethnic/minority focus unit as a training site in transcultural psychiatry. Acad Psychiatry 15:218–225, 1991

CHAPTER 12

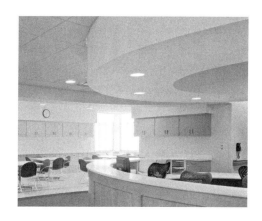

THE FORENSIC UNIT

Michael A. Norko, M.D.
Charles C. Dike, M.D., M.P.H., M.R.C.Psych.

The forensic unit is presented with the same clinical challenges that are addressed on acute or long-term care units in general psychiatric hospitals. In addition to those challenges, the forensic unit must be able to manage the mostly mandated nature of the care provided and the dual nature of forensic treatment (i.e., serving both the care needs of the individual patient as well as the security/safety needs of the facility and the society in which it operates). Because of the nature of this work, the forensic unit is positioned in the middle of the many competing and often adversarial postures of various agents.

Forensic units regularly admit acutely ill patients—who are often psychotic and agitated—under several forms of legal status (discussed later). Patients, particularly those found not guilty by reason of insanity, may also stay many years on forensic units because of concerns about their risk management.

Although much of general inpatient treatment is mandated in some way (e.g., civil commitment, requirements of employment, strong urging of spouse), forensic inpatient treatment may also be mandated by criminal courts—often to the displeasure of individual

patients. Clinicians providing such mandated treatment do not need to feel apologetic about care delivered in such circumstances, but they do need to attend to the special circumstances created by these special mandates (Zonana and Norko 1993).

The dual nature of forensic treatment means that all staff members on a forensic unit (including security staff) need to attend to both treatment and safety/security concerns, because effective treatment can never be delivered in an environment in which people feel unsafe or security is compromised. A collaborative model usually works best in balancing treatment and safety/security concerns (Scales et al. 1989).

Even when such balance is achieved, however, forensic clinicians find themselves practicing in the cross fire of multiple adversarial agents. When treatment is ordered through criminal court, prosecution and defense may both focus attention in court on the care provided and decisions reached by the hospital treatment teams, even though the team members are not retained by either party. Because of the inherently mandated nature of most forensic treatment, legal advocates pay particularly close attention to the rights of these patients, often arguing for treatment that conflicts with the unit's responsibility to courts and local and public safety. Because forensic patients are doubly stigmatized, discharge planning often places the forensic unit in the middle of controversies argued publicly among officials representing defense, prosecution, advocacy, and public safety concerns, all while attempting to maintain hope and the momentum of personal development for the patients.

Admission Criteria

Patients are admitted to forensic units generally under one of four categories: restoration of competency to stand trial; evaluation/treatment of insanity acquittees (those found not guilty, or not criminally responsible, by reason of mental disease or defect); transfers of inmates from correctional facilities for evaluation, acute care, or placement at end of sentence; and civil patients (either voluntary or involuntary) admitted due to agitation and risk of assault that cannot be managed in other environments.

Although many jurisdictions permit outpatient competency restoration, most often this work is accomplished in secure inpatient settings due to concerns about custody as well as treatment compliance. These defendant-patients are sent to the forensic unit by order of a criminal court because they have been found not competent to stand trial. They may have severe psychosis, severe affective disorders, dementia, or cognitive effects of substance abuse or mental disorders caused by medical conditions. The goal of treatment for these patients is to restore the individual's abilities to understand the legal proceedings and to assist in the defense process. This means that this treatment is not directed at holistic or "client centered" goals, because as soon as the relevant capacities are restored, the individual is returned to court. This does not mean, however, that forensic units do not have to do adequate discharge planning, because many defendants (e.g., those with low-level charges) may be released from custody or even have their charges disposed at the time that they are found restored to competence by the court; they are thus returned to the community where they will need ongoing services to help them maintain their health and functioning. It also does not mean that the forensic unit is relieved of the responsibility for providing services to meet immediate needs that are not directly related to competency to stand trial; for example, the unit may have to provide for long-neglected psychiatric, medical, or even surgical interventions.

Insanity acquittees may be brought to the forensic unit for evaluation and/or treatment and custody in a secure environment. This also requires a criminal court commitment after a finding that the individual has met the jurisdiction's legal criteria for a successful insanity defense. In some jurisdictions, the processes for release of acquittees invite even misdemeanor defendants to pursue the defense, whereas in other jurisdictions a strongly conservative statutory approach skews this population to a select group of those charged with only the most serious offenses. Despite the fact that a successful insanity defense requires that the individual both admit the criminal act and prove a serious mental illness, the successful acquittee will often arrive at the hospital denying both propositions emphatically (Zonana and Norko 1993). This complicates therapeutic engagement and treatment planning. Periods of potential commitment may be quite long (e.g., decades), creating challenges for instilling hope for recovery and release.

Patients are referred from correctional settings to forensic units to provide acute hospital-level psychiatric care that cannot be adequately provided in the prison or jail. Such patients are often experiencing acute psychosis, mania, or depression with suicidal thoughts/actions and may well be agitated and have a history of violence both in the community and in correctional environments. They are also sometimes referred for various statutorily created evaluations as part of the criminal justice process. Often inmates with continuing serious psychiatric disabilities may be referred for admission to forensic units upon completion of their prison sentence. Correctional transfer patients may arrive on a voluntary admission or an involuntary admission (including emergency admission processes), often separate from usual civil processes, but with parallel provisions due to constitutional requirements. These admissions are best accomplished through a collaborative approach between mental health colleagues in the hospital forensic unit and the correctional settings.

Finally, the forensic unit is used in many jurisdictions as a tertiary referral cite for civil patients whose aggressive behavior is difficult to manage in other inpatient settings. This happens because forensic units are generally more secure, have increased security staffing, and have experience in dealing with aggressive behaviors among individuals admitted through various stages of the criminal justice system. Civil patients are often admitted under emergency provisions of civil statutes and maintain their civil status while admitted to the forensic unit. Their admission most often also prompts additional scrutiny by legal advocates because admission to forensic units may entail additional curtailment of liberties, invite increased stigma, subject the civil patient to an environment of criminally committed patients, and delay or deter later successful discharge to the community.

Diagnostic Workup

The diagnostic process in a forensic psychiatric inpatient unit is necessarily comprehensive. It involves not only an assessment of the psychiatric condition but also an ongoing assessment of needs and risks. Therefore, a multidisciplinary team approach to diagnosis is emphasized and advocated.

Immediately after an initial admission process involving assessments by psychiatry and nursing (and sometimes social work, psychology, and rehabilitation therapy if the admission occurs during regular hours), a presumptive diagnosis is made. Thereafter, the various disciplines—psychiatry, nursing, psychology, rehabilitation therapy, occupational therapy, social work, and sometimes physical therapy—begin an intense period of discipline-specific assessment of needs that will culminate in the development of a more comprehensive treatment plan within a few days of the admission. A thorough medical assessment also occurs within this period and includes a recommended set of admission laboratory investigations and other special investigations as needed.

Every team member is involved in the assessment of risks, which includes assessing risk-relevant needs and deficits of the individual, so that interventions can be delivered to target those needs and enhance protective factors (Dvoskin and Heilbrun 2001). The patient's behavior is closely monitored on and off the unit and in group settings for risks of suicide, violence, or elopement. "Patients' preferences" can be noted and documented in a special section in the chart. This is a record of how a patient would like to be managed during periods of agitation or loss of control, including ways in which the staff can be most helpful to the patient during these times as well as those steps the patient can directly take to moderate the negative state. These might include time spent alone in a quiet area, listening to music, talking to others, or walking outside in the courtyard.

Obtaining collateral information is generally an important element of formulating diagnosis, but it is even more so in a forensic psychiatric hospital. Patients often arrive directly from court, sometimes with minimal documentation of psychiatric history or current mental state. Important information includes whether the patient was living in the community (in a private residence or program) before the admission or is arriving directly from a correctional setting (prison or jail). If the admission is directly from corrections, it is helpful to note if the patient had been involuntarily medicated, had attempted suicide, or received any "tickets" for disciplinary problems. This information is helpful in the immediate assessment of the severity of psychiatric disorder and current risk of suicide or violence.

A problem often encountered during off-hours admissions from the courts is the unavailability of records. Most of these patients were in jail or prison before going to court and often arrive at the forensic hospital late at night due to the logistics of transport by court marshals. It is often difficult to contact health care workers from the other agencies at such a late hour. Even when this is accomplished, the exaggerated fear that other colleagues hold of breaching patients' confidentially, even when treater-to-treater exemptions to confidentiality are explained to them, prevents disclosure of important, and sometimes life-saving, medical and psychiatric information to the staff of the admitting forensic unit. Risks of not only suicide and violence but also serious medical or surgical problems that require close monitoring and treatment may be overlooked.

Later in the assessment process, a decision is made about the necessity for psychological or neuropsychological testing to assess malingering, personality characteristics, intelligence, cognitive disorders, mood disorders, or psychosis.

Treatment

The most effective treatment utilizes a multidisciplinary approach and involves biological, psychological, and social models of treatment. In addition, the spiritual dimensions of patients' lives are taken into account, and provisions are made, as much as possible, to allow patients to engage in their religious practices. Pastors, imams, priests, and rabbis are incorporated in treatment, especially where there is a religious element to a patient's illness. Furthermore, specific cultural issues that might have an impact on treatment are addressed by inviting specialists in the culture. Despite the mandated nature of treatment on forensic units, opportunities to employ principles of recovery in the work with individual patients should be sought.

Medication Treatment

In terms of biological treatment, psychotropic medication treatments are the most common, but occasionally, electroconvulsive therapy and hormonal therapy are indicated and prescribed. Antipsychotic medications, mood stabilizers, and antidepressants are the most common medications prescribed. Antipsychotics are commonly used, not only for psychosis but also for agitation (Zimbroff 2003), mood stabilization, aggression, and impulsivity (Glancy and Knott 2003). In turn, mood stabilizers are prescribed for agitation, aggression, impulsivity (Glancy and Knott 2002), and augmentation of antipsychotic and antidepressant medications in addition to mood stabilization. Antidepressants are used for depression, anxiety disorders, sexual disorders, and compulsivity/impulsivity (Coccaro and Kavoussi 1997). All three groups of medications are sometimes used for their sleep-inducing side effect potential. Hormonal therapy is indicated for sex offenders (Saleh and Guidry 2003), which includes antiandrogens (e.g., medroxyprogesterone acetate), synthetic gonadotropin-releasing hormone analogues, and oral estrogens. The use of antipsychotic medications and mood stabilizers for aggression and impulsivity is not approved by the U.S. Food and Drug Administration (FDA). Likewise, antidepressants and hormones are used off-label for treating sex offenders.

As noted earlier, the population of patients on a forensic unit is varied, although some treatment resistance is a feature common to many patients. The high prevalence of refractory psychiatric disorders and aggression fosters the use of high dosages of psychotropic medications as well as antipsychotic polypharmacy, despite limited evidence of its usefulness (Stahl 2002). As a result, the prevalence of side effects of medications, such as involuntary motor movements and metabolic syndrome, is high. A relatively sedentary lifestyle imposed by a combination of the patients' illnesses and the structure and nature of forensic units, compounded by the tendency of patients to indulge in excessive eating (food being one of the few pleasures readily available to them), complicate the problem by worsening or maintaining obesity, a common side effect of psychotropic medications. Likewise, the risk of drug–drug interactions is high. Common examples of such interactions include serotonergic syndrome secondary to a combination of medications that increase central nervous system serotonin and increased risk of seizures due to a combination of clozapine and bupropion.

Close monitoring of the metabolic profile of patients through regularly scheduled blood tests and weight documentation would hopefully lead to early detection of abnormalities and prompt treatment. In addition, abnormal involuntary movement should be regularly assessed using the Abnormal Involuntary Movement Scale with patients given antipsychotic medications.

In some instances, however, potentially dangerous side effects or drug–drug interactions may limit medication choices available for vigorously treating psychosis or aggression. The risk of physical aggression to other patients and staff due to inadequate treatment must then be balanced against the dangers of treatment to the patient. This is a complicated process that should be carefully considered and openly discussed with the treatment team members, the patient, and the patient's chosen advocate/representative (or appointed guardian or conservator) as needed. On some occasions, patients admitted for restoration to competency have been recommended to the courts as not competent to stand trial and not restorable because concerns of side effects or adverse drug interactions have made adequate treatment impossible.

A unique characteristic of forensic units that affects medication use is the wide age range of the unit population, from the late teens to the geriatric. Some acquittees spend decades in the hospital, and as they get older, particular attention should be paid to the dosages of their psychotropic medications. Dosages should be adjusted for age as patients move from adulthood to geriatric age in order to avoid gradual toxicity that may sometimes appear to be sudden and inexplicable. In addition, treatment for multiple medical problems resulting from old age may not only complicate psychiatric disorders but also cause dangerous drug–drug interactions.

On a positive note, forensic psychiatric hospitals are exempt from the pressures exerted by insurance companies that lead to quick, and sometimes precipitous, discharges of patients from the hospital. Except for situations when the need to quickly manage aggression dictates otherwise, treatment teams have a unique opportunity to slowly titrate or taper dosages of medications and to try various combinations that may be beneficial for their patients.

Psychotherapies

Psychotherapeutic techniques include individual and group therapy. Commonly used and available individual psychotherapeutic treatments include cognitive-behavioral therapy, behavioral therapy, psychoanalysis, supportive therapy, and various other forms of dynamic psychotherapy. Few forensic units have sufficient resources to offer individual psychotherapy to every patient, nor would it be indicated, so patients are selected for individual therapy on the basis of assessed need and likelihood of efficacy.

Unlike individual therapy, every patient is involved in group therapy sessions. The more basic or routine groups include groups for anger management, social skills training, symptom management, apartment living, money management, medication education, relaxation training, and substance abuse (e.g., Alcoholics Anonymous or Narcotics Anonymous, cognitive-behavioral therapy groups). There are also specialized groups such as dialectical behavior therapy groups that target patients with emotional/behavioral dysregulation related to personality disorder. In addition, patients participate in groups that are specifically germane to a forensic unit, such as competency to stand trial education, not guilty by reason of insanity, family homicide (individuals who have killed family members), legal education, and problem sexual behavior/sex offender groups.

Forensic psychiatry patients often have a long history of institutionalization and have either lost their social skills or never developed them. Anger is usually a big problem, and a history of childhood trauma is common. Group therapy provides an opportunity for patients to learn from their peers and instructors, get support from their peers, and also get feedback on the impact of their behavior on others.

Another psychotherapeutic intervention crucial to managing difficult personality disorders, refractory psychosis, mental retardation, and aggression is behavior therapy. Rewards and reinforcements (positive and negative), as well as clear consequences for inappropriate or intolerable behavior, are used to shape behavior to socially acceptable standards. Although behavioral interventions are very effective, consistent application of behavioral plans through all shifts is difficult. This may be due to staff vacations (especially of trained staff), frequent use of float (work-off) staff who are unfamiliar with the plans, and the reluctance of staff to fully engage in the program. Behavioral plans are often more involved than routine care and require vigilance and active participation of staff to be effective. The relative scarcity of behaviorally trained psychologists further compounds the problem. Therefore, despite research that clearly shows the effectiveness of behavioral interventions in controlling difficult behaviors, behavioral techniques are often not utilized nearly as much as they could be.

Patient and Family Education

The goal of patient and family education on a forensic unit is not only to provide education for family members of forensic patients but also to provide support to them. Often, family members are confused about the differences between a forensic unit and a prison, especially in situations when they have to pass through metal detectors to get to the units. Family members also get frustrated when they are told they cannot bring certain food items or other seemingly innocuous materials that most other hospitals gladly welcome and have difficulty appreciating the potential danger the materials pose. Therefore, family education is necessarily broad in scope and includes an understanding of specific major mental illnesses as well as the special processes and external reviewing agencies that dictate certain special activities of a forensic unit.

In the Whiting Forensic Division of Connecticut Valley Hospital, social workers run the family support group once a month. In addition to providing educational materials covering major mental illnesses, they also invite certain individuals to speak to the family members. Speakers have included the director of the Psychiatric Security Review Board, which reviews movement of insanity acquittees; a public defender assigned specifically to defend insanity acquittees; the director of the forensic units; and an attending psychiatrist on one of the units. In other situations the meetings have a social flavor, and in that context information is shared informally among attendees.

The supportive role these meetings have for family members cannot be overemphasized. They provide opportunities for family members to mutually support each other, share experiences, and offer advice. Those whose relatives have been hospitalized for years share insights with others relatively new to the process. It is believed that the more equipped and the more confident family members feel, the more helpful they will be to both the treatment team and their loved ones.

Rehabilitation and Recreational Therapies

Recreational therapies are used to treat and maintain the physical, mental, and emotional well-being of patients through a variety of techniques, including music, relaxation, arts, sports, games, dance, drama, and community outings. These therapies help individuals reduce depression, stress, and anxiety; develop better social skills; and become more confident. The goal is for patients to express their feelings in a therapeutic setting and to experience meaningful and pleasurable activities despite the limitations of their mental illness.

In addition, therapists help long-stay patients reintegrate into the community by teaching them how to use community resources and recreational activities.

Community trips are planned for patients who have progressed through the maximum security units to less secure units and who have low risks of aggression or elopement. Patients are taught how to utilize relaxation techniques to relieve anxiety. They are also encouraged to develop adaptive leisure activities and hobbies. Leisure activities, especially structured group programs, are particularly helpful not only to maintain patients' general health and well-being but also to decrease opportunities for aggressive behavior.

When patients are involved in structured activities, they may be less likely to grow bored and to intentionally or unintentionally provoke each other out of the frustration of inactivity. Exercise and sports programs help in dissipating energy and in generating an overall feeling of well-being. Through team sports patients learn to work collaboratively with others to achieve a common goal. These activities also provide opportunities for therapists to teach patients anger management and appropriate methods of coping with frustration. For certain patients, especially those with communication difficulties, art therapy may provide an avenue for self-expression, and pet therapy may help the patient establish a connection not only with the pet but also with the staff handler.

In some facilities, forensic patients may have access to a library, computers, and vocational rehabilitation activities such as woodcraft, leather shop, sewing and mending, and cooking. A schoolteacher may be available for those patients who want to pursue further education to obtain a general education diploma. Female patients may be provided special sessions on grooming, including the use of makeup. Due to the potentially dangerous materials available in these activity centers, patients need to attain a certain level of trust in order to be allowed to participate in them. In addition, an agency security officer is always present to ensure patients do not secrete dangerous objects on their persons.

Other rehabilitation therapies, such as physical therapy, occupational therapy, and speech therapy, are available as necessary to help patients achieve their highest level of function.

Other Modalities

Other modalities of treatment include electroconvulsive therapy, which is very effective for treating severe depression and resistant mania. It has also been used to treat chronic and refractory psychosis, but its effectiveness for chronic psychosis is questionable (Tang and Ungvari 2003).

Sex offender treatment is another modality offered on a forensic unit. Most of these individuals have a primary diagnosis of paraphilia, or paraphilia with comorbid psychotic disorder or substance misuse disorders. A growing trend in forensic psychiatry is the admission of sex offenders to forensic units after completion of their sentences in prison. Unfortunately, currently available treatments for sex offenders—hormones, antidepressants, and sex offender groups—have not been proven conclusively to be effective at reducing recidivism; findings of positive effect remain controversial and await further definitive study (Collaborative Outcome Data Committee 2007).

Milieu Management

In addition to the usual requirements of maintaining an effective therapeutic milieu on an inpatient unit, the staff and managers of forensic units must attend to the special demands of milieu management related to safety and control of aggression. Forensic patients have often committed horrifying acts of violence as the basis of their referral, and many exhibit ongoing aggressive behavior that may have been unresponsive to management in other settings. In addition, patients transferred from correctional settings may bring with them pro-criminal attitudes and a prison mentality (including, for example, the perceived need to create and maintain a weapon, or involvement with gangs).

In such an environment it is easy for staff and patients alike to experience fear. The most common reaction to fear is anger, which then potentiates the eruption of violence (Maier et al. 1987). It is thus important to manage fear in order to mitigate staff countertransference and patient aggression. Direct care staff will feel a need to create structure through rules, schedules, and regulations in order to manage safety, although patients often experience this as an excess of staff control (Caplan 1993).

There are several steps to be taken in managing the milieu on a forensic unit in order to maintain safety and promote effective treatment. The first is to acknowledge this task explicitly and programmatically through training of both clinical and security staff. All staff must understand the importance of being mindful of safety and security as well as the need to achieve the therapeutic goals of the unit. Ongoing discussions between treatment and security staff may help keep both these tasks operationalized in practice (Scales et al. 1989).

One of the ways in which security concerns are operationalized by all staff is by attention to the environment. This begins with specific attention to the safety of furniture, mirrors, building materials, hardware, windows, electricity, bathroom facilities, and so on. It also includes regular searches for contraband and weapons in all areas accessible to patients. Items that can be used for cutting, creating fire, or as a weapon should be identified as nonpermitted items, and this information made available to patients and visitors in writing (Kaltiala-Heino and Kahila 2006).

Room and common area inspections also include searching for broken items, missing screws or other hardware, and missing components of appliances, including batteries. Both security and clinical staff participate in such searches, but caution must be exercised to prevent a "guard mentality" from emerging (Phillips and Caplan 2003). The goal is the therapeutic effect of maintaining a safe milieu, not the exercise of control, per se.

On forensic units in which both male and female patients are treated, attention must not only be given to the environmental factors of separated shower and toilet facilities but also to the management of this mixed population. Female patients may feel particularly isolated and vulnerable if they are only one or two among many more male patients on a unit. Thus, sometimes it becomes necessary to group female patients due to gender concerns, despite legal status, diagnosis, or other considerations. The presence of male patients who have histories of sexual aggression or physical assault on females must also be considered in placement decisions.

Performance improvement activities may also be utilized to identify environmental root causes of times or places of increased incidents of aggression. In one facility, the dining rooms were identified as a focus of increased patient aggression. An action plan was created in which utensils were changed, music was provided, some patients were allowed to leave the area earlier, food service workers received extra training in therapeutic communication, and courtyard and gym areas were kept open during this time (Hunter and Love 1996). It is also common that assaults occur more frequently from mid-afternoon through the evening, when available activities often decline. Special attention should be given to extending therapeutic and recreational activities (as well as the requisite staffing) into this higher-risk time period.

Staffing in general is a significant component of effective milieu management in the forensic unit. It is often perceived that higher staffing ratios should generally be available on forensic units (Kaltiala-Heino and Kahila 2006). Direct care staff members feel more comfortable when lower staff-to-patient ratios are main-

tained, and patients perceive a higher level of staff control of the environment under such conditions (Phillips and Caplan 2003). Patients' perception that the environment is safe and well controlled has a calming effect on the unit by decreasing fears and negative stimulation. Too great a perception of rigid control, however, increases the sense of hostility among patients and decreases safety. Effective communication among staff and patients in community meetings is important to maintaining this delicate balance of a controlled environment while permitting individuals to experience some needed levels of privacy and freedom.

Programmatic interventions can also play a major role in the development and maintenance of a therapeutic milieu in forensic environments. For example, behavioral programming can be very effective when it rewards nonaggressive behavior, improvement in social skills and cooperation, and participation in treatment and educational activities. Social learning programs have been instituted effectively in several forensic settings, reducing aggression and use of restraint and seclusion and leading to improvements in milieu management and discharge success (Beck et al. 1991; Goodness and Renfro 2002; Menditto et al. 1991). Although these programs require a significant investment in staff training and maintenance of program integrity, they provide a model of staff intervention that is interactive, continuous, and positive and that contributes to recovery.

Finally, it is worth recognizing that even when the physical environment is safely maintained, staffing levels are adequate, and effective program models are utilized, staff members must still cope with a group of individuals with seriously disturbed behavior and histories of extraordinary violence. Providing settings in which staff can safely unload the effects of chronic stress and exposure to negative thoughts and feelings can be very helpful (Kuhlman 1988).

Management of Suicidal and Aggressive Behaviors

The mix of patients on a forensic unit makes it inherently a high-risk environment. Some patients are transferred directly from correctional settings, some from maximum-security or "super-max" prisons, with a history of being in segregation for violent behaviors or with multiple "tickets" for aggression. These patients are suddenly placed onto units with patients who may be in the early phase of their legal entanglement (sent for restoration to competency) or still trying to make sense of their current legal situation and who are vulnerable by virtue of serious mental illness or developmental disability. In addition, patients who present unmanageable risks of suicide in general hospitals are sometimes sent to forensic hospitals for management because forensic hospitals are more secure and stricter about the availability of dangerous materials with which suicidal patients might harm themselves. Staff in forensic units must therefore be more vigilant to cues that indicate high potential for suicide or physical aggression in their patients.

With regard to suicide, specific interventions to decrease risk include a combination of pharmacological treatment, environmental manipulation, and close monitoring. The presence of depression should be carefully evaluated and vigorously treated, and personality traits that include impulsivity and careless disregard for safety should be noted. Past history of suicide attempts should be thoroughly explored to understand triggers for acting out in such a manner. Family history of suicide or parasuicide is important, but even more so is the patient's opinion regarding the suicide or suicide attempt.

With regard to the physical plant or environmental manipulation, careful attention should be paid to sturdy and standing structures around which vulnerable patients could tie sheets or clothing for hanging. Bathrooms should have detachable shower heads, and the divider between toilet stalls should not provide access to exposed poles, wooden or otherwise. Rooms of acutely suicidal individuals should be stripped of all potentially dangerous materials such as sharp objects, and bed sheets should be replaced by "strong blankets" that cannot be tied together or tied around an object. There should be no access to windows, especially on upper floors, in order to prevent patients from jumping to their death.

Depending on the degree of risk of suicide, patients are often placed under a level of observation. For patients on continuous observation, it might be necessary to include in the physician's orders that the patient should be continuously observed even when using the bathroom. Tragedies can occur when staff members try to protect the privacy of suicidal patients by not observing them closely while in the bathroom/toilet. There should be open and clear communication between the unit leadership and the line staff, including staff members working off-unit who may not fully appreciate the risks involved.

Management of aggression also includes pharmacotherapy, psychotherapy, and environmental manip-

ulation. Pharmacotherapeutic techniques used for treating aggressivity include mood stabilizers, antipsychotics, and antidepressants. These often need to be combined with behavioral interventions to be successful. Sometimes the mere change of a patient's bedroom to a room in a quiet hallway, away from the other patients, may decrease aggression.

For the agitated patient in conflict with his or her peers, a short period of solitude in a time-out room may help de-escalate the situation more quickly. Such use of time-out must be voluntary and may be one of the actions listed by the patient on the patient preferences list. However, there are times when an agitated and angry patient is unable to utilize voluntary time-out but remains threatening and imminently dangerous. Taking such a patient involuntarily to a time-out room may be effective at immediately decreasing agitation, but the intervention would then be considered seclusion because it is no longer a voluntary time-out procedure.

The use of seclusion and restraints to manage aggression (both self- and other-directed) on a forensic unit has become controversial in recent years. The Joint Commission and the Centers for Medicare and Medicaid Services have announced standards that restrict the use of restraints and seclusion to emergency situations in which there is imminent risk that the individual may physically harm himself or others. It is intended that restraints are to be used only as a last resort and to be discontinued as soon as the imminent risk is resolved. These developments were stimulated by the investigative reports of Connecticut's *Hartford Courant* in 1998, which revealed a large number of deaths nationwide during restraint procedures (Appelbaum 1999). The president of the Joint Commission concluded, "These standards underscore the importance of applying great care in using interventions that can harm or even kill patients" (Medscape Medical News 2000). Not only are there restrictions on the initial application of restraint, there are also tighter policies regarding duration in restraints, monitoring of restrained or secluded patients by a licensed independent practitioner, and monitoring of the physical health of the patient during and after restraints/seclusion.

Advocates for some continued use of restraints and seclusion maintain that there are certain situations when a patient loses control and becomes imminently dangerous to self and others, during which the use of restraints and seclusion is appropriate to maintain safety (Liberman 2006). Opponents argue that there are absolutely no indications for the use of restraints and seclusion to manage aggression. They suggest that the best practice is to train line staff in verbal de-escalation methods, mediation techniques, and conflict resolution and to detect aggressive behavior in its early phases and hopefully mitigate it before it becomes uncontrollable (Curie 2005). A balanced approach may seek to reduce the use of seclusion and restraint maximally via programmatic developments and staff training, yet still recognize that, particularly in environments faced with the challenge of violent patients who have been refractory to interventions in other settings, some use of these procedures may still be necessary.

For forensic patients with high risk of aggressive behavior, the unit staff should generate a list of behavioral cues that indicate increasing agitation or psychosis that have historically been associated with violence for the individual. Early detection of these behavioral cues could lead to immediate removal of the patient from the aggravating situation or allow the utilization of the patient's preferred method of decreasing his agitation as recorded in the patient preferences form. Training of line staff on verbal de-escalation techniques is useful. For some patients, the early use of medications for agitation, in addition to interventions discussed earlier, is successful at decreasing aggression. The development of social learning programs, or other behavioral models, can have a significant impact on reducing the risk of aggression by rewarding behaviors that increase communication, cooperation, and conflict resolution and thus increase skills.

Discharge Planning

Involvement of Community Providers, Resources, and Significant Others

As with all inpatient units, discharge planning on the forensic unit ideally begins at the time of admission, when strengths and supports available to the patient in the community are assessed and the trajectory of care is being plotted. There are many special variations of discharge planning within a forensic setting, however.

Patients transferred from correctional settings may well be returned to those settings so that issues of housing, employment, insurance, and availability of health care are not immediate concerns. For these patients, the collaborative relationships that have been built with health care colleagues in the correctional settings are important to successful continuity of care.

Patients restored to competency to stand trial will be returned to court; for serious charges, they will likely be returned to correctional settings, so the comments just made about relationships with correctional colleagues still apply. However, the forensic unit staff can never know what might become of a defendant returned on less serious charges, so they must usually prepare contingency discharge plans. If the patient-defendant is returned to corrections, the treatment staff there will be provided with necessary information for follow-up care. If the individual is released from court, there must be community plans in place for residence, aftercare, and other supports as needed.

When insanity acquittees are discharged to the community, it is often the result of a great deal of work with community providers to craft a detailed plan for appropriate monitoring and delivery of treatment services. Often this follows experience with graded exposures to the community through therapeutic passes or conditional releases. Family, friends, and community providers are involved in the coordination of these carefully constructed plans.

An element of this planning that is unique to this population is the need to overcome the fears and special concerns of community providers, or even the public, that may accompany the release of a well-known insanity acquittee who caused great anguish for the community. These fears will often limit the range of placement opportunities normally available to patients with chronic psychiatric disabilities and often require skillful negotiations on the part of social work staff and other clinicians and managers to assuage fear and promote willingness to engage with a notorious acquittee. Patients labeled "forensic," especially those who have been treated in maximum security facilities, face significant obstacles to successful discharge planning.

Transition to Next Level of Care

For those forensic patients not being returned to correctional settings, it is precisely in the transitioning that the key to successful discharge planning lies. When risk-relevant needs and deficits have been identified and interventions delivered to target them, it is through "demonstration data" of success in graded steps that risk is best managed and plans evolved for the transition process (Dvoskin and Heilbrun 2001). Successful transitioning requires the elaboration of a relapse-prevention plan, detailing measures to avoid circumstances leading to potential harm, contingencies for containing risk when those circumstances are encountered, and strategies for reducing harm should containment plans fail (Dvoskin 2002).

In all of this planning, it is necessary to be mindful of an ethics of risk assessment and management practices. Clinicians must be vigilant to focus their concerns on the clinical care of their patients, avoiding the all-too-easy lapse into becoming agents of social control. Paul Mullen (2000) has expressed this concern poignantly: "Risk assessments…are the proper concern of health professionals to the extent that they initiate remedial interventions that directly or indirectly benefit the person assessed…. Confining and containing offenders as punishment, or simply to prevent further offending, may be legitimate for a criminal justice system but should have no place in a health service" (p. 308).

Special Burden of the Forensic Unit

The dual mandate of the forensic unit to provide clinical care of the individual and protection of the public can often be successfully negotiated by providing good treatment that is focused on the patients' clinical needs. This is most likely to occur when the patients are appropriately admitted for treatable psychiatric conditions that are the source of the risk to the community.

Clinical administrators of forensic units must try to guard against the admission of individuals who pose risk by virtue of criminality and antisocial personality because there is no credible end point for hospitalization of such individuals. The admission of some such individuals is often politically and legally unavoidable, but their presence is debilitating to the therapeutic milieu and staff morale. The misuse of forensic units for preventive detention of dangerous individuals who would otherwise not require hospital-level care contributes to the stigma of mental illness and wastes the finite resources available to treat people with serious mental illness who require conditions of enhanced security. The barriers to discharge (and demands on staff time) of inappropriately placed individuals are extraordinary and contribute to poor bed utilization and patient flow to aftercare placements.

Conclusion

The forensic unit is similar to other inpatient psychiatric units in the diagnoses of patients and the modalities of treatment provided. Forensic units must provide acute care to some individuals and often extended care to other individuals whose psychiatric disabilities are refractory to treatment.

What distinguishes the forensic unit are the explicit specialization in the management of aggression; a patient population composed of individuals who have exhibited often extraordinary levels of violence and destruction; and the need to balance treatment and recovery concerns for patients with security and safety concerns for patients, staff, and visitors to the facility and the outside community. Forensic units can be challenging places to work, especially when staff members find themselves at the center of various competing advocacies and adversarial processes. When balanced approaches are taken to the special tasks of the forensic unit, and when productive teamwork can be fostered, the work can nonetheless be very rewarding.

References

Appelbaum PA: Seclusion and restraint: Congress reacts to reports of abuse. Psychiatr Serv 50:881–885, 1999

Beck NC, Menditto AA, Baldwin LJ, et al: Reduced frequency of aggressive behavior in forensic patients in a social-learning program. Hosp Community Psychiatry 42:750–752, 1991

Caplan CA: Nursing staff and patient perceptions of the ward atmosphere in a maximum security forensic hospital. Arch Psychiatr Nurs 7:23–29, 1993

Coccaro EF, Kavoussi RJ: Fluoxetine and impulsive aggressive behavior in personality-disordered subjects. Arch Gen Psychiatry 54:1081–1088, 1997

Collaborative Outcome Data Committee: Sexual Offender Treatment Outcome Research: CODC Guidelines for Evaluation. Ottowa, Canada, Public Safety Canada, 2007. Available at: http://www.publicsafety.gc.ca/res/cor/rep/codc-en.asp#1. Accessed May 1, 2007.

Curie CG: SAMHSA's commitment to eliminating the use of seclusion and restraint. Psychiatr Serv 56:1139–1140, 2005

Dvoskin J: Knowledge is not power—knowledge is obligation. J Am Acad Psychiatry Law 30:533–540, 2002

Dvoskin JA, Heilbrun K: Risk assessment and release decision-making: toward resolving the great debate. J Am Acad Psychiatry Law 29:6–10, 2001

Glancy GD, Knott TF: Psychopharmacology of violence, part II: mood stabilizers. Newsl Am Acad Psychiatry Law 27:14, 2002

Glancy GD, Knott TF: Psychopharmacology of violence, part III. Newsl Am Acad Psychiatry Law 28:14, 2003

Goodness KR, Renfro NS: Changing a culture: a brief program analysis of a social learning program on a maximum-security forensic unit. Behav Sci Law 20:495–506, 2002

Hunter ME, Love CC: Total quality management and the reduction of inpatient violence and costs in a forensic psychiatric hospital. Psychiatr Serv 47:751–754, 1996

Kaltiala-Heino R, Kahila K: Forensic psychiatric inpatient treatment: creating a therapeutic milieu. Child Adolesc Psychiatr Clin N Am 15:459–475, 2006

Kuhlman TL: Gallows humor for a scaffold setting: managing aggressive patients on a maximum-security forensic unit. Hosp Community Psychiatry 39:1085–1090, 1988

Liberman RP: Elimination of seclusion and restraint: a reasonable goal? Psychiatr Serv 57:576, 2006

Maier GJ, Stava LJ, Morrow BR, et al: A model for understanding and managing cycles of aggression among psychiatric inpatients. Hosp Community Psychiatry 38:520–524, 1987

Medscape Medical News: Joint Commission releases revised restraints standards for behavioral healthcare. Medscape Medical News, 2000. Available at: http://www.medscape.com/viewarticle/411832. Accessed April 27, 2007.

Menditto AA, Baldwin LJ, O'Neal LG, et al: Social-learning procedures for increasing attention and improving basic skills in severely regressed institutionalized patients. J Behav Ther Exp Psychiatry 22:265–269, 1991

Mullen PE: Forensic mental health. Br J Psychiatry 176:307–311, 2000

Phillips RTM, Caplan C: Administrative and staffing problems for psychiatric services in correctional and forensic settings, in Principles and Practice of Forensic Psychiatry, 2nd Edition. Edited by Rosner R. London, Arnold Publishing, 2003

Saleh FM, Guidry LL: Psychosocial and biological treatment considerations for the paraphilic and nonparaphilic sex offender. J Am Acad Psychiatry Law 31:486–493, 2003

Scales CJ, Phillips RTMP, Crysler D: Security aspects of clinical care. Am J Forensic Psychol 7:49–57, 1989

Stahl SM: Antipsychotic polypharmacy: squandering precious resources? J Clin Psychiatry 63:93–94, 2002

Tang W-K, Ungvari GS: Efficacy of electroconvulsive therapy in treatment-resistant schizophrenia: a prospective open trial. Prog Neuropharmacol Biol Psychiatry 27:373–379, 2003

Zimbroff DL: Clinical management of agitation. Medscape Psychiatry Clinical Update, April 2003. Available at: http://www.medscape.com/viewprogram/2311_pnt. Accessed July 11, 2007.

Zonana HV, Norko MA: Mandated treatment, in Clinical Challenges in Psychiatry. Edited by Sledge WR, Tasman A. Washington, DC, American Psychiatric Press, 1993, pp 249–291

CHAPTER 13

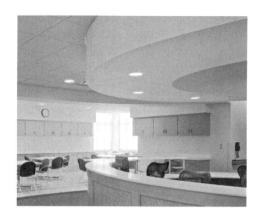

THE STATE HOSPITAL

Brian M. Hepburn, M.D.
Lloyd I. Sederer, M.D.

History and Nosology of Inpatient Psychiatric Service in the United States

State hospital psychiatry has changed dramatically over the past 50 years. With these changes, differences have evolved in hospitals from state to state. As the expression goes, "if you have seen one state hospital system, you have seen one state hospital system." Differences among the states are the rule, not the exception.

For well over a century, the state hospitals in the United States provided the great predominance of inpatient services for individuals with severe mental illness (Geller 2000; Goldman et al. 1983; Talbott 2004). However, since the introduction of community mental health and of Medicare and Medicaid in the 1960s, there has been a dramatic increase in inpatient services at acute general and private psychiatric hospitals. In fact, these settings now provide the predominance of hospital care. The state hospitals have thus come to serve the severely and persistently ill population who cannot be managed in or gain access to the private sector, in addition to individuals with forensic

or other special containment needs. State hospitals generally also represent the safety net for individuals who are uninsured and whose illness does not respond to briefer forms of intervention.

Figure 13–1 illustrates the dramatic change in state hospital beds between 1970 and 2002. In 1970 there were 413,066 state hospital beds, and in 2002 there were 57,263 (Foley et al. 2002, Table 19.2). This was an 85% decrease. In 1970, 33% of all hospital beds were psychiatric beds. By 2002, this was reduced to 14% (National Institute of Mental Health 1970).

Figure 13–2 shows the steady decrease in the number of state hospitals from 310 to 222 (Foley et al. 2002, Table 19.1). Private psychiatric hospitals increased from 150 to 253 (after peaking above 400 hospitals between 1990 and 1998). Nonfederal general hospitals with separate psychiatric units increased from 664 to 1,232 (after peaking at 1,600 hospitals between 1990 and 1998).

Figure 13–3 illustrates changes in psychiatric admissions between 1969 and 2002. State hospital admissions were reduced from 486,000 to 239,000, whereas private psychiatric hospital admissions increased from 92,000 to 477,000, and general hospital psychiatric admissions increased from 478,000 to

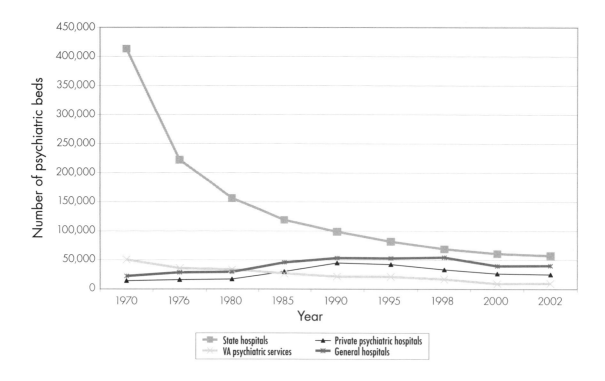

FIGURE 13–1.   Distribution of psychiatric beds by type of hospital, 1970–2002.

Source.   Prepared by Ted Lutterman, National Association of State Mental Health Program Directors Research Institute, using public-domain data from Foley et al. 2002.

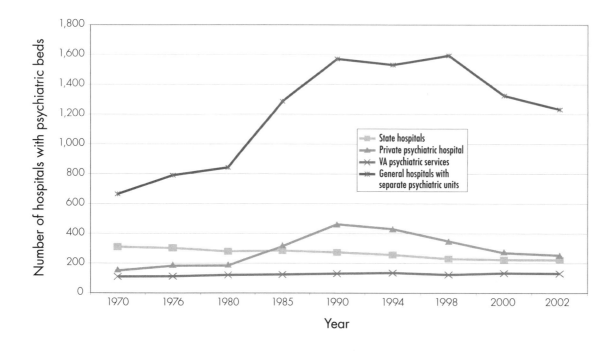

FIGURE 13–2.   Number of hospitals with psychiatric beds, 1970–2002.

Source.   Prepared by Ted Lutterman, National Association of State Mental Health Program Directors Research Institute, using public-domain data from Foley et al. 2002.

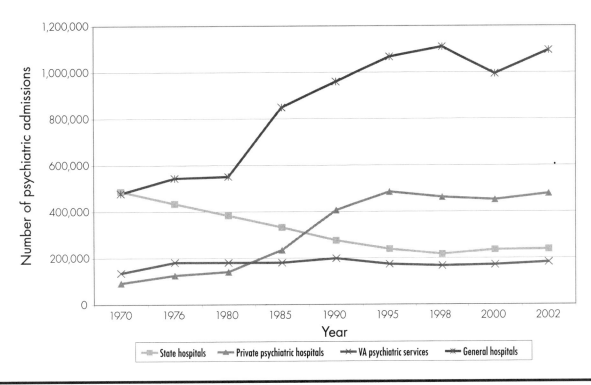

FIGURE 13-3. Admissions to psychiatric beds by type of hospital, 1970–2002.

Source. Prepared by Ted Lutterman, National Association of State Mental Health Program Directors Research Institute, using public-domain data from Foley et al. 2002.

1,095,000. There were approximately 1.2 million psychiatric admissions in 1969 and 2 million admissions in 2002 (Foley et al. 2002, Table 19.3). Current state hospital bed utilization is 0.63 per 1,000 persons, with rates steady for the past 3 years (Center for Mental Health Services 2005). Almost every state operated a psychiatric hospital in 2006 (National Association of State Mental Health Program Directors Research Institute 2006c). In 2005, 81% of individuals in state hospitals were adults ages 21–64. Twenty years ago, persons more than 64 years old made up more than 25% of the state hospital population. Today, they make up only 4%. Women compose 37% of the state hospital population, and men compose 63% of the population (Center for Mental Health Services 2005). The races and ethnicities of the adults in state hospitals are identified in Figure 13–4. These data compare with those of the general adult population: white 74%; African American 11%; Hispanic 11%; American Indian/Alaskan Native 1%; and Asian/Pacific Islander 4% (Schacht and Higgins 2002b). The majority of the adults in state hospitals have serious mental illnesses, such as schizophrenia and affective disorders. In facilities serving adults, approximately 35% of inpatients have co-occurring substance abuse disorders (Schacht and Higgins 2002a).

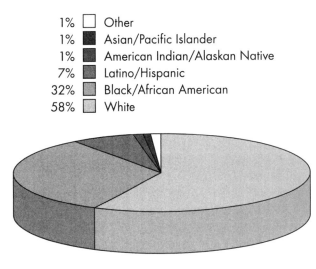

1%	Other
1%	Asian/Pacific Islander
1%	American Indian/Alaskan Native
7%	Latino/Hispanic
32%	Black/African American
58%	White

FIGURE 13-4. Racial/ethnic makeup of state hospitals.

Source. Public-domain data from Schacht and Higgins 2002b.

Types of State Hospital Units

Although there is variation between states depending on the number of state psychiatric hospitals and the number of beds, state hospital units may be identified as follows (Santoni and Sundeen 2007):

- *Acute units* are admission and evaluation units where intensive intervention and treatment and discharge planning occurs.
- *Continuing care units* are units in which nursing and rehabilitation services are provided in addition to treatment for individuals who require inpatient care beyond the acute phase of their mental illness.
- *Medical–surgical units* are hospital units designed to provide medical and nursing services for co-occurring acute and chronic physical illness in addition to hospital-level mental health treatment.
- *Forensic admission units* are secure acute units to which individuals are admitted for pretrial and posttrial evaluations and for treatment after a court adjudication of an individual as "not criminally responsible."
- *Forensic residential units* are secure units treating and housing those members of the population identified in forensic admission units with service needs similar to individuals treated in continuing care nonforensic units.
- *Forensic discharge units* are minimum-security units that treat and house forensic patients who are in the process of leaving inpatient care. In some states, the civil status and forensic populations are evaluated and treated separately, and in other states they are combined on the same unit.

Civil Status Population

The civil status population in state hospitals is made up of individuals identified as dangerous to self or others as a result of mental illness. They may be voluntary or certified. The determination of dangerousness has become controversial as legal standards regarding imminent danger to self or others have been established. Consequently, individuals may be certified in one state but not another. This may result in individuals not getting treatment because they are not yet an imminent danger. The trend in state hospitals is to only admit certified individuals. Seventy-five percent of this population is discharged within 30 days (National Association of State Mental Health Program Directors Research Institute 2006d; Figure 13–5).

If an individual does not stabilize on an acute unit and is not able to leave the hospital, then he or she is typically transferred to a longer-term or specialty unit. Those individuals who have stable community supports and resources will generally be able to leave the hospital sooner. Both acute and long-term units focus

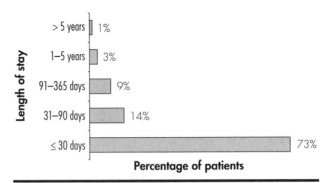

FIGURE 13–5.   Lengths of stay for patients with civil admission status.

Source.   Public-domain data from National Association of State Mental Health Program Directors Research Institute Web site (www.nri-inc.org).

on stabilization, medication treatment, individual and group therapies, and discharge planning (including finding stable housing and securing entitlements). One of the important changes in state inpatient care has been the inclusion of rehabilitation services in addition to traditional treatment services. Rehabilitation services aim to improve communication, work capability, and daily living skills (Dhillon and Dollieslager 2000).

Child and Adolescent Population

Some states do not provide state hospital services to individuals younger than 21 years. However, across the country, individuals younger than 21 years make up 15% of the individuals in state hospitals (Center for Mental Health Services 2005). Figure 13–6 shows the racial/ethnic distribution of these youth in 2001. These data compare with those for individuals younger than 21 years in the general population: white 64%; African American 15%; Hispanic 16%; American Indian/Alaskan Native 1%; and Asian/Pacific Islander 4% (Schacht and Higgins 2002b). Most have mental disorders such as attention-deficit/hyperactivity disorder, conduct disorder, oppositional defiant disorder, or affective disorders. This group had a rate of co-occurring substance abuse of 14%. The rate of co-occurring mental retardation or developmental disorders was 10% (Schacht and Higgins 2002a).

Crisis intervention with rapid stabilization and reintegration into the community continues to be the primary focus of child inpatient treatment. Diagnostic assessment, symptom management, and community reintegration require collaboration between parents and/or guardians, the educational setting, and other agencies. In addition to crisis management, state-

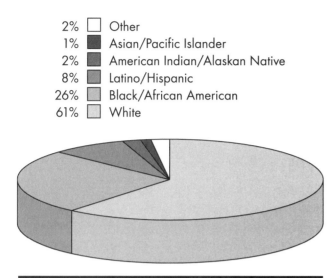

2% ☐ Other
1% ■ Asian/Pacific Islander
2% ▨ American Indian/Alaskan Native
8% ▨ Latino/Hispanic
26% ▨ Black/African American
61% ☐ White

FIGURE 13–6. Racial/ethnic distribution of individuals younger than 21 years admitted to state hospitals in 2001.

Source. Public-domain data from National Association of State Mental Health Program Directors Research Institute Web site (www.nri-inc.org).

operated child units provide the opportunity for more extensive diagnostic evaluations, complex medical management, and coordination of care with other state agencies (dosReis et al. 2003).

Similar to those for the adult population, the public inpatient mental health facilities for children and adolescents have moved in the direction of providing court-ordered evaluation and/or treatment. A recent change in the use of public psychiatric child and adolescent units is their role in determining competence. Youth found to be not competent are referred to competency restoration services, which may be inpatient. After an inpatient stay and restoration of competency, these individuals are then referred back to the court (Grisso 1997).

Forensic Population

Many state hospitals have responsibility for court-ordered evaluations of criminal defendants' competency to stand trial or to determine criminal responsibility (legal "insanity"). Many of these individuals will initially be placed on an acute unit for evaluation. However, individuals charged with higher-level crimes, such as murder, rape, arson, armed robbery, kidnapping, or carjacking, may be evaluated on a secure forensic unit or in a maximum-security hospital.

Individuals admitted for evaluation may be offered treatment during their stay, but medications ordi-

narily may not be forced except in an emergency. The evaluation is done on the forensic unit, and the evaluators' reports are then submitted to the court. The court determines whether the individual is competent to stand trial. Criminal responsibility is also determined at trial (Simon and Shuman 2008). In many states, the large majority of pretrial evaluations are conducted on an outpatient basis in the community, and the defendant is committed only if found incompetent to stand trial or not criminally responsible. If an individual is found not criminally responsible, he or she may be committed to a state hospital for inpatient care or treatment (if dangerous because of a mental disorder), released (if not dangerous), or placed on "conditional" release (if safe to be in the community with services in place and other conditions imposed). Individuals who have been committed will have periodic review hearings with a court or an administrative authority. In most states, only the court may release the individual. In some states, an agency or facility-based forensic review board will review the treatment team's findings and advise the state hospital regarding its opinion for the court on the individual's readiness for release or conditional release. Although the legal and security issues are prominent, it is important to note that the focus of the treatment team and the forensic review board is on the patient's psychiatric illness and rehabilitation needs.

Nearly all state mental health authorities (SMHAs) provide forensic mental health services (National Association of State Mental Health Program Directors Research Institute 2005). Seventy-six percent of states use their psychiatric hospitals to provide services to forensic patients. Fifteen percent of individuals discharged from state hospitals in 2005 had forensic status, and 40% of residents in state hospitals at the end of 2005 had forensic status.

One of the more recent areas of involvement for public mental health has been working with the forensic population referred by the courts after conviction for a sexual offense (Fitch and Hammen 2003). Nineteen states have laws providing for the special civil commitment of sex offenders, called *sexually violent predators* in some states (National Association of State Mental Health Program Directors Research Institute 2005). Generally, these laws provide for commitment after an individual has completed his or her criminal sentence and is about to be released. Although the SMHA is typically responsible for evaluation and treatment, at times it may also provide or administer the facility or purchase security services. The treatment of sexually violent individuals is similar to other state hospital patients when an underlying severe psychiatric illness exists. However, only a small percentage of these individuals have severe mental illness, whereas the majority are diagnosed with paraphilias and personality disorders (Becker and Johnson 2008; Berlin 2003). The main reason for their commitment is related to community safety. These individuals receive postsentence commitment that may result in indefinite confinement with little opportunity to return to the community. Their confinement may take resources away from the mental health system and further stigmatize the individuals with mental illness. For a more extensive discussion of this important subject, which is beyond the scope of this chapter, please see Prentky et al. (2003).

Impact of the State Hospital in the Overall Continuum of Care for Civil Status and Forensic Patients

State hospitals are generally an important part of the continuum of psychiatric care and affect the overall health care system. The reduction of state hospital beds in addition to the recent declines in the number of general hospital and private psychiatric hospital beds has resulted in 80% of states reporting a shortage in psychiatric beds (National Association of State Mental Health Program Directors Research Institute 2006d). Emergency departments report taking twice as long to place individuals for inpatient psychiatric care as for inpatient physical health care (Committee on the Future of Emergency Care in the United States Health System 2007).

An additional complicating factor is the increasing number of uninsured individuals with substance abuse problems using the emergency department for their health care. In March 1996 Congress passed Public Law 104–121, which terminated Social Security and Social Security Disability benefits to individuals disabled primarily by drug addiction and alcoholism because of the perception that having these benefits contributed to the individuals' drug use. Many of these individuals may need psychiatric services and, in some cases, inpatient psychiatric services. However, some individuals appear to be using psychiatric symptoms, including threat of suicide, as a way of gaining access to services they are unable to access for their substance abuse problem (Lambert 2002). This has put additional demand on emergency departments, the acute inpatient system, and state hospitals, where 35% of

adults have a diagnosis of substance abuse (Schacht and Higgins 2002a). The state hospitals have become the safety net for this additional population at a time when the supply of beds is decreasing.

In addition to the increased emergency department pressure, the limited availability of state hospital beds has created problems for the court system and jails. The longer waits for admission into state hospitals add to the crowding of jails with people who would be more appropriately served in clinical settings. Some states have responded by setting up diversion strategies, crisis intervention teams, and mental health courts, but the problem is far reaching and too few alternatives exist (Boothroyd et al. 2005; Kanapaux 2002).

The relationship between state hospital and community services varies among the states. Across the country, 70% of expenditures of SMHA are for community services, and approximately 30% are for state hospitals (National Association of State Mental Health Program Directors Research Institute 2006c). Despite greater funding for community services, there continues to be a shortage of community services. As indicated previously, 70% of civil admissions are discharged within 30 days; these represent people the state hospital has been able to discharge to community providers. The remaining 30% are significantly more difficult to return to the community because of persistent psychiatric symptoms, the need for intensive levels of community services (e.g., assertive community treatment), housing, and/or other complicating social issues.

The lack of psychiatric beds puts pressure on community providers, emergency departments, jails, and the judicial system. Until recently, the impact of the reduction of state beds was buffered by the increase in private-sector beds. However, the decrease in private-sector beds and resulting bed crisis has illustrated the importance of including the state hospitals in the planning for the health care system.

Accreditation, Patient Rights, and Legal Issues

Joint Commission Accreditation and Performance Measurement

Since 1971, the Joint Commission on Accreditation of Hospital Organizations has been evaluating organizations that provide mental health services, including state hospitals. In 2006, 90% of state psychiatric hospitals were accredited by the Joint Commission (National Association of State Mental Health Program

Directors Research Institute 2006b). Two of the primary areas of the Joint Commission's focus are performance and safety.

In February 1997, the Joint Commission began its ORYX initiative to integrate outcomes and other performance measurement data into the accreditation process. However, reporting of data for behavioral health organizations, including state hospitals, was deferred until core measures were identified. The Joint Commission and various mental health organizations have worked together to identify and implement a test set of core performance measures (Joint Commission 2008). To date, agreement has been reached on testing the following measures: assessment of violence risk, substance use disorder, trauma, and patient strengths; hours of restraint use; hours of seclusion use; patients discharged on multiple antipsychotic medications; and discharge assessment and aftercare recommendations sent to the next level of care providers upon discharge. A final set of measures to meet Joint Commission performance measurement requirements is expected for state hospitals in the fall of 2008.

The purpose of the Joint Commission's National Patient Safety Goals is to promote specific improvements in patient safety, including in state hospitals (Joint Commission 2007). The Joint Commission emphasizes goals that focus on systemwide solutions. Examples of these types of goals for state hospitals include improved communication with consumers and families and early identification of suicide risk.

State Regulatory Accreditation and Quality Monitoring

Each state has a government office that licenses and regulates hospitals and health-related institutions. This office typically monitors quality of care and compliance with both state and federal regulations. This office also generally undertakes complaint investigations. For those state hospitals that do not have Joint Commission accreditation, the state office performs regular inspections. This office also is responsible for inspection and certification of state hospitals participating under the deemed compliance authority from the Centers for Medicare and Medicaid Services. The office may initiate administrative action against state hospitals that violate state rules and regulations, and then it coordinates its actions with the Joint Commission and the Centers for Medicare and Medicaid Services. When hospital quality of care is in question, hospitals perform a root cause analysis (RCA) as required by the Joint Commission. The RCA focuses primarily on systems and processes, not individual performance. The state hospital identi-

fies risks and contributing factors for problem recurrence and determines what improvements are needed.

Protection and Advocacy for Individuals With Mental Illness

In 1975, the U.S. Department of Health and Human Services established a program to protect and to advocate for the rights of persons with disabilities (Protection and Advocacy for Individuals with Mental Illness [PAIMI] program; http://mentalhealth.samhsa.gov/cmhs/P&A). In 1986, Congress passed the Protection and Advocacy for Individuals with Mental Illness (PAIMI) Act (Center for Mental Health Services 2003). Protection and advocacy systems are authorized to access consumers and records for the purpose of conducting independent investigations of abuse, neglect, and rights violations in various types of public and private facilities, including state hospitals. PAIMI-eligible individuals are those diagnosed with a significant mental illness who were abused, neglected, or had their rights violated or were in danger of abuse, neglect, or rights violations while receiving care or treatment.

Court Oversight, Receivership, and Decrees

Court decisions have had a major impact on state hospitals. The *Wyatt v. Stickney* decision (Byrne 1981) gave patients the right to receive treatment that would result in a cure or would improve their mental condition. This landmark decision resulted in increased funding for state hospitals and also contributed to the movement to have treatment in the community. In some jurisdictions, the court decisions have resulted in mental health systems being put into receivership (Johnson 2001). In others, there have been more limited decisions. For example, in Maryland there is a program for the protection of patients' rights in the state psychiatric hospitals, the Resident Grievance System, which was established as part of the negotiated settlement of a class-action lawsuit (*Coe v. Hughes*, et al. [see Maryland Department of Health and Mental Hygiene 1998]). The settlement established an administrative process to protect patient rights and also established legal assistance providers to provide legal assistance to state hospital patients. Court decisions and mental health law continue to reflect the tension between the interests of the mentally ill and the community's fear of the mentally ill (Appelbaum 2006). Major legal areas continuing to face state hospital psychiatry include the right to refuse treatment, the insanity defense, and confining sex offenders postsentence.

Summary

In summary, the accreditation, regulatory, and legal environment has gained prominence in state hospitals over the past decades. State hospitals are under substantial scrutiny in all of these areas and need to effectively staff offices to attend to these oversight requirements. Although there may be concern on the part of state hospital clinicians and administrators that there is too much oversight and the additional monitoring takes needed resources from clinical care, there is no indication that this will change in the near future.

Consumers, Advocates, Providers, and the State Hospital

There continues to be debate within the mental health community regarding state hospitals. Consumer groups, family organizations, employees, unions, community providers, mental health associations, and disability law advocacy organizations have differing opinions on state hospitals. There is not a consensus on the future role of state hospitals among these organizations.

In the 1950s, nearly 35% of private-sector employees were union members, and public employees in unions were almost nonexistent (Barone 2005). However, by 2005 about 8% of private-sector employees were union members and between 30% and 40% of public employees were union members, making public sector unions a powerful voice in the future of state hospitals. State hospital employees and unions have expressed concern at the trend toward state hospitals providing care for an increasingly forensic population at the same time as there is pressure to stop the use of restraint and seclusion. They are concerned the state hospitals are becoming unsafe for employees and patients. They also express concern at the shortage of staff and the lack of training for staff in dealing with forensic patients. There has also been criticism from others that some public-sector employees and unions have become obstacles to change and have created a system that is not responsive to consumer needs (Schatz 2007).

The National Alliance on Mental Illness (NAMI; http://www.nami.org) position is that state psychiatric hospitals play an important role in the recovery of people with severe mental illness. NAMI regards state hospitals as an important part of the continuum of care, especially for those who need a longer time to recover. It supports involuntary care when safety is at stake and for those who will not agree to treatment because their illness impairs their judgment. NAMI also holds a similar position regarding involuntary medication: people should have a choice about medications, although there are times when individuals who are severely mentally ill are not able to act in their own best interest. NAMI also expresses concern that incarceration or victimization may result if an individual does not get needed state hospital treatment.

Some community providers argue that there is too much funding going to a small number of individuals who are in state hospitals. They assert that if there was more funding for community supports, rehabilitation, supported employment, and housing, there would be far less need for state hospitals. The U.S. Psychiatric Rehabilitation Association (http://www.uspra.org) maintains that psychiatric rehabilitation services enable independent living and socialization and produce a 65% reduction in hospital stays, a 70% decline in homelessness, 70% fewer incarcerations, and an 80% increase in employment.

Mental Health America (http://www.mentalhealthamerica.net) is a strong advocacy group dedicated to improving the quality of life for individuals with severe mental illness. It also advocates for an end to seclusion and restraint, except in rare circumstances. They are in favor of Consumer Satisfaction Teams working with state hospitals (see http://www.thecst.com). They support state hospitals being included as part of the continuum of care but also support vigorous adherence to the U.S. Supreme Court decision *Olmstead v. L.C.* (1999) that allows individuals with mental illness to live in the community with adequate supports.

Most states have consumer organizations. Twenty years ago, the consumer organization in Maryland (On Our Own of Maryland; http://www.onourownmd.org) called for the closure of the largest state hospital. However, since then they have called for the gradual downsizing to smaller hospitals. Consumer organizations vary in their positions regarding state hospitals. Some call for immediate closure, whereas others are in favor of gradual downsizing and having state hospitals as part of the continuum of care. They are generally against restraint, seclusion, coercion, and involuntary medication. They are in favor of Consumer Satisfaction Teams working with state hospitals to embrace the recovery model.

The Disability Law Center advocacy organizations are private, nonprofit organizations staffed by attorneys and paralegals to ensure that people with disabilities are accorded the full rights and entitlements afforded to them by state and federal law. They may seek the closure of state hospitals and assert that individuals' rights are not being protected in state hospitals. For example, they may argue that restraint and seclusion are used punitively and for the convenience of the staff. They argue that individuals with mental illness can be successfully treated in the community if appropriate resources are in place. Their advocacy agendas generally include removing barriers to independence; preventing seclusions and/or restraint of children, adolescents, or adults in state psychiatric hospitals; protecting the rights of persons diagnosed with a mental illness to refuse psychotropic medications; and advocating the enforcement of the right of persons diagnosed with a mental illness to live in the community with adequate supports, as set forth by the *Olmstead* decision (see Bazelon Center for Mental Health Law [http://www. bazelon.org/index.html] and Maryland Disability Law Center [http://www.mdlcbalto.org/mentalhealth.htm]). The tension between individual rights, family rights, and community safety is often played out in discussions between legal advocacy and other stakeholders.

The stakeholders in the mental health community hold varied views regarding the role of state hospitals. Some argue for the current status, some for state hospitals to be downsized but continue to be part of the continuum of mental health care, and others for the closure of state hospitals. However, state hospitals appear to be an essential part of the continuum of care in most states. Therefore, it will be important for stakeholders and the SMHA to reach consensus about the transformation of state hospitals and work toward a best-practice model.

Budget and Legislative Issues

Since World War II, state hospitals have been seen as very costly, and there has been a trend to close hospitals and use the savings to reduce government spending and support community-based care. The budgets for state hospitals decreased from $3.8 billion to $2 billion from fiscal year 1981 to fiscal year 2004. Community expenditures increased from $2 billion to $5 billion during the same time period (National Association of State Mental Health Program Directors Research Institute 2006a). These figures are based on 1981 dollars.

The majority of state hospital costs are covered by the states. However, several strategies have been used to maximize Medicaid reimbursement through the Disproportionate Share Hospital (DSH) program, payments to age groups outside of the Institution for Mental Disease (IMD) exclusion, and through managed care waivers to the IMD exclusion. In 1981, Congress established the Medicaid DSH program (Mechanic 2004) for hospitals that serve a significant number of low-income patients with special needs. DSH programs became a major source of funding for the nation's state hospitals (Kaiser Family Foundation 2007). In 2002, 15% of the DSH payments (~$1.5 billion) went to state hospitals. The "Medicaid IMD exclusion" has been part of federal Medicaid law since its 1965 enactment (42 CFR § 431.620 [1979]). The IMD exclusion refers to the rule that Medicaid will not pay for the inpatient treatment of individuals between ages 22 and 64 in "institutions for mental diseases," defined as any hospital, nursing facility, or other institution with more than 16 beds that is primarily engaged in providing diagnosis, treatment, or care of persons with mental diseases, including medical attention, nursing care, and related services. Individuals younger than 21 years make up 15% of the state hospital population, and individuals older than 64 years make up 4% of the state hospital population. State facilities can collect from Medicaid for these two age groups. In addition, a growing number of states have used federal Medicaid managed care waivers to bill for patients ages 22–64 years. This has allowed those states to receive Medicaid payments for hospital care in an IMD. Approximately one-third of the funding for state psychiatric hospitals is estimated to come from Medicaid. These important DSH and Medicaid trends face reductions, however, as DSH payment limits are implemented and as IMD managed care waivers are eliminated in fiscal year 2008. These factors will put additional pressure on the financing of state hospital operations (Buck 2003; Draper et al. 2003; Kate 2003).

Pharmacy has been a budget item that has grown dramatically in state hospitals. The new-generation antidepressants and antipsychotic medications as well as polypharmacy have increased costs. One response has been the introduction of preferred drug lists as well as efforts to influence the behavior of prescribers (Patrick et al. 2006) to reduce polypharmacy and higher-than-needed dosing. Standardization protocols have been introduced to improve quality and control costs (e.g., the Texas algorithm project; Kashner et al. 2006). The protocols have generally assumed the superiority of the new generation of antipsychotics. This may change as a result of the recent Clinical Antipsychotic Trials in Intervention Effectiveness studies of the new-generation antipsychotics (National Institute of Mental Health 2006). Operating cost concerns have also led to the development of buying groups (e.g., Minnesota Multi-State Contracting Alliance for Pharmacy [MMCAP; http://www.mmd.admin.state.mn.us/mmcap/current_vendors.htm]) that negotiate with manufacturers and wholesalers for the best price. There are currently 43 states participating in the MMCAP.

An additional major cost to state hospital systems has been the growing population of individuals who are postsentence and civilly committed as sexually violent predators. The cost of operating secure facilities for such individuals in the United States in 2004 was estimated at $224 million annually. Each sexually violent predator in hospital care costs on the average more than $200,000 per annum (Leib and Gookin 2005). Only a small number of individuals actually are discharged from these programs, so the costs will continue to increase. There is concern that the United States may be moving in the same direction as England in moving dangerous persons with severe personality disorders into psychiatric facilities when they finish their prison sentences (Appelbaum 2005). The stigma to individuals with mental illness is a concern, and costs will escalate and may end up decreasing funding for individuals with severe mental illness.

The cost of funding state hospitals continues to be problematic. States have been successful at collecting Medicaid dollars for state hospital services. However, there are indications that they may collect less from Medicaid in the future. There continues to be growth in the costs of state hospitals and little interest in most states to increase the state hospital budget appropriation.

The Future of State Hospitals

The future of state hospitals has been debated for decades. The hospitals are often demonized and looked upon as archaic relics of an embarrassing past, despite the fact that 90% are Joint Commission accredited, and they often provide the safety net function for uninsured severely mentally ill individuals in addition to providing inpatient care to the mentally ill forensic population. There is no indication that state hospitals are going to disappear in the near future. Perhaps the focus should be on how they need to work with stakeholders to provide services consistent with today's science and consistent with a recovery-based model following the goals set out by the President's New Freedom Commission on Mental Health (2003; see

also Hogan 2003). In order to meet the goals of the New Freedom Commission as they apply to state hospitals, the following will need to happen for each New Freedom Commission goal:

1. *Americans understand that mental health is essential to overall health.* This goal addresses stigma and health care parity. It calls for greater anti-stigma efforts so that more individuals will get their mental health needs addressed in the community with less shame and discrimination. It also calls for parity of services and benefits with those that physical health care now receives. Major work lies ahead to remove the stigma of state hospitals and for those individuals coming out of state hospitals. Lessening or eliminating stigma for this population will require great efforts by consumers, family members, mental health professionals (including state hospital employees), and advocacy groups. The integration of the state hospital with community mental and physical care will be needed for this to happen.

2. *Mental health care is consumer and family driven.* This means that consumers substantively advise on those matters that are most important to them, including job, home, relationships, and improving quality of life. The goal is to ensure that consumers and families have choices in the care they are receiving in state hospitals, including involvement in treatment and aftercare planning. It also means involving consumers and families fully in orienting the state hospital toward a recovery model as well as introducing self-help, peer support, consumer satisfaction teams, consumer education programs, and family education programs. This will be a special challenge for state hospitals serving individuals with forensic involvement, which appears to conflict with giving consumers and families more choice.

3. *Disparities in mental health services are eliminated.* The uninsured disproportionately end up in state hospitals. Part of this is by design, because of the safety net function of the state hospitals. However, it is also because the uninsured often do not access community services and tend to wait until a crisis has occurred. To the extent that disparities are reduced in benefits and services, more people will obtain preventive care and obtain treatment early in the course of their illnesses, thereby helping to reduce the use of state hospitals. Reductions in the uninsured and benefit disparities will also improve access to services for those leaving state hospital care. Another important disparity is the fact that there are twice as many African Ameri-

cans in state hospitals as compared with their representation in the general population (Schacht and Higgins 2002b). There needs to be improved and expanded culturally competent state hospital and community services for this population.

4. *Early mental health screening, assessment, and referral to services are common practice.* There is a growing trend for patients in state hospitals to have co-occurring substance abuse disorders. Co-occurring substance abuse has been identified in approximately 35% of individuals in state hospitals (Schacht and Higgins 2002a). The early identification of co-occurring substance abuse enables proper treatment and far better chance for recovery.

5. *Excellent mental health care is delivered, and research is accelerated.* In order for state hospitals to provide quality care, there needs to be adequate staff that is well trained and participating in the recovery model. Mental health workforce issues are at a critical point (Hoge et al. 2005). State mental health systems are moving toward clinical guidelines and evidence-based practices to improve the quality of care (Drake et al. 2006; Lehman et al. 2004). Public academic partnerships may facilitate the move toward improved care in state hospitals, for example, to reduce seclusion and restraint and increase trauma-informed care (see the Center for Mental Health Services' National Center for Trauma-Informed Care [http://mentalhealth.samhsa.gov/nctic]; University of Maryland School of Medicine's Evidence-Based Practice Center [http://medschool.umaryland.edu/Psychiatry/services_research/centers_ebpc.asp]; and Substance Abuse and Mental Health Services Administration 2006). In addition, the partnership promotes the use of training sites in state hospitals for various disciplines. The advantage to the state is that it is better able to have high-quality professional staff, with university appointments, providing services in state facilities. In addition, these facilities serve as important sites from which to recruit trainees into public service (Douglas et al. 1994; Goetz et al. 1998; Talbott 1991). Public academic partnerships also allow an opportunity for the evaluation and treatment of individuals who are not responding to treatment as well as to provide opportunities for clinical research (see Maryland Psychiatric Research Center [http://www.mprc.umaryland.edu/treatment.asp]; Nathan S. Kline Institute for Psychiatric Research [http://www.rfmh.org/nki]; and New York State Psychiatric Institute [http://nyspi.org/Kolb/index.htm]). Telemedicine may be a way of improving communica-

tions between academia and state hospitals, especially in rural areas or for hospitals that will not be able to have an on-site academic presence. It may also help with the challenge of workforce development.

6. *There is a need for SMHAs, state hospitals, and community providers to serve a critical role in the physical health care of people with serious mental illness.* People with severe mental illness die significantly younger than their age counterparts (National Association of State Mental Health Program Directors Medical Directors Council 2006). They smoke, eat poorly, and have sedentary lifestyles that can lead to chronic illnesses such as heart disease, chronic pulmonary disease, and diabetes, and their medications may produce metabolic disorders (National Association of State Mental Health Program Directors Medical Directors Council 2006). State hospitals are uniquely positioned to promote wellness and early detection of these chronic diseases. This may include making state facilities entirely smoke free.

7. *Technology is used to access mental health care and information.* State hospitals must increasingly use modern technology. Electronic prescribing and electronic medical records are essential next steps for safety and quality of care. Twenty-two states reported they are implementing electronic medical records in their state psychiatric hospitals (National Association of State Mental Health Program Directors Research Institute 2006d). There is a vital need to link hospital records with the community and other government and service agencies to enhance continuity of care. Telemedicine may also help for workforce issues, conferences, second opinions, and the growing links with academic settings and the private sector. Thirty-five SMHAs are engaged in activities to promote the use of telemedicine to provide mental health services (National Association of State Mental Health Program Directors Research Institute 2006d).

Conclusion

Currently, state hospitals are an important part of the continuum of mental health care in each state. They vary in the amount of civil and forensic populations under their care and in the amount of acute and long-term care that is provided. In some discussions, transformation assumes an end to state hospitals, with a view that everyone will be maintained in the community and close to their natural supports. However, the limits of science today, coupled with the gravity of disorder in a small but enduring proportion of people with mental illness, will require secure and longer-stay environments for some individuals. In addition, because state hospitals are being used for forensic care, they serve as an essential element in a full spectrum of state-supported services. There is an opportunity for state psychiatric hospitals to become tertiary care sites, where consumers and families turn when high levels of expertise are needed for extended periods of time. The state hospital, in effect, becomes part of the continuum of care from ambulatory to acute to tertiary care and is integrated into the full spectrum of care needed by all large communities. The future may hold a valued and distinguished role for these facilities, not unlike the role these hospitals had in the era of moral therapy almost 200 years ago (Sederer 1977).

References

Appelbaum PS: Law and psychiatry: dangerous severe personality disorders. England's experiment in using psychiatry for public protection. Psychiatr Serv 56:397–399, 2005

Appelbaum PS: Law and psychiatry: twenty-five years of law and psychiatry. Psychiatr Serv 57:18–20, 2006

Barone M: Public employee unions rule—or do they? US News & World Report, August 12, 2005. Available at: http://www.usnews.com/blogs/barone/2005/8/12/public-employee-unions-rule151or-do-they.html. Accessed April 22, 2007.

Becker JV, Johnson BR: Gender identity disorders and paraphilias, in The American Psychiatric Publishing Textbook of Clinical Psychiatry, 5th Edition. Edited by Hales RE, Yudofsky SC, Gabbard GO. Washington, DC, American Psychiatric Publishing, 2008, pp 729–753

Berlin FS: Sex offender treatment and legislation. J Am Acad Psychiatry Law 31:510–513, 2003

Boothroyd RA, Mercado CC, Poythress NG, et al: Clinical outcomes of defendants in mental health court. Psychiatr Serv 56:829–834, 2005

Buck JA: Medicaid, health care financing trends, and the future of state-based public mental health services. Psychiatr Serv 54:969–975, 2003

Byrne G: Wyatt v Stickney: retrospect and prospect. Hosp Community Psychiatry 32:123–126, 1981

42 CFR § 431.620 (1979)

Center for Mental Health Services: Protection and Advocacy for Individuals With Mental Illness (PAIMI) Program. Washington, DC, Center for Mental Health Services, Division of State and Community Development Systems, State Planning and Systems Development Branch, 2003. Available at: http://mentalhealth.samhsa.gov/cmhs/P&A/about.asp. Accessed April 22, 2007.

Center for Mental Health Services: 2005 CMHS Uniform Reporting System Output Tables. Washington, DC, Substance Abuse and Mental Health Services Administration, 2005. Available at: http://mentalhealth.samhsa.gov/cmhs/MentalHealthStatistics/URS2005.asp. Accessed April 22, 2007.

Committee on the Future of Emergency Care in the United States Health System: Hospital-Based Emergency Care: At the Breaking Point (Future of Emergency Care series). Washington, DC, National Academies Press, 2007

Dhillon AS, Dollieslager LP: Rehab rounds: overcoming barriers to individualized psychosocial rehabilitation in an acute treatment unit of a state hospital. Psychiatr Serv 51:313–317, 2000

dosReis S, Barnett S, Love RC, et al: A guide for managing acute aggressive behavior of youths in residential and inpatient treatment facilities. Psychiatr Serv 54:1357–1363, 2003

Douglas EJ, Faulkner LR, Talbott JA, et al: A ten-year update of administrative relationships between state hospitals and academic psychiatry departments. Hosp Community Psychiatry 45:1113–1116, 1994

Drake RE, Becker DR, Goldman H, et al: Best practices: the Johnson and Johnson–Dartmouth Community Mental Health Program. Disseminating evidence-based practice. Psychiatr Serv 57:302–304, 2006

Draper D, McHugh M, Achman L, et al: Medicaid Financing of State and County Psychiatric Hospitals (DHHS Publication No. SMA 03-3830). Rockville, MD, U.S. Department of Health and Human Services, 2003. Available at: http://download.ncadi.samhsa.gov/ken/pdf/SMA03-3830/CMHS11A.pdf. Accessed April 22, 2007.

Fitch LF, Hammen D: The new generation of sex offender commitment laws: which states have them and how do they work? in Protecting Society from Sexually Dangerous Offenders: Law, Justice, and Therapy. Edited by Winick BJ, La Fond JQ. Washington, DC, American Psychological Association, 2003, pp 27–39

Foley DJ, Manderscheid RW, Atay JE, et al: Highlights of organized mental health services in 2002 and major national and state trends, in Mental Health, United States, 2004. Edited by Manderscheid RW, Berry JT. Rockville, MD, U.S. Department of Health and Human Services, 2002, pp 200–236. Available at: http://mentalhealth.samhsa.gov/publications/allpubs/SMA06-4195/chapter19.asp. Accessed April 21, 2008.

Geller JL: The last half-century of psychiatric services as reflected in Psychiatric Services. Psychiatr Serv 51:41–67, 2000

Goetz R, Cutler D, Pollack D, et al: A three-decade perspective on community and public psychiatry training in Oregon. Psychiatr Serv 49:1208–1211, 1998

Goldman HH, Adams N, Taube CA: Deinstitutionalization: the data demythologized. Hosp Community Psychiatry 34:129–134, 1983

Grisso T: Juvenile competency to stand trial: questions in an era of punitive reform. Criminal Justice, Vol 12, Fall 1997. Available at: http://www.abanet.org/crimjust/juvjus/12-3gris.html. Accessed April 22, 2007.

Hogan MF: The President's New Freedom Commission: recommendations to transform mental health care in America. Psychiatr Serv 54:1467–1474, 2003

Hoge MA, Morris JA, Daniels AS, et al: Report of recommendations: the Annapolis Coalition Conference on Behavioral Health Work Force Competencies. Adm Policy Ment Health 32:651–663, 2005

Johnson NH: Order accepting final plan for Department of Mental Health. DC Watch, April 2, 2001. Available at: http://www.dcwatch.com/govern/mental010402.htm. Accessed April 22, 2007.

Joint Commission: 2007 National Patient Safety Goals. Oakbrook Terrace, IL, The Joint Commission, 2007. Available at: http://www.jointcommission.org/PatientSafety/NationalPatientSafetyGoals/07_npsgs.htm. Accessed April 22, 2007.

Joint Commission: Performance Measurement Initiatives: Hospital-Based, Inpatient Psychiatric Services (HBIPS) Candidate Core Measure Set, last updated February 15, 2008. Oakbrook Terrace, IL, The Joint Commission, 2008. Available at: http://www.jointcommission.org/PerformanceMeasurement/PerformanceMeasurement/Hospital+Based+Inpatient+Psychiatric+Services.htm. Accessed April 22, 2008.

Kaiser Family Foundation: Kaiser State Health Facts. Washington, DC, Kaiser Family Foundation, 2007. Available at: http://www.statehealthfacts.org. Accessed April 22, 2007.

Kanapaux W: Criminal Justice Primer for State Mental Health Agencies, September 2002. Alexandria, VA, National Technical Assistance Center for State Mental Health Planning, 2002. Available at: http://www.nasmhpd.org/nasmhpd_collections/collection5/publications/ntac_pubs/reports/Primer.pdf. Accessed April 22, 2007.

Kashner TM, Rush AJ, Crismon ML, et al: An empirical analysis of cost outcomes of the Texas Medication Algorithm Project. Psychiatr Serv 57:648–659, 2006

Kate M: States find creative ways to fund public-sector care. Psychiatric News 38:10, 2003

Lambert MT: Seven-year outcomes of patients evaluated for suicidality. Psychiatr Serv 53:92–94, 2002

Lehman AF, Lieberman JA, Dixon LB, et al: Practice guideline for the treatment of patients with schizophrenia, 2nd edition. Am J Psychiatry 161 (suppl):1–56, 2004

Leib R, Gookin K: Involuntary Commitment of Sexually Violent Predators: Comparing State Laws. Olympia, Washington State Institute for Public Policy, 2005. Available at: http://www.wsipp.wa.gov/rptfiles/05-03-1101.pdf. Accessed April 22, 2007.

Maryland Department of Health and Mental Hygiene: Residence Grievance System. Baltimore, Maryland Department of Health and Mental Hygiene, 1998. Available at: http://www.dhmh.state.md.us/yourrights. Accessed April 22, 2007.

Mechanic RE: Medicaid's Disproportionate Share Hospital Program: Complex Structure, Critical Payments (National Health Policy Forum Background Paper). Washington, DC, National Health Policy Forum, 2004. Available at: http://www.nhpf.org/pdfs_bp/BP_MedicaidDSH_09-14-04.pdf. Accessed April 22, 2007.

National Association of State Mental Health Program Directors Medical Directors Council: Morbidity and Mortality in People With Serious Mental Illness. Alexandria, VA, National Association of State Mental Health Program Directors, 2006. Available at: http://www.nasmhpd.org/nasmhpd_collections/collection4/meeting_presentations/Summer%202006%20commish/NASMHPD%20Morbidity%20and%20Mortality%20Slides%20071006.pdf. Accessed April 22, 2007.

National Association of State Mental Health Program Directors Research Institute: State Forensic Mental Health Services. State Profile Highlights, September 30, 2005. Alexandria, VA, National Association of State Mental Health Program Directors Research Institute, 2005. Available at: http://www.nri-inc.org/projects/Profiles/Profiles04/Forensic2004.pdf. Accessed April 22, 2007.

National Association of State Mental Health Program Directors Research Institute: Final Report: Funding Sources of State Mental Health Agencies: Fiscal Year 2004. Alexandria, VA, National Association of State Mental Health Program Directors Research Institute, 2006a. Available at: http://www.nri-inc.org/projects/Profiles/RE04.cfm. Accessed April 25, 2007.

National Association of State Mental Health Program Directors Research Institute: Implementation of Electronic Health Records and Health Information: 2006. State Profile Highlights (No. 06-2), November 21, 2006. Alexandria, VA, National Association of State Mental Health Program Directors Research Institute, 2006b. Available at: http://www.nri-inc.org/projects/Profiles/Profiles05/EMR2006.pdf. Accessed April 22, 2007.

National Association of State Mental Health Program Directors Research Institute: State Mental Health Agency Organization and Structure: 2006. State Profile Highlights (No. 06-3), November 21, 2006. Alexandria, VA, National Association of State Mental Health Program Directors Research Institute, 2006c. Available at: http://www.nri-inc.org/projects/Profiles/Profiles05/2006SMHAOrganization.pdf. Accessed April 22, 2007.

National Association of State Mental Health Program Directors Research Institute: State Psychiatric Hospitals: 2006. State Profile Highlights (No. 06-4), November 21, 2006. Alexandria, VA, National Association of State Mental Health Program Directors Research Institute, 2006d. Available at: http://www.nri-inc.org/projects/Profiles/Profiles05/2006StateHospital.pdf. Accessed April 22, 2007.

National Institute of Mental Health: Distribution of Psychiatric Beds by Geographic Division (Statistical Note No. 45). Bethesda, MD, National Institute of Mental Health, 1970

National Institute of Mental Health: Studies offer new information about treatment choices for schizophrenia (phase 2 results). Science Update, April 1, 2006. Available at: http://www.nimh.nih.gov/press/catie_phase2.cfm. Accessed April 22, 2007.

Olmstead v L.C., 527 U.S. 581 (1999)

Patrick V, Schleifer SJ, Nurenberg JR, et al: Best practices: an initiative to curtail the use of antipsychotic polypharmacy in a state psychiatric hospital. Psychiatr Serv 57:21–23, 2006

Prentky RA, Janus ES, Seto MC: Introduction. Human sexual aggression. Ann N Y Acad Sci 989:ix–xiii, 2003

President's New Freedom Commission on Mental Health: Achieving the Promise: Transforming Mental Health Care in America. Rockville, MD, President's New Freedom Commission on Mental Health, 2003. Available at: http://www.mentalhealthcommission.gov/reports/Finalreport/FullReport.htm. Accessed April 22, 2007.

Santoni T, Sundeen S: Staffing Study. Baltimore, Maryland Department of Health and Mental Hygiene, 2007

Schacht LM, Higgins KM: NRI Behavioral Healthcare Performance Measurement System Public Report: Diagnostic Profile of Clients Served. Alexandria, VA, National Association of State Mental Health Program Directors Research Institute, 2002a. Available at: http://www.nri-inc.org/reports_pubs/2002/DxProfileMay2002.pdf. Accessed April 22, 2007.

Schacht LM, Higgins KM: NRI Behavioral Healthcare Performance Measurement System Public Report: Race/Ethnicity of Clients Served in State Hospitals. Alexandria, VA, National Association of State Mental Health Program Directors Research Institute, 2002b. Available at: http://www.nri-inc.org/reports_pubs/2002/RaceEthnicity ProfilesSept2002.pdf. Accessed April 22, 2007.

Schatz T: Public-sector unions are a major obstacle to fighting waste, abuse. Budget & Tax News, February 1, 2007. Available at: http://www.heartland.org/Article.cfm?artId=20476. Accessed April 22, 2007.

Sederer LI: Moral therapy and the problem of morale. Am J Psychiatry 134:267–272, 1977

Simon RI, Shuman DW: Psychiatry and the law, in The American Psychiatric Publishing Textbook of Clinical Psychiatry, 5th Edition. Edited by Hales RE, Yudofsky SC, Gabbard GO. Washington, DC, American Psychiatric Publishing, 2008, pp 1555–1599

Substance Abuse and Mental Health Services Administration: Action Plan: Seclusion and Restraint, Fiscal Years 2006 and 2007. Rockville, MD, Substance Abuse and Mental Health Services Administration, 2006. Available at: http://www.samhsa.gov/Matrix/SAP_seclusion.aspx. Accessed April 22, 2007.

Talbott JA: The Pew Project: a national effort to improve state–university collaborations. Hosp Community Psychiatry 42:70, 1991

Talbott JA: Deinstitutionalization: avoiding the disasters of the past. Psychiatr Serv 55:1112–1115, 2004

CHAPTER 14

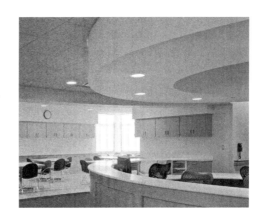

THE VETERANS HOSPITAL

Anne M. Stoline, M.D.

"The Veterans Hospital": for some, this phrase conjures an image of dim corridors lined with wheelchairs of hollow-eyed men. Yet U.S. Department of Veterans Affairs (VA) hospitals no longer are treatment options of last resort; most instead are modern facilities offering care at least comparable with that in the private sector. Care in the VA may surpass that in other health care systems, not only because of the strong academic interface through research and clinical training but also due to the VA's vast computerized information network and electronic patient record. Through this system, clinicians at the bedside have access to a broad range of patients' historical and current clinical information.

VA inpatient psychiatric care resembles in most respects that in community, university, and other public hospitals. Inpatient care is provided by multidisciplinary treatment teams just as in the state and private sectors. Though a nationwide system, VA hospitals too are subject to state laws. However, other variables dif-

ferentiate VA from other health care systems, such as its annual discretionary federal funding, its vast and complex administrative infrastructure, and as mentioned, its computerized patient clinical information system. Psychosocial factors as well, such as high rates of homelessness, limited social supports, unemployability—some attributable to veterans' institutional dependence from years spent in highly structured military life—set the VA patient population apart from patients in other settings. Clinical needs are broader than those in the civilian population, because veterans also have conditions unique to military service such as combat exposure and battle injuries. Veterans' psychiatric symptoms range from time-limited problems to chronic mental illnesses, and many patients are chronically hospitalized. As such, a VA inpatient psychiatric unit today may be caring for a 21-year-old just home from Iraq and a 50-something Vietnam veteran still coping with sequelae of his war experience alongside a World War II veteran with dementia.

Department of Veterans Affairs System

With earlier roots in health care for disabled soldiers dating back to the 1700s, the Veterans Administration was established in 1930. The system at that time comprised 54 hospitals, 31,600 employees, and 4.7 million living veterans. The scope of the VA has broadened since then, with the addition of Federal Benefits in the 1950s and the National Cemetery Administration in the 1970s. In 1989, the VA was renamed the Department of Veterans Affairs and was elevated to Cabinet status; it is currently the second largest of the 15 Cabinets under the leadership of the Secretary of Veterans Affairs. It operates nationwide programs for health care, financial assistance, and burial benefits. In fiscal year 2007, VA health care spending was estimated at nearly $35 billion. Of the estimated 24 million U.S. veterans, nearly 5.5 million received VA health care in 2006 (U.S. Department of Veterans Affairs 2007a).

As of December 2007, the VA health care system had locations in all 50 states, the District of Columbia, and Puerto Rico, encompassing 155 medical centers, 132 of which provide inpatient psychiatric care. Outpatient mental health services and in-home services are available in nearly 700 clinics located in hospitals or outpatient clinics (U.S. Department of Veterans Affairs 2007c). In addition, there are more than 200 Vet Centers providing outpatient counseling and individual and group therapy. All services are available free of charge to veterans who served in a combat zone during wartime or anywhere during a period of armed hostilities and to their families (see http://www.vetcenter.va.gov). Forty-five residential rehabilitation treatment programs, 108 home health service programs, and 135 nursing homes complete the spectrum of care. Programs for the homeless and vocational rehabilitation are other sources of help (U.S. Department of Veterans Affairs 2007a).

Veterans Affairs Workforce

The VA now is the largest health care provider in the nation. In 2006 approximately 250,000 employees, including about 16,000 physicians, cared for more than 5 million people (U.S. Department of Veterans Affairs 2007a). Through the VA's association with medical schools and university hospitals, veterans benefit from care provided by faculty physicians and physicians-in-training who rotate through VA hospitals. In fact, VA is the largest provider of health care training in the United States, with more than 90,000 health professionals receiving VA training annually. More than half of U.S. physicians today have received some part of their training at a VA site (U.S. Department of Veterans Affairs 2007a).

Millions of dollars from both VA and non-VA sources fund extensive research activity as well. The VA nationwide network makes possible large-scale, multicenter trials that would be daunting in smaller systems. Historical accomplishments in mental health attributed to VA research and development initiatives include advances in understanding the genetic underpinnings of schizophrenia and dementias and frontier work on chronic pain, posttraumatic stress disorder (PTSD), and other conditions. Current research continues in those and many other areas, including neuroimaging techniques (U.S. Department of Veterans Affairs 2008d).

National pride, patriotism, and veteran loyalty are among the factors fueling the VA volunteer workforce, the largest volunteer program in the federal government. Volunteers provide a variety of comfort and ancillary services, such as ward recreational activities and community transportation to VA appointments. Recent statistics show more than 90,000 people nationwide participated in VA Voluntary Services, logging 13 million hours of service in 2004 alone (U.S. Department of Veterans Affairs 2008a).

Veterans' Health Benefits

Financing the VA's mandate to provide medical benefits to veterans depends on appropriations annually determined by Congress and the president. This discretionary process means that the VA is not "fully funded,"[1] in contrast to other programs such as Social Security. Understaffing during periods of monetary shortfall may translate into reduced scope of services and long waiting times for care over and above the bureaucratic delays inherent in any large and complex system. Given the high demand for VA medical benefits, budget constraints also lead to delays and limits in the enrollment process. To maintain enrollment manageable with available fiscal resources, the qualifications to receive benefits are evaluated annually for

---

[1] Money for a fully funded program is set aside to meet the program's projected costs over time. No such reserves are created for non–fully funded programs.

necessary criteria modifications. Over time, more stringent enrollment criteria have been implemented. As one might expect, this budget-balancing strategy is highly politicized, because the argument can always be made that resources should be available to meet demand, not vice versa. Some of the major adjustments to enrollment criteria are described later.

An honorable discharge is required to qualify for VA health benefits, although certain exceptions apply. Length of service criteria require (again, with certain exceptions) 24 months of active duty to qualify for VA benefits (U.S. Department of Veterans Affairs 2007b). A major enrollment restriction was implemented in 2003, limiting guaranteed enrollment only to the period 2 years after military discharge, a change affecting veterans who served in the Afghanistan and Iraq conflicts.[2] Although soldiers who develop psychological or psychiatric symptoms during active duty can transition directly from military health care to VA care, the clinical impact of this limit is obvious for conditions such as PTSD, which often does not manifest until years after the trauma. Another change in 2003 created a priority system for VA enrollment including Priority Group 8: "not allowed to enroll for VA benefits" (Albano 2007). Although reserved for those veterans with other opportunities for access to health care, such as those in higher income brackets or with other insurance such as Medicare, these various limitations have been politically controversial. Many hope that when political tides shift, restrictions will be lifted.

Spending and Revenue Adjustments

In 1995 Congress passed legislation requiring psychiatric deinstitutionalization, one goal of which was cost savings through the transition to less intensive levels of care. As part of that process, the national VA health care system was divided into 22 VA Integrated Service Networks (VISNs) intended to consolidate resources, avoid duplication of services, and optimize access to services at the appropriate level of care. In 2002, VISNs 13 and 14 were merged into a new network, VISN 23 (U.S. Department of Veterans Affairs 2002). Figure 14–1 shows the VISN organization by state. Deinstitutionalization and decentralization to VISNs necessitated creation of a continuum of care from inpatient to outpatient, as well as community residences, outreach, and support for those no longer in-

stitutionalized. Although this mental health care system is in place, VISNs continue to provide regional and local leadership and oversight, reporting to the national administration.

Patient cost-sharing through copays and deductibles adds to VA health care revenue. Copay rates for services and pharmacy benefits are calculated using factors such as service connection and national income standards adjusted for regional differences. These adjustments too can be politically controversial, as some feel that veterans should not have to pay anything for VA medical care. VA bills private insurance companies for services provided to their insured veterans.[3] Not surprisingly in light of this interface with the private insurance sector and managed care, VA has implemented private-sector models for determining aspects of care such as acuity criteria and length of stay, monitored closely by its utilization review program. As a result, clinicians in many acute-care settings are held to standards as strong as any in the private sector. Results are reflected in data obtained in the VA Maryland Health Care System in VISN 5, where the average length of stay on the acute inpatient psychiatric units in 2006 was less than 5 days.

Information Technology

Compared with other branches of medicine, psychiatry is not typically a high-technology specialty. Yet psychiatry joined with the other medical specialties in 1996 when VA successfully integrated computer technology into routine clinical care. Termed VistA (Veterans Health Information Systems and Technology Architecture), the system includes among its many applications the Computerized Patient Record System (CPRS).

CPRS links computer terminals at points of clinical care with associated services such as laboratory and radiology. Laboratory results, vital signs, and progress notes are entered into the system. CPRS facilitates daily tasks such as entering orders, requesting consultations, reviewing radiographic images, monitoring vital signs, scheduling laboratory services, and a host of other tasks that can be completed electronically. Local VistA and CPRS systems store visual images, including pathology slides, X-rays, and computed tomography and magnetic resonance imaging studies. The system is fast, eliminates errors due to handwriting confusion, and alerts clinicians to possible errors such as ordering

---

[2] Operation Enduring Freedom and Operation Iraqi Freedom.

[3] Conversely, under some circumstances VA is obligated to reimburse for care in the private sector for psychiatric services unavailable in the VA system, such as eating disorders, after patient and clinician demonstrate the necessity of such care.

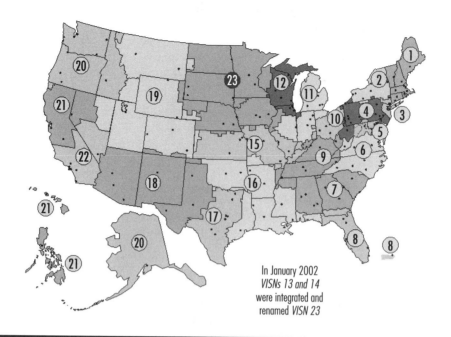

In January 2002
VISNs 13 and 14
were integrated and
renamed VISN 23

FIGURE 14–1.   **Veterans Integrated Service Networks (VISN) organization map by states.**

VISN 1: VA New England Health Care System (Boston, MA); VISN 2: VA Health Care Network Upstate New York (Albany, NY); VISN 3: Veterans Integrated Service Network (Bronx, NY); VISN 4: VA Stars & Stripes Health care Network (Pittsburgh, PA); VISN 5: VA Capitol Health Care Network (Baltimore, MD); VISN 6: The Mid-Atlantic Network (Durham, NC); VISN 7: The Atlanta Network (Atlanta, GA); VISN 8: VA Sunshine Health Care Network (Bay Pines, FL); VISN 9: Mid South Veterans Health Care Network (Nashville, TN); VISN 10: VA Health Care System of Ohio (Cincinnati, OH); VISN 11: Veterans Integrated Service Network (Ann Arbor, MI); VISN 12: The Great Lakes Health Care System (Chicago, IL); VISN 13: VA Upper Midwest Health Care Network (Minneapolis, MN); VISN 14: Central Plains Health Network (Omaha, NE); VISN 15: VA Heartland Network (Kansas City, KS); VISN 16: Veterans Integrated Service Network (Jackson, MS); VISN 17: VA Heart of Texas Health Care Network (Dallas, TX); VISN 18: VA Southwest Health Care Network (Phoenix, AZ); VISN 19: Rocky Mountain Network (Denver, CO); VISN 20: Northwest Network (Portland, OR); VISN 21: Sierra Pacific Network (San Francisco, CA); VISN 22: Desert Pacific Health Care Network (Long Beach, CA).
Note.   In January 2002, VISNs 13 and 14 were integrated and renamed VISN 23 (VA Midwest Health Care Network [Minneapolis, MN]).

Source.   U.S. Department of Health and Human Services Web site (http://www.hhs.gov/healthit/ahic/materials/09_07/ce/nazi_files/images/image5.png). Accessed May 10, 2008.

duplicate tests or attempting to prescribe an agent listed as a patient allergy. CPRS enhances preventive care by posting reminders for health screening such as annual mammograms, pap smears, and tuberculosis test screens. CPRS also provides standardized screening questionnaires for conditions such as trauma, depression, and suicide attempt history.

VistA also links every VA facility nationwide. Clinical information is recorded back to 1995, and paper charts hold earlier patient information as well as ongoing legal paperwork, ambulance transfer reports, and so on. Through the "remote access" feature, the clinician can review hospitalizations, progress notes, laboratory results, medications prescribed, and a host of other variables in every other VA facility. This capability proves invaluable in obtaining medical history, tracking the course of an illness, reviewing past medi-

cation trials, and providing clinical information such as laboratory results. The use of computer information technology increases the quality of VA health care by improving the efficiency, efficacy, and comprehensiveness of services. Its application to the inpatient psychiatry unit opened a new era in administrative management and patient care. The next information technology achievement is an electronic interface between the veteran him- or herself and the VA system. This tool, called MyHealtheVet (available at http://www.myhealth.va.gov), went online in 2005. MyHealtheVet is designed to enable veterans to refill prescriptions online, check scheduled appointments, view copay balances, and view some parts of their electronic medical record. Using the Track Health tool, veterans can record and track personal health data, including blood pressure, weight, and other medical information.

National Drug Formulary

As in any hospital setting, VA prescribers choose medications from a drug formulary. Until January 2007, hospitals and VISNs made their own formulary choices. At that time, the VA began transitioning to a National Formulary, at the completion of which every VA hospital in the country will have the same list of outpatient prescriptions and inpatient medications. Hospital and VISN pharmacy committees still retain authority to impose dosage or indication restrictions and to authorize nonformulary agents on a case-by-case basis. For example, in the VA Maryland Health Care System in VISN 5, approval of duloxetine requires a prior trial of venlafaxine (excepting preexisting cardiovascular complications), and a review of the potential complications of metabolic syndrome is required before an atypical antipsychotic can be prescribed. The VA gains cost advantages through use of generic substitutes, volume pricing, and its large market share. The psychopharmacological armamentarium as of April 2008 is listed in Table 14–1.

VA Clinical Population

The VA psychiatric patient population differs in several respects from the general U.S. psychiatric population. For example, some veterans are affected by experiences not found among civilians, such as basic training, deployment far from home, and combat exposure. Some clinical conditions, such as substance abuse, are not exclusive to veterans but occur more frequently in this population. Again using the VA Maryland Health Care System in VISN 5 as an example, the top five primary admission diagnoses in 2006 were alcohol dependence, alcohol withdrawal, opioid dependence, paranoid schizophrenia, and schizoaffective disorder (VA Maryland Health Care System 2006).

Inappropriate Enlistees

Military recruitment and enlistment procedures of course influence the VA patient population. For example, the VA cares for some patients with conditions that would have disqualified them from military service at other recruitment phases. Lax recruiting decisions result in some veterans with disqualifying conditions such as intellectual disability, disabling social and/or interpersonal skills, conduct disorders, affective illness, or psychosis. With these conditions, such soldiers are often unable to adapt to military service; not an insignificant number of VA psychiatric patients failed to complete basic training or had very short stints in the military but then require lifelong care in the VA. Even more unfortunate are those ill-suited soldiers who also have been exposed to combat or other trauma; these are some of the most functionally and psychologically compromised veterans in the VA patient population.

Major Mental Illness

Some psychiatric disabilities are unrelated to military service; the major mental illnesses that manifest in young adulthood develop in young adult soldiers as well. However, veterans who can demonstrate the onset of major mental illness during active duty or within 1 year of separation from the military are likely to be awarded service-connected[4] disability benefits as well as lifelong medical and psychiatric care. Others qualify despite later disease onset. With the VA continuum of care, these veterans receive comprehensive treatment and services for conditions such as schizophrenia, schizoaffective disorder, and bipolar disorder. Resembling trends in the private and other public sectors, in the 3 years following the 1995 deinstitutionalization policy, the number of veterans with major mental illnesses who were treated as inpatients decreased by 30% (National Mental Health Association 1999). Reactions to this change varied; some viewed it as an abandonment of the neediest veterans (particularly before the VA outpatient and community infrastructure was in place), whereas others lauded the emancipation of institutionalized veterans to community settings. Some staff on long-term units saw these patients as family members and grieved their discharge, fearing that they would not receive comparable nurturance in the community. However, once an adequate continuum of care was in place, the shift from institutional to community living certainly benefited many deinstitutionalized patients.

---

[4] A "service-connected" disability is a condition incurred during or exacerbated by military service. Disabilities are rated from 0% to 100%, reflecting loss of earning capability. As of April 2008, a 100% service-connected veteran receives at least $2,527 annually in tax-free compensation (U.S. Department of Veterans Affairs 2007d). Not surprisingly, given the stakes involved, at times an active claim for service-connected disability can influence a patient's clinical presentation.

TABLE 14–1. VA National Formulary psychopharmacological agents: April 2008

Category	Approved agents
Antidepressants	Amitriptyline, bupropion, citalopram, clomipramine, desipramine, doxepin, duloxetine, fluoxetine, imipramine, mirtazapine, nortriptyline, paroxetine, phenelzine, selegiline, sertraline, tranylcypromine, trazodone, venlafaxine
Mood-stabilizing agents	Carbamazepine, divalproex sodium, lamotrigine, lithium, valproic acid
Neuroleptics	Aripiprazole, chlorpromazine, clozapine, fluphenazine, droperidol, haloperidol, loxapine, molindone, olanzapine, perphenazine, pimozide, quetiapine, risperidone, thioridazine, thiothixene, trifluoperazine, ziprasidone
Benzodiazepines	Alprazolam, chlordiazepoxide, clonazepam, diazepam, lorazepam, temazepam
Aids to substance abuse recovery	Buprenorphine, buprenorphine/naloxone, disulfiram, methadone, naloxone, naltrexone, nicotine gum and patches, varenicline
Dementia treatments	Donepezil, galantamine, memantine
Miscellaneous	Buspirone, chloral hydrate, dextroamphetamine, gabapentin, methylphenidate, topiramate, zolpidem

Source. U.S. Department of Veterans Affairs 2008b.

Geriatric Psychiatry

Comorbid psychiatric conditions typically manifesting in older adults also are reflected in the VA patient population. Included in this group are patients with dementia; those with the long-term psychiatric sequelae of alcohol and other substance abuse; and those with intractable psychoses, affective disorders, and/or PTSD. Elderly veterans who have treatment-refractory behavioral disturbances (e.g., physical or verbal aggression) that render them unsuitable for in-home services, community assisted-living facilities, or nursing home care instead remain in long-term-care psychiatric units. As the number of aging veterans increased, VA forecast a time when veterans' need for services would exceed the system's resource capacity. As a result, in January 2003 the VA suspended new enrollment of veterans in Priority Group 8—those without service connection or compensable disability whose income exceeds the VA income threshold (U.S. Department of Veterans Affairs 2008c). This was an unfortunate fiscal consequence for senior veterans who had not consumed VA resources earlier in adulthood yet perhaps counted on access to medical and nursing home care in their senior years, when they would need it most.

Traumatic Brain Injury

Some of the most challenging clinical conditions result from traumatic brain injury (TBI). Soldiers are particularly vulnerable to injury during rigorous training exercises, exposure to weapons, and, of course, battle. Modern warfare technology such as improved body armor and helmets reduce the chance of death in combat, but survivors of blows and jolts to the head have greatly increased the VA TBI population (U.S. Government Accountability Office 2008). It is estimated that the percentage of survivors with TBI injured in Afghanistan and Iraq will be much higher than in previous military conflicts, which already carried TBI estimates as high as 20% (G.J. Adams 2007). In a study reported by the Defense and Veterans Brain Injury Center (see http://www.dvbic.org/cms.php?p= Blast_injury), more than half of all injured soldiers screened at Walter Reed Army Medical Center were positive for TBI. Many TBI insults are obvious, but mild and moderate TBI resulting from insults such as repeated proximity to explosions may go undetected, delaying appropriate treatment (G.J. Adams 2007). Psychiatric sequelae of TBI can include attentional deficits, poor impulse control, dementia, affective syndromes, organic psychotic symptoms, and behavioral disturbances that result in occupational and interpersonal deficits. In response to this growing need, legislation has been put forth to expand VA TBI care. The proposed TBI treatment units will afford both clinical services and research opportunities to advance the care of TBI in areas including diagnosis and assessment, psychological interventions, psychopharmacology, behavior therapy, cognitive retraining, family education and therapy, and psychosocial supports (Michaud 2007).

Combat Trauma

The major distinguishing feature of VA psychiatric care is treatment of trauma disorders. Military service entails a variety of situations traumatic for even the staunchest individuals, from arduous training exercises (such as prisoner of war training), to threat of imminent death in combat, to developing the ability to kill another person and being called to do so in the line of duty. Soldiers suffer grief from the death of comrades, separation from family, possible physical mutilation, and countless other hardships. To meet the broad range of personal thresholds for experiencing trauma, VA trauma services range from outpatient counseling to long-term inpatient and residential treatment.

From acute "shell shock" to chronic disabling symptoms, PTSD is a consequence of military service for some veterans. The National Center for PTSD was legislated into existence in 1989 to address the treatment of Vietnam War veterans. The number and severity of affected veterans brought the condition to light, and the syndrome is now recognized as a consequence of all types of trauma. Although not exclusive to soldiers, PTSD today is more common in war veterans than any other group. Estimates of the incidence of PTSD in veteran populations vary widely as a result of sample differences and screening methods, but one study estimates that 10%–20% of Vietnam War veterans experienced ongoing PTSD symptoms 20 years after the war (Prigerson et al. 2002). In fact, to this day Vietnam War veterans are admitted to the inpatient psychiatric unit with conditions related to undiagnosed and/or untreated PTSD; this phenomenon may be related to the unmasking through retirement or sobriety of symptoms managed through the diversions of work or substance abuse during earlier adulthood.

As the result of lessons learned in the post-Vietnam era, the U.S. Department of Defense and VA are very invested today in screening soldiers and veterans for PTSD and referring them for treatment. Postdeployment transitional programs are now in place and designed to educate new veterans and their families about the signs and symptoms of PTSD and other sequelae of military service. It is hoped that these preventive efforts will lead to early treatment interventions and minimize comorbidities. Nonetheless, the VA is preparing to handle the expected influx of new cases.

Sexual Trauma

Sexual crimes can be perpetrated anywhere, but they are among the worst adversities of military service in war or peacetime for both men and women. Military sexual trauma (MST) is defined by law as "sexual harassment, sexual assault, rape, and other acts of violence." It is estimated that nearly one-third of sexual trauma victims develop PTSD (U.S. Department of Veterans Affairs 2007a). Traumatic consequences in the military can be compounded when victims often must live and work alongside their attacker, face indifference to attack by superior officers, or suffer career disruption if they relocate to move away from their attacker. Although the majority of civilian sexual crimes go unreported, military conditions further intensify the potential shame, intimidation, and stigma for soldiers reporting these events (Wolfe et al. 1998).

Despite its frequency, MST received little notice until the early 1990s. Yet with the increasing number of women in the military, the official recognition of MST as a valid and important issue, and the reduced social stigma for reporting these crimes, the number of reported incidents of MST has reached staggering proportions. In 2006 nearly 3,000 soldiers reported assault or rape by fellow soldiers. It has been estimated that 20% of female VA patients and 1% of male VA patients have been victims of sexual trauma, with rates of incidents of harassment much higher (Goldzweig et al. 2006; Public Broadcasting Service 2007; U.S. Department of Veterans Affairs 2007e).

In 1992, VA implemented a Military Sexual Trauma Program for men and women, addressing the psychological and physical sequelae of MST (U.S. Department of Veterans Affairs 2007e). The length of service requirement is waived for MST victims to receive treatment and/or disability compensation. In addition to standard inpatient psychiatric care and outpatient individual and group therapy, when necessary veterans can be referred for admission to one of several VA residential MST programs nationwide (see Appendix for links). Separate programs for men and women are available.

Substance Abuse

More than 55,000 VA admissions annually are related to substance abuse; as noted previously, three of the top five admission diagnoses in one VA survey were substance abuse–related (VA Maryland Health Care System 2006). Although alcohol is the most frequently abused agent (68%), cocaine (15%) and opiate addictions (8%) are significant as well (Substance Abuse and Mental Health Services Administration Office of Applied Studies 2001, 2003). VA substance abuse treatment services include outpatient methadone and buprenorphine programs, group therapy, intensive outpatient programs, acute detoxification admissions, and residential treatment programs. VA has

developed an array of psychosocial services to interface with substance abuse treatment services.

Women's Health Services

Eligibility for women in military service began in
1947 and was limited to nurses; enrollment opened to
women in the general population starting in 1948. At
that time, the enrollment of women was capped at 2%
of the soldier population, and strict ceilings existed on
rank attainment and approved assignments for
women. The intervening years brought progressively
more lenient regulations for women, allowing them
to progress in rank and broaden their scope of service
(Women's Research and Education Institute 2007).

In 1973 the draft ended, and the U.S. military became a voluntary force. To encourage enlistment, military pay was raised (and became comparable with
civilian wages), and other improvements such as sub-
sidies for education were implemented. Military service provided the opportunity for gender equity in job
performance as well as opportunities to progress in
rank, other factors appealing to women (Quester and
Gilroy 2007). Reflecting these changes, the percentage
of women in the active duty military rose from 2.5% in
1973 to nearly 15% in 2004 (Klein 2005).

More women in military service translates into
more women veterans, although women still represent
only 6%–8% of the veteran population (Klein 2005).
Because a higher percentage of female than male veterans use VA health care services, approximately 10%
of the veteran patient population is female. Statistics
demonstrate that a growing percentage of substance
abuse admissions are women (6% in 2000, up from 4%
in 1995; Substance Abuse and Mental Health Services
Administration Office of Applied Studies 2003).

An office to address women's health issues was
established by the VA in 1988. VA treatment for gen-
der-specific conditions such as gynecological care and
mammograms began in 1992 with nationwide implementation of Women's Health Programs (see Appendix). Although in the minority on general psychiatric
units, women veterans may also be treated in the several women-only VA programs across the country for
treatment of MST and PTSD.

Vocational Rehabilitation

Veterans with psychiatric illnesses may be underem-
ployed or unemployed and face more serious barriers

to stable employment than the civilian population. As
a result, vocational rehabilitation is an important part
of the VA continuum of care. With roots dating back to
World War II, VA's program for service-connected veterans now is called the Vocational Rehabilitation and
Employment Program. This program has developed
into a complex assessment and treatment network interfacing extensively with community businesses (Vocational Rehabilitation and Employment Services, San
Diego VA Regional Office 2008). Through job training, sheltered employment, and other work arrangements, important therapeutic gains can be attained.

For veterans receiving sustained inpatient psychiatric care, work therapy assignments can provide both
an important structure to daily activity and a significant source of patient satisfaction. Stable inpatients
also participate in Compensated Work Therapy or Incentive Therapy. These programs prepare veterans for
further vocational rehabilitation in the community
and provide a source of spending money for chronically hospitalized veterans. For less impaired veterans
who are outpatients, Compensated Work Therapy and
Transitional Work positions may provide critical financial support or enable return to full employment.
Veterans may live in VA residential housing during
this phase of their recovery.

Homeless Program

Veterans make up a significant percentage of the
homeless male population; although only 34% of the
general adult population are veterans, they compose
40% of the homeless population. Homeless veterans
are more likely than housed veterans to be admitted
for psychiatric and substance abuse diagnoses (J. Adams et al. 2007). As a result, discharge decisions not
infrequently hinge on the availability of appropriate
outpatient housing.

Various factors render veterans vulnerable to homelessness, including unemployability, substance abuse
and/or major mental illness, and treatment noncompliance. Studies have shown that soldiers from the
late-Vietnam and post-Vietnam eras have higher rates
of homelessness than those who participated at the
height of the Vietnam War (Rosenheck et al. 1996).
"These veterans had little exposure to combat but appear to have increased rates of mental illness and addiction disorders, possibly due to recruitment patterns" (National Coalition for the Homeless 2007).
Along these lines, one might speculate that soldiers'
lack of independent living experience as adults while

living in strict military organization may have deprived them of critical developmental milestones to achieve stable work and housing after military service. Veterans coping with prolonged and severe war memories may have loosened or cut their ties to friends and family, and this social isolation may predispose to homelessness; however, studies have shown that homeless veterans are *less* likely to have combat experience than the nonhomeless (Rosenheck et al. 1996). For others, military skills may not be readily transferred to civilian jobs.

The VA provides a safety net for those unfortunate veterans who are unable to afford or otherwise maintain shelter. In 1987, the VA Homeless Program (see Appendix) was begun in order to create locally based medical care programs, residential programs, and other benefits to homeless veterans. A variety of services fall under this program's rubric, from homeless outreach, to subsidy of community shelter beds specifically for veterans, to domiciliary settings, to long-term recovery programs for homeless veterans with substance abuse.

Conclusion

VA hospital psychiatry today is a unique blend of traditional care and soldier-specific treatments. State-of-the-art information technology, including an electronic patient record, improves efficiency and effectiveness. Every VA hospital benefits to some extent from VA research and education programs. The patient population spans adults of all ages with widely varying conditions, with the care of many further complicated by challenging psychosocial situations. VA provides specialty treatment for conditions not found in civilian treatment settings, such as combat-related PTSD and MST. From acute inpatient stays to sustained and even permanent hospitalizations, the VA hospital psychiatrist depends on multidisciplinary collaboration and a full continuum of services to an extent unavailable to most in the private sector. All told, the VA may offer the most varied clinical experience in U.S. hospital psychiatry today.

References

Adams GJ: Incidence of traumatic brain injury in the military. EzineArticles.com, September 26, 2007. Available at: http://ezinearticles.com/?Incidence-Of-Traumatic-Brain-Injury-In-The-Military&id=752358. Accessed May 10, 2008.

Adams J, Rosenheck R, Gee L, et al: Hospitalized younger: a comparison of a national sample of homeless and housed inpatient veterans. J Health Care Poor Underserved 18:173–184, 2007

Albano T: Veterans group seeks mandatory VA funding. People's Weekly World: October 4, 2007

Goldzweig CL, Balekian TM, Rolon C, et al: The state of women veterans' health research: results of a systematic literature review. J Gen Intern Med 21 (suppl):S82–S92, 2006

Klein RE: Women Veterans: Past, Present and Future. Washington, DC, Department of Veterans Affairs, Office of the Actuary, 2005

Michaud M: House expected to pass Michaud bill to improve traumatic brain injury treatment and screening today (5/23/07). Congressman Mike Michaud Web site, 2007. Available at: http://michaud.house.gov/article.asp?id=420. Accessed May 10, 2008.

National Coalition for the Homeless: Homeless Veterans (NCH Fact Sheet #14). August 2007. Available at: http://www.nationalhomeless.org/publications/facts/veterans.html. Accessed May 13, 2008.

National Mental Health Association: NMHA leads the fight for better health care for veterans: seeks $64 million in community reinvestments. NMHA Legislative Alert, May 3, 1999. Available at: http://www1.nmha.org/newsroom/system/lal.vw.cfm?do=vw&rid=111. Accessed May 10, 2008.

Prigerson HG, Maciejewski PK, Rosenheck RA: Population attributable fractions of psychiatric disorders and behavioral outcomes associated with combat exposure among US men. Am J Public Health 92:59–63, 2002

Public Broadcasting Service: Military sexual trauma. Now, September 7, 2007. Available at: http://www.pbs.org/now/shows/336. Accessed May 10, 2008.

Rosenheck R, Leda CA, Frisman LK, et al: Homeless veterans, in Homelessness in America: A Reference Book. Edited by Baumohl J. Phoenix, AZ, Oryx Press, 1996, pp 97–108

Quester AO, Gilroy CL: Women and minorities in America's volunteer military. Contemp Econ Policy 20:111–121, 2007

Substance Abuse and Mental Health Services Administration Office of Applied Studies: Veterans in Substance Abuse Treatment. The DASIS Report. Rockville, MD, Substance Abuse and Mental Health Services Administration, 2001

Substance Abuse and Mental Health Services Administration Office of Applied Studies: Veterans in Substance Abuse Treatment, 1995–2000. The DASIS Report. Rockville, MD, Substance Abuse and Mental Health Services Administration, 2003

U.S. Department of Veterans Affairs: Statement of the Honorable Anthony J. Principi, Secretary of Veterans Affairs, Before the Committee on Veterans' Affairs, United States Senate, May 13, 2002. Available at: http://www.va.gov/oca/testimony/svac/13my02TP.asp. Accessed April 26, 2008.

U.S. Department of Veterans Affairs: Fact Sheet: Facts About the Department of Veterans Affairs. December 19, 2007a. Available at: http://www1.va.gov/opa/fact/vafacts.asp. Accessed April 25, 2008.

U.S. Department of Veterans Affairs: Health Eligibility and Enrollment. January 16, 2007b. Available at: http://www.va.gov/healtheligibility/eligibility/DetermineEligibility.asp. Accessed June 13, 2008.

U.S. Department of Veterans Affairs: Mental Health: About the VA Mental Health Group. September 27, 2007c. Available at: http://www.mentalhealth.va.gov/mentalhealth/vamentalhealthgroup.asp. Accessed May 13, 2008.

U.S. Department of Veterans Affairs: VA Compensation and Pension Payment Rates: Veterans Compensation Benefits Rate Tables—Effective 12/1/07. November 27, 2007d. Available at: http://www.vba.va.gov/bln/21/Rates/comp01.htm. Accessed April 26, 2008.

U.S. Department of Veterans Affairs: Women Veterans Health—Military Sexual Trauma Program. April 5, 2007e. Available at: http://www1.va.gov/wvhp/page.cfm?pg=20. Accessed May 10, 2008.

U.S. Department of Veterans Affairs: Fact Sheet: VA Voluntary Service. February 7, 2008a. Available at: http://www1.va.gov/opa/fact/volsvcfs.asp. Accessed May 13, 2008.

U.S. Department of Veterans Affairs: Pharmacy Benefits Management Strategic Healthcare Group—National Formulary. April 14, 2008b. Available at: http://www.pbm.va.gov/NationalFormulary.aspx. Accessed April 26, 2008.

U.S. Department of Veterans Affairs: Public and Intergovernmental Affairs—Current Benefits. April 28, 2008c. Available at: http://www.va.gov/opa/vadocs/current_benefits.asp. Accessed May 10, 2008.

U.S. Department of Veterans Affairs: VA Research and Development—Historical Accomplishments. April 23, 2008d. Available at: http://www.research.va.gov/about/history.cfm. Accessed May 13, 2008.

U.S. Government Accountability Office: Report to Congressional Requesters: Mild Traumatic Brain Injury Screening and Evaluation Implemented for OEF/OIF Veterans, but Challenges Remain (GAO-08-276). February 2008. Available at: http://www.gao.gov/new.items/d08276.pdf. Accessed May 10, 2008.

VA Maryland Health Care System: Mental Health Clinical Center, Acute Inpatient Services. June 1, 2006. Available at: http://www.maryland.va.gov/services/mhcc/subproduct/acute.htm. Accessed May 6, 2008.

Vocational Rehabilitation and Employment Services, San Diego VA Regional Office: History of Veteran's Vocational Rehabilitation. March 12, 2008. Available at: http://www.vba.va.gov/ro/sandiego/vre/history.html. Accessed May 10, 2008.

Wolfe J, Sharkansky EJ, Read JP, et al: Sexual harassment and assault as predictors of PTSD symptomatology among US female Persian Gulf War military personnel. J Interpers Violence 1:40–57, 1998

Women's Research and Education Institute: Chronology of Significant Legal and Policy Changes Affecting Women in the Military: 1947–2003. Arlington, VA, Women's Research and Education Institute, 2007. Available at: http://www.wrei.org/WomeninMilitary.htm. Accessed May 13, 2008.

APPENDIX

Online Resources for Veterans

Defense and Veterans Brain Injury Center: http://www.dvbic.org

Fact Sheet: Facts About the Department of Veterans Affairs: http://www1.va.gov/opa/fact/vafacts.asp

Fact Sheet: VA Voluntary Service: http://www1.va.gov/opa/fact/volsvcfs.asp

Homeless Veterans: http://www1.va.gov/homeless

Military Sexual Trauma Program: http://www1.va.gov/wvhp/page.cfm?pg=20

MyHealtheVet: http://www.myhealth.va.gov

National Coalition for the Homeless: http://www.national-homeless.org

Office of Public and Intergovernmental Affairs: http://www1.va.gov/opa

Pharmacy Benefits Management Service: http://www.pbm.va.gov

Programs for Women Veterans: http://www1.va.gov/wvhp/page.cfm?pg=26

Research and Development: http://www.research.va.gov/about/history.cfm

VA Careers: http://www.vacareers.va.gov

VA Mental Health Group: http://www.mentalhealth.va.gov/mentalhealth/vamentalhealthgroup.asp

Veterans Health Information Systems and Technology Architecture (VistA): http://www.va.gov/vista_monograph

Vocational Rehabilitation and Employment Program: http://www.vba.va.gov/ro/sandiego/vre/history.html

Women's Mental Health Center: http://www.women-vetsptsd.va.gov

CHAPTER 15

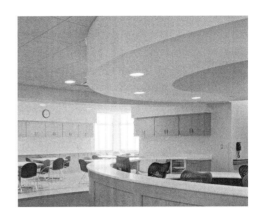

CONSULTATION–LIAISON PSYCHIATRY

Lucy A. Epstein, M.D.
Philip R. Muskin, M.D.

Consultation–liaison (CL) psychiatry, also known as psychosomatic medicine, is a subspecialty of psychiatry in which professionals focus their clinical, research, and teaching efforts on the intersection of medicine and psychiatry. CL psychiatrists prescribe psychotropic medication and practice psychotherapy, but they also may engage in making medical decisions on which patients' lives may depend. CL psychiatrists practice in many settings, including hospital medical floors (Kornfeld 1996b), medical–psychiatric inpatient units (Kathol and Stoudemire 2002), and outpatient facilities (Unutzer et al. 2002). Because their field is interdisciplinary in nature, CL psychiatrists also are uniquely positioned to participate in broader arenas, such as medical student education, residency training, and medical ethics (Kornfeld 1996a, 2002). Research also is integral to CL psychiatry; however, resource limitations have challenged research opportunities (Ilchef 2006).

The field of CL psychiatry is dynamic and expanding; in 2003, psychosomatic medicine was recognized as a subspecialty by the American Board of Psychiatry and Neurology (ABPN) and approved by the American Board of Medical Specialties. The first certification examination was given in 2005. As of 2007, 583 psychiatrists have qualifications in psychosomatic medicine from the ABPN (www.apbn.com). In 2004, the American Psychiatric Association (APA) formed a Council of Psychosomatic Medicine. As of 2000, almost 800 psychiatrists have received specialized training in psychosomatic medicine, and almost 3,000 psychiatrists in the United States devote at least part of their practice to CL psychiatry (Gitlin et al. 2004; Noyes et al. 1992). In addition to the APA, international organizations such as the Academy of Psychosomatic Medicine provide an organizational "home" for psychiatrists who practice this subspecialty.

As CL psychiatry has evolved, so has its nomenclature (Gitlin et al. 2004). The term *psychosomatic medicine,* the official designation of the subspecialty, describes the broad spectrum of clinical, research, and teaching activities of the CL psychiatrist. Many clinicians still refer to themselves as *consultation* psychiatrists to emphasize the interaction between their practice and medical and surgical disciplines. The term *liaison* in this context refers to work that focuses on the clinical needs of a specific medical team, such as an intensive care unit. Medical staff can benefit from the presence of a psychiatrist they may have come to know and trust (Lipowski 1986). Unfortunately, in part due to an inhospitable reimbursement environment, in recent years liaison activities have transformed into a less fixed and more consultation-based relationship (Ramchandani et al. 1997).

CL psychiatrists are essentially physicians who are prepared to diagnose and treat psychiatric illness in a medical context. (Table 15–1 presents a list of common clinical scenarios for consultation.) Consultations generally fall into one of several categories, as described by Lipowski (1967). First, CL psychiatrists treat psychiatric manifestations of medical illness or its treatment. They may, for example, discover that the patient who appears depressed actually has lupus cerebritis or a frontal brain mass. Second, they treat psychiatric complications of medical illness or its treatment, such as behavioral change after herpes encephalitis or mania secondary to treatment with steroids. Third, they treat medical complications of psychiatric illness or its treatment. For example, they may treat a patient with anorexia nervosa and bradycardia, or a patient who has overdosed on lithium. Last, consultants may use their knowledge of psychotherapeutic principles to assist with psychological reactions to medical illness.

At any one time, the treatment strategy may include pathophysiological, pharmacological, and psychodynamic approaches. Most importantly, the CL psychiatrist aims to think on each of these levels simultaneously. She or he also takes into account the needs of the individual patient, the patient's loved ones, the medical staff, and the larger health care system (Miller 1973a, 1973b). The CL psychiatrist may sometimes feel as though she or he is "treating the entire floor" or "containing the affect of the unit" (Mozian and Muskin 2008). At times, this is exactly what is going on. The specialized training of the CL psychiatrist, throughout residency and fellowship, is crucial for the effective management of the intense emotions involved in these difficult cases.

History

Physicians have been curious about the mind–body problem since the early days of medicine. René Des-

TABLE 15–1. Common clinical scenarios for psychiatric consultation

Condition

Delirium

Affective illness

Anxiety disorders

Psychosis

Dementia

Substance intoxication or withdrawal

Suicidal/homicidal ideation

Axis II disorders

Management of aggression

Neuropsychiatric presentations

Eating disorders

Coping with medical illness

Somatoform disorders

Factitious disorders/malingering

Pain

Capacity evaluations/ethics

Population

Child/adolescent

Perinatal

Geriatric

Cardiac

Burns

Transplant

HIV/AIDS

Rehabilitation

Cancer/palliative care

cartes (1637) famously introduced the mind–body split (*cogito ergo sum*). The Dutch philosopher Baruch Spinoza (1632–1677) and the English physician William Harvey (1578–1657) rejected this idea and proposed the integration of mind and body (Lipsitt 2006). Johann Christian Heinroth is credited with coining the term *psychosomatic* as a description of the unconscious processes that influence the health of the body (Heinroth 1818). Other influential thinkers of the eighteenth century include George Ernst Stahl, who described a "vital force" integrating physiological events with dynamic psychological phenomena, and Johann Christian Reil, who called for humanistic treatment of the mentally ill in Germany (Lipsitt 2006). In the nineteenth century, the works of Benjamin Rush helped to lay the foundation of modern psychosomatic medicine (Rush 1811); Rush, the father of American psychiatry, is credited with writing the first psychiatric textbook and founding the APA (Lipowski 1996; Lipsitt 2006).

The early twentieth century witnessed significant development in theory, research, and practice. During this time, psychosomatic medicine was heavily influenced by psychoanalytic theory, as exemplified by Franz Alexander, who focused on the somatic impact of psychodynamic conflict (Hackett et al. 2004). Others, such as Walter Cannon, Morton Prince, and Felix Deutsch (the latter coined the term *psychosomatic medicine*), were influential in further development of theory and practice during the early twentieth century (Lipsitt 2006). Flanders Dunbar, at Columbia–Presbyterian Medical Center, embraced an organic synthesis perspective, which aimed to merge physiology with psychoanalytic principles (Hackett et al. 2004). Dunbar conducted research on the impact of psychological factors in a large cohort of patients with medical illness (Dunbar et al. 1936) and founded both the journal *Psychosomatic Medicine* (1939) and the American Psychosomatic Society (1942) (Lipsitt 2006). Adolf Meyer, another influential figure of this time, developed an important center for psychosomatic medicine at Johns Hopkins University Hospital and later became the president of the APA (Lipsitt 2006). His work emphasized a psychobiological model with a holistic orientation (Lipsitt 2006). A significant upsurge in interest in psychosomatic medicine occurred in the middle of the twentieth century, with greater emphasis placed on the social aspects of psychiatric illness, such as the health effects of combat-related stress in World War II veterans (Lipsitt 2006).

The twentieth century also heralded the development of formal CL psychiatry services in general medical hospitals. Lipowski's (1996) book is highly recommended for a comprehensive overview of the historical development of this field. James Jackson Putnam and Joseph Pratt were important figures in the "Boston group," which served as a focal point for the emergence of CL psychiatry (Lipsitt 2006). George Henry, who wrote the first article on CL psychiatry (Henry 1929–1930), inaugurated the first formal consultation service in 1929. Edward Billings, who created the CL service at the University of Colorado, was the first to term these services "liaison psychiatry" (Billings 1939). Crucial financial support allowed CL psychiatric practice to flourish. From 1934 to 1935, funding by the Rockefeller Foundation (with Alan Gregg at the helm of its Division of Medical Sciences) strengthened both consultation–liaison and general psychiatry across the nation (Lipowski 1996). As a result, by the 1960s, almost 75% of all psychiatric programs in the United States included CL services (Mendel 1966). During the 1970s, the vision and leadership of James Eaton from the National Institute of Mental Health (Eaton et al. 1977) helped to expand CL psychiatry as a field (Hackett et al. 2004). Some of the National Institute of Mental Health funding included training grants for CL fellowships, which significantly increased the number of psychiatrists specializing in psychosomatic medicine (Gitlin et al. 2004). Flagship consultation services were founded at Massachusetts General Hospital (under the direction of Stanley Cobb, followed by Erich Lindemann, Avery Weisman, and Thomas Hackett), Beth Israel Hospital in Boston (Grete Bebring), University of Rochester (John Romano and George Engel), University of Colorado (Edward Billings), and Mount Sinai (M. Ralph Kaufman) (Lipowski 1996). Limited funding, comparative lack of evidence-based practice, and other challenges have been important issues for organized CL psychiatry in recent years (Ilchef 2006). The recent establishment of psychosomatic medicine as a subspecialty, with field-specific interdisciplinary collaboration and clinical research, has served to consolidate knowledge and to encourage future work.

Consultation Process

There is no "method" for performing a consultation, because it is a process. Certain fundamental principles are central to performing an effective consultation (Goldman et al. 1983; Pasnau 1985). However, each case is unique, and flexibility is key. Many of the typical components of psychiatric practice, such as a private space, a set appointment time, and a physically and cognitively healthy patient, cannot be taken for granted (Querques and Stern 2004). At times, patients may not even know that they have been referred to a psychiatrist (Shakin Kunkel and Thompson 1996); informing patients about the consultation process and the psychiatrists' role in the medical setting may help to engender trust (Smith et al. 2005).

An effective consultation comprises a series of stages, as described by Querques and colleagues (Querques and Stern 2004; Smith et al. 2005). A crucial first step is to talk directly with the person requesting the consultation. Consultation requests are notoriously vague and may reflect conflicts surrounding the patient, inexperience of the person requesting the consultation, or confusing messages within the medical team. A CL psychiatrist will be attuned to both the implicit and the explicit meanings underlying a team's requests (Smith et al. 2005). The various medical services have specific expectations and questions for the consultant, which may range from a capacity evaluation to a plan for disposition to an explanation of the psychosocial aspects of the patient's presentation (Shakin Kunkel and Thompson 1996). The consultant next gathers collateral information by perusing the patient's current and prior medical record, laboratory findings, and any other available data. Close inspection of the medication list (including dosing, timing, and route of administration) is crucial. Nursing, occupational therapy, and physical therapy notes also may contain a wealth of information about the patient's behavior (Smith et al. 2005). As with all psychiatric consultations, talking with the patient and his or her family is the core of the process. A full psychiatric interview should be conducted when possible; however, medically ill patients may be too physically uncomfortable or fatigued to tolerate a long discussion. Expressing empathy for a patient's physical suffering can help to establish an alliance (Smith et al. 2005). The psychiatrist then makes a preliminary diagnosis, which may be psychiatric, medical, or both, recognizing that it may evolve with time. Direct communication to the team about the diagnosis and proposed treatment is essential (Popkin et al. 1981). It is important to tailor recommendations based on the team's specific needs (Shakin Kunkel and Thompson 1996). The final step is to write a complete, but succinct, note. Regular follow-up is essential to ensure that the diagnostic and treatment plan is correctly instituted (Shakin Kunkel and Thompson 1996). Last, a wise psychiatric consultant knows the value of signing off on the case (with communication to the team) when the patient has stabilized and/or the consultation question has been answered completely.

Diagnostic Strategies

One of the consultant's most important goals is to provide an accurate diagnosis for the change in the patient's affect, behavior, or cognition. Because many medical conditions can have psychiatric presentations, the consultant's job will be to correlate or newly identify these conditions in order that they be addressed and treated.

Case Example

A 23-year-old man was admitted to the surgery service after a C7 spinal cord injury that resulted in near quadriparesis and a complicated hospital course. When sedation was lifted, he was unusually "quiet"

per his mother, who described him as a previously gregarious and athletic college student. The psychiatry team was consulted for "depression." The consultant felt that it was unclear whether the patient could either understand or communicate with the team and recommended magnetic resonance imaging, which revealed chronic intracranial bleeding and communicating hydrocephalus, resulting in mutism. A ventriculoperitoneal shunt was placed, resulting in immediate improvement in the patient's language and motor skills. He was subsequently discharged to a rehabilitation facility in improved condition.

History

There is no more important aspect of the consulting psychiatrist's job than to gather the essential and complete history from the patient, if possible. Ideally, the psychiatric consultant will gather a full history of psychiatric symptoms, including timing, severity, frequency, nature, precipitants, and any known relationship to current medical illness. The consultant should perform a psychiatric review of systems, asking questions regarding the affective, anxiety, and psychotic realms. A substance abuse history can often be the turning point of a confusing medical presentation, as patients may be unwilling or unable to reveal their use.

Case Example

An elderly woman was admitted for neurological evaluation. She was confused, disoriented, and disinhibited. Her family reported that she never drank alcohol. The woman had been functioning well until 3 days before the admission, when she became agitated and confused. She reported taking no medications except for a "Centrum" at bedtime. Her daughter brought in two shopping bags of medications the patient kept under her bed, which included several empty bottles of Centrax (prazepam). The patient's encephalopathy resolved when she was started on a regular dosage of a benzodiazepine, from which she was slowly withdrawn over the following week.

Patients should be asked about current suicidal or homicidal ideation. No other person may have asked such questions, fearing that the question will "induce" the thoughts. Patients may follow the "don't ask, don't tell" philosophy about such thoughts, but they will talk about them if asked in the appropriate manner. Information regarding past psychiatric history, such as prior suicide attempts, hospitalizations, medication trials, and current therapy, should be gathered. Close attention should be paid to the current medical illness, past medical history, home medications, and allergies. The consultant should obtain a detailed family and social history, which may be particularly important for those consultations that are focused on the challenges of coping with medical illness.

Examination

A mental status examination is a detailed observation of a patient's behavior, speech, language, affect, and cognition. Because this examination is hierarchical in nature, it is important to perform it meticulously (Hyman and Tesar 1994; Smith et al. 2005). Ideally, the mental status examination would allow someone unfamiliar with the patient to pick him or her out of a group of people. Sometimes this can be done quickly, creating an accurate "snapshot" description of the patient.

Case Example

A consultant receives the following page: "You are needed immediately on the inpatient internal medicine unit. Please don't delay." After alerting security, the consultant finds a highly agitated young woman who is screaming, disoriented, and confused. She is trying to tear the electrocardiogram electrodes off her skin and the intravenous line out of her arm. It is impossible to interview her. All that is known is that the laboratory results indicate diabetic ketoacidosis. After a small intramuscular dose of an antipsychotic medication, the patient is calm enough for the medical team to address her medical needs. When the patient again becomes agitated later in the day, the mental status examination provides a quick reference point for checking her serum glucose and electrolytes before administering more of the antipsychotic.

The physical examination, which is not a typical part of an outpatient psychiatrist's examination, adds important information. Attention to vital signs, cardiac abnormalities, gastrointestinal symptoms (e.g., stigmata of liver disease), and other subtleties, aids immensely in the diagnostic process. Knowledge of the neurological exam and an ability to recognize focal neurological deficits are essential (Smith et al. 2005). Perhaps the most important part of the physical exam is testing for evidence of frontal lobe dysfunction, which may result in significant behavioral abnormalities. Tasks to elicit frontal lobe function include tests of motor sequencing (e.g., asking a patient to reproduce a sequence of hand gestures), language production (e.g., asking the patient to name as many animals as possible in 1 minute), and abstraction (e.g., listing differences between an apple and an orange) (Smith et al. 2005). The Mini-Mental State Examination (Folstein et al. 1975) can provide an impression of the patient's cognition. It is most useful as a concise scan of the patient's cognitive functions (including attention, memory, language, visuospatial, and executive functioning), but it has limited sensitivity or specificity for a given diagnosis. Indications that the patient is "A&O×3" (alert and oriented to person, place, and time) should be held suspect until the consultant has talked with the patient. Confusion and disorientation may have a variety of etiologies, but no accurate diagnosis can be made without knowing if the patient is or is not intact cognitively.

Laboratory Tests

Some diagnostic tests are particularly useful for the CL psychiatrist; the specific tests ordered depend on the concern(s). (Table 15–2 lists common laboratory tests that may be useful during the course of a consultation.) For example, for a patient with a sudden change in mental status, life-threatening causes must be ruled out first (e.g., by a lumbar puncture for suspected meningitis or a toxicology screen for a suspected overdose). A standard battery of tests used by the CL psychiatrist includes a complete blood count, a metabolic panel, and levels of thyroid-stimulating hormone, vitamin B_{12}, folate, and rapid plasma reagin. Specialized tests (e.g., HIV serology, electrocardiogram, imaging study, electroencephalogram) may also be useful, depending on the clinical situation. The consultant maintains the focus that the *cause* of the behavioral dyscontrol must be discovered, even if the behavior itself dissipates (Muskin et al. 1998). The psychiatrist may bring a fresh eye to a complicated case, and tactful suggestions regarding the diagnostic evaluation may expand the differential diagnosis and change the medical course.

Imaging

Imaging can be helpful to the differential diagnosis, although imaging alone does not typically confirm a diagnosis (Dougherty and Rauch 2004). There are several imaging options that are easily accessible, efficient, and useful. Computed tomography (CT) is an imaging method that provides rapid assessment of anatomic structures. Although it does not provide high resolution of structural abnormalities, a CT scan shows gross changes, such as the presence of an acute hemorrhage stroke, subdural hematoma, or large mass lesion. Magnetic resonance imaging (MRI) with angiography can provide high-level resolution of both parenchymal and vascular structures. It is the imaging modality of choice for acute stroke (if a facility is available in a timely fashion) as well as for the visualization of subtle changes. Psychiatric syndromes that are most likely to produce abnormalities detected by MRI in-

TABLE 15–2. Common diagnostic tests in psychiatric consultation

Complete blood count

Chemistry panel

Liver function tests

Thyroid-stimulating hormone (thyrotropin) concentration

Vitamin B_{12} (cyanocobalamin) concentration

Folic acid (folate) concentration

Human chorionic gonadotropin (pregnancy) test

Serum and urine toxicology panel

Serological tests for syphilis

Urinalysis

Antinuclear antibody

HIV serology

Chest X ray

Electrocardiogram

Computed tomography scan

Magnetic resonance imaging scan

Electroencephalography

Neuropsychological testing

Source.   Adapted from Smith FA, Querques J, Levenson JL, et al: "Psychiatric Assessment and Consultation," in The American Psychiatric Publishing Textbook of Psychosomatic Medicine. Edited by Levenson JL. Washington, DC, American Psychiatric Publishing, 2005, pp 3–14.

clude dementia, vasculitides, infectious processes, and mass lesions. Electroencephalography (EEG) is another useful imaging modality. Findings are normal in patients with depression, mania, and psychosis, but not in patients with delirium, dementia, and ongoing seizures. One limitation is that EEG may not detect deep brain activity (such as in the temporal region); thus, an absence of an abnormality does not necessarily mean that electrical dysrhythmias are not present. Single photon emission computed tomography (SPECT) and positron emission tomography (PET) scans are not available in every institution but offer an option to assess abnormalities of metabolism in different areas of the brain.

Neuropsychological Testing

It can be useful to ask for neuropsychological testing in certain clinical situations. These tests are divided into two main categories: cognitive and projective. Examples of cognitive tasks include the 100-point Modified Mini Mental State (3MS) examination (Teng and Chui 1987), which follows a similar format to the

Mini-Mental State Examination (Folstein et al. 1975) but with more extensive and detailed questioning, and the Trail Making Test Part B (Army Individual Test Battery 1944), which assesses mental agility, executive decision making, and planning. These tests might be most useful in documenting the degree of cognitive decline in a patient with subacute changes in mental status, such as with a dementing process. Projective testing, which can both detect the presence of underlying psychiatric illness and provide a window into the patient's coping style, can be useful in certain settings.

Case Example

A 75-year-old woman was referred for treatment of "dementia." She was depressed and psychotic, maintaining that someone had entered her new home and stolen important papers. Her symptoms began after moving to an apartment following 50 years of living in the same house. Neuropsychological tests revealed superior intellectual functioning, depression, and psychosis. Although the woman was reluctant to take medication, after confrontation with her test results and her symptoms, she adhered to treatment with an antidepressant and antipsychotic. Her symptoms resolved over the next 2 months. When she was taken off medication 1 year later, fully recovered, she was able to admit that she was "out of my head."

Consultation/Collaboration With Other Services

At times, the psychiatric consultant may suggest that the primary care team request the expertise of other medical services. This may be particularly useful in clinical situations that lie on the interface of more than one discipline. When multiple consultation services are involved, difficulties can sometimes arise, stemming from differences in the history, culture, and diagnostic strategies of the various disciplines (Caplan et al. 2008). A collaborative spirit and direct communication allow for effective teamwork. Even if there are disagreements, the psychiatric consultant should avoid "chart wars" and the debasing of other services' recommendations.

Principles of Treatment

Biological Management

One of the most important decisions for the CL psychiatrist is whether to start, continue, taper off, hold, or discontinue a patient's psychotropic medication. The first consideration is the certainty of the diagnosis. For example, what appears to be "flat affect" could actually be apathy due to a frontal lobe lesion or the masked facies that is a characteristic of Parkinson disease. At the same time, while the underlying cause is being determined, it is important to treat its consequent behaviors. For example, treating an agitated, delirious patient empirically with an antipsychotic has several benefits. The calming effect of the medication increases the ability of the patient to cooperate with the evaluation, and it may shorten the length of the hospital stay by permitting a more rapid diagnostic and therapeutic process.

The selection of an optimal medication for the medically ill patient is an important, though complicated, task. The pharmacokinetics of the medication needs to be carefully considered, including its absorption, distribution, metabolism, and excretion, any of which may be abnormal in a patient with physical illness (Querques and Stern 2004). For example, a patient with end-stage cirrhosis may have increased side effects from medications that are extensively metabolized by the liver, and adjustments in dose and/or the choice of an alternative agent may be necessary. Drug–drug interactions are important to consider, as medically ill patients are often on a long list of medications (Querques and Stern 2004). For example, linezolid, a systemic antibiotic that has weak monoamine oxidase–inhibiting properties, can potentially interact with serotonergic agents (Lavery et al. 2001). In these cases, it can be useful to review cytochrome enzyme substrates and catalysts to determine whether potential interactions could be averted (Cozza et al. 2003). Psychotropic medications also can produce deleterious effects in medically ill patients. For example, multiple psychotropic and systemic medications (each of which can impact repolarization of the myocardium) can prolong the QT interval and make the patient vulnerable to arrhythmia (Glassman and Bigger 2001).

Psychological Management

A CL psychiatrist utilizes a biopsychosocial approach to understanding a patient's problem and formulating the treatment. Understanding the coping skills available to patients when they are medically ill provides a framework for many of the interventions in the hospital (M.A. Groves and Muskin 2005). Two considerations that factor into whether or not a consultation will be requested are what the patient thinks about his or her illness and how the patient behaves in accordance with those health beliefs. How the psychiatrist chooses to help a patient handle a problem will be based on what works most efficiently for the particular

issue. Psychodynamic, cognitive-behavioral, interpersonal, or systems-based approaches all have utility depending on the patient, the problem, and the time frame. Financial and social resources available to the patient and physician are important considerations in determining what approach is practical (Miller 1973a, 1973b).

Medical illness and hospitalization is, by its nature, a regressive experience. Illness places the individual in a situation of dependency, which replicates the developmental stresses of childhood (Strain and Grossman 1975). Regression to less reality-based and adaptive coping is to be expected (Field 1979; M.A. Groves and Muskin 2005). The defensive structure prior to medical illness is the starting point for each patient; the lower this point, the more primitive the defensive structure to which the patient may regress (Muskin 1995). Simultaneously, patients react to this regression and attempt to return to their baseline level of function and control. These attempts are frequently the reason for psychiatric consultation (Muskin 1995). A particular challenge for the CL psychiatrist is caring for the "difficult" patient, who can elicit strong countertransference reactions from staff (J.E. Groves 1975, 1978; Mozian and Muskin 2008). How productively the patient–psychiatrist dyad utilizes both the regression and its reaction determines the outcome of the consultation (Rosnick 1987).

PSYCHODYNAMIC STRESSORS

As Strain and Grossman (1975) noted, "The vast majority of patients are able to cope and to assume the role of the patient without difficulty, and this is extraordinary in itself when one considers the magnitude of these stresses." According to these authors, there are seven categories of psychodynamic stress faced by the hospitalized patient (Strain and Grossman 1975).

1. *Threat to narcissistic integrity.* Medical illness poses a direct threat to healthy narcissism, which is an integral part of human functioning. To function effectively in the world, an individual must be able to trust in basic principles of bodily integrity and self-sufficiency. Medical illness, with its inherent uncertainty, indignity, and lack of control, undermines this healthy defense. Physicians may then become the object of a patient's frustration that the infantile fantasy of omnipotent parents (who will ensure the child's pleasurable and protected existence) will not be met, which may manifest as disruptive behavior (Muskin 1995).

2. *Fear of strangers.* Hospitalized patients, by necessity, put their well-being in the hands of relative strangers. Highly intimate processes (e.g., venipuncture, nasogastric tube feeding, urine collection, pelvic examination) occur commonly. The daily changes in nursing staff and the multitude of relative strangers who conduct business in the patient's room may add to this disquieting experience. This situation can be a particular challenge for patients whose psychiatric illness leads to a difficulty in trusting others, whether due to paranoia or personality disorders (e.g., borderline personality disorder) (Muskin 2001). In addition, patients with trauma histories (especially sexual or physical abuse) may be fearful of harm from others whose intent is benign. Staff continuity, discretion, and explicit explanations of procedures can be helpful measures for the consultant to suggest in these situations.

3. *Separation anxiety.* Psychological health does not occur in a vacuum but in a series of overlapping spheres of family, community, and environment. When patients are hospitalized, they are separated from what is familiar and comfortable in their daily lives. The noise, lights, disruptions, and lack of privacy of the hospital can be deeply unsettling. This situation is particularly problematic for patients who need to rely on routine in order to function, such as patients with dementing illnesses (Muskin 1995).

4. *Fear of loss of love and approval.* Many of the stresses that accompany physical illness, such as loss of a part of one's physical self (e.g., mastectomy), may elicit fear of loss of love and approval. A patient whose hospital course is complicated may subconsciously feel that he or she has failed the doctor by not being a good patient who gets well with treatment. In contrast, a patient who had disappointing caregivers in the past may be more likely to express ongoing discontent, which is then externalized to the physician (Ciechanowski et al. 2001).

5. *Fear of loss of control of developmentally achieved functions.* One of the most fundamental premises of childhood development is mastery over developmental tasks, such as the ability to urinate, regulate one's bowels, change clothing, and clean oneself. Physical illness can threaten a person's ability to perform these functions, and unresolved conflicts stemming from these functions can also flare under duress (Muskin 1995). The ability to regulate more primitive emotions, such as rage, may be compromised by severe physical illness, altered mental status, or medical conditions or treatments that directly affect the central nervous system (Muskin 1995).

6. *Fear of loss or injury to body parts.* Loss of integrity of bodily function may promote deep-seated anxieties surrounding mutilation or castration. Many early childhood memories are somatic; to feel safe, an infant needs to have his or her bodily needs met (to be fed, held, and soothed). In later developmental stages, feelings of potency emerge when the young child can master some of his or her own physical universe (Muskin 1995). Medical illness, with its many manifestations of physical vulnerability and potential loss of power, may result in profound anxiety about having basic safety needs addressed (Muskin 1995).

7. *Reactivation of feelings of guilt and shame and accompanying fears of retaliation for previous transgressions.* It may be inevitable that at some point a patient wonders why he or she has become ill. Some patients, such as the lifelong smoker who develops lung cancer, may feel guilt about perceived transgressions (Muskin 1995). Others might fear they are being punished by an outside force. For yet others, the connection may be less clear, but the feelings of guilt remain.

PATIENT COPING STYLES

Just as regression is an inherent part of hospitalization and medical illness, so are attempts to cope with these challenges. Each patient has a particular manner (or character style) in which he or she addresses an illness. Several schemas have been developed that describe basic coping mechanisms common to most patients (Groves and Muskin 2005). One framework, suggested by Kahana and Bibring (1964), is strongly recommended reading for the psychiatric consultant. In this schema, personality categories (including dependent, obsessive, histrionic, masochistic, paranoid, narcissistic, and schizoid) are described, with predictions as to how patients in each category might cope with medical illness.

Case Example

A 56-year-old accountant is hospitalized for surgery for colon cancer. Consultation is requested when the patient is reported to be asking incessant questions about his situation. Upon interview, the patient, who has a laptop next to him, states that he has read virtually everything about his illness on the Internet but still feels he does not know enough about what will happen to him in the hospital. The consultant recognizes the obsessive nature of this patient's coping style and recommends that staff provide pragmatic and straightforward information to the patient and allow him to participate actively in treatment planning.

Although published descriptions of coping mechanisms provide a useful guide for the CL psychiatrist, each person is unique. At times, a patient's coping style can take on pathological features. In such cases, the consultant should aim not to overemphasize a particular "diagnosis" (Geringer and Stern 1986) but rather to assess how each person's internal resources can be mobilized most effectively.

PHYSICIAN COPING STYLES

Each physician, like each patient, has a unique coping style (Muskin 1995). Physicians bring their own strengths, weaknesses, and challenges to the medical setting—a circumstance perhaps best exemplified by Gabbard's (1985) profile of the compulsive, overly responsible physician plagued by guilt and doubt. As physicians traverse the highly intensive training process—which entails sleep deprivation, continually shifting priorities, constant work, and disconnection from family and friends—they rely on their own defensive structures to negotiate these stressors (Lurie et al. 1989; Muskin 1995). The CL psychiatrist can provide insight into the dyadic nature of the doctor–patient relationship and help his or her physician colleagues to understand how the process of countertransference can either augment or detract from patient care (Muskin 1995).

Behavioral and Safety Interventions

A CL psychiatrist is often asked to help manage the patient whose behavior is disruptive to a hospital unit. For example, a behavioral plan may benefit the patient who repeatedly leaves the floor (possibly to use illicit substances), does not cooperate with recommendations, or acts in ways that violate the hospital's cultural norms (such as by participating in sexual activity in the hospital bathroom). At times, the CL psychiatrist may need to intervene actively to maintain the safety of the patient and unit employees. Patients whose behavioral dysregulation results in imminent risk of harm to self or others may require a stepwise series of interventions, which may include verbal redirection, use of antipsychotic and/or sedative medications, enlistment of security staff, and/or physical restraint (if all behavioral interventions have failed). Because many physicians have received little or no training in the use of behav-

ioral interventions or in safe, time-limited, effective, and approved restraint techniques, the consultant will aim to educate them on the use of the least restrictive method to manage behavior safely.

Case Example

A 59-year-old woman with cirrhosis is admitted to the medical service with hepatic encephalopathy. Over the course of the evening, she becomes highly agitated. She is found screaming incoherently and running down the hospital corridor. The overnight medical intern requests physical restraint after medication has demonstrated little effect. The on-call psychiatrist, noting that the restraint is increasing the patient's agitation, recommends a full-time sitter instead, resulting in immediate improvement in her symptoms.

Social Interventions

CL psychiatrists commonly interact with the many people who surround the patient, such as family, partners, and friends. The highly charged countertransference responses some patients evoke in staff may require the psychiatrist to intervene with hospital staff (J. E. Groves 1978). Knowledge of group processes, such as splitting, scapegoating, and triangulating, can be essential to effective management. CL psychiatrists may often find themselves "holding the affect of the unit," so that they can appropriately metabolize it in a way that patients stay safe and continue to get the care they need. The psychiatrist also can serve to bridge communication gaps among family members and the patient. In addition, the CL psychiatrist can provide expertise in managing situations laden with intense affect, such as complicated end-of-life issues or pain management for patients with substance dependence.

Future Challenges for Psychosomatic Medicine

Psychosomatic medicine faces several important challenges in the future. One of these challenges involves the artificial separation of the fields of psychiatry and medicine. Psychiatric conditions are an inherent part of medical illness, and vice versa. Patients are differentially vulnerable to psychiatric disorders based on a complicated interplay of genetic, environmental, and other factors that have yet to be elucidated. Because many psychiatric disorders do not yet have clearly defined pathophysiology, some physicians may discount the importance of the CL psychiatrist in the care of the patient. The attitude that "It's all in the patient's head" can be a demeaning and devaluing view of the patient and of the psychiatric consultant.

A second challenge is the need for increased resource allocation for CL psychiatrists in general hospitals. In 2004, approximately 24% of all adult admissions in community hospitals involved affective, psychotic, or other mental health or substance use–related disorders; an even higher percentage occurred among uninsured patients (Owens et al. 2007). Almost 10 times as many patients with mental health or substance abuse disorders were seen in community hospitals as in psychiatric facilities (Owens et al. 2007). Psychiatric comorbidity results in worse medical outcomes, longer hospital stays, and increased hospital and aftercare costs (Francis and Kapoor 1992; Katon 1996; Koenig and Kuchibhatla 1998; Levenson et al. 1990; Saravay and Lavin 1994; Saravay et al. 1991). At the same time, psychiatric interventions on medical services have been shown to decrease the length of hospital stays and increase the likelihood of returning home (Levitan and Kornfeld 1981; Strain et al. 1991). The current system is extremely underresourced. Suggested solutions have included a reinstatement of federal funding for clinical fellowships in CL psychiatry to increase the number of highly trained practitioners of psychosomatic medicine, and better training in psychiatric principles for nonpsychiatric physicians. Access to psychiatric care is quite limited for many patients with medical illness in the outpatient setting, as is access to medical care for psychiatric outpatients (Kathol et al. 2006).

A related challenge is inadequate funding for the treatment of hospitalized patients with mental health or substance abuse disorders. Reimbursement for psychiatric consultations does not adequately support CL services. For example, for the 7.6 million patients with mental health or substance abuse disorders hospitalized in community settings in 2004, about 60% of the costs were billed to the government (approximately 50% to Medicare and 18% to Medicaid) (Owens et al. 2007). Patients hospitalized primarily for mental health or substance abuse disorders were the most likely group to be uninsured (Owens et al. 2007). CL psychiatrists also are grappling with the financial ramifications of the managed care era (Goldberg and Stoudemire 1995). The survival of psychiatric CL services is jeopardized by a combination of immense patient need and lack of parity for reimbursement of psychiatric services, as compared to other medical services. A large proportion of the patients in need of psychiatric consultation have little or no reimbursement. Many services are in the process of strengthening their financial capabilities, by such means as streamlining information systems, administrative processes, and billing functions (Hall et al. 1996; Schuster 1992). Insurers who carve out behavioral health services in an effort to save money actually increase the ultimate health care expenditures for patients in need of integrated care (Kathol et al. 2006). The need for integrated medical and psychiatric services emerges as a crucial challenge to be overcome in order to provide patients with the best possible care.

Conclusion

The focus of a CL psychiatrist's expertise is on the evaluation and management of the affective, behavioral, and cognitive aspects of patients who are experiencing medical illness. Practitioners of psychosomatic medicine have an overarching view of the complex interplay of medical and psychiatric diseases from both a psychopharmacological and psychodynamic perspective. Their work is by nature multidisciplinary, interactive, and collaborative. The theory, research, and practice of psychosomatic medicine and CL psychiatry continue to evolve. Psychosomatic medicine, in its modern form, is well positioned to lead clinical, research, and educational efforts in medical psychiatric practice.

References

Army Individual Test Battery: Manual of Directions and Scoring. Washington, DC, War Department, Adjutant General's Office, 1944

Billings EG: Liaison psychiatry and intern instruction. J Assoc Am Med Coll 14:375–385, 1939

Caplan JP, Epstein LA, Stern TA: Consultants' conflicts: a case discussion of differences and their resolution. Psychosomatics 49:8–13, 2008

Ciechanowski PS, Katon WJ, Russo JE, et al: The patient-provider relationship: attachment theory and adherence to treatment in diabetes. Am J Psychiatry 158:29–35, 2001

Cozza KL, Armstrong SC, Oesterheld JR: Drug Interaction Principles for Medical Practice, 2nd Edition. Washington, DC, American Psychiatric Publishing, 2003

Dougherty DD, Rauch SL: Neuroimaging in psychiatry, in Massachusetts General Hospital Psychiatry Update and Board Preparation, 2nd Edition. Edited by Stern TA, Herman JB. New York, McGraw-Hill, 2004, pp 227–232

Dunbar FH, Wolfe TP, Rioch JM: Psychiatric aspects of medical problems. Am J Psychiatry 93:649–679, 1936

Eaton JS, Goldberg R, Rosinski E, et al: The educational challenge of consultation-liaison psychiatry. Am J Psychiatry 134 (suppl):20–23, 1977

Field HL: Defense mechanisms in psychosomatic medicine. Psychosomatics 20:690–700, 1979

Folstein MF, Folstein SE, McHugh PR: "Mini-Mental State": a practical guide for grading the cognitive state of patients for the clinician. J Psychiatr Res 12:189–198, 1975

Francis J, Kapoor WN: Prognosis after hospital discharge of older medical patients with delirium. J Am Geriatr Soc 40:601–606, 1992

Gabbard GO: The role of compulsiveness in the normal physician. JAMA 254:2926–2929, 1985

Geringer ES, Stern TA: Coping with medical illness: the impact of personality types. Psychosomatics 27:251–261, 1986

Gitlin DF, Levenson JL, Lyketsos CG: Psychosomatic medicine: a new psychiatric subspecialty. Acad Psychiatry 28:4–11, 2004

Glassman AH, Bigger JT: Antipsychotic drugs: prolonged QTc interval, torsade de pointes, and sudden death. Am J Psychiatry 158:1774–1782, 2001

Goldberg RJ, Stoudemire A: The future of consultation-liaison psychiatry and medical-psychiatric units in the era of managed care. Gen Hosp Psychiatry 17:268–277, 1995

Goldman L, Lee T, Rudd P: Ten commandments for effective consultation. Arch Intern Med 143:1753–1755, 1983

Groves JE: Management of the borderline patient on a medical or surgical ward: the psychiatric consultant's roles. Int J Psychiatry Med 6:337–348, 1975

Groves JE: Taking care of the hateful patient. N Engl J Med 298:883–887, 1978

Groves MA, Muskin PR: Psychological responses to illness, in The American Psychiatric Publishing Textbook of Psychosomatic Medicine. Edited by Levenson JL. Washington, DC: American Psychiatric Publishing, 2005, pp 67–90

Hackett TP, Cassem NH, Stern TA, et al: Beginnings: psychosomatic medicine and consultation psychiatry in the general hospital, in Massachusetts General Hospital Handbook of General Hospital Psychiatry, 5th Edition. Edited by Stern TA, Fricchione GL, Cassem NH, et al. Philadelphia, PA, CV Mosby, 2004, pp 1–7

Hall RC, Rundell JR, Hirsch TW: Economic issues in consultation-liaison psychiatry, in The American Psychiatric Press Textbook of Consultation-Liaison Psychiatry. Edited by Rundell JR, Wise MG. Washington, DC, American Psychiatric Press, 1996, pp 24–37

Heinroth JC: Lehrbuch der storungen des seelenlebens. Leipzig, Germany, FCW Vogel, 1818

Henry GW: Some modern aspects of psychiatry in general hospital practice. Am J Psychiatry 86:481–499, 1929–1930

Hyman SE, Tesar GE: The emergency psychiatric examination, including the mental status examination, in Manual of Psychiatric Emergencies, 3rd Edition. Edited by Hyman SE, Tesar GE. Boston, MA, Little, Brown, 1994, pp 3–11

Ilchef R: Diamonds in the coalface: new research in consultation-liaison psychiatry. Curr Opin Psychiatry 19:175–179, 2006

Kahana RJ, Bibring GL: Personality types in medical management, in Psychiatry and Medical Practice in a General Hospital. Edited by Zinberg N. New York, International Universities Press, 1964, pp 108–123

Kathol RG, Stoudemire A: Strategic integration of inpatient and outpatient medical-psychiatry services, in The American Psychiatric Publishing Textbook of Consultation-Liaison Psychiatry. Edited by Rundell JR, Wise MG. Washington, DC, American Psychiatric Publishing, 2002, pp 871–888

Kathol R, Saravay SM, Lobo A, et al: Epidemiological trends and costs of fragmentation. Med Clin N Am 90:549–557, 2006

Katon W: The impact of major depression on chronic medical illness. Gen Hosp Psychiatry 18:215–219, 1996

Koenig HG, Kuchibhatla M: Use of health services by hospitalized medically ill depressed elderly patients. Am J Psychiatry 155: 871–877, 1998

Kornfeld DS: Clinical ethics, an important role for the consultation-liaison psychiatrist. Psychosomatics 38:307–309, 1996a

Kornfeld DS: Consultation-liaison psychiatry and the practice of medicine. The Thomas P. Hackett Award lecture given at the 42nd Annual Meeting of the Academy of Psychosomatic Medicine, 1995. Psychosomatics 37:236–248, 1996b

Kornfeld DS: Consultation-liaison psychiatry: contributions to medical practice. Am J Psychiatry 159:1964–1972, 2002

Lavery S, Ravi H, McDaniel W, et al: Linezolid and serotonin syndrome. Psychosomatics 42:432–434, 2001

Levenson JL, Hamer RM, Rossiter LF: Relation of psychopathology in general medical inpatients to use and cost of services. Am J Psychiatry 147:1498–1503, 1990

Levitan SJ, Kornfeld DS: Clinical and cost benefits of liaison psychiatry. Am J Psychiatry 138:790–793, 1981

Lipowski ZJ: Review of consultation psychiatry and psychosomatic medicine, II: clinical aspects. Psychosom Med 29:201–224, 1967

Lipowski ZJ: Consultation-liaison psychiatry: the first half century. Gen Hosp Psychiatry 8:305–315, 1986

Lipowski ZJ: History of consultation-liaison psychiatry, in The American Psychiatric Press Textbook of Consultation-Liaison Psychiatry. Edited by Rundell JR, Wise MG. Washington, DC, American Psychiatric Press, 1996, pp 3–11

Lipsitt DR: Psychosomatic medicine: history of a "new" specialty, in Psychosomatic Medicine. Edited by Blumenfeld M, Strain J. Philadelphia, PA, Lippincott Williams & Wilkins, 2006, pp 3–20

Lurie N, Rank B, Parenti C, et al: How do house officers spend their nights? N Engl J Med 320:1673–1677, 1989

Mendel WM: Psychiatric consultation education—1966. Am J Psychiatry 123:150–155, 1966

Miller WB: Psychiatric consultation, part I: a general systems approach. Int J Psychiatry Med 4:135–145, 1973a

Miller WB: Psychiatric consultation: part II: conceptual and pragmatic issues of formulation. Int J Psychiatry Med 4:251–271, 1973b

Mozian SA, Muskin PR: The difficult patient, in The Approach to the Psychiatric Patient. Edited by Barnhill JW. Washington, DC, American Psychiatric Publishing, 2008, pp 192–196

Muskin PR: The medical hospital, in Psychodynamic Concepts in General Psychiatry. Edited by Schwartz HJ. Washington, DC, American Psychiatric Press, 1995, pp 69–88

Muskin PR, Haase EK: Personality disorders, in Textbook of Primary Care Medicine, 3rd Edition. Noble J, editor in chief. Philadelphia, PA, CV Mosby, 2001, pp 458–464

Muskin PR, Stevenson EM, Levin FR: A multiple diagnostic approach to behavioral symptoms in medically ill patients. Journal of Practical Psychiatry and Behavioral Health 4:356–362, 1998

Noyes R, Wise TN, Hayes JR: Consultation-liaison psychiatrists: how many are there and how are they funded? Psychosomatics 33:128–133, 1992

Owens P, Meyers M, Elixhauser A, et al: Care of adults with mental health and substance abuse disorders in US community hospitals, 2004 (HCUP Fact Book No. 10; AHRQ Publication 07-0008). Rockville, MD, Agency for Healthcare Research and Quality, 2007

Pasnau RO: Ten commandments of medical etiquette for psychiatrists. Psychosomatics 26:128–132, 1985

Popkin MK, Mackensie TB, Callie AL: Improving the effectiveness of psychiatric consultation. Psychosomatics 22:559–563, 1981

Querques J, Stern TA: Approach to consultation psychiatry: assessment strategies, in Massachusetts General Hospital Handbook of General Hospital Psychiatry, 5th Edition. Edited by Stern TA, Fricchione GL, Cassem NH, et al. Philadelphia, PA, CV Mosby, 2004, pp 9–19

Ramchandani D, Lamdan RM, O'Dowd MA, et al: What, why, and how of consultation-liaison psychiatry: an analysis of the consultation process in the 1990s at five urban teaching hospitals. Psychosomatics 38:349–355, 1997

Rosnick L: Use of a long-term inpatient unit as a site for learning psychotherapy. Psychiatric Clinics of North America: Intensive Hospital Treatment 10:309–323, 1987

Rush B: Sixteen Introductory Lectures. Philadelphia, PA, Bradford & Inskeep, 1811

Saravay SM, Lavin M: Psychiatric co-morbidity and length of stay in a general hospital. Psychosomatics 35:233–252, 1994

Saravay SM, Steinberg MD, Weinschel B, et al: Psychological co-morbidity and length of stay in the general hospital. Am J Psychiatry 148:324–329, 1991

Schuster JM: A cost-effective model of consultation-liaison psychiatry. Hosp Community Psychiatry 43:330–332, 1992

Shakin Kunkel EJ, Thompson TL: The process of consultation and organization of a consultation-liaison psychiatry service, in The American Psychiatric Press Textbook of Consultation-Liaison Psychiatry. Edited by Rundell JR, Wise MG. Washington, DC, American Psychiatric Press, 1996, pp 12–23

Smith FA, Querques J, Levenson JL, et al: Psychiatric assessment and consultation, in The American Psychiatric Publishing Textbook of Psychosomatic Medicine. Edited by Levenson JL. Washington, DC, American Psychiatric Publishing, 2005, pp 3–14

Strain JJ, Grossman S: Psychological Care of the Medically Ill. New York, Appleton-Century-Crofts, 1975

Strain JJ, Lyons JS, Hammer JS, et al: Cost offset from a psychiatric consultation-liaison intervention with elderly hip fracture patients. Am J Psychiatry 148:1044–1049, 1991

Unutzer J, Katon W, Callahan CM, et al: Collaborative care management of late-life depression in the primary care setting: a randomized controlled trial. JAMA 288:2836–2845, 2002

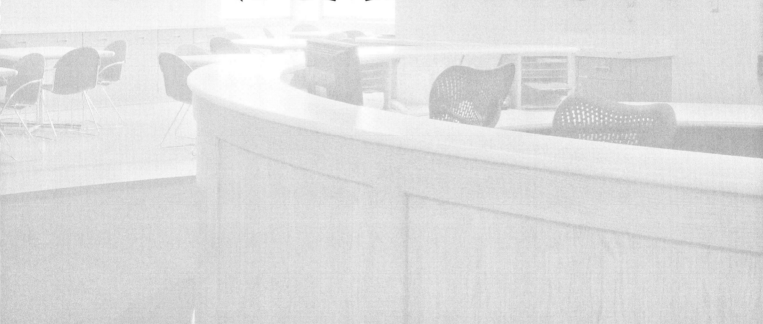

Part II

SPECIAL
CLINICAL ISSUES

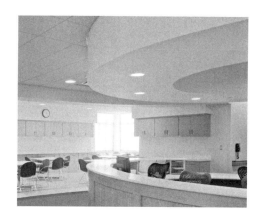

CHAPTER 16

FROM WITHIN

A Consumer Perspective on Psychiatric Hospitals

Lisa J. Halpern, M.P.P.
Howard D. Trachtman, B.S., C.P.S.
Kenneth S. Duckworth, M.D.

The Hospital on the Hill

"Lisa, I think it's time to take you down to the unit," was how the psychiatrist I had been seeing as an outpatient for about 3 months suggested it was time to try hospitalization. The catalyst was my story of being in a local subway station with a date and feeling frozen by fear. I had started weeping but had sucked in my sobs to try to avoid embarrassment. I kept closing my eyes because the lights were flashing too brightly and covering my ears to shut out the squealing noise of antiquated trains—trains that I was convinced had been transported back to 1940s-era Nazi Germany and were going to the concentration camps. I knew that if I got on a red-line train I was going to die. Green—go. Red—Stop! Blood! Die! Over and over again in my head: Red—Die! Die! Die!

My doctor's suggestion to "use the hospital" came across as just that—a suggestion or recommendation of action, rather than a declaration, which I likely would have resisted because of my lack of trust in psychiatric systems. I reasoned that my hospitalization was merely the next hurdle my doctor and I must jump over together to get to a future place that we both saw as worth fighting to reach. The notion of "using the hospital" as a tool means viewing hospitalization as a point along a circular continuum of care, not a nadir of failure like the low rung on a ladder. The concept of vertical versus circular care allowed me to accept the use of hospitalization when needed as an integral part of treatment.

My first hospitalization, on the short-term unit (STU) at a private psychiatric hospital, began with a strip search—a rather frightening introduction, coming with no explanation of what, for example, the searcher was looking for, and thus exacerbating my paranoia. My outpatient psychiatrist was separated from me when I became an inpatient, and there was no time to get to know the doctor assigned to me in the STU. What I did learn of him I didn't like. This new doctor had a very combative, aggressive, curt style—he scared me (not a tough task considering that I believed many people, including my landlord and former classmates, wanted me dead and were actively working to complete that end). When he came by for rounds, he chided me for "not answering his questions promptly" and wondered out loud if my reticence was because "I was biting my tongue until it bleeds." Then he declared, "I have no time for people like you" and left the room. I was so perplexed and offended by this doctor, I was even further frozen into silence and determined (although not quite sure how to go about it) to leave the STU quickly no matter what I had to do, or say, to get out.

Once leaving the STU became my goal, I began to learn a bit about the privilege system that determines where one walks, how often one goes outside, and with what frequency one is checked on. The sum total of all these items sort of equaled how quickly one was discharged, or at least this was how it appeared to me. No clear explanation was available for me to follow, so I tried to figure it out on my own. For example, if you want to get higher privileges on a scale of 1 through 4, you had to go to groups, make an effort to speak up in groups, and make eye contact with staff and other patients at groups. This undertaking can be incredibly difficult, and I remained a "2 w/no s/f" (Level 2, not allowed sharps or flames) for days not because I was violent or uncooperative but because I didn't understand, and no one told me, that one of the main ways to get an increase in privileges was to attend groups.

Beyond group attendance, the primary way to go about increasing hospital inpatient privileges seemed to be to ask the psychiatrist in charge to change them. Looking "normal" seemed to help too. When I was first hospitalized I would wrap towels around my head to try to stop the voices from attacking my brain. To me, placing towels over my head was a harmless way to try to dull the painful thoughts I was hearing, and my outpatient psychiatrist allowed me to place towels over my head for sessions so I could endure visits with him. However, what my private psychiatrist had tolerated ("I would much rather see you in session and have you here even if you want to cover your eyes—at least you're here!"), hospital nurses and mental health workers would not. The staff made it clear, without telling me why, that until the towels came off I would not progress toward my goal of climbing the privilege-level ladder and getting out of the hospital.

Once I figured it out—make eye contact with everyone (no matter how that affects you), go to groups, talk at groups (Say anything! Just talk!), and lose the turban look—I got out of the STU in a couple of days, but found myself rehospitalized in a psychotic disorders unit at the same private hospital within a couple of months. I believe this revolving-door effect occurred because at the STU I concentrated what depleted brain power I had left on getting out of the hospital at any cost, rather than learning how to live a recovered life outside the hospital. I didn't take the hospitalization seriously but saw it as a bunch of hoops to jump through, starting with entry and triumphing with exit. I left the hospital with a medication whose severe side effects I wasn't ready for.

During my admittance to the STU, I was so sick that I believed my family wanted ill for me. I only contacted my parents in California (who took the red-eye immediately to be by my side, meet my doctors, and offer assistance) when hospital employees threatened to contact my parents to tell them that I was in the hospital. I also figured my discharge would come sooner if I could show a good family relationship. Although I didn't trust her and didn't want any human (physical) contact, I assumed staff would be watching my reaction, so I gave my mom a big hug when she arrived. By the time of my second hospitalization, my family had become an integral, omnipresent, positive support in my life and with my illness. During my admittance to the psychotic disorders unit, my mom was with me the entire time—there was no strip search or mention of one—and my goal was to get better, not just get out.

This time when I was admitted as an inpatient, steps were taken to see that my outpatient, regular psychiatrist would remain part of my inpatient team via consultation and daily visits. I don't know whether it was his influence, a difference in approach because it was a longer-term unit, because the doctors on staff were more understanding, or other influences coming together that made the difference, but this time I was a member of the team and was included in discussions about my treatment. I remember sitting in a circle and listening to the lead doctor say, "Clozaril is not an easy medicine to take, but nothing in your life's path has shown us that you choose to take the easy way out, ever." I signed the papers to begin Clozaril that day and left the hospital soon after.

A key factor in why my second hospitalization "stuck" whereas the first made me a "repeat visitor" is the amount of time doctors spent listening to me and trying to determine the difference between natural personality and interwoven illness. This is no small feat when there is an inherent lack of trust. How does one (the doctor) gain the trust of one (the patient) who does not trust? My answer? Time and effort. The doctor or provider needs to put in the time listening to another person's story and find ways to communicate around the obstacles inherent in a brain disorder that scrambles communication, such as schizophrenia.

In my opinion, my two hospitalizations shared certain positive qualities—short stay, goal oriented, clear understanding of purpose, long-term impact (no repeat visits since then). My first hospitalization centered upon the goal of getting me—unmedicated at the time—to take some type of psychotropic medication at a therapeutic level on a regular basis. My second hospitalization focused on taking me off the medications I was on and starting me on Clozaril. "Using the hospital" when needed, as one of many options available within the comprehensive system of psychiatric care, made it possible for me to move forward and focus on living a full life in recovery.

—Lisa J. Halpern

My Experience With Psychiatric Hospitals

Prior to my multiple admissions to psychiatric hospitals, I knew very little about mental health, psychiatric treatment, and what happens in a hospital. My "knowledge" was based on what I had seen on television and in movies such as *One Flew Over the Cuckoo's Nest.* As a young person, I recall being told that a friend of mine had jumped into Niagara Falls, ending his life. This was triggered by a breakup with his girlfriend. At the time I couldn't understand why a person would want to end his life. Now I know.

I have been interested in computers all my life and knew that Massachusetts Institute of Technology (MIT) was the best place for me to learn artificial intelligence and build robots. I became a freshman at MIT right after my sixteenth birthday in 1983. One of my professors told me about visiting an MIT student who was catatonic in a psychiatric unit. I didn't think I would ever be a patient myself.

One day during my freshman year, a friend left a 20-page suicide note in my room. Bewildered, I was advised to see an MIT psychiatrist to get this person help. The psychiatrist thought I also needed help, but I don't recall receiving a diagnosis or any medication being suggested. I do remember being told that if matters got worse I should go to a particular private hospital.

Just before my eighteenth birthday, I was up all night at the MIT Artificial Intelligence Laboratory. I became convinced that artificially intelligent computers were taking over the world and that I needed to flee to my parents in Buffalo. While waiting to change planes, I started thinking that some planes were going to heaven and others were going to hell. I knew I needed to read the Bible. Because I was acting strangely, the police brought me to a crisis center. When the doctor asked me if I heard voices, I answered "yes" because I thought I was just being asked if I could hear people talking. As a result I was placed in four-point leather restraints and injected with Haldol.

My parents flew up in the morning, and I was discharged to their custody. We flew home, but I was still in crisis and immediately walked out of the house, barefoot, looking for a Bible. My parents initially had difficulty having me admitted to a hospital, but once they mentioned that I thought I was Jesus Christ, I was admitted to a short-term unit in a private hospital. Although I spent several weeks there and was pre-

scribed Thorazine, I was told little about my condition. I was not given a diagnosis, received little therapy, and was not told the importance of remaining on medication. I spent most of the time reading and watching television and very little time speaking to mental health workers, nurses, or doctors.

I returned to Boston shortly after my nineteenth birthday, and soon I was again up all night. I actually called 911, and the police brought me to an emergency department. I was placed in four-point restraints and told I was being sent to a private hospital. I felt betrayed when the ambulance brought me to a state hospital. I was assigned a psychiatrist who wore black boots. Coupled with her power over me at the hospital, at times I was convinced she was a Nazi.

I ended up spending 9 months on the admissions unit, a coed floor with three large dormitory-style rooms. Every so often as the male–female balance changed, we would be moved from one room to another. There were only two groups a week: privilege group and group therapy. Initially patients were restricted to the unit, but once a week in the privilege group, you could ask for the next level of freedom. It took quite a while for me to move up the privilege ladder because I was never told how a person graduated to the next level. Several months elapsed before I reached the first level, a staff pass that would, for example, enable me to be on the grounds accompanied by a staff person. The next level, a mutual pass, allowed one patient to take another patient out on the grounds. The third level was being allowed on the grounds by oneself. The final level was being allowed off the grounds. My first time with a mutual privilege level, I went with another patient who disappeared on me. When I returned to the unit, I was informed I had lost all my privileges and would have to start over. This was a major setback to me.

Group therapy met for 1 hour a week. The staff must have liked me, because after a few months I was given my own therapist for an extra hour a week, which I found very helpful. Otherwise, most of my time was wasted playing games and watching television. I really hated not having constructive activities and learning skills to keep me out of the hospital.

Life on the unit was traumatic. One patient kept trying to persuade me to have sexual relations with him. One night the staff announced he had hanged himself on the grounds. Another time, while I was in bed, a patient assaulted me.

There was a hallway of quiet/seclusion rooms where the difficult patients would be placed, some spending most of their time in those rooms. The original idea was that people wouldn't be exposed to too much stimulation while in these rooms, but to me it seemed like punishment, just like being in restraints felt like torture. When I would be sequestered I would frequently push the door open to get fresh air, only to have the door pushed back and locked—locked-door seclusion. Once a week I would be asked to sign the required paperwork for being secluded.

It was never explained to me that if I didn't open the door they would not have locked it and I would have been let out much sooner. Now some state hospitals have consumers whose job it is to debrief all instances of restraint and seclusion and work to prevent future episodes. I wish that had existed back then. I also wonder why, when I was my sickest during those 9 months in the state hospital, restraints were never used, but later, in several private hospitals, I was frequently put into restraints. Only once in the state hospital was I given an injection to calm down. Several friends of mine have stated they received better care in state hospitals than in private facilities.

One lesson I learned at the state hospital was what I now know is called "learned helplessness." When I realized I needed dental care, I went to the hospital dental office, made an appointment, and kept it. When I returned to my unit following the appointment, the staff was angry that I did this on my own.

I formed friendships with some of the people on the unit. We would play games or go for walks together on the campus. Most Fridays we played bingo. I was popular and was elected president of the unit, which perhaps foreshadowed my future role as a leader of the consumer empowerment movement. I organized a car wash at the hospital to raise money for a pizza party.

One day my parents came to take me out on a pass. I became very anxious, acted out, and feared I would lose my opportunity to be with them. However, the doctor gave me some Ativan and allowed me to go off the grounds with them. Her understanding touched me and enhanced my respect for her.

A few months into my state hospitalization, I was told I was being considered for discharge and would move into an adolescent group home. However, a fellow patient convinced me that my medications were bad for me, and I experimented with tonguing (pretending to take them and then throwing them out). This set my treatment back several months. On the day of my discharge I was taken to the Social Security office to apply for disability benefits; soon after, I was required to apply for welfare and Medicaid. The message I received was that I was profoundly disabled and would never be able to work. I also met my new therapist, whom I kept continuously for more than 18 years. I developed a solid rapport with him and can only say good things about not having to continually look for a new therapist.

After discharge, even as I became medication compliant, I continued to require hospitalizations, all of which were in private facilities. Although I was able to maintain a relationship for several years, my housing situation changed a few times, and I felt like ending my life. I went to be evaluated and told the doctor I wanted to kill myself. She noted I didn't have any previous attempts and sent me home. I took a major overdose later that night.

Eventually, after several hospitalizations, I was prescribed clozapine and required no further hospitalizations for 6 years. I also discovered the consumer empowerment movement, which became essential in my recovery. Although I learned much from my peers, actually doing advocacy work was a tremendous boost. I was mentored by many people and discovered I had something to offer by helping other people both individually and systemically.

After those 6 quality years on clozapine, I experimented with functioning without medication, but soon required additional hospitalizations. Seven years ago I resumed clozapine as part of a cocktail of various medications. My outpatient psychiatrist tapered me off the additional medications, and I have remained out of the hospital since then. In 2005 I cofounded the Boston Resource Center, a consumer-run program that connects people with support, information and referral, and vocational opportunities. Last year I completed a training program for peer specialists and passed my written and oral examinations to become a certified peer specialist.

—Howard D. Trachtman

Nothing About Us Without Us

Psychiatric hospitals serve a crucial role in the lives of individuals with psychiatric crises; yet until recently these specialized hospitals rarely involved their patients' experience and feedback in conceptualizing, designing, or improving care. Goal 2 of the President's New Freedom Commission on Mental Health (2003) defines an exemplary mental health system as one in which input and participation from consumers (those who use the mental health system) and family members inform clinical care at all levels of the mental health service system, including psychiatric hospital units. As the culture of welcoming consumer input, evaluation, and design of services continues to take hold, material progress can be made toward the commission's vision.

What's in a Name?

Psychiatric hospitals have unique power dynamics. The power differential between the people holding the keys, issuing orders, and deciding on passes and privileges and the people in a locked ward who may be there against their will is a structural fact of inpatient psychiatric care, and language can reflect this differential. Even words like *patient* or *chronic*, which can be benign to doctors, may be quite charged for people receiving psychiatric services who connect being a "chronic" mental "patient" with very low status or minimal prospects for improvement.

The way we speak about people can reflect the beliefs we have about them on many levels. Referring to people with disabilities by the name of the disability—for example, a schizophrenic, a paraplegic—implies that the disability is their defining characteristic. One remedy for defining people by their illness is the use of the less limiting "person first" language—for example, a *person living with* schizophrenia or *someone with* paraplegia. Accepting that people may call themselves *consumers* or *peers* (our terms for this chapter), *residents* (of a living situation), *members* (of a clubhouse), *survivors* (of perceived abuse in the system), or even *prosumers* (consumers who work professionally in the system) gives a glimpse into the varying ways people think about their relationship to the work of recovery and to the care system. Hope and dignity are key elements of recovery, and language needs to reflect that spirit.

Prior to a few years ago, when the philosophy and ideology of recovery began to weave its way throughout the mental health paradigm, consumers were left to attempt to foster ideas of hope and well-being and recovery in a mental health system that "viewed serious psychiatric disorders as harbingers of doom" (Corrigan and Ralph 2005). Pessimistic views of the course of the conditions in psychiatry, coupled with societal prejudice and language, have historically added to the burden of having a major mental illness. Unlike a shortened length of stay or a crisis in access to inpatients beds, language is fully under the control of those who use it.

Human rights is an all-encompassing category that incorporates basic human rights within the hospital, efforts to minimize restraint and seclusion use, efforts to provide access to outdoors to inpatients, and efforts made to make a psychiatric hospital consumer friendly and treatment focused. Consumers who find themselves in psychiatric hospital environments are at a vulnerable point in their lives, and service design and delivery need to be mindful of this. Although clinical and human needs are usually met in a healthy and dignified environment and lives are saved, the Civil Rights Division of the U.S. Department of Justice, pursuant to the Civil Rights of Institutionalized Persons Act, has recounted horrors of care in their state psychiatric hospital investigations in multiple states. Breakdowns of safety systems, excessive use of restraint and seclusion (e.g., as punishment), abuse, inadequate medical care, and poor environmental conditions are among the most common concerns mentioned in their annual reports. Failures of leadership and funding, variables that are out of the control of consumers, are key elements in the difference between respectful and compassionate or grossly defi-

cient care. Consumers understandably feel safer with guarantees of basic rights and processes to ensure them.

In 1997 Massachusetts' consumer advocates celebrated the Act to Protect Five Fundamental Rights for all persons receiving services from programs or facilities operated by, licensed by, or contracted with the Massachusetts Department of Mental Health. The guaranteed rights include "reasonable access" to a telephone to make and receive confidential calls; the right to send and receive "sealed, unopened, uncensored mail"; the right to receive visitors of one's "own choosing daily and in private, at reasonable times"; the right to a humane environment, including living space that ensures "privacy and security in resting, sleeping, dressing, bathing and personal hygiene, reading, writing, and in toileting"; and the right to access legal representation (Massachusetts General Laws, Chapter 123, Section 23). However, penalties for violating the law were not specified, and many consumers report violations of these basic rights (Rice 2007).

After a 1998 *Hartford Courant* investigative series (Weiss et al. 1998) exposed the large number of deaths nationwide resulting from the misuse of restraint and seclusion, consumer advocates and policy makers combined their efforts to reduce the use of these treatment modalities. Although people vary in their descriptions of their experiences, a range of difficult experiences, including "torture," are described in a National Alliance on Mental Illness (NAMI; 2000) report entitled *Cries of Anguish*. Even patients and staff who witness restraint and seclusion can themselves become traumatized, especially patients who already have a trauma history.

As in other areas, consumers are at the forefront in working to reduce, and even eliminate, restraint and seclusion for inpatients. NAMI's Consumer Council created a Restraint and Seclusion Committee, and consumers are active in each state's Protection and Advocacy for Individuals with Mental Illness Advisory Council, mandated by federal statute to address abuse and neglect as a top priority. Gayle Bluebird, a consumer who is a registered nurse, has championed the conversion of seclusion rooms into comfort or quiet rooms that function as sanctuaries where patients eagerly choose to go to take a break from unit activities (Bluebird 2005). With extensive occupational therapy input, hospitals in many states have designed similar consumer-friendly spaces to help people calm themselves (Champagne 2006).

Access to outdoor space, a right taken for granted in most correctional settings, is a recent addition to basic human rights for inpatients of psychiatric hospitals. Consumers who are denied access to the outdoors report feeling demoralized and contained, which can result in an increase in symptoms, leading in turn to an increased length of stay. Because some hospitals have allowed only smokers the "privilege" of going outside, some individuals have tragically started smoking while an inpatient because it is the only means for them to achieve outdoor access (Mello 2007). Consumers feel that fresh air is good for the body and soul, decreasing depression, stifling aggressiveness, and ultimately leading to better therapeutic results.

Making hospitals more consumer friendly can also improve outcomes. Some suggestions are as simple as having a quiet space for being interviewed at intake. The distress of another patient nearby may be easier for the professional to tune out than the consumer. Also, having a distraught, disoriented person tell his or her story multiple times to multiple people and complete reams of paperwork upon entry is counterproductive. Although printed information is helpful, having a peer orally and visually orient a person to the unit and its rules is far more effective in reducing stress. Psychiatric hospitals might even emulate some practices of general hospitals that strive to attract patients who have a choice about where to go by such small gestures as offering toiletries or care packages to those arriving without luggage or having snacks available between meals.

Most importantly, because hospital care is treatment focused, it is essential to involve patients in their treatment planning. Forming a treatment alliance with shared decision making, while treating patients with respect and courtesy, helps demonstrate that the individual has value. Such valuation should continue through supportive outpatient/transitional care planning to confirm that the hospital has optimism for the patient's future.

Consumer Evaluation of Hospital Services

Consumers of psychiatric services deserve and desire high-quality services to assist them in recovery and in leading meaningful and productive lives. Although many psychiatric institutions have at least one person responsible for quality and/or risk management, the consumer advocacy movement has identified the utilization of consumers themselves as catalysts for system transformation (Substance Abuse and Mental Health Services Administration 2005). Consumer-

controlled entities (organizations whose boards of directors consist of a minimum of 51% consumers and whose employees are primarily people in recovery from mental illness and/or addictions) have formed to monitor and improve the quality of psychiatric services. The organizations, frequently called *Consumer Satisfaction Teams*, are able to be effective by utilizing consumers across the full spectrum of roles: as interviewers, researchers, report writers, and executive directors. The first such team in the United States was created by consumers and family members in Philadelphia, Pennsylvania, in response to the closure of the state-run psychiatric hospital in 1990. They, as well as advocates and the city of Philadelphia, wanted to ensure that not only the needs but also the preferences of people discharged from the hospital be considered in the design and delivery of community services (Pearson et al. 2003).

In Massachusetts, consumer advocates also wanted a greater role in improving the quality of public mental health services. In 1998, the state Division of Medical Assistance created a financial performance incentive for the state managed care carve-out organization to implement a Consumer Satisfaction Team process. The new consumer-run organization (now called Consumer Quality Initiatives) quickly partnered with other organizations to further strengthen the consumer voice in the quality of mental health services in the state (www.cqi-mass.org).

By having consumers interview other consumers face to face with a qualitative and quantitative instrument, valuable and unique data can be collected; respondents can and do reveal information that they would not share with a nonconsumer staff person or on a sterile survey instrument. Because consumers are the most important stakeholders in hospital quality, consumer researchers are best able to identify areas for improvement and advocate for the system transformation that needs to occur. More recently, organizations that started as satisfaction teams have grown to utilize Community-Based Participatory Action Research, deliver white papers on quality improvement, and work on service planning and needs assessment.

Alternatives to Hospitalization

Being proactive about one's life includes preventing hospitalization whenever possible. From their start in the mid-1800s and continuing through the modern movement beginning in the 1940s, consumer-run self-help and advocacy groups have operated outside the formal mental health system and have been a means to avoid hospitalization. In recent decades there has been increasing support and pressure to establish and legitimize consumer-operated settings as either adjuncts or alternatives to traditional, professionally run services as part of the continuum of care offered by public mental health systems. As professionals continue to accept the involvement of consumers, the culture will face significant stresses and outstanding opportunities.

It is estimated that more than 25 million Americans have participated in a mutual-help group at some point over their lifetimes and that groups for individuals with mental illness are the second most frequented type of group; only groups for people with substance abuse troubles have a higher membership (Kessler et al. 1997). Mutual-help groups function according to a belief system that lived experience with mental illness is paramount (Borkman 1990). As a result of the inherent value placed on lived experience and experiential knowledge, mutual-help groups are structured to reflect the assumption that all group participants have something of value to contribute.

Such groups currently offer support to avoid hospitalization in programs such as warm lines and crisis hotlines, peers in the emergency department, personal care assistant services, crisis respite, transitional respite, crisis stabilization units, urgent care walk-in, programs for assertive community treatment teams, and so on. Proactive alternatives like Mary Ellen Copeland's Wellness Recovery Action Plan can often avoid inpatient care and maximize independence for consumers who know their risk factors and supports and have clear communication with their outpatient caregivers. Advance directives for care follow the same guidelines.

Conclusion

Hospitals that rely solely on the medical model tend to focus primarily on pathology and disease (Mead et al. 2001) and to define *recovery* as a set of predetermined outcomes that emphasize symptom elimination and a return to premorbid functioning. This model of illness can be defeatist because it undermines hope, which has been described by advocates and consumer leaders as "one of the cornerstones of recovery" (Deegan 1988). Consumers of mental health services face many challenges in terms of social attitudes, low social status, and prejudice, yet attitudes are improving

and so is knowledge that anyone can have a psychiatric illness at any time in their lives. The challenge for us all is to integrate the best of the consumer movement into the medical service model. The resulting synthesis can continue to improve the quality and experience of care at psychiatric hospitals.

References

Bluebird G: Comfort rooms: reducing the need for seclusion and restraint. Residential Group Care Quarterly 5(4):5–6, 2005 (Available at: http://www.cwla.org/programs/groupcare/rgcqspring2005.pdf)

Borkman TJ: Experiential, professional and lay frames of reference, in Working With Self-Help. Edited by Powell TJ. Silver Spring, MD, National Association of Social Workers Press, 1990, pp 3–30

Champagne T: Creating sensory rooms: environmental enhancements for acute inpatient mental health settings. Mental Health Special Interest Section Quarterly 29:1–4, 2006

Corrigan RW, Ralph RO: Introduction: recovery as consumer vision and research paradigm, in Recovery in Mental Illness: Broadening Our Understanding of Wellness. Edited by Corrigan RW, Ralph RO. Washington, DC, American Psychological Association, 2005, p 4

Deegan PE: Recovery: the lived experience of rehabilitation. Psychiatr Rehabil J 11:11–19, 1988

Kessler RC, Mickelson KD, Zhao S: Patterns and correlates of self-help group membership in the United States. Soc Policy 27(3):27–46, 1997

Massachusetts General Laws, Chapter 123, Section 23 (Rights of persons receiving services from programs or facilities of department of mental health)

Mead S, Hilton D, Curtis L: Peer support: a theoretical perspective. Psychiatr Rehabil J 25:134–141, 2001

Mello F: Right to fresh air sought for patients. Boston Globe, July 8, 2007 (Available at: http://www.m-power.org/right_to_fresh_air_sought_for_patients)

National Alliance on Mental Illness: Cries of Anguish: A Summary of Reports of Restraint & Seclusion Abuse Received Since the October 1998 Investigation by *The Hartford Courant* (pamphlet). Arlington, VA, National Alliance on Mental Illness, 2000

Pearson S, Sabin J, Emanuel E: No Margin, No Mission: Health Care Organizations and the Quest for Ethical Excellence. Oxford, England, Oxford University Press, 2003

President's New Freedom Commission on Mental Health: Achieving the Promise: Transforming Mental Health Care in America. Final Report (DHHS Publ No SMA-03-3832). Rockville, MD, U.S. Department of Health and Human Services, 2003

Rice P: Incommunicado: mental health wards restrict access to email. Spare Change News, February 5, 2007 (Available at: http://www.m-power.org/mental_health_wards_restrict_access_to_email)

Substance Abuse and Mental Health Services Administration: Consumer-Directed Transformation to a Recovery-Based Mental Health System (NMH05-0193). Rockville, MD, Substance Abuse and Mental Health Services Administration, 2005

Weiss EM, Altimari D, Blint DF, et al: Deadly restraint: a nationwide pattern of death. The Harford Courant, October 11–15, 1998, p 1

CHAPTER 17

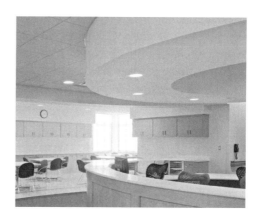

WORKING WITH FAMILIES

Lisa B. Dixon, M.D., M.P.H.
Aaron B. Murray-Swank, Ph.D.
Bette M. Stewart, B.S.

Family members play an integral role in the lives of most persons with serious mental illness (SMI), and the importance of family involvement in the treatment of these persons is widely recognized. The recent President's New Freedom Commission on Mental Health (2003) report calls for a care system that is "consumer and family centered." Moreover, in a large number of randomized trials, family psychoeducation programs have demonstrated robust effects in reducing patients' rates of relapse (Murray-Swank and Dixon 2004). Best-practice treatment guidelines of the American Psychiatric Association (2004) and other professional organizations strongly recommend family involvement in treatment as a critical element of quality care for persons with SMI.

The inpatient phase of care may be an especially critical time to involve family members in the treatment process. During acute periods of illness and crisis, family members often "ramp up" the level of involvement they have with the patient. During these times, family members may provide emotional support and practical assistance (e.g., housing, transporta-

tion) and are often involved in arranging for the patient to go to the hospital. During the hospitalization, family members may frequently visit the patient and may be an integral part of the patient's support system on discharge.

In this chapter, we first focus on common themes and issues for clinicians to appreciate in working with families in the inpatient setting. Next, we discuss a number of potentially disruptive issues and challenges that clinicians may encounter in their efforts to involve patients' families in the treatment process. This chapter is focused on families of competent adults who are hospitalized. The issues involved in working with family members of child patients, of geriatric patients who have substituted consent, and of other specialized patient groups may differ. We also want to emphasize that we write this chapter as family members of people living with mental illness in addition to our professional roles as mental health clinicians and researchers who focus on the delivery of services for patients with SMIs—such as schizophrenia, schizoaffective disorder, bipolar disorder, and depression—and their families. In this chapter, we offer our perspectives grounded in our experience as spouses, siblings, parents, and children of people with mental illness. By considering this topic from the dual vantage points of both family members and professionals, we hope to provide a useful road map to navigate clinicians' work with families.

Working With Families in Inpatient Settings: Common Themes and Issues in the Family Experience of Mental Illness

The family experience of mental illness varies substantially depending on the family members' relationship to the patient (e.g., parent, spouse, sibling) as well as the patient's diagnosis and phase of illness. However, we would like to highlight several typical themes in the family experience among families who experience the psychiatric illness and hospitalization of a loved one. In this section, we discuss four common themes that are critical to appreciate for clinicians who work with families in the inpatient setting.

Range of Emotional Responses

As family members, we have experienced the "roller coaster" of emotional responses that accompany an acute phase of illness requiring inpatient treatment. Family members often experience profound fear, shock, and trauma related to their relatives' illness and its impact on family life. When their loved one has become ill and requires hospitalization, this is likely to be a time of instability and chaos in the life of the family. Coupled with this tremendous stress, family members may feel a sense of relief that their loved one has "landed somewhere" with admission to the hospital.

When interviewing family members, clinicians should be attuned to their emotional state and make active efforts to acknowledge and normalize what they might be feeling. Techniques such as reflection (e.g., "It sounds like you are feeling frustrated") and summarizing statements can help family members feel heard and understood. Another way for a clinician to communicate this message could be to say things such as "I realize that you have really been through a lot during this time—you may be feeling anxious, worried, overwhelmed, angry, or maybe a combination of many different feelings—this is certainly understandable, normal, and to be expected as you are dealing with everything going on with [patient's name]."

It is also important to realize the impact on family members of visiting a loved one on an inpatient psychiatric unit. One of us recalled first seeing our loved one hospitalized: "I burst into tears…it was worse than I could have imagined." This initial impact can be particularly jarring for family members who have been involved in the involuntary commitment of their loved one. Confronted with the realities of a locked inpatient unit, the family member can be filled with guilt and second thoughts about "Did I do the right thing?" Guilty feelings can also arise from worries family members often have about whether they did "something wrong" to cause the illness, or worries that they passed on "bad genes" to their child. A reassuring comment at the right moment can be greatly comforting, by showing understanding of the family's concerns (e.g., "naturally it can be disturbing to see [name] in the hospital"); reassuring them that hospitalization was the right course (e.g., "I just want to emphasize that you really did the right thing bringing [name] into the hospital, even though he didn't want to come in. I think you might have saved his life. It took real courage and love to do what you did. He is very lucky he has you, and that you were there to do what needed to be done to help him."); and emphasizing that their loved one will receive adequate care and attention (e.g., "we are going to do everything we can to help him get better").

We also have found it useful to have an awareness of the setting's unique impact on all family members as they become familiar with the unit. For instance, it can be helpful to inquire about family members' experiences when first meeting them in the inpatient context. A clinician might say something such as, "Thanks so much for making the time to meet with me today. We believe that your participation in the treatment process is really important. I'm wondering if you have had the opportunity to meet with inpatient staff when [name] has been hospitalized in the past." It also can be helpful to learn what the family's experience has been like in the past, to provide a sense of how they may be experiencing the current inpatient setting. For example, the clinician might say, "I'm also wondering if you have had any particularly good or particularly bad experiences with inpatient programs before." This can also be a point at which the clinician can orient the family to the unit and the hospital. Such an orientation and introduction can put family members at ease and help the clinician understand "where the family is at" as they are entering the often unfamiliar (and, at times, chaotic and frightening) world of inpatient psychiatric treatment.

Intense Unmet Needs for Information

Research has consistently documented that family members of people with SMI report strong, and often unmet, needs for information and support related to their loved one's psychiatric disorder (Tessler and Gamache 2000). In our experience as family members, we have felt the desperation of not knowing "where to turn" in coping with the mental illness of our loved ones. A lack of knowledge, combined with societal stigma regarding psychiatric disorders, often leaves family members feeling profoundly isolated in dealing with the many challenges they face related to their loved one's disorders.

It is important for clinicians to keep in mind that family members may have varying levels of knowledge about mental illness. Some families may have a great deal of information about psychiatric disorders, whereas others may have little knowledge. It is important, therefore, to avoid making assumptions about family knowledge (or to assume a lack of knowledge). At this point, in building an alliance with families, we have found it helpful to meet the family "where they are" by first supporting the family's desire to be involved and then asking some introductory questions to assess family members' understanding of their relative's problems. For example, one could begin by saying, "Thanks for meeting with me today about [name's] treatment. To begin, it would be helpful to get your thoughts about the problems that [name] is seeking treatment for. If it is OK with you, I would like to ask you a couple questions to get your input and learn about your understanding of things. Can you tell me a little bit about what you think about [name's] problems?" Follow-up inquiries can include more focused questions such as, "What do you think has caused [name] to have these problems?"; "Has anybody ever given you a diagnosis for [name's] problems?" (if they have been given a diagnosis, it is useful to follow up with, "What is your understanding of what that diagnosis means?"); "Are there things that make things better for [name]?"; and "Are there things that make things worse?"

Questions such as these can help the clinician learn about family members' views of their relative's psychiatric problems. In addition, such questions can provide useful information to inform the patient's treatment. For example, family members often have valuable observations about prodromal symptoms that signal a risk for relapse in the patient. Note that these inquiries avoid using the terms *illness, disorder*, or other psychi-atric terminology. It is best to avoid using this language and to hold off on offering educational information until the interviewer has a good understanding of the family members' views of the patient's problems.

Varying (and Sometimes Unrealistic) Expectations

Families may have a wide variety of expectations of hospitalization and treatment. Particularly in the initial years of illness, family members may have unrealistic expectations that hospitalization will "fix" the problem and return their loved one back to normal on discharge. It is often frustrating for clinicians to encounter such beliefs, and we have certainly felt these frustrations when working with families in our professional roles. At the same time, it is critical to realize that families' unrealistic expectations are typically not rooted in a willful "denial" of their loved one's illness. Instead, families' beliefs often reflect a lack of information coupled with an emotional coping process of trying to come to terms with the painful reality of their relative's illness.

In addressing families' expectations, it can be helpful to provide an orientation to the current context of inpatient care at some point during the family interview. The following is an example of how a clinician may explain the current situation:

> "It is important for you to know what we do here on the inpatient unit, and the role that we play in [name's] treatment. Typically, the purpose of hospitalization is to help get people through a crisis when their symptoms get worse, to provide an environment to ensure their safety, and to make sure they are linked up with outpatient care as they are discharged. Nowadays, extended periods of hospitalization are pretty unusual for people with mental illness. Instead, the emphasis is more focused on helping people get back to the community when they are safe and able to return to their living environment. I know this can be difficult for family members, who sometimes experience a sense of relief when their loved ones are hospitalized. It can be frustrating for all of us to deal with the limits of what we can accomplish while [name] is in treatment here. However, we do hope that we can work with you as we help [name] get her illness more under control. We also hope to address your needs for information about [name's] illness and treatment and her plan for care while she is hospitalized here."

This may also serve as a point of entry to discuss sources of support for family members, including professional family services as well as other education programs and avenues of support. For example, some inpatient units have educational family programs that provide a forum for family members to learn about their loved one's illness. Community resources, such as family education programs offered by the National Alliance on Mental Illness, can offer another place to refer families for education and support. As a practical matter, we have found it helpful for staff who work with families to have a current, well-organized repository of information about mental illness and such resources so that information can be provided rapidly and smoothly to families.

Differing Family Organization and Member Roles

It is important for clinicians who work with families to recognize ways in which families are organized and the roles that different family members of the patient may play. One common theme is that one family member may be the designated "spokesperson" for the family when the patient is hospitalized. It is critical to take the time to make a positive bond with this spokesperson, because his or her translations of your message may be the only information from which the family makes its impression of the care. Also, it is important to appreciate that the patient's illness often prompts a reshuffling of roles in the family.

Moreover, as time passes, there may be generational transitions, such that siblings or other family members may assume a more active role as the patient's parents age. The key point for clinicians is to assess and be sensitive to who in the family are the central figures in the life of the patient. For example, interviewers may inquire, "Who is usually involved in helping [name] when he has difficulties?" In addition to appreciating these common themes in the family experience, it is important to acknowledge and address potentially disruptive issues and barriers to working with families in the inpatient settings.

Potential Barriers and Challenges for Clinicians Working With Families in the Inpatient Setting

In this next section, we describe common barriers and obstacles that clinicians encounter in working with families and offer strategies for clinicians to overcome these challenges and establish an effective working alliance with family members. In general, these challenges can be broken down into clinician-level barriers (e.g., lack of time, confidentiality issues), patients'

concerns about involving their family in their treatment, and family-level barriers (i.e., difficulty engaging families and dealing with differences of opinion between family members and clinicians).

Clinician-Level Barriers: Time Limitations and Confidentiality

Contact between clinicians and families may occur in a variety of ways in the inpatient context. Family meetings may be planned during the course of hospitalization. We have often found that contact with families happens through a variety of more informal avenues: during family visits to the patient, family phone calls to the unit, and phone calls from the treatment team to the family. In this section we examine two areas that sometimes can create stress between staff and family: 1) time and 2) confidentiality.

For clinicians, the first difficulty is time—not enough of it. In a common scenario, family members may visit and request an unplanned meeting with their loved one's physician or other staff on the unit. Frequently, it is not possible for staff to "drop everything" and make time for such a meeting. However, in building an alliance with families, we believe that it is critical to communicate the message that family input and involvement in treatment is valued by the clinical team. As family members, we have found it frustrating to be "brushed off" by clinical staff completing paperwork or attending to other duties on the unit. Thus we believe that it is important for staff to be attentive to families, within the context of their limited time and other demands. For example, a busy psychiatrist with only 10 minutes to meet with a visiting family could explain that their input is valuable and that talking with them is important, but that he or she has limited time at the moment, for example, "I only have 10 minutes right now, so let's set priorities in how we might use our time. Perhaps you could tell me about your main questions and concerns, and we can come up with a plan to make sure you are included in the treatment process while [name] is being treated here."

Issues of confidentiality can pose particular challenges to clinicians in working with families in the inpatient setting. Professional ethics and organizational policies appropriately require clinicians to obtain the consent of patients before releasing specific information about their treatment to family members (although there can be specific exceptions when safety issues, such as suicide and homicide, are active). This consent is typically documented in a written "release of information" form. Marsh (1998) provided useful guidelines for organizational policy and clinical practice concerning issues of confidentiality, designing appropriate forms, and working with families of patients with SMI.

Perhaps one of the most difficult and common scenarios is when a family member contacts clinicians asking for information about the patient's treatment, and the patient has not provided permission to release information to family. In such situations, we feel it is important for clinicians to first reinforce the family members' interest in the patient's treatment and to recognize their effort to make contact; for example, "I am so glad that you called, and that you are interested in learning more about [name's] treatment here."

Next, the clinician should provide a straightforward explanation to the family member regarding the relevant confidentiality issues; for example, "As you probably know, medical information is private and protected. Therefore, I can't share any specific information about [name's] treatment at this time without her permission. I know it's hard for family members in these kinds of situations; it is difficult for us, too, because we really value the opportunity to include patients' families as part of the treatment whenever we can. What I can do is talk with [name] the next chance that I get to try to get her permission to talk with you more about her treatment."

It can then be helpful to ask the family member about his or her needs and offer information that *can* be shared, such as answering general questions about psychiatric illness, treatment programs, and resources for family members. For example, "Although I can't share specific information about [name's] treatment, I would be happy to answer more general questions you might have at this time. Do you have any general questions about our unit, or about psychiatric illness, that I might be able to help with?" Some types of information that can be helpful for families include a description of the inpatient unit, other treatment resources in the community, programs to support family members of people with mental illness, and general information about psychiatric illness and treatment. Written materials can also be sent to family members to provide them with this type of information (e.g., brochures or booklets about mental illness, Internet-based information, flyers about specific programs).

Patients' Concerns About Involving Family Members in Their Treatment

To initiate contact with families, it is necessary to ask the patient to identify members of his or her family and to obtain the patient's permission to speak with them. Although the primary focus of this chapter is on working with families, this work will be brief or nonexistent unless the clinician has done a good job of talking with the patient about involving his or her family members in the treatment process. Furthermore, the involvement of family in treatment should be guided by patient's preferences and views about his or her family and the potential role they may play in the treatment process. Consequently, we would like to devote attention to the issue of talking with patients about involving their family in their treatment.

Patients may have a wide range of family experiences and preferences in regard to family involvement in their mental health care. As an initial starting point, it is important to assess who the patient considers to be their "family support system" and what role these individuals may play in helping them manage their psychiatric disorder (if any), for example, "I would like to ask you some questions to better understand your family relationships and support system. Do you have people you would consider to be your family or 'like family' to you? Who would those people be for you?"

For many patients, significant "family" and potential allies in treatment may include members of the support network who are not relatives (e.g., friend, pastor, 12-Step group sponsor). After identifying the key members of the support network, it is helpful to learn about the patient's level of contact with these individuals, for example, does the patient live with a family member? If not, how close do family members live? How often does the patient talk, e-mail, or get together with family members? Next, it is important to understand the role that these individuals play in supporting the patient, including any involvement in their mental health treatment, for example, "So, you have said that you are closest to your two brothers, whom you get together with every couple of weeks. I'm wondering if your brothers have been supportive as you have been dealing with your mental illness?"

Patients may have a variety of experiences with family in relation to their illness. Interviewers should use techniques such as summaries and reflections to gain an understanding of the patient's experience and help him or her feel supported. Finally, if it not yet known, the interviewer can assess the degree to which family has been involved in the patient's mental health treatment in the past and the patient's preferences with regard to involving family at this time. For example,

1. "Have your brothers been involved in your mental health treatment by coming in to meet with your doctor(s)?"

2. "Have they ever attended any kind of educational programs or groups?"
3. "Would you like to have your brothers involved in your mental health treatment?"
4. "What might be the possible benefits?"
5. "What, if any, are your concerns about having them involved?"

Overall, the goals of this discussion are to help the patient identify family members who could be allies in his or her treatment, consider the potential advantages of family involvement in treatment, and identify concerns the patient might have about family participation.

In some instances, the patient may be ambivalent about involving the family. This is understandable, given the complexity of family relationships and the possibility of the presence of abusive family members, as well as the personal nature of mental health treatment. When patients experience mixed feelings about involving family in their mental health care, the primary task of the clinician is to help them explore the potential value of family involvement and to make informed choices, considering the potential advantages and disadvantages of family involvement in care. At times, the patient may refuse family involvement, even when the clinical team feels that such involvement would be in his or her best interest. In these situations it is important for the clinician to revisit the issue during the course of treatment, especially if the patient was acutely ill or in a state of crisis when first asked about involving the family.

It is always a good practice to talk with patients and obtain their consent before speaking with their family. However, there are special situations in which safety or other imminent concerns may create the need to speak with family members without the consent of the patient. In these cases, the appropriate practice *may* be to involve family members in the treatment even if the patient has not consented to such involvement. Clinicians should know and follow their relevant local rules and policies in such cases, adhere to principles of good clinical practice, and always try to work as collaboratively with the patient as possible in such circumstances.

At times, the patient's unwillingness to involve family in treatment may be due to acute symptoms that he or she is experiencing, such as active psychotic symptoms, withdrawal, or disorganization. In these situations, we have found that the family may be a particularly valuable source of information and can often provide useful guidance to the clinical team about how to effectively interact with the patient. Thus special effort is often warranted to get the family involved.

When encountering this type of resistance, clinicians should use a range of clinical skills to effectively negotiate issues of family involvement. Sometimes, certain members of the clinical team may be more connected with the patient and may be more likely to get them to agree to family involvement. It is often helpful to remember that involving the family is rarely an "all or none" proposition. It can be useful to present a range of options and to encourage choices with regard to how the family can be involved. It is also important to carefully consider all potential family members in the patient's support system (as well as other people who are "like family" to the patient). Many patients may be hesitant to involve certain family members in their treatment but very willing to allow others to be involved.

Even in cases in which patients are interested in their family being involved, considerable challenges can arise in engaging and working with families. In the next section, we focus on two common challenges—difficulties initiating work with family members and addressing situations in which the family has differences of opinion with the clinical team. For a more detailed discussion of clinical intervention with families of persons with SMI (e.g., "family psychoeducation"), see McFarlane (2002), Anderson et al. (1986), and Mueser and Glynn (1999). These excellent treatment manuals provide a detailed description of strategies to initiate work with patients' families as well as evidence-based models to provide ongoing therapeutic intervention.

Family-Level Barriers: Difficulties With Engagement and Differences of Opinion With Family Members

Engaging families as allies in the treatment process can be a challenge. It is important to recognize that family members may have reservations about meeting with their loved one's mental health clinicians or participating in family services. For example, family members may be concerned about intruding on their relative's privacy or may be worried that such participation will add additional caregiving demands. Practical barriers, such as limited time, child care needs, and lack of transportation, may also prevent family members from participating in services. Unfortunately, some family members may have past negative experiences with the mental health system or "family therapy," given prior outdated theories that emphasized the family environment as a causative influence on mental disorders (e.g., "the schizophrenogenic mother").

In this regard, clinicians should appropriately communicate the message that the illness is not the family's fault and provide educational information about what is known about the etiology of psychiatric disorders. For example, when given the opportunity, a clinician can explain thus:

> "Relatives often have questions about why their loved one developed schizophrenia. Although the causes are not completely understood, we know that genetics play a big part in determining who is most likely to develop schizophrenia. Also, we know that stressful life events play a role in triggering episodes of the illness. Research has shown that schizophrenia is an illness of the brain. In other words, the symptoms of the illness are caused when certain areas of the brain are not functioning properly, and the chemicals that the brain uses to communicate are out of balance. I want to emphasize that schizophrenia is not caused by parenting or family behaviors. In fact, some of the most loving parents I have ever met have had children who go on to develop schizophrenia. On the other hand, we do know that families can play an important role in helping their loved ones manage and cope with this difficult illness."

To engage families, clinicians must communicate the value of family involvement to both patients and their relatives. Shea (1998) described a variety of interviewing techniques that can help address the underlying fears family members may bring to the initial meeting. In one technique, the clinician openly acknowledges the immense value of the family member's firsthand longitudinal knowledge of both the patient and the patient's care to date; for example, "One of the things I want to emphasize early on is how important your input and background information are in our helping [name]. There is no one in the world who knows [him/her] better than you. We are dependent on your input. I also really want to know what you think has worked and what you think hasn't."

In their discussion of how to best engage families, Mueser and Glynn (1999) offered three useful strategies that clinicians can use to enhance engagement: 1) letting family know they are not alone, 2) providing support and allowing relatives to vent, and 3) instilling hope for change. In addition to these strategies for interacting with family members, persistence and flexibility are important ingredients in the effort to engage family members as allies in treatment.

Perhaps one of the most challenging scenarios for clinicians is when the family has views that are in direct contrast to the current biopsychosocial under-

standing of psychiatric disorders. For example, family members may believe that the patient just needs to pull him- or herself "up by the bootstraps" in dealing with his or her problems, believing that psychiatric medications are not needed. In these types of situations, it is helpful to attentively listen and understand the family members' perspectives. To the extent that it is appropriate, it is useful to first validate the family member's concerns or points of view. However, the clinician should follow with respectful and culturally appropriate educational information. If the family member opposes medication and believes that the patient just needs to try harder, the clinician can acknowledge this perspective, for example, "I agree that it's almost always true that people do better if they try harder and believe they can be successful. So, it would be really great if [name] could try harder at cleaning up around the house. But one of the things we are learning about the illness of schizophrenia is that chemical changes in the brain change a person's ability to plan and be organized. It can also reduce a person's ability to feel satisfied and proud of completing a task. All of these problems limit someone's ability to pull themselves up."

With regard to medication, an example dialogue may go as follows:

> *Clinician:* I completely understand your hesitation about medication. Can you help me further understand what your concerns are about [name] taking the medicine?
>
> *Family member:* Well, every time he comes in, it seems like they add more medicines for him to take! And the more medicines you take, the more problems you get—and I don't see any of them helping.
>
> *Clinician:* I'm glad you raise these questions about the medicines he is on, and how they might be affecting him. Let me also say that I know it's frustrating to see such limited progress—I wish we had more effective ways to help people get better quicker. Let's talk more about the role that medications might play in helping [name] at this time. The overall goal of the medications is to help reduce the symptoms that are part of schizophrenia—things like developing unusual beliefs, not making sense, hearing voices. When he gets sick, these are the kind of symptoms that get worse for him.
>
> *Family member:* Yeah, he acts pretty crazy sometimes.
>
> *Clinician:* For most people, the medicines can help control these kinds of symptoms. Although they won't make everything better, controlling these kinds of symptoms is an important first step. You also raised a concern about the number of medicines he is on and the possible side effects they might have. Let me tell you a little bit about each

of his medications, and the possible side effects to watch out for. *[Clinician provides appropriate information about specific medications.]* I'm so glad that you raised these questions—things usually work best when we can all work together—[name], you, and I—to find the medicines that work best for him and have the fewest negative side effects.

Conclusion

In summary, effectively working with families requires a cross between the clinical skills required for working with patients and the communication skills necessary for interacting effectively with colleagues. In many ways, clinicians are best viewed as consultants to family members, who are often faced with multiple stresses and challenges and can benefit tremendously from practical information, guidance, and support. By establishing an effective working alliance with patients' family members during inpatient hospitalization, clinicians can substantially improve the quality of care, enhance treatment outcomes following hospital discharge, and improve quality of life for both patients and their family members.

References

American Psychiatric Association: Practice Guideline for the Treatment of Patients With Schizophrenia, 2nd Edition. Washington, DC, American Psychiatric Publishing, 2004

Anderson CM, Reiss DJ, Hogarty GE: Schizophrenia and the Family. New York, Guilford, 1986

Marsh D: Serious Mental Illness and the Family: The Practitioner's Guide. New York, Wiley, 1998

McFarlane WR: Multifamily Groups in the Treatment of Severe Psychiatric Disorders. New York, Guilford, 2002

Mueser KT, Glynn SM: Behavioral Family Therapy for Psychiatric Disorders, 2nd Edition. Oakland, CA, New Harbinger Publications, 1999

Murray-Swank AB, Dixon LB: Family Psychoeducation as an evidence-based practice. CNS Spectr 9:905–912, 2004

President's New Freedom Commission on Mental Health: Achieving the Promise: Transforming Mental Health Care in America (DHHS Publication No. SMA-03-3832). Rockville, MD, U.S. Department of Health and Human Services, 2003

Shea SC: Psychiatric Interviewing: The Art of Understanding, 2nd Edition. Philadelphia, PA, WB Saunders, 1998

Tessler R, Gamache G: Family Experiences With Mental Illness. Westport, CT, Auburn House, 2000

CHAPTER 18

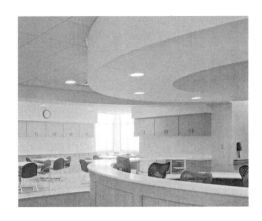

IMPROVING SAFETY IN MENTAL HEALTH TREATMENT SETTINGS

Preventing Conflict, Violence, and Use of Seclusion and Restraint

Kevin Ann Huckshorn, R.N., M.S.N., C.A.P., I.C.A.D.C.
Janice L. LeBel, Ph.D.

Violence in Mental Health Settings: Issues and Costs

Violence in mental health settings has a significant impact on quality of care, the safety of service users and staff, staff morale, and staff retention (Joint Commission on Accreditation of Healthcare Organizations 2002; Owen et al. 1998). Research supports the growing acknowledgment that violent incidents are often preceded by behavioral signs but that these signs are often difficult for untrained staff to note (Duxbury 2002). Owen et al. (1998) identified the need to combine evidence on patient propensity (individual characteristics) for violence with environmental triggers in order to prevent conflict and aggression in inpatient settings, with a focus on improving safety for all.

Seclusion is defined as "the involuntary confinement of a person in a room where they are physically prevented from leaving or think they are" (National Executive Training Institute 2007). *Physical restraint* is defined as a "manual method or mechanical device, material, or equipment attached or adjacent to the patient's body that he or she cannot easily remove that restricts the patient's freedom or normal access to one's body" (National Executive Training Institute 2007).

Seclusion and restraint are used in mental health settings to "manage" aggressive behaviors and have been the object of increased interest, oversight, and regulatory attention by legislators and policy makers since 1998 (Substance Abuse and Mental Health Services Administration 2004; U.S. General Accounting Office 1999). This interest appears to be due to increasing awareness of the short- and long-term physical and emotional consequences of these procedures on both patients and staff (Honberg and Miller 2003).

The Hartford Courant Series

In 1998, The Hartford Courant, a newspaper in Connecticut, released a series of reports titled "Deadly Restraint: A Nationwide Pattern of Death" (Weiss et al. 1998). Driven by the tragic death of an 11-year-old boy, this investigative series cataloged the largely unregulated and unreported deleterious effects of seclusion and restraint on children and adults (Busch and Shore 2000). These publications sent tremendous reverberations throughout the mental health system in the United States (National Association of State Mental Health Program Directors 1999a, 1999b, 2001; U.S. General Accounting Office 1999).

The investigative team (Weiss et al. 1998) interviewed health care officials, federal and state regulatory agencies, consumers, family members, advocacy organizations, and other stakeholders to piece together a picture of violence and the use of seclusion and restraint in mental health and intellectual disability care settings. The reporters canvassed 50 states and the District of Columbia regarding the propensity of violence and the use of seclusion and restraint. From 1988 to 1998, 142 deaths were attributed to restraint or seclusion. Harvard University's Center for Risk Analysis reviewed these findings and estimated that 50–150 deaths occur annually as a result of these practices.

The Courant noted that seclusion and restraint–related deaths were occurring in a variety of venues, including hospitals, residential facilities, group homes, and other types of inpatient settings. These reports revealed the disproportionate number of deaths of children for merely refusing to obey staff orders, such as to move to another seat or to give up a contraband family photograph (Weiss et al. 1998). Finally, this series detailed the deaths of a medically ill woman after 558 hours of restraint, a 15-year-old girl who used a pencil to threaten staff, and 33 others who died by asphyxiation after being restrained face down (U.S. General Accounting Office 1999).

Most troubling were the lack of formalized reporting of seclusion and restraint use, the lack of standardized federal regulations guiding practice, the lack of a national database recording serious injuries and deaths, and the lack of accountability for use, injuries, or deaths in health provider organizations (Lieberman et al. 1999). The Hartford Courant's findings were subsequently substantiated and expanded in a Congress-commissioned study on seclusion and restraint use by the U.S. General Accounting Office (1999).

Consequences of Seclusion and Restraint Use

When conflict leads to violence and seclusion or restraint, the result can be physical and emotional injury to all parties (Robins et al. 2005; U.S. General Accounting Office 1999). Restraint interventions alone are estimated to cause up to 1,240 deaths or serious injuries among service users each year in the United States, according to the Joint Commission (Joint Commission on Accreditation of Healthcare Organizations 2005). The incidence of staff injury has been less studied, but one survey, conducted in three states, reported 26 injuries for every 100 mental health technicians (Love and Hunter 1996). This reported injury rate surpassed those found in the lumber, construction, and mining industries and highlighted the safety problems in inpatient mental health environments (Love and Hunter 1996). The legal consequences of inappropriate physical containment have led to increasingly frequent court findings of civil damages, administrative sanctions, and criminal prosecution (Haimowitz et al. 2006). Seclusion and restraint procedures are believed to be high risk and potentially dangerous for both clients and staff and have resulted in federal, state, and legal mandates to significantly reduce or eliminate use (Centers for Medicare and Medicaid Services 2006; Health Care Finance Administration 1999, 2001; Substance Abuse and Mental Health Services Administration 2004).

Factors in Conflict and Violence Causality

National and international literature reviews have identified the inconsistent and often idiosyncratic decisions that are frequently present when seclusion and restraint are used (Busch and Shore 2000; Duxbury 2002; Hinsby and Baker 2004; Smith et al. 2005). These research studies suggest that cultural and facility-specific biases affect the decision to use seclusion and restraint. Patient characteristics such as gender, race, age, staff perceptions, and administrative attitudes inform these practice choices and are often valued as more important variables than other factors, such as understanding actual antecedents to conflict (Busch and Shore 2000; Legris et al. 1999). Current research demonstrates that conflict and violence causality goes beyond the traditional focus on patient characteristics and that conflict and violence frequently emerge as a result of environmental factors such as staff attitudes and facility cultures (Duxbury 2002; Hinsby and Baker 2004).

It is important that medical leaders understand the internal and external factors that may contribute to conflict and violence. These include patient factors such as having a history of violence and/or being in seclusion or restraint in the past as well as environmental and agency norms (Okin 1985; Ray and Rappaport 1995). It is telling that several studies have found very dissimilar practices in very similar settings (LeBel et al. 2004; Steinert and Needham 2007).

Similarly, it is imperative that leadership appreciates the tangible impact of violence in health care settings. The use of seclusion and restraint derails treatment and day-to-day unit operations. These violent episodes translate into significant disruptions, staff time away from service users, longer lengths of stay, higher staffing costs, greater staff turnover, and absenteeism (LeBel and Goldstein 2005). On-unit violence has a direct impact on clinical care, service quality, and the fiscal "bottom line" (LeBel and Goldstein 2005).

Mental health care clinicians, especially physicians, must become better educated about their roles in improving workplace safety and use that knowledge to practice in a manner that prevents normal conflict from escalating to violence (Joint Commission on Accreditation of Healthcare Organizations 2002). This is key to workforce retention; a study conducted by the American Nurses Association reported that more than 40% of nurses had been injured on the job, and 17% had been the target of physical assaults (as cited in Joint Commission on Accreditation of Healthcare Organizations 2002). Safety has been cited as a key factor in staff retention; without efforts to improve the safety of the work environment, staff will leave direct-care settings, and safety will further deteriorate (Joint Commission on Accreditation of Healthcare Organizations 2002).

The Call to Transform Mental Health Care

Long before *The Hartford Courant* published its series, some organizations had started to reduce the use of se-

clusion and restraint in their respective facilities. A few of these programs and facilities were highlighted in the report by the U.S. General Accounting Office in 1999 and are examples of what could happen given leadership, creativity, and the will to change practice patterns. These include model programs in Pennsylvania, Massachusetts, and New York. Many of these projects were co-led by physicians.

Following the *Courant* series, federal regulators promulgated policy and regulatory revisions in an attempt to ensure the safer use of seclusion and restraint practices (Centers for Medicare and Medicaid Services 2006; Health Care Finance Administration 1999, 2001). However, the latter regulations did not specifically address the prevention of conflict or violence and are considered minimum standards, not best practices (L. Norwalk, Director, Centers for Medicare and Medicaid Services Behavioral Health Standards, personal communication, January 18, 2007). In 1999, the National Association of State Mental Health Program Directors (NASMHPD) unanimously approved a policy statement committing to the reduction and eventual elimination of seclusion and restraint, and its Medical Directors Council authored a series of technical reports on seclusion and restraint use with recommendations for change (National Association of State Mental Health Program Directors 1999a, 1999b, 2001).

The President's New Freedom Commission Report on Mental Health Care was published in 2003. In 2005, the Institute of Medicine published its report titled "Improving the Quality of Health Care for Mental and Substance-Use Conditions." These works provide strong support for transformative change in the delivery of mental health care that includes significant attention to the reduction of conflict, violence, and coercive measures.

The United States is not alone in the growing concern about use of coercive interventions. International standard-bearing organizations have explicitly articulated the essential rights of people who receive mental health care and experience seclusion and restraint. The United Nations adopted a resolution titled *Principles for the Protection of Persons With Mental Illness and for the Improvement of Mental Health Care* in 1991 and outlined inviolable basic rights recognized by the international community, including 1) the right to be protected from harm or abuse and 2) the right to be free from restraint or seclusion unless it is used as the "only means available to prevent immediate or imminent harm to the patient or others" (United Nations 1991). Despite these and other fundamental protective covenants adopted by the European Union and other countries, harm to individuals in psychiatric settings persists nationally and internationally (Declaration of Dresden Against Coerced Psychiatric Treatment 2007; Mental Disability Advocacy Center 2003).

Mental health consumers and advocates have been concerned about the use of coercive interventions in mental health settings for years (Bluebird 2004). In recent decades, the mental health advocacy movement has grown beyond its modest beginnings, and groups of ex-patients became more organized, holding conferences, publishing newsletters, and lobbying legislators for recognition of their issues (Bluebird 2004). The mental health consumer movement is now well established in the national arena; it is recognized as a significant, viable, and effective stakeholder group. Many states have added consumer affairs staff to their state mental heath agencies, and most states now host peer-run drop-in centers. Peer specialists are now in 30 states, and in 6 states Medicaid has approved reimbursement for this role (Goldberg 2007). Mental health providers are recognizing peer support, peer-provided services, paid peer staff, and self-help as critical in recovery-oriented systems of care (National Executive Training Institute 2007).

The involvement of service users as full partners is still limited in the private and public sectors due to a combination of fear, distrust, and discomfort (Bluebird 2004). However, as noted in the President's New Freedom Commission on Mental Health (2003) report and the Institute of Medicine (2005) report, the sincere and meaningful inclusion of consumers and advocates in every component of the service system not only is absolutely critical but also is a mandatory best practice that distinguishes the new mental health system from the old.

Consumer and Staff Experiences

It has become clear to clinical and policy experts that it is incumbent upon the mental health system to listen and give value to "self-reports" by people who have personally experienced violence in health settings as well as to staff who are expected to use these procedures (National Executive Training Institute 2007). Personal vignettes provide a picture of individual experiences that should not and cannot be minimized or ignored, even though they may not reach the level of empirical research.

The following experiences were recorded from people who were involved in violent events in mental health settings and the staff who were expected to use these procedures (National Executive Training Institute 2007):

"I would just like to say that I only jumped in the restraint because, in my eyes, staff were hurting a patient and it brought back memories for when I was being hurt by people and no one was there to help me, but I figured that patient might have thought no one was there to help her, but I was." (Female patient, age 16 years)

"One of the things that doesn't get talked about very much is the trauma of the staff. We talk about the trauma paradigm for our clients or people in recovery. But not very often in my 20 years of work in the field of mental health have I heard much about what happens to us, the workers, and I think that's an area where we need to do some work. I've seen some pretty traumatic things from when I first started 20 years ago. Some of those things still haunt me that I've seen." (Female direct-care staff member)

"It became a 'war of words' all about who had the power. I was restrained and forcibly injected. I did not speak to anyone for the next 2 days, and developing any sort of trusting relationship was seriously delayed." (Male patient, age 32 years)

"I got put in the quiet room for pulling the alarm. I pulled the alarm because my grandma did not visit with me so I felt really bad and did not know what to do." (Male patient, age 16 years)

"I had never seen such a thing...a blue mattress with restraints. They strapped me in face down. I have a memory that they also gave me an injection, but that might have been from another time. I remember whispering to the nurse, 'What happens now?' I was petrified because all their behavior and equipment seemed so weird. She said, 'Just try to sleep.'" (Adult female patient)

"The first time that I helped with a restraint, a four-point restraint, I walked out of the room in tears because it was one of the most horrible things I had ever seen." (Female direct-care staff member)

"I've been injured from time to time. Nothing severe. I have bruises, yeah, sometimes I get headaches. I get shaky." (Male direct-care staff member)

Some unexpected vignettes also identified practices that appeared to help individuals cope with being put in restraints or seclusion, in the aftermath of the event.

"She asked if I would be safe if she took off the restraints, and I said yes. She said, 'Well, that is a good safe.' When she took the restraints off of my wrists and

legs, I was unable to move my right hand and shoulder. It was very swollen. She couldn't believe how swollen I was and immediately called for medical attention. It was her passion and conviction about the fact that I had not received any medical attention. She was screaming to whoever it was. Then she got me up and helped me take a shower and got me food. In her face I could see that she cared for me and also in her voice." (Adult female patient)

"It was a Palm Sunday and I wanted to go to Mass. It was a Catholic hospital. The nurse let me go though she knew that I was expressing suicidal thoughts. When I came back one and a half hours later, I was put in seclusion. The nurse did not talk to me. Nobody talked to me. I was on a little mat in the room. When my doctor (psychiatrist) came back 2 days later after being gone on a long weekend, he was furious. He talked to the nurse and told her, 'You had no right doing that.' He got me out of seclusion. He then spent time with me." (Adult female patient)

Principles Underlying Trauma-Informed Systems of Care

A core construct believed to be critical in reducing the use of seclusion and restraint is the emerging science of trauma-informed care. The implementation of the principles of trauma-informed care is a "universal precaution" when attempting to prevent conflict or violence (National Executive Training Institute 2007). These principles have been developed and studied by clinicians and researchers for two decades but have only now begun to receive significant attention (Moses et al. 2003; National Association of State Mental Health Program Directors 2005).

Mental health literature reports are now replete with studies on the high prevalence of traumatic life experiences in the general public as well as in the lives of adults and children in the public mental health system (Cusack et al. 2004; Mueser et al. 1998; Saxe et al. 2003). *Traumatic life events* are defined as those that involve a direct threat of death, severe bodily harm, or psychological injury that the person, at the time, finds intensely distressing (Rosenberg et al. 2001). *Trauma* and *traumatic events* are defined as "the personal experience of interpersonal violence including sexual abuse, physical abuse, severe neglect, loss and/or the witnessing of violence" (National Executive Training Institute 2007).

Epidemiological studies estimate that between 36% and 81% of the general population has experienced some kind of significant traumatic event, and the rates are even higher for people who seek clinical services from public mental health and substance abuse providers (Cusack et al. 2004; Mueser et al. 1998). Kessler et al. (1995) conducted a nationally representative study of the general population in the United States. In face-to-face interviews with 5,877 people ages 15–54 years, 60% of men and 51% of women reported at least one traumatic event at some time in their lives.

In a widely cited report titled "Origins of Addiction: Evidence From the Adverse Childhood Experiences Study," Felitti (2003) found that the "compulsive use of nicotine, alcohol and injected street drugs increases proportionally in a strong, graded, dose–response manner that closely parallels the intensity of adverse childhood experiences" (p. 3) in a population-based study of more than 17,000 middle-class American adults. The impact of traumatic life events, characterized by subjectively perceived threats of harm, has also been clearly defined and linked positively to posttraumatic stress disorder (PTSD), acute stress disorder, poor treatment outcomes, and personal distress (Jennings 2004).

Individuals who experience trauma sometimes develop PTSD, a clinical disorder characterized by stress and anxiety-related acute and chronic signs and symptoms (Frueh et al. 2000). PTSD is considered to be chronic and debilitating and to have serious adverse effects on social, familial, and occupational functioning. Studies demonstrate a high prevalence rate of PTSD in people with mental illness (up to 43%) and even higher rates of traumatic exposure in the same population (51%–98%) (K.J. Cusack, B.C. Frueh, T.G. Hiers, et al., "The Impact of Trauma and Posttraumatic Stress Disorder Upon American Society: Report to the President's Commission on Mental Health," unpublished paper, 2003; Kessler et al. 1995; Mueser et al. 1998). Other studies have found trauma prevalence rates of 52%–90% in persons who have schizophrenia, schizoaffective disorders, major depression, and co-occurring disorders (Cusack et al. 2004; Frueh et al. 2002; Green et al. 2000; Mueser et al. 1998). Leading researchers have concluded that the syndrome of PTSD is associated with significant psychiatric and medical comorbidity, social maladjustment, and poor quality of life (Frueh et al. 2006). Current research on the neurobiology of PTSD indicates that although it is strikingly similar to major depression, PTSD has several distinctive features, including hyperactivity of the hypothalamic-pituitary-adrenal system and hypersecretion of corticotropin-releasing factor in the presence of normal to low cortisol levels

(Newport and Nemeroff 2003). There is also considerable evidence that early traumatization is associated with adoption of high-risk behaviors, substance abuse, revictimization, reduced treatment adherence, poor quality of life among HIV-infected individuals, and increased morbidity (Whetten et al. 2006). On balance, the literature regarding PTSD is compelling. This complex psychiatric disorder not only results in emotional distress but also has far-reaching effects, including impaired social and work functioning, negative life-course consequences, increased likelihood of repeat traumatic experiences, and often a duration of many years (Kessler 2000).

The significance of trauma in the lives of the people with mental conditions cannot be ignored in mental health environments. The following principles of trauma-informed systems have been identified as critical in preventing adverse events and in reducing the use of seclusion and restraint (Fallot and Harris 2002; National Executive Training Institute 2007):

1. An understanding of the neurological, biological, psychological, and social effects of trauma and violence in human experience.
2. An appreciation of the high prevalence of traumatic experience in the lives of the people who receive mental health services.
3. The use of a standardized, early, and thoughtful trauma assessment on admission to any mental health service or setting, with positive results informing treatment.
4. A recognition and sincere attempt to minimize the fact that mental health treatment environments are often traumatizing, both overtly and covertly.
5. Valuing the consumer in all aspects of care, including highly individualized treatment planning and shared decision making.
6. The use of neutral, objective, supportive "person first" language in policy, procedure, and daily usage.
7. Workforce development activities that seek to increase staff awareness and understanding of trauma in the lives of people served. This principle also includes ongoing reviews of organizational rules, practices, and policies that are possibly homogenizing, demeaning, disrespectful, confusing, or worse.
8. Organization-wide practices that seek to minimize the use of coercive practices such as seclusion, restraint, punishment, consequences, and forced medication.

In some settings, the implementation of these principles alone has completely transformed the culture of care and reduced or eliminated the use of seclusion and restraint (National Executive Training Institute 2007). These principles are believed to be not only a universal precaution against conflict and violence in our treatment settings but also a core component in creating a recovery-based service system as articulated by the President's New Freedom Commission on Mental Health (2003) and the Institute of Medicine (2005).

Effective Strategies to Prevent Violence and Improve Safety

Facilitating recovery, independence, and illness self-management is the goal of a transformed mental health service system (Institute of Medicine 2005; President's New Freedom Commission on Mental Health 2003). Implicit in the recovery model are principles and values that require a reduction of coercive, violent, and involuntary procedures done to persons with mental illness as part of a major shift in practice. The National Consensus Statement on Mental Health Recovery was developed by the Center for Mental Health Services (2004) and describes the recovery process and explicates key principles. Simply stated, transformed systems of care that are recovery focused and trauma informed are not characterized by rigid rules, coercive practices, or "one size fits all" treatment. As such, these principles are important in understanding the rationale for preventing violence and improving safety.

Preventing Violence Through a Formal Plan

In order for a mental health facility to begin a conflict and violence prevention effort, including a reduction in the use of seclusion and restraint, a facility-specific strategic action plan should be developed and structured to include tasks that identify the responsible parties, due dates, and expected outcomes. Conceptually, the plan should address the "Six Core Strategies" identified in the NASMHPD approach, because this model continues to integrate effective strategies from across the country (National Executive Training Institute 2007). These strategies form the training curriculum that has been developed to assist psychiatric facilities in preventing both violence and the use of seclusion and restraint. The curriculum was designed for use with mental health populations; however, the strategies have been successfully adapted and applied to other populations and care settings as well. These strategies are not meant to replace evidence-based and other clinical approaches, meaningful treatment activities, or effective pharmacological management, but rather are designed to be used in conjunction with these methods. The "Six Core Strategies" to improve workplace safety are paraphrased from the National Executive Training Institute (2007) and are described in detail in the sections that follow.

1. LEADERSHIP TOWARD ORGANIZATIONAL CHANGE

This strategy outlines the role of the executive director or facility administrator and other executive staff. Reduction of the use of seclusion and restraint must start with clear, focused leadership. Leaders must define and articulate a mission and philosophy about seclusion and restraint reduction and outline the roles and responsibilities of all staff in the facility (Huckshorn 2006). The development and implementation of the prevention plan are leadership responsibilities that require full and consistent participation by a facility administrator or chief executive officer who is firmly committed to this effort. The reduction plan should be presented in a continuous quality improvement framework that understands that culture change takes time and that we "learn as we go."

A core activity included in this strategy is elevating the oversight of every seclusion and restraint event by executive management. This requires that a very different level of attention be paid to these events than historically practiced. It ensures a timely (minimum weekly) senior administrative review of all incidents that captures detailed information valuable in determining necessary prevention activities. It takes advantage of the fact that facility leaders can implement policy changes quickly due to their organizational position, power, and influence.

Leadership strategies include the development of a facilitywide policy statement that outlines the prevention/reduction approach relative to the use of seclusion and restraint for all staff, determines data-driven goals to reduce use, announces a "kickoff" event and routinely celebrates successes, identifies seclusion and restraint reduction champions at all levels of the organization, and assigns these staff to specific prevention roles. The leadership strategy also includes supporting staff practice change, with frequent communication and hospital rounds done by executives (Hardenstine 2001). Another effective action step is voluntarily raising the minimum standards of practice—for example, reducing the maximum seclusion or restraint orders from 4 hours to 2 hours.

Leadership must also ensure the inclusion of consumers, family members, and advocates in all aspects of the effort and create mechanisms so that this involvement will happen, be understood by staff, and be viewed in a positive manner (Bluebird 2004). The key issue with this strategy, based on real reduction experiences, is that leadership is essential. If leaders are committed to the effort, significant organization-wide culture change will occur; if not, it will fail. In summary, the critical function of organizational leadership is to take an active, visible role; prioritize the initiative; "preach and teach"; and hold people accountable for all aspects of the plan.

2. USE OF DATA TO INFORM PRACTICE

This strategy uses facility-specific seclusion and restraint data in a nonpunitive manner, provides for healthy competition among facility units or wards, and elevates the general oversight and knowledge of seclusion and restraint use in real time for everyone involved (Hardenstine 2001; Huckshorn 2006). It encourages the administration to identify successful staff and specific units so that effective seclusion and restraint prevention practices can be shared.

Using data in this way includes an analysis of facility seclusion and restraint usage by unit, shift, day, and staff member involved, although this latter strategy needs to be recorded confidentially for identifying individual staff training and supervisory needs and not for disciplinary actions in general (Huckshorn 2006). The facility also needs to highlight seclusion and restraint use by graphing and posting these data on all units so that they are clearly visible for staff and consumers.

It is also important, initially, to identify the facility's baseline use of seclusion and restraint so that performance improvement goals can be set, use can be monitored over time, and progress (or lack thereof) can be tracked (Hardenstine 2001). This includes setting data-driven goals and communicating these goals to staff. Reducing seclusion and restraint through the thoughtful use of data includes tracking core measures such as seclusion and restraint episodes and hours and also tracking supplemental measures that include the use of emergency, involuntary (usually intramuscular) medication administration; incidence of both consumer and staff injuries; and qualitative reports of consumer and staff satisfaction (Bluebird 2004).

3. WORKFORCE DEVELOPMENT

The workforce development strategy focuses on the creation of a treatment environment where policies, procedures, and practices are based on the knowledge and principles of recovery and the characteristics of trauma-informed systems of care (Huckshorn 2006). This strategy is implemented primarily through staff training, education, and human resources development activities. It provides guidelines for choosing seclusion and restraint application training vendors, particularly vendors who have data demonstrating success in seclusion and restraint reduction using their particular model.

This strategy ensures that staff are given the opportunity to develop and practice individualized treatment planning and practice skills that integrate seclusion and restraint prevention strategies for persons served. Included are activities that ensure adequate staff education about the experiences of consumers and staff with seclusion and restraint, address the common myths associated with use, introduce the rationale and characteristics of trauma-informed care, educate about the neurobiological and psychological effects of trauma, and describe a prevention-based approach to reduction.

Also included is facility leadership's understanding that many seclusion and restraint events occur because of win–lose conflicts set up by facility rules and staff roles in enforcing these rules. Because of this institutionally driven risk issue, leadership must understand the value of allowing staff to "suspend" institutional rules and procedures, when necessary, to avoid or resolve conflicts when addressing individual needs (Huckshorn 2006). Examples of this important construct are rigid policies regarding attendance at activities, wake and sleep times, curfews, smoke breaks, mealtimes, and other rules designed to keep order that do not take into account individual needs or the signs and symptoms of mental illness.

Other important activities include discussing the facility's seclusion and restraint reduction plan in new-hire interviews and incorporating expectations in job descriptions, performance evaluations, and new staff orientation activities (Huckshorn 2006). It is the job of senior management to ensure that the seclusion and restraint prevention plan is communicated early and is consistently reinforced, that staff clearly understand their important role in the plan, and that they are supervised throughout the process so that learning can occur.

4. USE OF SECLUSION AND RESTRAINT PREVENTION TOOLS

This strategy reduces the use of seclusion and restraint through a variety of preventive tools and risk assess-

ments that are integrated into hospital policy and procedure and each individual consumer's treatment plan. This intervention includes using tools to identify risk for violence (including previous seclusion and restraint history), tools to identify persons with medical risk factors for death and injury, and tools to identify persons with psychological risk factors that would be informed by a trauma assessment; developing and using de-escalation or safety plans (including psychiatric advance directives); creating sensory-based interventions to teach self-calming and soothing; making changes to the physical environment (including the development of comfort and/or sensory rooms); and implementing daily meaningful treatment activities.

Each of these tools has a specific purpose and associated goals, such as identifying people who are at higher risk for seclusion and restraint use based on past incidents and those who are at higher risk for injury or death due to conditions such as obesity, respiratory disease, cardiac anomalies, medication side effects, recent ingestion of food, prone positioning, and past trauma histories. De-escalation or safety plans assist the service recipient in learning illness self-management by identifying emotional triggers and developing awareness of interpersonal or environmental stressors that could lead to conflict or emotional dyscontrol. Proactive strategies can be practiced in advance of a crisis. A behavior scale can offer a set of guidelines to staff to ensure that staff responses are appropriate to the behavior being demonstrated by the service recipient. This helps to ensure that behavior truly meets the criterion of imminent dangerousness prior to the implementation of seclusion and restraint. Many seclusion and restraint incidents are initiated prematurely before the level of "imminent danger" occurs, often because staff do not know any other approach to use.

One of the most promising practices to aid in seclusion and restraint reduction efforts and the creation of alternatives to containment is the use of sensory interventions. Sensory interventions can be applied across the range of milieu-based services. This approach requires knowledge of occupational therapy; an assessment of each service user's "sensory diet" (Ayers 1979); an understanding of specific sensory needs (sensory seeking or avoiding); and creation of person-centered care plans based on that knowledge. Applying these concepts to clinical service leads to meaningful, creative therapeutic activities; sensory education and intervention practice; greater instruction in self-calming and soothing techniques; and consideration of unit environments. Implementing sensory interventions at the environmental level shifts the focus from "unit space" to "unit place." The former indicates physical location and boundaries, whereas the latter connotes therapeutic meaning and purpose within the environment (Hasselkus 2002). This can be readily achieved through thoughtful attention to the full range of sensory experience throughout the unit by attending to color, sound, aroma, lighting, furniture placement, plants, murals—the "softscape"—or creating specific rooms to experience calm, such as comfort rooms or sensory rooms, or simply creating quiet areas or smaller seating arrangements that offer greater privacy, sanctuary, and an opportunity to restore. The use of sensory rooms and interventions have been attributed to decreased perceived distress, reduced maladaptive behavior, and enhanced participation and task performance among consumers in treatment settings (Ashby et al. 1995; Champagne 2006; Champagne and Sayer 2003; Hutchinson and Haggar 1991). Moreover, sensory room/comfort room development has been identified as an integral component to many successful restraint reduction efforts in psychiatric facilities throughout the country (Champagne and Stromberg 2004; LeBel and Goldstein 2005; National Executive Training Institute 2007). Some hospitals reported significant reductions (54%–91%) in restraint and seclusion use as this preventive alternative was implemented (Champagne and Stromberg 2004; LeBel and Goldstein 2005).

5. Full Inclusion of Consumers and Advocates

The full and formal inclusion of consumers or "persons in recovery," as well as family members and external advocates, in a variety of roles in the organization assists in the reduction of seclusion and restraint (Bluebird 2004). These roles can be developed by converting vacant positions and hiring consumers into full- or part-time jobs such as the director of advocacy services, peer specialist, drop-in center director, and consumer advocate. These roles are immeasurably valuable if the facility and staff understand and are open to the depth and breadth of knowledge that consumers bring to an organization.

It is necessary that these roles and their importance be defined for staff and that consumer staff report to managers who understand and support these roles. The new role of a consumer in an inpatient facility can be daunting, intimidating, and difficult. It is essential that all staff clearly understand this role and that attention be given to orienting and training people who undertake these new roles. It is equally important that inclusion is real and consumers are empow-

ered to do their jobs, including making mistakes or receiving additional training (Bluebird 2004). Similarly, the inclusion of family members and external advocates can be extremely valuable and very necessary in children's units where service recipients are too young to participate in these kinds of roles. Inviting the local protection and advocacy organization to be involved can be very helpful in preventing problems and developing a transparent organization committed to quality improvement.

6. Rigorous Debriefing Activities

The final strategy uses event debriefing procedures (defined as rigorous analysis) to reduce the use of seclusion and restraint through knowledge gained from a careful review of seclusion and restraint events. This knowledge is then used to inform policies, procedures, and practices to avoid repeats in the future (Huckshorn 2006). A secondary goal of this strategy is to attempt to mitigate harm and the potentially traumatizing effects of a seclusion and restraint event for involved staff and consumers and for all witnesses to the event. Debriefing activities are separated into two distinct but equally important activities that follow a seclusion and restraint event.

The first is an immediate postevent discussion that is led by a nursing supervisor or a senior staff person who was not involved in the event. The purpose is to ensure the safety of all involved parties, review the documentation, interview staff and others who were present, and attempt to return the unit to the precrisis milieu. The use of an interview guideline and the documentation of activities immediately following the event are highly recommended.

The second debriefing activity is more formal and occurs 24–48 hours later. It includes the treatment team, the attending psychiatrist, and a representative from management. It uses rigorous problem-solving methods such as root-cause analysis procedures to review and analyze the event. The purpose of this activity is to identify what happened and what can be changed to avoid an event in the future and to ensure that, as much as possible, traumatic sequelae are mitigated for everyone involved.

The inclusion of the consumer's perspective is critical here. It is potentially intimidating to expect a recently secluded or restrained individual to attend a large meeting, and alternatives are recommended. The service recipient's perspective can be included and represented by a staff advocate if the service user is comfortable with this plan and is able and willing both to agree and to communicate his or her perspective.

This alternative is not meant to patronize or otherwise assume inability of the service recipient to participate; it is intended only to make facility staff aware of the possibility of a patient's covert feelings of coercion or helplessness in the face of a group of professionals. In addition, establishing and maintaining a nonpunitive environment are essential to creating a safe space for staff to share their thoughts and feelings.

In summary, the "Six Core Strategies" (National Executive Training Institute 2007) are presented for use as part of a comprehensive performance improvement plan to reduce both conflict and the use of seclusion and restraint (Huckshorn 2006). They are focused on prevention and incorporate the most current and effective approaches known. These strategies have been substantiated in the literature and appear to be a common thread in successful projects (Donat 2003; Hardenstine 2001; Jonikas et al. 2004; National Executive Training Institute 2007; Visalli and McNasser 2000).

A Prevention Framework

The avoidance of conflict and violence starts with the use of prevention tools that train staff in best practices (Huckshorn 2006). An obvious place to start this effort is to focus on the reduction of the use of seclusion and restraint procedures. This is an attainable goal that has been achieved by many facilities throughout the United States and is well within the reach of every committed organization. Changing these practices is much more than rethinking the use of coercive procedures. The essence of this effort is about transforming practice, changing treatment cultures, reflecting on how we *think* about the people we serve and how to educate the staff who serve them. At its core, this work is about improving safety and using every preventive technique that is known and effective.

Traditional mental health practices have most often placed the reasons for conflict and the use of seclusion and restraint on the shoulders of the consumer—attributing acts of aggression in isolation from the environment, devoid of environmental triggers. A prevention approach is one way for physicians to take a lead role in reorganizing agency operations and can change the way that violence in mental health settings is currently viewed.

In physical health, the public health prevention model is a model of disease prevention and health promotion and is a logical fit with a practice issue such as seclusion and restraint (National Association of State Mental Health Program Directors 1999a). The applicability of this model focuses on identifying risk factors for conflict and violence along with early intervention strategies so that violence can be prevented. This approach directs efforts to anticipate conflicts, immediately resolve situations when they arise, and learn new prevention strategies from an analysis process when these events do occur. This model is best understood by the constructs of primary prevention, secondary prevention, and tertiary prevention to guide the development of reduction activities (National Executive Training Institute 2007).

Primary prevention interventions speak to the development of treatment environments that anticipate the potential for conflict to occur. Strategies include the implementation of visions, values, and principles of care that are trauma informed; a thorough analysis of organizational values to ensure they are reflected in current practices; and an ongoing revision of policies and procedures and early individualized assessments of a variety of risk factors for violence, injury, or death.

Secondary prevention activities speak to the immediate and effective use of early interventions to mitigate conflict or aggression when these do occur. These interventions include staff training focused on attitudes and behaviors when faced with a conflict situation, competency-based negotiation and de-escalation skills, and the use of individually developed crisis plans that assist in teaching emotional self-management (National Executive Training Institute 2007).

Tertiary prevention interventions address the most effective ways to minimize the damage done to consumers, staff, and others witnessing a seclusion and restraint event once it occurs. These strategies include rigorous problem-solving activities in event analyses and include the mandatory involvement of the involved service recipient. These types of interventions are also focused on identifying people who may require specific treatment for trauma.

Conclusion

Were seclusion and restraint regulated substances, the U.S. Food and Drug Administration would probably have banned their use, given the number of people who have died and continue to die from these procedures. Consumers are not the only victims; staff have also died or been seriously injured while engaged in implementing these practices (National Executive Training Institute 2007). The advantage to reports of seclusion and restraint deaths is that these publicized sentinel events often spur calls for practice reforms, and such reforms are now occurring domestically and internationally (Department of Health 2005; Mental Disability Advocacy Center 2003; National Executive Training Institute 2007). Despite well-codified local and worldwide human rights and patient protections, the harm to service users and staff who serve them persists (Declaration of Dresden Against Coerced Psychiatric Treatment 2007; Mental Disability Advocacy Center 2003).

The good news is that the knowledge about how to do this work is readily available and is in the public domain. Many "success story" facilities provide contemporary testaments to transformed mental health services and lived recovery experiences. None of these stories could be told without courageous leaders who are willing to take an unpopular stand, manage staff anxieties, weather perpetual challenges, and seriously commit to this initiative. Mental health facilities are encouraged to develop their own individualized safety plan. Documenting a safety improvement plan that includes violence prevention objectives is an important first step. Adopting prevention-oriented and trauma-informed principles by implementing NASMHPD's "Six Core Strategies" will help facilitate an organizational culture change process if committed medical and administrative leaders are willing to chart and stay the course and commit time and personal capital to the mission.

References

Ashby M, Lindsay W, Pitcaithly D, et al: Snoezelen: its effects on concentration and responsiveness in people with profound multiple handicaps. British Journal of Occupational Therapy 58:303–307, 1995

Ayers JA: Sensory Integration and the Child. Los Angeles, CA, Western Psychological Services, 1979

Bluebird G: Redefining consumer roles: changing culture and practice in mental health settings. J Psychosoc Nurs Ment Health Serv 42:46–53, 2004

Busch AB, Shore MF: Seclusion and restraint: a review of recent literature. Harv Rev Psychiatry 8:261–270, 2000

Center for Mental Health Services: National Consensus Statement on Mental Health Recovery. Washington, DC, U.S. Department of Health and Human Services, Substance Abuse and Mental Health Services Administration, 2004. Available at: http://mentalhealth.samhsa.gov/publications/allpubs/sma05-4129/. Accessed April 9, 2008.

Centers for Medicare and Medicaid Services: Final Rule, Medicare and Medicaid Programs. Hospital Conditions of Participation: Patients' Rights (42 CFR Part 482, Section 13). Baltimore, MD, U.S. Department of Health and Human Services, 2006

Champagne T: Creating sensory rooms: environmental enhancements for acute inpatient mental health settings. American Occupational Therapy Association, Mental Health Special Interest Section Quarterly 29:1–4, 2006

Champagne T, Sayer E: The effects of the use of the sensory room in psychiatry, 2003. Available at: http://www.ot-innovations.com/images/stories/PDF_Files/qi_study_sensory_room.pdf. Accessed September 18, 2007.

Champagne T, Stromberg N: Sensory approaches in inpatient psychiatric settings: innovative alternatives to seclusion and restraint. Psychosoc Nurs Ment Health Serv 42:35–44, 2004

Cusack KJ, Frueh BC, Brady KT: Trauma history screening in a community mental health center. Psychiatr Serv 55:157–162, 2004

Declaration of Dresden Against Coerced Psychiatric Treatment: The Declaration of Dresden Against Coerced Psychiatric Treatment Consensus Statement of the World Network of Users and Survivors of Psychiatry, European Network of Ex-Users and Survivors of Psychiatry, Bundesverband Psychiatrie-Erfahrener, and MindFreedom International. Presented at the World Psychiatric Association thematic conference, "Coercive Treatment in Psychiatry: A Comprehensive Review." Dresden, Germany, June 2007

Department of Health: Delivering race equality in mental health care: an action plan for reform inside and outside services and the government's response to the independent inquiry into the death of David Bennett. London, Crown, 2005. Available at: http://www.dh.gov.uk/en/Publicationsandstatistics/Publications/PublicationsPolicyAndGuidance/DH_4100773. Accessed January 10, 2007.

Donat DC: An analysis of successful efforts to reduce the use of seclusion and restraint at a public psychiatric hospital. Psychiatr Serv 54:1119–1123, 2003

Duxbury J: An evaluation of staff and patient views of and strategies employed to manage inpatient aggression and violence on one mental health unit: a pluralistic design. J Psychiatr Ment Health Nurs 9:325–337, 2002

Fallot RD, Harris M: The trauma recovery and empowerment model (TREM): conceptual and practical issues in a group intervention for women. Community Ment Health J 38:475–485, 2002

Felitti VJ: Origins of addictive behavior: evidence from a study of stressful childhood experiences [German]. Prax Kinderpsychol Kinderpsychiatr 52:547–559, 2003. English translation available at: http://www.acestudy.org/files/OriginsofAddiction.pdf. Accessed April 10, 2008.

Frueh BC, Dalton ME, Johnson MR, et al: Trauma within the psychiatric setting: conceptual framework, research directions, and policy implications. Adm Policy Ment Health 28:147–154, 2000

Frueh BC, Cousins VC, Hiers TG, et al: The need for trauma assessment and related clinical services in a state-funded mental health system. Community Ment Health J 38:351–356, 2002

Frueh BC, Cusack KJ, Grubaugh AL, et al: Clinicians' perspectives on cognitive-behavioral treatment for PTSD among persons with severe mental illness. Psychiatr Serv 57:1027–1031, 2006

Green BL, Goodman LA, Krupnick JL, et al: Outcomes of single versus multiple trauma exposure in a screening sample. J Trauma Stress 3:271–286, 2000

Goldberg C: Mental patients find understanding in therapy led by peers. Boston Globe, June 8, 2007, final edition. Available at: http://www.boston.com/news/local/articles/2007/06/08/mental_patients_find_understanding_in_therapy_led_by_peers/. Accessed July 13, 2007.

Haimowitz S, Urff J, Huckshorn KA: Restraint and seclusion: a risk management guide. Alexandria, VA, National Association of State Mental Health Program Directors, 2006

Hardenstine B: Leading the Way Toward a Seclusion and Restraint–Free Environment: Pennsylvania's Success Story. Harrisburg, PA, Office of Mental Health and Substance Abuse Services, Pennsylvania Department of Public Welfare, 2001

Hasselkus B: The Meaning of Everyday Occupation. Thorofare, NJ, Slack, 2002

Health Care Finance Administration: Interim Final Rule, Medicare and Medicaid Programs. Hospital Conditions of Participation: Patient's Rights (42 CFR Part 482, Section 13). Baltimore, MD, U.S. Department of Health and Human Services, 1999

Health Care Finance Administration: Interim Final Rule, Medicaid Program. Use of Restraint and Seclusion in Psychiatric Residential Treatment Facilities Providing Psychiatric Services to Individuals Under Age 21 (42 CFR Parts 441 and 483). Baltimore, MD, U.S. Department of Health and Human Services, 2001

Hinsby K, Baker M: Patient and nurse accounts of violent incidents in a medium secure unit. Psychiatr Ment Health Nurs 11:341–347, 2004

Honberg R, Miller J: Seclusion and Restraint: Task Force Report of the NAMI Policy Research Institute. Arlington, VA, National Alliance on Mental Illness, 2003. Available at: http://www.nami.org/Template.cfm?Section=Policy_Research_Institute&Template=/ContentManagement/ContentDisplay.cfm&ContentID=10979. Accessed April 9, 2008.

Huckshorn KA: Re-designing state mental health policy to prevent the use of seclusion and restraint. Adm Policy Ment Health 33:482–491, 2006

Hutchinson R, Haggar L: The Whitinghall Snoezelen Project. Chesterfield, Derbyshire, England, North Derbyshire Health Authority, 1991

Institute of Medicine: Improving the Quality of Health Care for Mental and Substance-Use Conditions (Prepublication copy, uncorrected proofs). Quality Chasm Series. Washington, DC, National Academies Press, 2005

Jennings A: The Damaging Consequences of Violence and Trauma: Facts, Discussion Points, and Recommendations for the Behavioral Health System. Alexandria, VA, National Association of State Mental Health Program Directors, National Technical Assistance Center, 2004

Joint Commission on Accreditation of Healthcare Organizations: Health Care at the Crossroads: Strategies for Addressing the Evolving Nursing Crisis. A JCAHO Public Policy Initiative. Oakbrook Terrace, IL, The Joint Commission, 2002. Available at: http://www.jointcommission.org/NR/rdonlyres/5C138711-ED76-4D6F-909F-B06E0309F36D/0/health_care_at_the_crossroads.pdf. Accessed July 14, 2007.

Joint Commission on Accreditation of Healthcare Organizations: The Joint Commission's sentinel event policy: ten years of improving the quality and safety of health care. Joint Commission Perspectives 25(5):1–5, May 2005

Jonikas JA, Cook JA, Rosen C, et al: A program to reduce use of physical restraint in psychiatric inpatient facilities. Psychiatr Serv 55:818–820, 2004

Kessler RC: Posttraumatic stress disorder: the burden to the individual and to society. J Clin Psychiatry 61 (suppl 5):4–12, 2000

Kessler RC, Sonnega A, Bromet E, et al: Posttraumatic stress disorder in the national comorbidity survey. Arch Gen Psychiatry 52:1048–1060, 1995

LeBel J, Goldstein R: The economic cost of using restraint and the value added by restraint reduction or elimination. Psychiatr Serv 56:1109–1114, 2005

LeBel J, Stromberg N, Duckworth K, et al: Child and adolescent inpatient restraint reduction: a state initiative to promote strength-based care. J Am Acad Child Adolesc Psychiatry 43:37–45, 2004

Legris J, Walters M, Browne G: The impact of seclusion on the treatment outcomes of psychotic in-patients. J Adv Nurs 30:448–459, 1999

Lieberman J, Dodd C, DeLauro R: Testimony to the Senate Committee on Finance. U.S. Senate proceedings, Washington, DC, March 1999

Love CC, Hunter ME: Violence in public sector psychiatric hospitals: benchmarking nursing staff injury rates. J Psychosoc Nurs Ment Health Serv 34:30–34, 1996

Mental Disability Advocacy Center: Cage Beds: Inhuman and Degrading Treatment in Four EU Accession Countries. Budapest, Hungary, Mental Disability Advocacy Center, 2003. Available at: http://www.mdac.info/documents/Cage_Beds.pdf. Accessed July 13, 2007.

Moses DJ, Reed BG, Mazelis R, et al: Creating Trauma Services for Women With Co-Occurring Disorders: Experiences From the SAMHSA Women With Alcohol, Drug Abuse and Mental Health Disorders Who Have Histories of Violence Study. Rockville, MD, Substance Abuse and Mental Health Services Administration, 2003. Available at: http://www.prainc.com/wcdvs/pdfs/CreatingTraumaServices.pdf. Accessed July 14, 2007.

Mueser KT, Goodman LB, Trumbetta SL, et al: Trauma and posttraumatic stress disorder in severe mental illness. J Consult Clin Psychol 66:493–499, 1998

National Association of State Mental Health Program Directors: Medical Directors Council Technical Report. Reducing the Use of Seclusion and Restraint: Findings, Strategies, and Recommendations. Alexandria, VA, National Association of State Mental Health Program Directors, 1999a

National Association of State Mental Health Program Directors: NASMHPD Position Statement on Seclusion and Restraint. Alexandria, VA, National Association of State Mental Health Program Directors, 1999b. Available at: http://www.nasmhpd.org/general_filesposition_statement/posses1.htm. Accessed July 14, 2007.

National Association of State Mental Health Program Directors: Medical Directors Council Technical Report. Reducing the Use of Seclusion and Restraint: Findings, Principles, and Recommendations for Special Needs Populations, Part Two. Alexandria, VA, National Association of State Mental Health Program Directors, 2001

National Association of State Mental Health Program Directors: Position Statement on Services and Supports to Trauma Survivors. Alexandria, VA, National Association of State Mental Health Program Directors, 2005. Available at: http://www.nasmhpd.org/general_files/position_statement/NASMHPD%20TRAUMA%20Positon%20 statementFinal.pdf. Accessed July 14, 2007.

National Executive Training Institute: Training Curriculum for Reduction of Seclusion and Restraint, 5th Edition. Alexandria, VA, National Association of State Mental Health Program Directors, National Technical Assistance Center, 2007

Newport DJ, Nemeroff CB: Neurobiology of posttraumatic stress disorder. Focus 1(3):313–321, 2003

Okin RL: Variation among state hospitals in use of seclusion and restraint. Hosp Community Psychiatry 36:648–652, 1985

Owen C, Tarantello C, Jones M, et al: Violence and aggression in psychiatric units. Psychiatr Serv 49:1452–1457, 1998

President's New Freedom Commission on Mental Health: Achieving the Promise: Transforming Mental Health Care in America. Final Report (DHHS Publ No SMA-03-3832). Rockville, MD, U.S. Department of Health and Human Services, 2003

Ray NK, Rappaport ME: Use of restraint and seclusion in psychiatric settings in New York State. Psychiatr Serv 46:1032–1037, 1995

Robins CS, Sauvageot JA, Cusack KJ, et al: Consumers' perceptions of negative experiences and "sanctuary harm" in psychiatric settings. Psychiatr Serv 56:1622, 2005

Rosenberg SD, Mueser KT, Friedman MJ, et al: Developing effective treatments for posttraumatic disorders among people with severe mental illness. Psychiatr Serv 52:1453–1461, 2001

Saxe G, Vanderbilt D, Zuckerman B: Traumatic stress in injured and ill children. PTSD Research Quarterly 14:1–7, 2003

Smith GM, Davis RH, Bixler EO, et al: Pennsylvania state hospital system's seclusion and restraint reduction program. Psychiatr Serv 56:1115–1122, 2005

Steinert T, Needham I: Seclusion and restraint in different European countries: incidence and interventions. Symposium presentation at the World Psychiatric Association thematic conference, "Coercive Treatment in Psychiatry: A Comprehensive Review." Dresden, Germany, June 2007

Substance Abuse and Mental Health Services Administration: SAMHSA Matrix: The Matrix Priority Programs: Addressing Unmet and Emerging Needs. Rockville, MD, Substance Abuse and Mental Health Services Administration, 2004. Available at: http://www.samhsa.gov/Matrix/brochure.aspx. Accessed July 14, 2007.

U.S. General Accounting Office: Mental Health: Improper Restraint or Seclusion Use Places People at Risk (GAO/HES-99-176). Washington, DC, U.S. General Accounting Office, 1999

United Nations: Principles for the Protection of Persons With Mental Illness and for the Improvement of Mental Health Care (Resolution 46/119). New York, United Nations General Assembly, 1991

Visalli H, McNasser G: Reducing seclusion and restraint: meeting the organizational challenge. J Nurs Care Qual 14:35–44, 2000

Weiss EM, Altimari D, Blint DF, et al: Deadly restraint: a nationwide pattern of death. The Hartford Courant, October 11–15, 1998

Whetten K, Leserman J, Lowe K, et al: Prevalence of childhood sexual abuse and physical trauma in an HIV-positive sample from the Deep South. Am J Public Health 96:1028–1030, 2006

CHAPTER 19

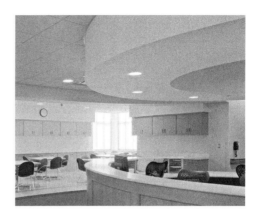

INPATIENT SUICIDE
Risk Assessment and Prevention

Robert P. Roca, M.D., M.P.H., M.B.A.
Laurie Hurson

> The estimation of suicide risk, at the culmination of the suicide assessment, is the quintessential clinical judgment, since no study has identified one specific risk factor or set of risk factors as specifically predictive of suicide or other suicidal behavior.
>
> American Psychiatric Association 2003

"Dangerousness to self" is among the most common precipitants of urgent psychiatric evaluation, and many inpatients are hospitalized because of a recent suicide attempt or current suicidal ideation and intent. Once patients are hospitalized, the risk of suicide often persists (Busch et al. 2003; Morgan and Priest 1991; Powell et al. 2000). Of the 30,000 suicides that occur annually in the United States, it is estimated that 1,500 take place in the hospital (American Psychiatric Association 2003), in some instances while patients are under the highest level of suicide observation (Busch et al. 2003). Of the "sentinel events" that have been reported to the Joint Commission[1] since 1995, only "wrong site surgery" has been reported

---

[1] A *sentinel event* is an unexpected occurrence involving death or serious physical or psychological injury, or the risk thereof. Serious injury specifically includes loss of limb or function. The phrase "or the risk thereof" includes any process variation for which a recurrence would carry a significant chance of a serious adverse outcome. Such events are called "sentinel" because they signal the need for immediate investigation and response (Joint Commission 2007).

more frequently than inpatient suicide (Joint Commission 2007).

Thus, it is extremely important that steps are taken to minimize the risk of suicide in the hospital. This requires building physical environments that are safe yet interpersonally warm, creating therapeutic milieus that provide support and restore hope, and performing suicide risk assessments to identify individuals at particularly high risk for suicide in the hospital so that special preventive measures can be instituted. These might be viewed as "universal precautions," that is, measures that are appropriate for all inpatient settings and all who are treated in them. The suicide risk assessment will identify individuals who need additional "special precautions" until imminent risk subsides.

Universal Precautions

Safe Physical Environments

Although it is impossible to create an absolutely suicide-proof environment, certain environmental features offer suicidal patients readily obvious opportunities to hurt themselves. These include standard glass mirrors that might easily be broken into sharp fragments that could be used for cutting, clothing hooks on walls or doors or bathroom fixtures from which hanging could be easily accomplished, windows that can be opened or penetrated and through which patients could jump, electrical outlets in bathrooms that could be used for self-electrocution, and storage of cleaning fluids and other poisonous compounds in places where patients might come upon and ingest them. It is helpful to inspect clinical spaces with the assistance of experienced clinicians and risk management professionals to look for particular features that pose unreasonable risk. It can also be useful to consult reviews such as the *Guidelines for the Built Environment of Behavioral Health Facilities* developed by the National Association of Psychiatric Health Systems (Sine and Hunt 2003) for ideas about how best to balance the sometimes competing values of safety and therapeutic warmth.

Safe and Effective Therapeutic Milieus

The reduction of suicide risk in the hospital depends on the mitigation of potentially remediable psychiatric factors that increase imminent risk. These include such symptoms as depression, agitation, anxiety, hopelessness, psychological pain, self-hatred, delu-

sions of guilt, and hallucinations advising suicide. The amelioration of these symptoms often depends at least in part on medical treatment (i.e., medications or electroconvulsive therapy) of the underlying psychiatric disorders. However, it also depends on the existence of a milieu that is respectful, affirming, hope inspiring, and attuned to discerning and responding to the changing states and particular needs of all patients. It may include special environments such as "comfort rooms" stocked with sensory modulation materials that may soothe patients who are experiencing unbearable psychological anguish (see Chapter 18, "Improving Safety in Mental Health Treatment Settings," by Huckshorn and LeBel). It may include group therapy using techniques such as dialectical behavioral therapy that have been shown to reduce suicidal thinking in selected populations (Linehan 1999). It is also a milieu in which staff are aware of the need to remain vigilant about the risk of self-harm and prepared to perform thorough suicide risk assessments when appropriate.

Suicide Risk Assessment

Suicide prediction is difficult for many reasons. This is in large measure because the community incidence in the United States is about 11 per 100,000 per year; at this rate, even an unrealistically effective predictor (e.g., one with false-negative and false-positive rates of 1%, respectively) would only correctly predict about 20% of suicides (MacKinnon and Faberow 1975). Even retrospective studies of in-hospital suicides have failed to identify risk indicators that would have allowed for the prediction and prevention of studied suicidal events (Powell et al. 2000).

Despite these odds it is necessary to try to identify persons at risk so that preventive measures can be instituted. Several demographic and historical factors have been shown to be associated with increased risk of suicide in studies of large populations. These factors include age (risk increases with age in the United States), sex (men commit suicide more often than women), race (Caucasians commit suicide more often than non-Caucasians), past suicide attempts, alcoholism, and a family history of suicide or suicide attempts (American Psychiatric Association 2003). These are of epidemiological interest and help identify cohorts of persons at an increased risk of dying by suicide at some point in the future. However, even large and complex instruments have limited predictive value (Pokorny 1983), and the task in the hospital of course is not to predict ultimate prognosis but to determine who is at special risk in the hospital during this admission. So what can be done by way of suicide risk assessment in the hospital?

Early risk assessment scales were inventories of demographic risk factors (Range and Knott 1997) with little, if any, documented reliability and limited demonstration of validity. The next generation of scales included some that were much more extensively researched. Prominent among these is the Scale for Suicide Ideation (Beck et al. 1979; Table 19–1). This scale shows excellent reliability as well as good discriminant, construct, and convergent validity. Predictive validity—what we are most interested in—is relatively weak; of all the items, only the hopelessness item predicted *eventual* suicide in a 10-year prospective study (Beck et al. 1985).

A number of other scales have been developed in research settings and have received variable levels of empirical validation (Linehan et al. 1983). Although useful research tools, they are too lengthy to be acceptable for routine use in most inpatient settings and in any case have not been shown to predict in-hospital suicide risk.

A handful of shorter instruments have the advantage of being potentially more practical for use in fast-paced treatment environments. These instruments include the SAD PERSONS scale (Patterson et al. 1983), the Nurses' Global Assessment of Suicide Risk (Cutcliffe and Barker 2004), the Positive and Negative Suicide Ideation Inventory (Osman et al. 2002), and the Scale for Assessing Suicide Risk of Attempted Suicide (Tuckman and Youngman 1968). The features of these scales are summarized in Table 19–1. Although they may prove helpful in various settings, it is important to recognize that the clinical utility of all such instruments is "limited [due to] high false positive and false negative rates and…very low positive predictive value…. As a result, such rating scales cannot substitute for thoughtful and clinically appropriate evaluation and are not recommended for clinical estimations of suicide risk" (American Psychiatric Association 2003, p. 11).

Sheppard Pratt Suicide Risk Assessment Instrument

The Sheppard Pratt Suicide Risk Assessment Instrument (SPSRAI; Figure 19–1) was designed not as a formal psychometric instrument but rather as a tool to remind clinicians to consider certain risk factors and protective factors in their decisions about observation levels for newly admitted inpatients. It does not dic-

tate clinical decisions; clinicians are left to use clinical judgment about the selection of interventions. However, it does ask them to make their judgments after taking these factors into account.

The risk factors are grouped into three categories: 1) expressed intentions (i.e., what the person is expressing explicitly by word or deed about suicidal intent), 2) mental status findings, and 3) aspects of history. Because each of these risk factors should come to light in the course of a thorough psychiatric evaluation (e.g., history and mental status examination), it is expected that the clinician will be able to answer most, if not all, of these questions after completing the evaluation and that little, if any, additional time will be required at the end of the interview to complete the SPSRAI.

Expressed Intentions

There are three expressed intentions questions on the SPSRAI: Has the person made a recent suicide attempt? Does the person have current suicidal intent? Does the person have an actionable plan? A recent suicide attempt is very common among inpatients; it is often the reason for admission. This factor is important because a history of a suicide attempt is one of the strongest predictors of subsequent attempts (American Psychiatric Association 2003).

Current intent and a plan to commit suicide that can be implemented in the hospital have undeniable face validity as clinical facts that should influence hospital management, especially the level of observation. Ordinarily the combination of current intent and an actionable plan should occasion the highest level of observation.

Mental Status Findings

The SPSRAI includes six mental status findings that are believed to have a bearing on risk. Of these, as noted earlier, hopelessness is the best-documented predictor of completed suicide (Beck et al. 1985). The rest of the features have face validity as predictors and are commonly cited as important modulators of risk but have limited empirical support as predictors of in-hospital risk. These include psychosis (Busch et al. 2003), a wish for death, self-hatred, agitation (Busch et al. 2003), and psychic pain. The latter two borrow from the insightful work of Schneidman (1999) and correspond to his notions of perturbation and "psychache." The presence of these factors should lead the clinician to consider instituting a more intensive level of observation even in the absence of expressed intentions to hurt oneself—because many patients who go

TABLE 19–1. Suicide risk assessment instruments

Overview	Design	Risk factors assessed	Scoring	Comment
Scale for Suicide Ideation				
This scale was developed to assess intensity of suicidal intentions.	19-item scale with an emphasis on psychological variables	Wish to live Wish to die Reasons for living/dying Desire to make active attempt Passive death wish Duration of ideation Frequency of ideation Attitude toward ideation Control over suicidal action Deterrents to active attempt Reason for attempt Planning for attempt Opportunity for attempt Capability to carry out attempt Anticipation of actual attempt Preparation for attempt Suicide note Final acts in preparation for death Concealment of contemplated attempt	Scores for each item range from 0 (lowest intensity of suicidal ideation) to 2 (highest intensity of suicidal ideation).	Higher total scores indicate more intense suicidal ideation and presumably greater suicide risk.
Nurses' Global Assessment of Suicide Risk				
This scale was developed in a mental health unit in the United Kingdom to help nurses, especially "novice nurses," evaluate suicide risk and determine the appropriate level of "engagement."	15-item observer-rated checklist of demographic, psychological, and social features that have been shown to modulate risk of suicide	Presence/influence of hopelessness* Recent stressful life event Persecutory voices/beliefs Depression/loss of interest/anhedonia* Withdrawal Warning of suicidal intent Suicide plan* Family history of serious psychiatric illness or suicide Recent bereavement or relationship loss* History of psychosis Widow/widower Prior suicide attempt* Socioeconomic deprivation Alcoholism/alcohol misuse Terminal illness	The presence of a risk factor followed by * earns 3 points; all others earn 1 point. 5 or less: Low risk 6–8: Intermediate risk 9–11: High risk 12+: Very high Higher levels of estimated risk call for greater "engagement" by clinical staff.	Face validity and content validity have been evaluated. Predictive validity has not been well studied as yet. It presently is used in inpatient settings in the United Kingdom and is part of the Tidal Model pilot assessment procedure.

TABLE 19–1. Suicide risk assessment instruments *(continued)*

Overview	Design	Risk factors assessed	Scoring	Comment
Positive and Negative Suicide Ideation (PANSI) Inventory				
The PANSI is intended to measure both "negative" (risk) and "positive" (protective) factors. Initial items were generated in part from adolescent and college-age men and women, with subsequent refinement using a more diverse population from a Midwestern university town.	14-item self-report scale (8 positive and 6 negative factors); time reference for rating items is "the past 2 weeks, including today"	*Positive Protective Factors:* "Felt you were in control" "Felt hopeful" "Felt excited" "Felt confident about abilities" "Felt life worth living" "Felt confident with plans" *Negative Risk Factors:* "Considered killing yourself" "Felt hopeless and wondered" "Felt unhappy" "Thought you could not accomplish" "Thought you could not find a solution" "Felt like a failure" "Thought problems were overwhelming" "Felt lonely"	A 5-point Likert scale is used: 1 (none of the time) to 5 (most of the time).	The development and validation of this scale predominantly utilized samples of adolescents and young adults residing in the Midwest; the findings may or may not be generalizable.
SAD PERSONS Scale				
This scale was designed to create a practical approach to assessing suicide risk that could be easily learned and remembered by medical students and nonpsychiatric physicians in general hospital settings.	10-item observer-rated scale	Sex (male) Age (≤19 or ≥45 years) Depression Previous attempts Ethanol abuse Rational thinking loss Social supports lacking Organized plan No spouse Sickness	The presence of a risk factor earns 1 risk point (e.g., 67-year-old man would receive 1 point each for sex and age).	Suggested interventions are as follows: 0–2 points: Allow the patient to go home and follow up with a clinician. 3–4 points: Do close follow-up and consider hospitalization. 5–6 points: *Strongly consider* hospitalization, depending on confidence in follow-up arrangements. 7–10 points: Definitely hospitalize.

TABLE 19–1.   Suicide risk assessment instruments (*continued*)

Overview	Design	Risk factors assessed	Scoring	Comment
Scale for Assessing Suicide Risk of Attempted Suicide				
This scale was devised to rate the risk of eventual completed suicide in individuals who attempted suicide. The sample consisted of 3,800 individuals who survived a suicide attempt between 1959 and 1966. Of these, 48 went on to commit suicide during the follow-up period.	17-item scale of mainly demographic features	Age ≥45 years Male White Separated, divorced, or widowed Living alone Unemployed, retired Poor physical health Psychiatric illness Medical care (within 6 months) Use of firearms, hanging, jumping, or drowning as method Attempt during warm month Attempt during day Attempt at home Immediate discovery No mention of intention Suicide note left Previous threat or attempt	The simple unweighted scoring method assigns a value of 1 to each risk factor.	In this study, the unweighted score was a good predictor of eventual suicide rate as expressed in suicides per 1,000 suicide attempters. Score (rate/1,000 attempters): 0–1: 0.00 2–5: 6.98 6–9: 19.61 10–12: 60.61

·*Sheppard Pratt*
A not-for-profit behavioral health system

ADDRESSOGRAPH

SUICIDE ASSESSMENT

This form should be completed:

1. Upon Admission as part of the nursing assessment

2. By the physician when a patient / resident on Intensive Suicidal Observation, Suicidal Observation, or Constant Observation (for suicidality) is assessed for change to a less restrictive status.

	CATEGORY	DESCRIPTION	YES	NO
1.	Recent suicide attempt?	Seriously attempted suicide immediately prior to hospitalization	❏	❏
2.	Imminent suicidal intent?	Currently expressing a desire to kill self in hospital	❏	❏
3.	Actionable plan?	Has specific plan that can be acted upon in the hospital	❏	❏
4.	Psychological pain or anguish?	Shows signs of extreme psychological discomfort	❏	❏
5.	Self-hatred?	Shows signs of extremely poor self-esteem and feelings of worthlessness and guilt	❏	❏
6.	Hopelessness?	Does not believe that he/she will ever feel better	❏	❏
7.	Agitation?	Is visibly restless and tense	❏	❏
8.	Psychosis?	Has delusions, especially delusional guilt, or hallucinations	❏	❏
9.	Wish for death?	Feels death would bring relief	❏	❏
10.	Family / Peer suicidal history?	Has a history of suicidal attempts or successful suicide by family members / friends	❏	❏
11.	Poor Social Support?	Lacks social support from:		
		1. friends and relatives;	❏	❏
		2. meaningful employment and/or school	❏	❏
		3. religious support systems	❏	❏
12.	Substance abuse?	Has recent history of substance abuse or dependence	❏	❏
13.	Recent severe stressor?	Has experienced a devastating loss, disappointment or threat	❏	❏

Questions 1 - 3 ask about the patient's intentions, expressed in words or behavior.

If the answer is Yes to items 1, 2, or 3, a high level of observation should be considered. If the answer is Yes to items 2 and 3, ISO should be ordered unless an equally intensive but more individualized plan is preferred; if so, the reasons for the choice should be clearly documented.

Questions 4 - 9 ask about features of the patient's mental status.

If the answer is Yes to one or several of items 4 - 9, a high level of observation should be considered even if the patient / resident denies suicidal thoughts.

Questions 10 - 13 ask about aspects of the patient's history.

If the answer is Yes to item 13, a high level of observation may be appropriate even if the patient / resident denies suicidal thoughts, especially if the answer is Yes to any of the items 4 - 9.

OBTAINING A "SAFETY CONTRACT" IS NEVER BY ITSELF AN ADEQUATE ASSESSMENT OF SUICIDE RISK.

Remember to document all interventions in the patient's / resident's medical record.

Print Name _____

Signature _____ Date _____

0101040 SPHS /R 11/01/20061

FIGURE 19–1. Sheppard Pratt Suicide Risk Assessment Instrument (SPSRAI).

Source. Copyright 2006, Sheppard Pratt Health System, Inc. All rights reserved.

on to commit suicide in hospitals show these painful symptoms but deny suicidal intentions when asked about them directly (Busch et al. 2003).

Selected Aspects of History

The selected aspects of history include a history of alcohol or drug abuse, a history of suicide in a friend or relative, a recent severe stressor, and the absence of social support from individuals, employment, or religious affiliation. Lack of support is really the absence of significant protective factors, because it is widely believed that social support from individuals, employment, and religion makes suicide less likely to occur (American Psychiatric Association 2003).

Use of the Instrument

The recommended practice in our hospital is that the assessment is performed at the time of admission and that staff are alert to changes in status along these dimensions during the hospitalization. There should be a formal reassessment whenever there is consideration of making the level of observation less intensive. Other times when it is important to perform and document such an assessment are when the patient's mental status changes suddenly and when acute psychosocial stresses come to light in the course of the hospitalization (American Psychiatric Association 2003).

Special Precautions

Frequency and Proximity of Observation

When the clinician performing the suicide assessment arrives at the judgment that the patient poses imminent risk of suicide in the hospital, the usual response is to place the patient under an intensive form of observation. Patients deemed at the highest level of risk may need the full attention of a staff member stationed no more than one arm's length away at all times; this is sometimes termed *one-to-one* or *intensive suicidal observation*. Patients presenting lower levels of risk may be placed under continuous observation (i.e., always directly in view of an assigned staff member) or may be subject to documented checks at intervals of no greater than 5, 10, or 15 minutes. Such checks should not occur at predictable times (e.g., not exactly every 5, 10, or 15 minutes) and should be documented as they occur.

Setting of Observation

Inpatients who pose imminent risk of suicide can generally be treated in the milieu. Under rare circumstances they may require separation from other patients, but under no circumstances should suicidal patients be left "in seclusion" alone and unobserved. Private rooms may be appropriate places for such observation, but it is important to be mindful of the risks associated with such commonplace features as windows (Can patients break through?), windowsills (Can patients stand on them and jump to the floor?), walls (Can patients strike them with their heads?), ventilation grating (Can metal elements be broken free and used for cutting?), wall-mounted fixtures (Can patients hang from them using cords, clothing, or bedding?), movable furniture (Can it be used as a barricade or as a platform on which patients can stand to get access to ceiling-mounted fixtures?), and doors (virtually every door is a potential gallows).

Access to Clothing and Belongings

Suicidal patients may harm themselves in countless ways; it is impossible to anticipate every conceivable method. Because hanging is a common method of inpatient suicide, it is important to control the access of suicidal inpatients to belts, ropes, cords, and even clothing that might prove a ready means of hanging. It is important to remember that belts, sheeting, and other forms of clothing can be used for self-asphyxiation even in the absence of a fixture from which to hang; self-asphyxiation may be accomplished by swallowing material in a manner that occludes the oropharynx or by tying a belt or article of clothing around the neck and cinching it tightly in a manner that holds it in place and effectively compresses the trachea. It is also important to be aware that inpatients may stockpile medications (administered but not swallowed) and hide them in mattresses, wadded paper in wastebaskets, and even body cavities and use them for suicidal overdoses.

Policies

Inpatient units must make decisions about the types of observation options to utilize, the settings in which to implement them, and the limitations on access to clothing and other belongings that should be applied when the clinician makes the judgment that the risk of suicide is high and immediate. These decisions should be formalized into policies with which staff members become familiar at the time of orientation and about which they receive regular in-service training.

Suicide-Prevention Contracts

Clinicians sometimes ask their inpatients to "contract for safety" or to commit to a "no-suicide contract"—that is, a promise to refrain from suicidal behavior and to inform the treatment team if they become unable to control the urge to engage in self-harm (Martin 1999). Such a measure may be a way of pursuing inquiry into the patient's intentions or a way of communicating concern for safety, particularly when there is a strong therapeutic alliance. However, because it only touches on a patient's intentions with regard to suicidal behavior (i.e., expressed intentions) and does not take into account relevant aspects of mental status or history, the safety contract does not in itself constitute a complete assessment of suicide risk. It also does not protect the clinician against potential liability in the event that the patient commits suicide. Thus, such a contract cannot be viewed as a substitute for the performance and documentation of a thorough suicide risk assessment (American Psychiatric Association 2003).

Conclusion

As many as 1,500 inpatient suicides may occur annually, and inpatient suicide remains one of the most commonly reported Joint Commission sentinel events. Because many persons receiving inpatient psychiatric care continue to be at risk of harming themselves after admission, certain measures (i.e., "universal precautions") are appropriate in virtually all hospital settings. These include physical environments that are free of ready access to common means of inpatient suicide, clinical milieus that provide timely relief of symptoms that may precipitate suicide attempts, and careful assessments of suicide risk that are made at the time of admission and at critical junctures thereafter. Although there is no scale or set of risk factors that reliably predicts inpatient suicide, it is generally agreed that a thorough suicide risk assessment includes consideration of the patient's expressed intentions, the presence of certain mental status findings, and certain psychosocial, demographic, and historical features. Many of these are aggregated in the SPSRAI, a tool that is designed to cue the clinician to consider all these factors—*not only expressed intentions*—in arriving at an estimation of suicide risk and a decision about which, if any, special suicide precautions may be necessary. *A "safety contract" by itself does not constitute an adequate suicide risk assessment.* When a patient is esti-

mated to pose high risk of suicide in the hospital, a variety of special precautions may be instituted; most often these include—at a minimum—intensive levels of observation, restricted access to personal belongings, and a reconsideration of the treatment plan. Unfortunately, such measures will not prevent all instances of inpatient suicide, but a systematic effort to create an "antisuicidal" environment and a therapeutic program, including thorough and timely suicide risk assessments, will reduce clinical risk and legal liability and will serve to reassure the staff that everything possible is being done to prevent this most tragic and demoralizing complication of psychiatric illness.

References

American Psychiatric Association: Practice Guideline for the Assessment and Treatment of Patients With Suicidal Behaviors. Washington, DC, American Psychiatric Publishing, 2003

Beck AT, Kovacs M, Weismann A: Assessment of suicide intention: the Scale for Suicide Ideation. J Consult Clin Psychol 47:343–352, 1979

Beck AT, Steer RA, Kovacs M, et al: Hopelessness and eventual suicide: a 10-year prospective study of patients hospitalized with suicidal ideation. Am J Psychiatry 142:559–563, 1985

Busch KA, Fawcett J, Jacobs DG: Clinical correlates of inpatient suicide. J Clin Psychiatry 64:14–19, 2003

Cutcliffe JR, Barker P: The Nurses' Global Assessment of Suicide Risk (NGASR): developing a tool for clinical practice. J Psychiatr Ment Health Nurs 11:393–400, 2004

Joint Commission: Sentinel Event Statistics. Oakbrook Terrace, IL, The Joint Commission, 2007. Available at: http://www.jointcommission.org/NR/rdonlyres/DB894476-8834-4798-AA11-77E4FC3F1D78/0/SE_Stats_033107.pdf. Accessed September 18, 2007.

Linehan MM: Standard protocol for assessing and treating suicidal behaviors for patients in treatment, in Harvard Medical School Guide to Suicide Assessment and Intervention. Edited by Jacobs D. San Francisco, CA, Jossey-Bass, 1999, pp 83–97

Linehan MM, Goodstein JL, Neilsen SL, et al: Reasons for staying alive when you are thinking of killing yourself: the Reasons for Living Inventory. J Consult Clin Psychol 52:276–286, 1983

MacKinnon D, Faberow NL: An assessment of the utility of suicide prediction. Suicide Life Threat Behav 6:86–91, 1975

Martin MC: Suicide-prevention contracts: advantages, disadvantages, and an alternative approach, in Harvard Medical School Guide to Suicide Assessment and Intervention. Edited by Jacobs D. San Francisco, CA, Jossey-Bass, 1999, pp 463–482

Morgan HG, Priest P: Suicide and other unexpected deaths among psychiatric inpatients: the Bristol confidential inquiry. Br J Psychiatry 158:368–374, 1991

Osman A, Barrios FX, Gutierrez PM, et al: The Positive and Negative Suicide Ideation (PANSI) Inventory: psychometric evaluation with adolescent psychiatric inpatient samples. J Pers Assess 79:512–530, 2002

Patterson WM, Dohn HH, Bird J, et al: Evaluation of suicidal patients: the SAD PERSONS scale. Psychosomatics 24:343–349, 1983

Pokorny AD: Prediction of suicide in psychiatric patients: report of a prospective study. Arch Gen Psychiatry 40:249–257, 1983

Powell J, Geddes J, Deeks J, et al: Suicide in psychiatric hospital inpatients. Br J Psychiatry 176:266–272, 2000

Range LM, Knott EC: Twenty suicide assessment instruments: evaluation and recommendations. Death Stud 21:25–58, 1997

Schneidman E: Perturbation and lethality, in Harvard Medical School Guide to Suicide Assessment and Intervention. Edited by Jacobs D. San Francisco, CA, Jossey-Bass, 1999, pp 83–97

Sine D, Hunt J: Guidelines for the Built Environment of Behavioral Health Facilities. Washington, DC, National Association of Psychiatric Health Systems, 2003. Available at: http://www.naphs.org/Teleconference/documents/REV9editedFINAL_001.pdf. Accessed September 18, 2007.

Tuckman J, Youngman WF: A scale for assessing suicidal risk of attempted suicide. J Clin Psychol 24:17–19, 1968

CHAPTER 20

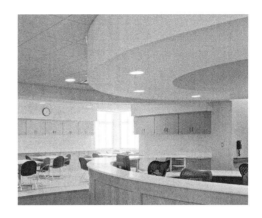

DISCHARGE DILEMMAS

John R. Lion, M.D.

Caretakers of today's hospitalized patients often find themselves uneasy about discharging those patients when insurance companies threaten to deny further care. Hospital stays have become very brief, thus affording acutely suicidal or homicidal patients little time for meaningful intrapsychic change. A week in-house may well remove the patient from a pathological family or relationship and relieve hostilities or despair, but the patient is apt to return to exactly what he or she left behind. A day hospital eases reentry, but not all patients are financially eligible for even this brief transition. Consequently, increasing numbers of patients are referred for consultation concerning the safety of discharge. Often this consultation is labeled "forensic," although rarely is there a legal problem. Instead, the issues at stake are clinical and pertain to dangerousness. Although the overt and recurring question posed is whether or not the patient is safe enough to leave the hospital, a persistent underlying anxiety pertains to a possible lawsuit and the clinician's major worry is that he or she will discharge a patient who will shortly thereafter harm him- or herself or others. Given the lack of intimate knowledge about the patient and his or her family, which could be

acquired by a lengthy hospital stay, staff face more unknowns. In a sense, the patient remains largely a stranger to those who observe him or her for only a few days or weeks. In past decades, relationships between doctors and nurses provided a measure of assurance when it came time to leave the hospital. Patients were weaned from the hospital slowly, first tested with overnight and weekend stays, and even allowed to have a job and return to the hospital at night. Graduated discharge of this sort has long passed as any standard of care. Yet even in these times of abbreviated stays, discharge from any psychiatric hospital is always a major psychological event. The hospital provides a nurturing milieu in sharp contrast to the homes and situations from which many patients come. Although the patient may clamor to be released, anxieties are high and expectations are frequently urgent and unrealistic.

On No Longer Being Suicidal

Assessing a patient's suicidality or intent to harm others is complex and cannot possibly be addressed by merely asking the patient a "yes" or "no" question. Yet this is the schematic whereby insurance providers allow or deny additional care. That a patient would come into the hospital because of an overdose and declare him- or herself no longer suicidal a few days later defies a certain credibility. True, the patient may no longer have the same lethal intent, but the profound underlying damaged self-esteem and rage toward the self still exist and are not eradicated by any pharmacological regimen or group therapy. They have merely, for the moment, subsided in strength. Unfortunately, the moment that patient professes to anyone that he or she no longer wants to commit suicide—and triggers a chart note to that effect—the discharge die is cast, even if the note is authored by the least trained member of the mental health staff. A reviewer is quick to seize upon such documentation. An attempt to undo such a statement requires a consultant with expertise in suicidal behavior. That consultant's report may be used as a bargaining chip to keep the patient longer, but too often the extension of stay is a token gesture of a few days. Although insurance companies may understand the prophylaxis of intensive treatment for heart or renal disease, they are not persuaded that the urge to die is deeply configured within the patient who considers or attempts it. In a sense, suicidality never fully disappears as a psychic agenda; it ebbs and flows, as does the urge to physically harm others. Unfortunately, the great pressure to admit and discharge patients from the hospital has obliterated the enormity of the problem. Some clinicians come to accept an insurance industry–driven view of mental illness to the point of being cavalier. They may have a secretary call to schedule the "forensic consult" as a mere perfunctory measure and be absent when it takes place. Other clinicians themselves call for the consultation and, more anguished about the fragility of discharge events, seek the consultant's view of existing risk factors such as a spouse who still wishes to leave the marriage, the patient's own motivation for therapy, the presence of delusions, and so forth. In the end, however, a decision must be reached as to whether the patient is acutely dangerous. *Acutely dangerous* generally invokes the concept of "imminent." Much has been written about the medicolegal complexity of this term (Simon 2006); in brief, one practical definition is that *imminent* means hours or days, not weeks or months. Thus having decided that a patient is not imminently dangerous, the clinician can presumably discharge the patient without worry about the long-term future. Yet does any time parameter really protect a caretaker from being sued? The matter is not simple. The greater the interval is between discharge and an

unfortunate event, the less likely it would seem that the clinician can be blamed for his or her decision to release the patient. In reality, doctors can be sued for the acts of their patients committed months and years later, even though the causality of events appears weaker and attendant publicity may be far less harsh. Sometimes, patients are generically classified as high or low risk on the basis of a checklist of behaviors such as previous violence, alcohol use, delusions, command hallucinations, and the like (Lion 2003). A high risk "score" leads to retention in the hospital, whereas a low risk justifies discharge. Risk factors are surely important on their own, but an actual description of what constitutes the specific danger is more clinically useful than assigning the patient a generic category. Besides, these days many patients are discharged with a significant degree of risk anyway, thus diluting the utility of the term.

Limitations of the Database

Risk assessment relies upon certain facts both observed by talking with the patient and obtained from information related by nurses and social work staff. Surprisingly, the medical record or chart is a limited source of information. This is because chart notes are often reductionistic and frequently redundant ("Patient doing better, interacted well on the unit, attended group therapy"). Under the pressure of time, process descriptions of patients' illnesses have given way to objective statements of behavior. The following case example illustrates these complexities.

> A mildly retarded adolescent was admitted after threatening to burn down the group home in which she resided. She had been in many homes and was often expelled from them for insubordinate behavior and fighting. She had made previous statements about burning down the places in which she had lived, but to the extent it could be determined, no fires had actually ever been set. She had been arrested once as a minor for a marijuana charge. Within the hospital, she was sullen and slept as much as she could. She participated minimally in any ward activities and steadfastly denied that she had ever threatened fires. She presented as a mildly angry young woman with no insight and an adamant desire to leave the hospital and return to the home from which she had come. The home agreed to take her back.

The issues here obviously pertain to the risk of a very dangerous behavior, but data to support the dangerousness were lacking. Given all the predictive factors available for the assessment of violence, the past history of violence still remains as a prime determinant (Monahan et al. 2001). Another factor is drug abuse. In this case, there is a history of cannabis use, but such usage is rarely accompanied by assaultive behavior, as opposed to alcohol, the substance ubiquitously associated with all forms of violence. Absent any demonstration of aggressiveness on the ward and only a chronically sullen demeanor, verbalized threats were the only data on which to base an assessment of risk. In such instances, staff impressions are important. The consultant can solicit various views of individual staff members or attend a staff meeting to gather a consensus. In the end, however, risk relates to where the patient is actually discharged. Discharging a patient in the community at large or to an uneducated family carries many unknowns. Lack of supervision is likewise itself a risk. When unsure, discharge to a structured setting such as day care or a halfway house allows for more observation and reduces risk. A group home, such as the one the patient ultimately went to, offers safeguards, albeit limited ones and for a short time only. The next case illustrates more dire circumstances associated with discharge in the face of limited data.

> An 18-year-old brain-damaged and immature man was admitted after threatening to assault the grandparents with whom he lived. He had destroyed property as well. Both grandparents left insistent messages on the social worker's phone to the effect that he was not safe to ever return home. Even the man's biological mother, who lived apart from her son, left such warnings. The man himself had been arrested for stealing a motorcycle and had a history of drug abuse. On admission, he had been paranoid and delusional. Suicidal threats had also been uttered, although on examination he denied both homicidal and suicidal urges. The man talked vaguely about having set a fire in his home but refused to elaborate, and no further information could be obtained.

This case posed more serious problems of risk, not only because of previous violence toward property but also because the patient had been psychotic as a result of his drug abuse. However, an overwhelming issue affecting risk was the massive rejection from his entire family. The fire-setting incident could not be investigated in the short time he remained on the ward, a rather typical occurrence unless the crime can be identified. Some states, such as Maryland, have public Web sites for criminal convictions. In light of the patient's prior history of homelessness, his apparent use of a drug that was thought to induce a psychotic state, and the repudiation of his grandparents and mother, it was obvious that he required some form of continued partial hospitalization. He was transferred to a quarter-way house but immediately eloped from that facility. Staff promptly wondered about seeking an emergency petition whereby he would be detained by the police and brought to a local emergency department for examination. In such situations, it is often useful to envision worst-case scenarios as a measure of dangerousness. For example, it was presented to the staff that the man could go to the very home in which he was not wanted, start an argument, and become homicidal. His rage could be fueled by illicit drugs. Liability appeared very great, particularly because family members had specifically told staff that they feared him and did not wish him back. In light of these considerations, it was decided that the hospital would be better served if staff acted proactively and filed an emergency petition. Fantasizing outcomes is an important process in risk assessment, although consultants must appreciate that discussions of worst-case scenarios may well evoke anxiety in staff. Still, under the pressure of discharge and the rapidity of patient turnover, treating clinicians may feel themselves to be mere triage agents who address the acute crisis only, leaving the patient to be followed by "someone else." Regrettably, finding a place to send a patient for further treatment is far more time-consuming than hospital treatment itself. Limited time also enters the equation when carefully documenting the reasoning for discharge in the face of certain dangers. Liability is generated when no record is made of a risk decision that goes awry. If, instead, the clinician notes the parameters of the risk and articulates the decision-making process, malpractice is far less apt to be successfully proven in a legal action. All too often, the chart may contain numerous admission entries regarding the patient's suicidal thoughts. Subsequent progress notes then benignly comment on the patient's behaviors within the hospital up to the time of discharge, without further mention of what happened to the patient's original desire to harm him- or herself; to the outside observer, the suicidal thoughts or intentions have simply evaporated or, far worse, been ignored by staff. For example, a discharge note should state: "Patient's threat to himself temporarily resolved by meetings with girlfriend. He is no longer acutely suicidal. Girlfriend more aware of hazards of ambivalence in her behavior toward patient. Weapons removed from home. Patient scheduled for visit with outpatient psychiatrist at end of week and will attend Alcoholics Anonymous. Risk factors and readiness for discharge reviewed by consultant."

Pathological Attachments

Cases in which the patient is admitted because he or she is suicidal or homicidal after the breakup of a romance are common and pose significant discharge problems. For one thing, the patient has been removed from the source of the agony and, for the moment at least, is not confronted with the rejection. Thus the hospital is not a true test of what will happen once discharge occurs and the patient returns to the community. Second, the rejecting lover may be ambivalent about ending the affair. Third, the mere fact that the rejection has spawned suicidality reflects the patient's own inner depletion and hopelessness. Thus the patient is already at risk for self-harm. Here the social worker member of the staff is most helpful to the evaluating consultant by advising him or her about the true finality of the breakup and whether rejector or rejectee are still in contact with one another. The following case illustrates these issues.

> A 31-year-old unmarried man was admitted for homicidal and suicidal ideation after he witnessed his prostitute girlfriend performing sex with another customer. The patient had fully recognized her profession, and he had been able to use denial in watching her enter cars and drive off with clients. However, when he actually saw what she did, his rage erupted. He hit her before police intervened to have him hospitalized, and he threatened her with his revolver. In the past, the patient had cut his wrists and overdosed. The girlfriend called him at the hospital to inquire how he was. On the ward, the patient denied any further desire to harm her and declared that he was ready to leave.

This patient had reached a certain tenuous equilibrium that, unfortunately, is the hallmark of today's criteria for discharge. His insurance company continually demanded to know if he was still dangerous and when told by the treating doctor that he indeed was, reluctantly granted him an additional few days of stay. Perhaps the chief utility of these added days was to arrange a meeting with the girlfriend to assess how aware she really was of the patient's dangerousness and what role her behavior played in the matter. Meetings of this sort remain crucial parameters to assessing the risk of discharge. When such a meeting is not possible or successful, and little dynamic change has occurred in either party, then the issue of a *Tarasoff* warning is always raised (Gellerman and Suddath 2007). Yet a formal warning is always clinically inferior to any insights that could be achieved through a therapy session involving the perpetrator and victim.

In this case, staff felt sufficiently hopeful in pointing out the pathological interactions between patient and girlfriend that discharge seemed possible. It should be stated that long-term abusive relationships pose particular discharge problems because the hospitalized patient is almost always quickly remorseful and as eager to return home as the victimized spouse is to have him back. The clinician must recognize that nothing has actually changed between both parties and that the possibility of violence remains high, even though it may not be acute. Thus, consideration should be given to discharging the patient to a partial care facility, always an unpopular choice in these circumstances, when both parties are so needful of one another.

Victims

The next two cases highlight the crucial matter of working with potential victims.

> A 30-year-old worker was angry with his manager for bypassing him in a promotion. He was a paranoid man and harbored vague thoughts of harming the manager. He owned a gun. The patient was not deemed to be acutely homicidal, but staff were still divided about how to handle the discharge. Some felt a formal warning to the manager was indicated, whereas others thought that such a tactic would worsen the situation by possibly leading the manager to fire the patient. The resolution appeared possible by having the patient call the manager himself, verbalizing how unfairly he felt he had been treated and asking how the situation could be remedied. This intervention proved successful by making the patient feel far less helpless.

A controversy existed as to whether having the patient confront the manager would be ameliorative of risk or worsen the situation. This is always an issue when little or nothing is known about how a victim would react. It is a compelling argument for supervised meetings within the hospital with staff present. Confrontations between patient and victim are best prepared by rehearsal, such as role playing, so that the patient can, to some extent, anticipate the would-be victim's negative reactions. Anxiolytic medication may be useful in preparation for the meeting or, in this case, the phone call. In some cases, this interaction with the victim almost entirely dictates the outcome of the case and the disposition at discharge. The following case example illustrates this principle of assessing dangerousness not by concentrating on the patient but by focusing on the victim's specific intentions at the time of discharge.

A 30-year-old woman with bipolar illness attempted to buy poison and was intercepted by the police when the merchant reported the act. Questioned by authorities, she related that she had intended to kill her husband because he had refused to help her reduce a large debt she had incurred during a manic episode. The husband's immediate reaction was to announce his intent to divorce her, but he reconsidered and, according to the patient, decided that he would accept her back home after hospitalization. The clinician caring for the patient asked for a consultation to determine the patient's safety for discharge. He had not met with the husband and considered the latter somewhat irrelevant to the problem of danger.

Here, much hinged upon the husband's decision, its lack of clarity, and the preciseness of his communication with the patient. The patient could certainly not be discharged outright to her home if the husband still harbored the decision to separate or divorce. On the other hand, an unmitigated decision on his part to take her back in the face of her homicidal intent seemed most unusual and would surely require exploration. Thus, much work needed to be done to evaluate the husband's mental state as well as the patient's, and some degree of finality about the marriage was a prerequisite to safe discharge. In any event, the patient needed to be discharged to a partial care facility that could monitor both her unstable mood disorder and her deranged thinking.

"Copycat" and Threat Cases

Highly notarized school shootings consistently evoke copycat threats in a small group of students who come to the attention of teachers or counselors and are urgently hospitalized. In most cases, the behaviors reflect the poverty of judgment associated with immaturity or a highly pathological need for attention which, although alarming, is not reflective of true dangerousness. However, a small percentage of this population represents difficult risk assessments because the student's preoccupation with violence appears excessive. The following case example illustrates this matter.

Following the Virginia Tech massacre of students, a 15-year-old student was hospitalized after stating that he wished more students had died. He further stated that he wanted to procure an assault rifle, and this prompted police intervention. His parents related a history of his mutilating animals and found a collection of news clippings from the Columbine killings. The patient himself presented with a chillingly flat affect and inappropriate smiling as he related his desire to block the doors of the school cafeteria to trap students he would then kill. He was ultimately discharged to a partial care facility.

The dismay of hospital staff caring for this patient was palpable, particularly in light of the fact that the college shootings had occurred only a month earlier. The boy himself had received a diagnosis of Asperger's syndrome, further alarming all concerned because they saw a patient who had few social skills and little empathy. Although well behaved within the hospital, he remained quite aloof on the ward and inappropriately related his story to anyone who would listen. His father owned weapons that, despite all that had occurred, were still in the home. This fact alone heightened the patient's dangerousness and is a variable about which inquiry should routinely be made. Contributing to the patient's high risk was his emotional coldness. Absent from the case was a "hit" list, as sometimes seen in would-be school shooting cases where students write down names of others they are angry with, or any bizarre drawings of mutilation or dismemberment, as are also sometimes found. The consultant should always ask about such items, because a preoccupation with the imagery of violence or the construction of a list of victims may represent a preparatory step to the actual act. It is also the task of the evaluating clinician to ascertain to what extent the threatener is physically capable of carrying out the act. In the case of bomb threats, for example, the student may have read about the construction of the device on the Internet but has not collected any of the necessary ingredients to make him or her an acute danger. A related problem occurs when students make threats to hurt teachers or harm school property and, upon examination, deny true intent or claim the threat to be a joke or prank. Here the consultant must remember that whether the threat is actual or not, the mere verbalization of it represents deviant judgment that must be explored. Meetings with parents or caretakers are almost always indicated. Although nowadays arranged with difficulty, psychometric assessment with an emphasis on projective testing can shed some light on both the primitiveness of the patient's thinking and his or her preoccupation with themes of violence.

Sexual Predatoriness

Patients who find their way into the hospital because of sexual concerns typically have comorbid illnesses such as mania or mental retardation. On rare occasions, an attorney may advise a client to enter the hospital to impress the court or as an alternative to incarceration.

Patients with a pure paraphiliac condition, such as pedophilia, should always be considered high-risk cases because the disordered behavior carries with it a high degree of recidivism (Laws and O'Donohue 1997). More passive criminal acts, such as exhibitionism, carry a smaller risk of escalating into predatory acts. On the matter of discharging patients to the police, this should be carefully orchestrated so that sufficient numbers of staff are present as a show of force. Occasionally, a patient may threaten suicide as a means of forestalling the arrest or detention that will occur upon discharge. To distinguish true intent from manipulativeness can be difficult, and it becomes untenable to keep the patient in the hospital indefinitely while incarceration looms as the inevitable outcome. Assuming there is no treatable depression, one strategy is to ultimately discharge the patient with a written communication to authorities that a suicidal threat has been made. Such threats are familiar to prison officials who have some skills in management. On occasion, a male patient may be admitted for assessment of risk in connection with some inappropriate touching that has occurred in an institutional setting, or the patient may have made inappropriate sexual remarks with content alluding to violence, such as rape. Admissions of this type are typically charged with high emotions. Veiled threats about the potential sequelae of premature discharge can be made by the potential victim and his or her family or spouse. Denial is apt to be the rule, and an absence of insight is almost invariably present. The following example is illustrative.

> A 13-year-old boy with Asperger's syndrome was urgently admitted after telephoning a neighbor's daughter and threatening to rape her and get her pregnant. On the hospital unit, he remarked to a pregnant staff member that he wished to cut out her fetus. He smiled as he related this incident and had virtually no awareness of the impact of his actions.

Had this boy been older, the risks of discharge would be considerably higher than they were. Nonetheless, staff were worried not so much about the physical act of rape but about his again threatening his victim, given his impoverished social skills and lack of introspectiveness. In meetings with staff, it became apparent that there existed some communication between the victimized girl's parents and the patient's parents. That being the case, the suggestion was made that the girl's parents obtain an unlisted phone number, a simple maneuver that would have a greater deterrent effect than any intervention with the patient. Additionally, discussion ensued regarding how the victim's family could somehow be included in a therapeutic meeting or otherwise be informed about the patient's condition without completely compromising privacy. These were admittedly unusual recourses, but they again emphasize the point that whenever the victim or victim's family can be brought into the picture, the better the clinical control becomes. Taking an adversarial stance in treating potentially dangerous patients by championing their privacy and excluding any intervention with a victim compromises a safe discharge.

Conclusion

Dangerousness is a common presenting behavior in today's hospitalized patients. The shortness of stay precludes the resolution of many conflicts that, at the time of discharge, remain worrisome. Rarely does suicidal or homicidal ideation simply disappear in the course of brief treatment. This, coupled with limited observational knowledge of the patient, imposes a higher level of stress on the hospital treatment team. Risk assessment encompasses not only the patient but also potential victims, and creative incorporation of the victim in discharge planning is important. Outright discharge is more the exception than the rule. Good documentation of the justifications for discharge is protective against litigation.

References

Gellerman DM, Suddath R: Violent fantasy, dangerousness, and the duty to warn and protect. J Am Acad Psychiatry Law 33:484–495, 2007

Laws DR, O'Donohue W (eds): Sexual Deviance: Theory, Assessment, and Treatment. New York, Guilford, 1997

Lion JR: A primer on workplace violence assessment for the front-line clinician. Clin Occup Environ Med 3:791–802, 2003

Monahan J, Steadman HJ, Silver E: Rethinking Risk Assessment: The MacArthur Study of Mental Disorder and Violence. Oxford, England, Oxford University Press, 2001

Simon R: The myth of "imminent" violence in psychiatry and the law. Univ Cincinnati Law Rev Winter:631–643, 2006

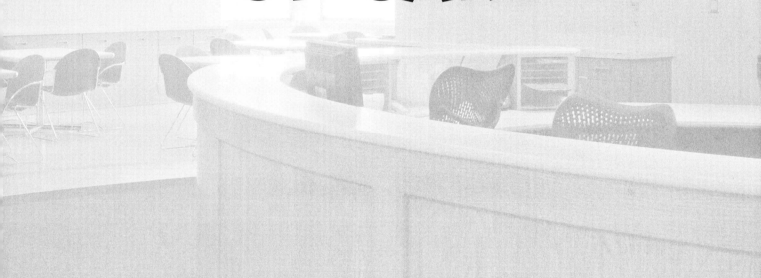

Part III

THE CONTINUUM OF CARE

CHAPTER 21

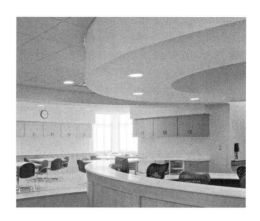

RESIDENTIAL PSYCHOTHERAPEUTIC TREATMENT

An Intensive Psychodynamic Approach for Patients With Treatment-Resistant Disorders

Edward R. Shapiro, M.D.
Eric M. Plakun, M.D.

Changes in Health Care and the Problem of Treatment Resistance

The transformation of both the delivery and funding of health care in the last part of the twentieth and early twenty-first centuries had a dramatic impact on the nature of hospital psychiatry. Increasing recognition of escalating health care costs led to the emergence of managed care, with a concomitant decrease in length of inpatient psychiatric stays, a shift in inpatient focus from definitive treatment to crisis intervention, more attention to biological treatments, and early discharge

planning aimed at moving patients quickly to less restrictive and usually outpatient settings. In response to these changes, a number of high-quality, long-term treatment centers closed their doors, patient readmissions to inpatient hospitals increased, and the doctor–patient relationship continued its transformation from an intimate encounter to a bureaucratically structured negotiation of the need and terms of treatment with third-party payers (Geller 2006; Plakun 1999; E.R. Shapiro 2001b).

Although many patients struggling with mental illness have benefited substantially from advances in biological treatments and short-term cognitive-behavioral interventions, available data indicate the limitations of these approaches. For example, perhaps one-third of patients with schizophrenia fail to respond or respond inadequately to antipsychotic medications (American Psychiatric Association 2004), whereas nearly 75% of patients in the Clinical Antipsychotic Trials in Intervention Effectiveness study discontinued the study medication regimen before 18 months of treatment (Lieberman et al. 2005). Between 15% and 50% of patients with mood disorders are treatment resistant (Foa and Davidson 1997; Thase et al. 2001), and only a minority of these fully recover on medications alone (Rush and Trivedi 1995). Results from the STAR*D trial of treatment for patients with major depressive disorder demonstrate that substantial numbers of patients fail to respond adequately either to initial treatment or various switch or augmentation strategies, including short-term cognitive-behavioral therapy (Thase et al. 2007). In adolescents with depression there are also significant rates of treatment resistance (Apter et al. 2005; Treatment for Adolescents With Depression Study Team 2003), and, for the subset of patients with chronic major depressive disorders and histories of serious childhood trauma or abuse, there is evidence that psychotherapy may be more effective than medication (Nemeroff et al. 2003).

For patients with bipolar disorder, the Systematic Treatment Enhancement Program for Bipolar Disorder study reports that only slightly more than half achieved recovery, and half of these had recurrences within 2 years (Perlis et al. 2006). Miklowitz et al. (2007) demonstrated that intensive longer-term psychosocial treatment as an adjunct to pharmacotherapy is more beneficial than brief treatment in enhancing stabilization from bipolar illness.

The presence of personality disorder—particularly borderline personality disorder—makes a significant contribution to treatment resistance in mood disorders. Data from the Collaborative Longitudinal Personality Disorder Study suggest that personality disorders adversely affect the prognosis of major depressive disorder and are in themselves significantly associated with persistent functional impairment, extensive treatment utilization, and significant risk of suicide (Bender et al. 2006; Skodol et al. 2005). It is not surprising, then, that treatment-resistant illnesses are expensive. The cost of treating patients with treatment-refractory mood disorders, for example, is 19 times higher than the cost associated with treating more responsive patients (Crown et al. 2002).

Patients with these treatment-resistant illnesses are often caught up in repeated and ongoing crises in their outpatient treatments with efforts to ward off the next suicide attempt or the need for another hospital stay. For some the risk of suicide has been the central issue keeping them in a state of crisis; for others it has been chronic inability to manage the transition from the role of child in the family to that of functioning and autonomous adult in the world.

In our own focus group discussions with graduating psychiatric residents and practitioners in New York City, Chicago, and Los Angeles, we heard the repeated view that patients with treatment-resistant illnesses were inevitably doomed to chronic crisis management. Many of these clinicians believed that there were no specialized resources for these patients beyond what they could find in their own urban setting or region.

Intensive Residential Treatment: The Austen Riggs Center

Longer-term treatment is generally utilized for those patients with disorders that fail to respond or respond inadequately to outpatient treatment and short-term inpatient settings or who have difficulty sustaining independent functioning. Several specialized inpatient settings offer longer-term treatment ranging from 1 to a few months (Menninger, Sheppard Pratt, McLean, and others), but for patients whose treatment-refractory disorders require a more extended period of treatment, residential programs with a continuum of care that allows progressive step-down in staffing intensity and cost, such as that provided at the Austen Riggs Center, are often required.

The range of available residential settings is fairly wide, including some programs offering primarily custodial care for patients whose illnesses fail to respond to usual treatment and have become chronic (often patients with psychotic spectrum or pervasive developmental disorders). Many of these programs are behaviorally focused, and some use token economies. Some longer-term residential programs offer a work environment with psychiatric support within a home, farm, or guesthouse milieu.

There is evidence, however, that for patients with severe personality disorders an extended residential treatment program with a psychodynamic focus and a continuum of care promotes social adaptation, reduces symptoms (including the frequency of self-harm and suicide attempts), and decreases the length and frequency of readmission (Chiesa et al. 2004). In addition, data from Austen Riggs (Fowler et al. 2004;

Plakun 2003; Perry et al., in press) suggest that longer-term psychodynamic residential treatment with step-down programs can be useful for that subset of patients with treatment-refractory Axis I disorders who have comorbid Axis II disorders—especially when there is a history of prominent early trauma, abuse, loss, deprivation, or neglect.

For this last group, treatment resistance is often a phenomenon related to personality pathology, ordinarily manifest in disturbances in interpersonal relatedness. Organizing treatment around these personality resistances offers a focused and precise intervention. This group of patients may be able to use a longer-term hospital or residential treatment that addresses these issues to overcome the chronic risk of suicide, achieve delayed age-appropriate role functioning, and take charge of their lives in a way that breaks the cycle of crisis and despair.

Intensive residential treatment for this population—offered at the Austen Riggs Center—adds to general psychiatric treatment a set of specialized and intensive individual, family, group, and milieu psychotherapeutic and psychosocial treatment components (Elmendorf and Parish 2007; Fromm 2006; Mintz and Belnap 2006; Muller 2007; Plakun 2006) intended to interrupt the often rageful cycles of failure these patients experience while providing an opportunity for them to take charge of their treatment and their lives in new ways.

The Patients

Who are these patients? The prospective, naturalistic, longitudinal Austen Riggs Center Follow-Along Study has been following 226 patients every 6–8 months during and after treatment at Riggs for a mean of 9 years. Our data indicate complex diagnostic comorbidity, with a mean of six Axis I and II disorders (Plakun 2003; Perry et al., in press). Fully 80% of the patients have treatment-refractory mood disorders that have failed to respond to standard interventions in inpatient and outpatient settings. More than 80% of patients also meet criteria for one or more personality disorders, most commonly borderline personality disorder. Two-thirds of patients have histories suggesting significant early adverse experiences of abuse, trauma, neglect, loss, or deprivation, and one-third meet criteria for posttraumatic stress disorder. Nearly half have substance use disorders complicating their clinical picture, and about one-quarter have symptoms of an eating disorder. About 15% present with psychotic spectrum disorders.

Beyond diagnosis, these patients typically have not been able to benefit from treatments of lesser intensity and have been unable to sustain functioning between outpatient sessions without the support of chronic crisis management. They demonstrate repeated struggles with authority deriving from early family dynamics, often presenting histories of family conflict around the management of relationships and generational role boundaries (Berkowitz et al. 1974; E.R. Shapiro 1982a; E.R. Shapiro and Freedman 1987; E.R. Shapiro et al. 1975). In response to problematic family dynamics, their struggles with authority contribute to considerable and frequently unconscious rage at clinicians who take up the authority role (Prelinger 2004; E.R. Shapiro 2004). Although this aggression can be a useful element for patients to learn about during the course of treatment, many outpatient clinicians do not have the specialized training or experience to notice, focus on, withstand, or productively engage these patients' rage at authority (Kernberg 1984; Plakun 2006; E.R. Shapiro 1982b; Winnicott 1949).

These patients often use actions rather than words for communication of intense and unbearable affect states; many have histories of recurrent self-injury and/or suicidal behavior. They have often been unable to adhere to prescribed medication regimens, are exquisitely sensitive to side effects, or induce countertransference reactions in the prescribers that confound treatment efforts (Mintz 2002). On admission to Austen Riggs, 50% of patients have made at least one potentially lethal suicide attempt, more than 40% have had six or more episodes of self-destructive behavior, and 60% have had three or more previous hospitalizations. Examination of patient histories indicates early trauma, abuse, neglect, loss, or deprivation in about 60%. A period preceding admission involving a downward spiral into chronic crisis management is typical, with repeated maladaptive patterns in relationships and behavior and multiple treatment failures involving medication trials and inpatient and outpatient treatment.

Nevertheless, these are also individuals with strengths. Many have had earlier life trajectories with academic, athletic, or artistic promise that collapsed as their symptom picture unfolded—often beginning during the period of late adolescence and early adulthood. Either the task of moving from the role of child in the family to that of adult in the world has been unmanageable during this developmental transition (Erikson 1964a, 1964b; R.L. Shapiro 1963) or later in life they fall apart when a long-standing adaptation crumbles in the face of a loss or life transition (e.g., parental death, the end of a long-term relationship, the repetition of abuse). These patients appear to have the capacity—although usually not the experience—for learning how to use words to describe their feelings while tolerating the associated affects. They indicate a readiness to learn how to delay acting on their impulses. Often they are at a point in their lives where they are poised between increasing desperation and readiness to change.

Basic Dilemmas in Constructing Treatment

These patients raise three central dilemmas for treatment:

1. *Alliance:* Because of difficult past experiences with caregivers, these patients fear and resist a treatment alliance. To engage them in an atmosphere that maximizes interdependency and engagement in the task of treatment requires an unremitting focus on their own authority and the importance of relationships.

2. *Limits:* In response to efforts by others (e.g., family, society, treaters) to set reasonable external behavioral limits and controls, these patients inevitably see the limits, because of their life experiences, as arbitrary, unempathic, and rigid. In response, they may attempt to defy limits and blame limit-setters for their own self-destructive behavior. To construct a treatment environment that puts them in charge and offers opportunities to gain perspective on their anger and the developmental context for their attack on limits—while helping them to remain safe—is a formidable task. When the patient's strengths allow it, treatment is optimally carried out in a completely open setting that requires careful negotiation and ongoing maintenance of a therapeutic alliance (Knight 1953), with differential authority for patients and staff. The staff's recognition of patient authority and the responsibility that goes with it create the basis for a therapeutic community. Interdependent and clearly defined role relationships in such a community emphasize the centrality of the commitment by both patients and staff to the treatment process (Kubie 1960).

3. *Behavior:* These patients tend to use actions to communicate rather than words. To construct a treatment in which they have the opportunity to recognize and acknowledge the meaning of their behavioral communications, translate their experience into language, bear the associated feelings, and put their feelings into historical perspective requires a therapeutic community with a focused

task. Such a community can focus on "examined living," providing feedback about the meaning and impact of behavior and allowing patients to develop a language for experience to bring into their individual psychotherapy and family work (Belnap et al. 2004; Elmendorf and Parish 2007; Fonagy et al. 2002; Fromm et al. 1986).

Determination of Suitability for Residential Care in an Open Setting

The program at Austen Riggs is predicated on these core notions; thus, the admission consultation explores them in detail. The prospective patient's capacity to take up his or her own authority in the admission negotiation, use the relationship with the admissions officer for learning, and open the possibility of finding meaning in symptoms determines the patient's suitability for treatment. Admission requires an explicit offer from the admissions officer after a 2-hour consultation with the patient alone and with relevant family members. The patient's interest in accepting the offer—however ambivalently—with acknowledgement of the anxiety that must inevitably accompany the freedom of the setting indicates the beginning of an alliance. Similarly, any third party who may be supporting the treatment financially, such as a relative or insurance company, must also agree to the conditions of treatment.

A central aspect of the admission consultation is a negotiation with the prospective patient and family (if available) about managing the risks of the open setting. When the patient's treatment-resistant illness is organized around a rebellion against authority, it may be manifest in an abdication of responsibility, with the expectation that those in authority will take over (and fail). This becomes apparent at admission when a patient's presentation seems to insist that it is the institution's job to keep him or her alive. Admissions officers regularly note with patients the way this implicit or explicit expectation is an impossible task.

Admission is dependent on patients beginning to recognize that it is their responsibility to manage their safety (or commit to inform staff if they become unsafe), while staff takes responsibility for overseeing the treatment process. Inevitably, engaging in and maintaining this negotiation is not possible for some—and 15%–30% of those admitted are ultimately not able to tolerate the responsibility sufficiently to sustain their treatment. Nonetheless, such an initial alliance—although often shaky and requiring ongoing vigilance—offers the best chance for a treatment process that patients can own as the first step in taking charge of their lives. This opening discussion with patients and their families also helps put family anxieties and unrealistic expectations in perspective and begins the process of defining clearer roles in treatment.

The following vignette illustrates some of these points. The case and treatment principles related to it are described in more detail elsewhere (Plakun 2003).

> Ms. A was a widowed woman in her 40s with treatment-resistant depression and a borderline personality disorder who was referred to the center because of recurrent suicidal ideation and behavior that kept her outpatient treatment chronically in crisis. Her insurance company agreed to support longer-term treatment because of the high cost to them of multiple previous short-term hospitalizations and in recognition of her high suicide risk. In the admission consultation Ms. A was able to engage with the admissions officer about the rage and despair beneath her recurrent suicidal threats and their link to an early history of sexual abuse and fears of abandonment, exacerbated by her husband's death several years earlier. She found the discussion of these issues and the tentative connections drawn between her symptoms and life history helpful and surprisingly calming, noting that she and her outpatient psychiatrist had rarely had the opportunity to explore anything but her response to medications and the level of her suicide risk. She felt able to contain her suicidal behavior if admitted, and admission was offered.
>
> Although the patient's insurance company was willing to support treatment 1 week at a time, it would not commit in advance to the minimum stay of 6 weeks. As a result, the patient, who had the resources, was asked to make the usual prepayment to secure the initial period of evaluation and treatment. On the day before admission the patient called to indicate her refusal to make the required prepayment, stating that if she were not offered admission anyway, she would carry out her suicide plan. The admissions officer noted her use of a suicide threat to get her way and reminded her of the work they had done to get an initial perspective on her struggles. He reminded her of her competence and determination in negotiating coverage with her insurance carrier and said it would be too bad if she threw away the chance for a treatment that might work. He then told her that he would not allow her to come in any way other than the one they had negotiated, which was the same for all patients admitted. Although initially enraged, Ms. A was also reassured by the holding of limits, made the prepayment, and was admitted.

Treatments

Many of these patients come from multiple short-term inpatient hospitalizations in locked settings in major cities. The Austen Riggs Center presents a striking contrast. A completely open residential treatment center in stately white buildings on the main street of the small New England village of Stockbridge, Massachusetts, the center offers a semirural setting for voluntary treatment. There are no privilege systems, no locked doors, and no explicit requirements to attend any treatments, although a lack of attendance inevitably leads to review of the patient's interest in treatment.

Patients are admitted for an initial 6-week period of intensive evaluation and treatment, although most stay longer. The median length of treatment in the continuum of care (from hospital level through step-down programs to outpatient care) is 6 months, with a range from 6 weeks to several years. In general, the effort is to interrupt the cycle of thwarted treatments by helping patients develop the capacity to express experience in language. This capacity increases the likelihood that after discharge patients will be able to manage outpatient psychotherapy without self-destructive behavior or other recurring crises interrupting the work and with new abilities to engage in adaptive social role functioning.

Although a brief-stay inpatient level of care is available for patients whose treatment alliance becomes uncertain during the course of treatment, the vast majority of patients enter a therapeutic community at one of two residential levels of care organized around the maximal exercise of patient authority and the possibility of turning to others for support. The more intensive residential program focuses on individual nursing care (often used with patients struggling to contain impulses to harm themselves or to use substances), whereas the other has less intensive nursing and relies more on peer groups. Having been screened at admission for their capacity to engage in a verbal psychotherapy, all patients begin and throughout their stay continue in four-times-weekly psychodynamic psychotherapy with a doctoral-level therapist. In addition, skill-based and symptom-focused groups are available in the community program. All patients have a psychopharmacologist who prescribes medication for sufficient symptom relief to allow the patient to participate fully in the range of treatments. Social workers—often with the individual therapist as family co-therapist—work with their families. The same interdisciplinary team that includes these clinicians and others follows the patient in transitions through various residences in the continuum of care—from hospital, to group residences in the main hospital building or elsewhere in Stockbridge and in the neighboring town of Lenox, to day treatment in patients' own apartments. The team works together over time to integrate a coherent view of the patient from different disciplinary perspectives.

> In a treatment team review of John, a 30-year-old man with major depressive disorder, narcissistic personality disorder, and substance use disorder, team members presented differing views of him. Nursing staff found him aloof and arrogant, challenging hospital policy and avoiding their efforts to engage him. Therapeutic community staff noted John's efforts to help younger female patients in distress, often encouraging them to speak up in community meetings. The female therapist reported John's deepening engagement in therapy and his increasing recognition of his defensive devaluation of her in the context of his beginning exploration of his vulnerability and anxiety about potential abandonment by women he depended on. The social worker reminded the team of John's younger sister's suicide in his youth—in the context of his parents' divorce—and his mother's worsening breast cancer. The discussion put John's confusing combination of defensively arrogant devaluation of older women and his caretaking efforts toward younger women in perspective, helping nursing staff to persist in their efforts to engage John and to help him see the defensive nature of his withdrawal. John began to recognize the historical determinants for his problematic relationships and the repetition of these patterns in his relationships with community members and his therapist.

There is an activities program, described by Austen Riggs staff as a nonclinical "interpretation-free zone," where patients take up the role of "student," working in visual media, ceramics, woodworking, fiber arts, and a greenhouse. The program includes a Montessori preschool for children from the local community where patients may serve as volunteer aides. There is also a community theater where patients collaborate with members of the outside community and a professional theater director to put on plays.

> Fran, a 36-year-old woman with an extensive history of childhood sexual abuse and multiple abusive adult relationships, was reading through a script for a planned play with a group of patients, Stockbridge residents, and the Austen Riggs theater director. Fran was to take the role of the wife of an army officer. In one scene, the woman dies and is carried offstage in the arms of the officer. As Fran read the stage directions, she gasped, saying, "I could never let a man touch me!" The theater director responded, "But you are dead!" Fran said, "Oh, that's right," and went on to do the play with great success, bringing her struggle around her experience into her psychotherapy.

The assessment phase culminates with a 2-hour case conference involving the entire clinical staff.

Chaired by the medical director, this conference invites the patient to bring his or her own treatment focus and questions into an interview with the medical director and staff. Often the patient's questions dovetail with the issues raised in the assessment, so that the group can reach a formulation and treatment plan relevant to the patient's stated goals.

Impact of the Setting

The open setting and the staff's reliance on patient authority meet and legitimize both autonomous functioning and dependency needs, including the need to belong. The structures of the program support patients' strengths instead of focusing relentlessly on psychopathology:

- The open setting leans on patients' capacities to manage themselves and, in a version of free association, gives patients room for and invites them to notice the choices they make each day.
- The therapeutic community authorizes patients' leadership capacities in elected positions.
- The activities program—which formally removes them for periods of time from the patient role—offers these "students" a space for creative expression and the mobilization of strengths and capacities, conceptualized as separate from treatment.
- The culture of the center is organized around patients developing the potential to take charge of their treatment and their lives.
- The staff is organized around the understanding that patient resistance—their "acting out"—is a form of communication that requires translation.

All of these supportive and progressive structures serve to counterbalance the inevitable regressive pulls that are an aspect of intensive and deepening individual psychotherapy.

The treatment focuses on three sustaining areas: *patient authority, meaning,* and *the importance of relationships.* These patients communicate through projective identification and enactment the meaning of their painful life experience. In other settings, where staff authority is exercised to ensure treatment compliance, the patient may only be able to take up a passive role. This may unwittingly and paradoxically foster "treatment resistance," when resistance to treatment is the only way left for a patient to exercise authority (Plakun 2006). Austen Riggs, through its freedom and structured examination of relationships, is designed to engage this difficulty through individual psychotherapy, family treatment, and the way individual transferences are enacted through relationships with other patients and staff (E.R. Shapiro and Carr 1987). In a therapeutic community of examined living, the resources are available to unpack these transferences, help tolerate them, and provide perspective (Muller 1999).

The community is constructed as a kind of theater in the round, a public opportunity for patients to live out—and begin to see—their difficulties with others. Managed by patients with staff consultation, the effort is to provide a structure for the translation of behavioral communication into words. Patient-led groups and a culture of ongoing interpersonal feedback communicate in different ways the impact that individual and group behavior has on others. For example, if a patient begins to get involved in an exclusive relationship with another patient, other patients inevitably feel envious and rejected. Public discussion of these reactions can illuminate how "pairing" is a group phenomenon (Bion 1961). If a patient is involved in self-destructive behavior, others inevitably become frightened, guilty, and worried. Discussion of these responses helps the particular patient feel less isolated and desperate. Characteristic individual defenses, ordinarily invisible to the individual, become powerfully visible in community life. Individuals—beginning to see themselves in the eyes of others—have the opportunity to take up authority and responsibility with others in a kind of participatory democracy (Elmendorf and Parish 2007).

Individual Psychodynamic Psychotherapy

Individual psychotherapy focuses on listening, making sense of transference experience, and an unfolding receptiveness to the patient's newly formulated experience (E.R. Shapiro 1982a). Many patients with severe personality disorders manage their unbearable experience through the creation of painful and anger-filled relationships. Using the psychological mechanism of projective identification (Kernberg 1975, 1984; Klein 1946; E.R. Shapiro and Carr 1991) to protect themselves from their internal experience, patients unwittingly transform their internal self-critical torment into stormy and provocative behavior with others.

These patients have acute sensitivity to vulnerabilities and blind spots in their therapist's character that they unconsciously use to evoke intense countertransferences (Prelinger 2004; E.R. Shapiro 2004). Detection and careful unpacking of the countertransference enactments in staff discussions (Kernberg 1984; Plakun 2001, 2007; E.R. Shapiro 1982b; E.R. Shapiro and Carr 1987)—and eventually in individual psycho-

therapy—are a frequent part of the unfolding of the treatment. This process helps patients to see the role of their self-hatred, rage, guilt, and shame in producing desperate acts of self-abuse (e.g., cutting, burning, parasuicidal and suicidal behaviors) and angry, provocative interpersonal behaviors.

The treatment environment at Austen Riggs helps contain the impact of this behavior, translating it into a language that allows patients to gain perspective on their own unconscious motivations. However, the work proceeds with the evolving recognition that there are two fallible human beings in the consulting room when a therapist and patient meet. The therapy staff has opportunities to consult with colleagues (both on and off the treatment team) to help bear the intense countertransference of the work and find their own contribution to some of the struggles.

Psychodynamic psychotherapy in such a program focuses on character issues, paying particular attention to repeated maladaptive patterns of behavior. These are assumed to be behavioral communications ("acting out") of inarticulate and painful childhood experiences. Interpretive work attempts to make sense of the problematic, usually negative, transferences that for many of these patients interfere with deepening relationships. The effort in psychodynamic treatment is to help patients put feelings into words, focusing on the contexts that evoke these behavioral patterns.

Family Treatment

A central context for the development of these difficulties for many of these patients is their families. Although parents do their best to love and support their children, they may also unwittingly bring into the family system powerful unconscious issues that can contribute to treatment resistance. Riggs invites families to participate in the treatment to help the patient and the clinicians both grasp the family's perceptions of the patient's development and begin to understand the family dynamics in which the patient's symptoms are embedded (E.R. Shapiro and Freedman 1987). These patients often have irrational roles in their families in which they are covertly invited through projective identification to carry problematic aspects of their parents' past experiences (Berkowitz et al. 1974; Fromm 2004, 2006; E.R. Shapiro et al. 1975; Zinner and Shapiro 1975). Family work aimed at unpacking these relationships places each member's history in perspective, freeing the individual patient to consider his or her own life without the pressures of family needs (Schwartz 2007; E.R. Shapiro 1982b; E.R. Shapiro and Carr 1991; E.R. Shapiro et al. 1979).

Bill, a brilliant and obsessive 32-year-old man, had failed at multiple attempts to complete his education. Unable to sustain a job because of frequent arguments with his male superiors, he had remained at home for years, isolated in his bedroom. Filled with hatred for his "cold, uncaring, and abusive" father, he insists that he remains home in order to protect his mother. On one occasion, confronted with his own inability to motivate his son, the father had said angrily to Bill, "I wish you'd never been born." These family tensions and Bill's periodic impulsive outbursts of rage led him to a potentially lethal suicide attempt that he survived only by accident.

When Bill was admitted to Austen Riggs, the therapist and social worker invited the family to a meeting. A rageful argument between father and son erupted, requiring the therapist to intervene. Turning to the silent mother, the therapist asked, "How do you stand this?" The mother responded, "I've given up." Both clinicians remarked to the mother that—given the potentially lethal outcome—she could not afford to withdraw. Recognizing how overwhelmed she was, they offered to assist her efforts to help her men discover their softer sides. This intervention opened for father and son the possibility of revealing their shared vulnerabilities and the ways they had deeply hurt each other. Their underlying love for one another, and the relationship of the father's angry withdrawal to his painful relationship with his own father, slowly emerged over months of work, allowing Bill some perspective on his family experience. His mother's increasing competence in engaging this discussion helped Bill to recognize her strength, allowing him to begin to separate his needs from hers.

Psychopharmacology

Treatment resistance is often manifest in the patient's relationship to the meaning of medication as much as in failure to respond to it. Mintz and Belnap (2006) described the practice of "psychodynamic psychopharmacology" with these patients, exploring the meaning that medications—and their side effects—have and the way these meanings may contribute to a "nocebo" (negative placebo) effect. These patients regularly experience caretakers as people likely to cause harm and react to prescribed medication as potentially harmful. This may interfere with medication adherence or may manifest as heightened sensitivity to even small doses. These adverse reactions evoke countertransference in the psychopharmacologist, contributing to the possibility of reactive irrational prescriptions that add multiple medications to respond to what is essentially a psychological problem. An interpretive treatment that includes team discussions between therapist and psychopharmacologist helps uncover such patterns; translating them into words can lead to a patient's im-

proved capacity to adhere to and tolerate potentially helpful medication regimens and engage more fully in treatment.

A second group of patients uses medications to replace relationships. Patients in this group experience their affects as "symptoms" and may use their clinical diagnoses and medications to reduce their responsibility for and engagement in life. Although patients in this group find medication helpful and necessary, they often do not appear to get better with them. Such patients at Riggs often find engagement in the therapeutic community to be an important stimulus for recognizing their own reactivity and responsiveness to others, opening the possibility of recognizing their affects as crucial information instead of pathological illness (Mintz and Belnap 2006).

Management of Financial Resources

In the traditional medical model, others—clinicians, managed care representatives, family members—ordinarily manage the financing of treatment on behalf of the patient. This leaves patients in a dependent position and creates an unfortunate incentive to do poorly in order to prove that treatment is needed. The wish to provide patients what they need in the face of resource limitations outside their control can lead clinicians to join patients in experiencing the "resource managers" in a shared projective way as bad, withholding, and unempathic (E.R. Shapiro 1997). Such collusion can both displace negative transference feelings from the therapy and interfere with rational collaboration around effective and appropriate use of inevitably limited resources.

Helping patients deal effectively with reality is an aspect of treatment. The cost of treatment and the limitations of financial resources must be faced in order to construct a secure and reliable treatment framework. Patients and families regularly have irrational emotional reactions to financial limitations, experiencing them through the filter of other limitations in life (emotional, security, health), making it difficult for them to think clearly. At Austen Riggs, a group of clinicians and business staff work with patients and families on resource limitations in order to help them grasp the actual financial facts and face the often conflicted feelings involved in using these funds (college funds, retirement assets, home equity loans) for treatment. When patients who value their treatment participate actively in discussions about the utilization of genuinely limited resources, they can emerge from a passive position and discover an incentive to manage themselves better so they can step down to a less expensive level of care to extend their treatment. Facing the limitations of resources provides opportunities for both patients and families to come to terms with anger, guilt, and grief about painful reality (Plakun 1996; E.R. Shapiro 1997).

Suicidal and Aggressive Behaviors in Treatment

The open setting allows a broad range of freedom and maintains a clear distinction between behaviors that are potentially lethal and those that are not (Plakun 1994, 2001). Patients may well choose to engage in non-life-threatening superficial cutting and burning and eating behaviors as inarticulate ways of managing (and expressing) their feelings or defining their boundaries (Elmendorf 2007; Gunderson 2001; Sacksteder 1989a, 1989b). These are ordinarily managed by nursing staff's bandaging or the local hospital's suturing when needed. Clinical staff members work with patients to understand the feelings, fantasies, and relationship events that lie behind these acts—and their impact on others—but recognize the futility of trying to take on the task of preventing them. These efforts over time begin to communicate to the patient that behavior is communication, often communication about unbearably painful feelings.

When self-destructive behaviors threaten the patient's life and the continuity of the treatment, the therapist immediately addresses the issue in relation to the alliance. Among other things, a suicide plan is a decision on the patient's part to end the treatment. It therefore reflects problems in the treatment relationship that must be explored, including, potentially, the therapist's unwitting contribution to that decision (Clarkin 2001, 2006; Kernberg 1984; Plakun 1994, 2001). Should a patient act with actual suicidal intent, the clinician assumes, in keeping with the clearly negotiated terms of admission, that the patient has chosen to end treatment at Austen Riggs. The patient is ordinarily then transferred elsewhere—to a locked setting—for emergency medical and psychiatric management. Often the patient returns to the center when safe, at which point the focus of the work of the patient, therapist, and treatment team is on carrying out a consultation over the next several weeks to determine why the patient chose to end treatment by ending his or her life, how the therapist may have unwittingly played a role in that choice, what the patient has learned in the event, whether the patient wishes to and is able to return to the kind of alliance needed to do the work, and whether the treatment can continue or has been damaged beyond repair. This process is often a powerful intervention that, when successful, has been associated with good outcome (Plakun 1991).

If patients engage in dangerous behaviors that suggest they are unable to adhere to the terms of the negotiated treatment alliance by keeping themselves safe, but they have not endangered their lives, they may step up to an open inpatient level of care at the center for relatively brief periods. During this time they negotiate with nursing staff the limits of their freedom (for example, turning in car keys or not leaving the hospital grounds) that make clinical sense while their treatment focuses intensively on monitoring their safety and determining whether they can repair their treatment alliance or need treatment elsewhere. The center does not use any restraint or seclusion unless acute psychotic or impulsive suicidal behavior requires temporary restraint prior to transfer. In such circumstances the police are called to help staff manage the situation. This happens rarely, because the culture of the community ordinarily helps patients turn to staff or to one another before they lose control.

Research

Wallerstein (1986) and Gabbard et al. (1999) presented cohort studies of patients treated at the Menninger Clinic suggesting the value of extended treatment for similar patients. Chiesa et al. (2004) provided evidence that extended psychodynamic residential treatment with a continuum of care was an effective treatment for patients with severe personality disorders, many of whom had significant Axis I comorbidity.

The Austen Riggs Center has been involved in studying this patient population since the 1950s, when Robert Knight (1954) wrote the seminal paper on borderline patients. Psychoanalytic theoreticians including Erik Erikson, David Rapaport, and Roy Schafer developed the field of ego psychology at Austen Riggs in the 1950s by working with this patient population (Erikson 1956, 1964a, 1964b; Rapaport 1959, 1967; Shafer 1999). Otto Will (1980) deepened his studies of schizophrenia at Austen Riggs, and several studies in the 1970s and 1980s focused on the outcomes of patients in treatment at the center (Blatt and Ford 1994; Plakun et al. 1985).

Recognizing that it had an opportunity to study this group of patients more intensively and in more depth than colleagues could in other settings—and that the clinical data included the family and social context—Austen Riggs decided that it had an obligation to the larger field. In 1994 it created the Erikson Institute for Education and Research to continue this learning and apply the concepts emerging from this work to other settings. Since that time the center has been engaged in the follow-along study described earlier, examining the progression of 226 patients (51% of the available sample) at 6-month intervals for 6–10 years. The hope is to learn about the natural progression of this difficult-to-treat group of patients.

The first paper from the study reports on the issue of suicide, showing an overall rate of completed suicide of 2.5% in discharged treatment-refractory patients (examining 100% of the patients discharged from Austen Riggs during the study period, including those who did not elect to participate in the study). Long-term results (a mean of 9 years of follow-up) suggest that study patients ultimately improved significantly in terms of suicide-related symptoms (Perry et al., in press). The data indicate that suicidal behavior remitted first, followed by self-destructive behavior, whereas suicidal ideation persisted longer. The findings are consistent with the hypothesis that this multimodal treatment approach helps patients with previously treatment-refractory illness, many of whom struggle with suicide, to begin to move from behavior into language to manage their painful experiences as they begin the process of taking charge of their lives.

In addition, the Erikson Institute has begun to apply the learning from Austen Riggs to some of the problems of the larger society, ranging from administration (E.R. Shapiro 2001a, 2001c), to the transgenerational transmission of trauma (Fromm 2004, 2006), to citizenship (E.R. Shapiro 2003, 2005; E.R. Shapiro and Carr 2006).

Conclusion

There is a subset of patients with treatment-resistant illnesses, often with comorbid mood and personality disorders and other comorbid disorders, for whom "resistance" to treatment is organized around unconsciously determined difficulty engaging in a treatment alliance in which they can find their own voice and authority. Recognizing that the alliance is the foundation that supports the treatment, the Austen Riggs Center has constructed a focused residential approach to these patients. The center places patients in charge of

themselves in an open setting in which authority is negotiated between staff and patients rather than assumed by staff. The negotiated agreement is to explore the patient's mind and the meaning of behavior and relationships. The patient's deviations from that agreement and the related acting-out behavior—when not threatening the patient's life or the treatment of others—are seen as opportunities for learning, because these patients tend to communicate their difficulties through behavior.

In this residential setting, attention to both the meaning of medication and its effects helps maximize its utilization. Individual psychodynamic psychotherapy is designed to help the patient focus on a deepening intimate relationship in which aspects of the past are relived and translated into language. Because these patients tend to split their transferences—often by idealizing one relationship and devaluing another—the capacity of the staff to sustain and examine the patient's relationships with all members of the treatment team allows the possibility of showing the patient how this phenomenon occurs while offering the possibility of reintegrating these split relationships within the individual therapy. At the same time, the experiences of examined living and constant feedback from a therapeutic community help the patient translate his or her behavior into language and meaningful experience. Concurrent family work gives the patient perspective on the developmental context of disturbance and helps to mobilize family relationships and resources for the treatment.

The constellation of resources available at Austen Riggs adds to contemporary general psychiatric treatment a diverse range of psychosocial treatments integrated by a psychodynamic understanding of personality functioning. These patients with treatment-resistant conditions may also be conceived of as delegates of their families and social contexts who are carrying potential learning about the unbearable difficulties of the interpersonal world and the larger society (Elmendorf and Parish 2007; Fromm 2004, 2006; E.R. Shapiro and Carr 1991). Far from being doomed to chronic crisis management, the evidence indicates that such patients are treatable and capable of finding their voices and a role in society.

Given the substantial problem of treatment resistance, it is important that this and similar comprehensive, integrative, psychodynamically based residential treatment centers continue to be available as part of the standard of care for these patients, who have so much to offer and from whom we have so much to learn. In addition, the insights developed from the intensive clinical work in this national referral center are applicable to other settings, including outpatient settings.

Patients with treatment-resistant illnesses emerge from our increasingly complex and stressful social contexts. Successful treatment of these illnesses requires a serious clinical commitment from the profession both to recognize how these struggles develop and to provide a sufficient biopsychosocial treatment space so that these patients might find their way to rejoin the larger society.

References

American Psychiatric Association: Practice Guideline for the Treatment of Patients With Schizophrenia, 2nd Edition. Washington, DC, American Psychiatric Publishing, 2004

Apter A, Kronenberg S, Brent D: Turning darkness into light: a new landmark study on the treatment of adolescent depression. Comments on the TADS study. Eur Child Adolesc Psychiatry 14:113–116, 2005

Belnap BA, Iscan C, Plakun EM: Residential treatment of personality disorders: the containing function, in Handbook of Personality Disorders: Theory and Practice. Edited by Magnavita JJ. New York, Wiley, 2004, pp 379–397

Bender DS, Skodol AE, Pagano ME, et al: Prospective assessment of treatment use by patients with personality disorders. Psychiatr Serv 57:254–257, 2006

Berkowitz DA, Shapiro RL, Zinner J, et al: Family contributions to narcissistic disturbances in adolescents. Int Rev Psychoanal 1:353–362, 1974

Bion WR: Experiences in Groups. London, Tavistock, 1961

Blatt SJ, Ford RQ: Therapeutic Change: An Object Relations Perspective. New York, Plenum, 1994

Chiesa M, Fonagy P, Holmes J, et al: Residential versus community treatment of personality disorders: a comparative study of 3 treatment programs. Am J Psychiatry 161:1463–1470, 2004

Clarkin JF, Foelsch PA, Levy KN, et al: Treatment of borderline patients with a psychodynamic approach: a preliminary study of behavioral change. J Personal Disord 15:487–495, 2001

Clarkin JF, Yoemans F, Kernberg OF: Psychotherapy of Borderline Personality: Focusing on Object Relations. Washington, DC, American Psychiatric Publishing, 2006

Crown WH, Finkelstein S, Berndt ER, et al: The impact of treatment-resistant depression on health care utilization and costs. J Clin Psychiatry 63:963–971, 2002

Elmendorf DM: Containment and the use of the skin, in The Embodied Subject: Minding the Body in Psychoanalysis. Edited by Muller JP, Tillman JG. New York, Rowman & Littlefield, 2007, pp 81–91

Elmendorf DM, Parish M: A view from Riggs: treatment resistance and patient authority, V: silencing the messenger: the social dynamics of treatment resistance. J Am Acad Psychoanal Dyn Psychiatry 35:375–392, 2007

Erikson E: The problem of ego identity. J Am Psychoanal Assoc 4:56–121, 1956

Erikson E: Identity: Youth and Crisis. Austen Riggs Monograph, No 7. New York, WW Norton, 1964a

Erikson E: The nature of clinical evidence, in Insight and Responsibility. New York, WW Norton, 1964b, pp 49–50

Fava M, Davidson KG: Definition and epidemiology of treatment-resistant depression. Psychiatr Clin North Am 19:179–200, 1997

Fonagy P, Gergely G, Jurist E, et al: Affect Regulation, Mentalization and the Development of the Self. New York, Other Press, 2002

Fowler JC, Ackerman A, Blagys M, et al: Personality and symptom change in treatment-refractory inpatients: evaluation of the phase model of change using Rorschach, TAT and DSM Axis V. J Personal Assess 83:306–322, 2004

Fromm M: Psychoanalysis and trauma: September 11 revisited. Diogenes 51:3–14, 2004

Fromm M: A view from Riggs: treatment resistance and patient authority, II: transmission of trauma and treatment resistance. J Am Acad Psychoanal Dyn Psychiatry 34:445–458, 2006

Fromm MG, Stern DA, Sacksteder JL: From coercion to collaboration: two weeks in the life of a therapeutic community. Psychiatry 49:18–32, 1986

Gabbard GO, Coyne L, Allen JG, et al: Evaluation of intensive inpatient treatment of patients with severe personality disorders. Psychiatr Serv 51:893–898, 1999

Geller JL: Avoiding extinction: successful private psychiatric hospitals in the opening decade of the twenty-first century. Psychiatry Q 77:189–201, 2006

Gunderson JG: Borderline Personality Disorder: A Clinical Guide. Washington, DC, American Psychiatric Publishing, 2001

Kernberg OF: Borderline Conditions and Pathological Narcissism. New York, Jason Aronson, 1975

Kernberg OF: Severe Personality Disorders: Psychotherapeutic Strategies. New Haven, CT, Yale University Press, 1984

Klein M: Notes on some schizoid mechanisms. Int J Psychoanal 27:99–110, 1946

Knight RP: Management and psychotherapy of the borderline patient. Bull Menninger Clin 17:139–150, 1953

Knight RP: Borderline states, in Psychoanalytic Psychiatry and Psychology: Clinical and Theoretical Papers (Austen Riggs Monograph No. 1). Edited by Knight RP, Friedman CR. New York, International Universities Press, 1954, pp 97–122

Kubie LS: The Riggs Story: The Development of the Austen Riggs Center or the Study and Treatment of the Psychoneuroses. New York, Paul B. Hoeber, 1960

Lieberman JA, Stroup TS, McEvoy JP, et al: Effectiveness of antipsychotic drugs in patients with chronic schizophrenia. N Engl J Med 35:1209–1223, 2005

Miklowitz DJ, Otto MW, Frank E: Psychosocial treatments for bipolar depression. Arch Gen Psychiatry 64:419–426, 2007

Mintz D: Meaning and medication in the care of treatment-resistant patients. Am J Psychother 56:322–337, 2002

Mintz D, Belnap B: A view from Riggs: treatment resistance and patient authority, III: what is psychodynamic psychopharmacology? An approach to pharmacological treatment resistance. J Am Acad Psychoanal Dyn Psychiatry 34:581–601, 2006

Muller J: The third as holding the dyad. Psychoanalytic Dialogues 9:471–480, 1999

Muller J: A view from Riggs: treatment resistance and patient authority, IV: why the pair needs the third. J Am Acad Psychoanal Dyn Psychiatry 35:221–241, 2007

Nemeroff CB, Heim CM, Thase ME, et al: Differential response to psychotherapy versus pharmacotherapy in patients with chronic forms of major depression and childhood trauma. Proc Natl Acad Sci 100:14293–14296, 2003

Perlis RH, Ostacher MJ, Patel JK, et al: Predictors of recurrence in bipolar disorder: primary outcomes from the Systematic Treatment Enhancement Program for Bipolar Disorder (STEP-BD). Am J Psychiatry 163:217–224, 2006

Perry JC, Fowler JC, Zheutlin B: Recovery from suicidal and self-destructive phenomena among adults with treatment-refractory disorders in the Austen Riggs follow-along study. J Nerv Ment Dis (in press)

Plakun EM: Prediction of outcome in borderline personality disorder. J Personal Disord 5:93–101, 1991

Plakun EM: Principles in the psychotherapy of self-destructive borderline patients. J Psychother Pract Res 3:138–148, 1994

Plakun EM: Economic grand rounds: treatment of personality disorders in an era of resource limitation. Psychiatr Serv 47:128–130, 1996

Plakun EM: Managed care discovers the talking cure, in Psychoanalytic Therapy as Health Care: Effectiveness and Economics in the 21st Century. Edited by Haley H, Eagle M, Wolitsky D. Hillsdale, NJ, Analytic Press, 1999, pp 239–255

Plakun EM: Making the alliance and taking the transference in work with suicidal borderline patients. J Psychother Pract Res 10:269–276, 2001

Plakun EM: Treatment refractory mood disorders: a psychodynamic perspective. J Psychiatr Pract 9:209–218, 2003

Plakun EM: A view from Riggs: treatment resistance and patient authority, I: a psychodynamic perspective. J Am Acad Psychoanal Dyn Psychiatry 34:349–366, 2006

Plakun EM: Perspectives on embodiment: from symptom to enactment and from enactment to sexual misconduct, in The Embodied Subject: Minding the Body in Psychoanalysis. Edited by Muller JP, Tillman JG. Lanham, MD, Rowman & Littlefield, 2007, pp 103–116

Plakun EM, Burkhardt PE, Muller JP: 14-year follow-up of borderline and schizotypal personality disorders. Compr Psychiatry 26:448–455, 1985

Prelinger E: Thoughts on hate and aggression. Psychoanalytic Study of the Child 59:30–43, 2004

Rapaport D: A historical survey of psychoanalytic ego psychology. Psychological Issues 1:5–17, 1959

Rapaport D: The theory of ego autonomy, in Collected Papers of David Rapaport. New York, Basic Books, 1967, pp 722–741

Rush AJ, Trivedi MH: Treating depression to remission. Psychiatr Ann 25:704–709, 1995

Sacksteder JL: Psychosomatic dissociation and false self development in anorexia nervosa, in The Facilitating Environment: Clinical Applications of Winnicott's Theories. Edited by Smith BL, Fromm MG. New York, International Universities Press, 1989a

Sacksteder JL: Sadomasochistic relatedness to the body in anorexia nervosa, in Masochism: The Treatment of Self-Inflicted Suffering. Edited by Montgomery JD, Greif AC. New York, International Universities Press, 1989b

Schwartz A: A view from Riggs: treatment resistance and patient authority, VI: working with family resistance to treatment. J Am Acad Psychoanal Dyn Psychiatry 35:607–625, 2007

Shafer R: Recentering psychoanalysis from Heinz Hartmann to the contemporary British Kleinians. Psychoanal Psychol 16:339–354, 1999

Shapiro ER: On curiosity: intrapsychic and interpersonal boundary formation in family life. International Journal of Family Psychiatry 3:69–89, 1982a

Shapiro ER: The holding environment and family therapy with acting out adolescents. Int J Psychoanal Psychother 9:209–226, 1982b

Shapiro ER: The boundaries are shifting: renegotiating the therapeutic frame, in The Inner World in the Outer World. Edited by Shapiro E. New Haven, CT, Yale University Press, 1997, pp 7–25

Shapiro ER: The changing role of the CEO. Organisational and Social Dynamics 1:130–142, 2001a

Shapiro ER: The effect of social changes on the doctor-patient relationship. Organisational and Social Dynamics 2:1–11, 2001b

Shapiro ER: Institutional learning as chief executive, in The Systems Psychodynamics of Organizations: Integrating the Group Relations Approach, Psychoanalytic and Open Systems Theory. Edited by Gould L, Stapley L, Stein M. New York, Karnac Press, 2001c, pp 175–195

Shapiro ER: The maturation of American identity: a study of the elections of 1996 and 2000 and the war against terrorism. Organisational and Social Dynamics 3:121–133, 2003

Shapiro ER: Discussion of Ernst Prelinger's "Thoughts on hate and aggression." Psychoanalytic Study of the Child 59:44–51, 2004

Shapiro ER: Joining a group's task: the discovery of hope and respect. Int J Group Psychother 55:211–227, 2005

Shapiro ER, Carr AW: Disguised countertransference in institutions. Psychiatry 50:72–82, 1987

Shapiro ER, Carr AW: Lost in Familiar Places: Creating New Connections Between the Individual and Society. New Haven, CT, Yale University Press, 1991

Shapiro ER, Carr AW: Those people were some kind of solution: can society in any sense be understood? Organisational and Social Dynamics 6:241–257, 2006

Shapiro ER, Freedman J: Family dynamics of adolescent suicide. Adolesc Psychiatry 14:191–207, 1987

Shapiro ER, Fromm MG: Erik Erikson's clinical theory, in Comprehensive Textbook of Psychiatry. Edited by Sadock BJ, Kaplan HI. New York, Williams & Wilkins, 1999, pp 2200–2207

Shapiro ER, Zinner J, Shapiro RL, et al: The influence of family experience on borderline personality development. Int Rev Psychoanal 2:399–411, 1975

Shapiro ER, Shapiro RL, Zinner J, et al: The borderline ego and the working alliance: indications for family and individual treatment in adolescence. Int J Psychoanal 58:77–87, 1979

Shapiro RL: Identity and the psychology of the ego. Psychiatry 26:77–87, 1963

Skodol AE, Gunderson JG, Shea MT, et al: The Collaborative Longitudinal Personality Disorders Study (CLPS): overview and implications. J Personal Disord 19:487–504, 2005

Thase ME, Friedman ES, Howland RH: Management of treatment-resistant depression: psychotherapeutic perspectives. J Clin Psychiatry 62 (suppl):18–24, 2001

Thase ME, Friedman ES, Biggs MM, et al: Cognitive therapy versus medication in augmentation and switch strategies as second-step treatments: a STAR*D report. Am J Psychiatry 164:739–752, 2007

Treatment for Adolescents With Depression Study Team: Treatment for Adolescents With Depression Study (TADS): rationale, design, and methods. J Am Acad Child Adolesc Psychiatry 42:531–542, 2003

Wallerstein RS: Forty-Two Lives in Treatment: A Study of Psychoanalysis and Psychotherapy. New York, Guilford, 1986

Will O: Schizophrenia: psychological treatment, in Comprehensive Textbook of Psychiatry III. Edited by Kaplan HI, Freedman AM, Sadock BJ. Baltimore, MD, Williams & Wilkins, 1980, pp 1217–1240

Winnicott DW: Hate in the countertransference. Int J Psychoanal 30:69–74, 1949

Zinner J, Shapiro ER: Splitting in families of borderline adolescents, in Borderline States in Psychiatry. Edited by Mack J. New York, Grune & Stratton, 1975, pp 103–122

CHAPTER 22

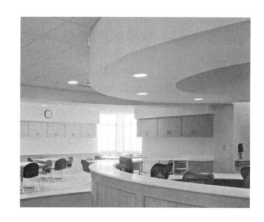

RESIDENTIAL TREATMENT FOR CHILDREN AND ADOLESCENTS

Michael A. Rater, M.D.
Alex Hirshberg, B.A.
Cynthia Kaplan, Ph.D.

Residential treatment for children and adolescents is a term describing a broad group of programs that differ in many fundamental ways but share the fact that the child or adolescent lives at the program in which he or she receives treatment (B. Kamradt, C. Connolly, "Re-Engineering Residential Treatment: Challenges and Opportunities for Purchasers and Providers," background paper for the Children in Managed Care Initiative Center for Health Care Strategies, April 2003; Leichtman 2006; Whittaker 2000). One subgroup of residential treatment programs is designed to treat more focal problems within a relatively brief time frame of 1 to several weeks. These are called "acute residential treatment programs" for the purposes of this chapter. Other programs are meant to treat more chronic situations that require the child to be taken out of the home for an extended period of time. These are designated "long-term residential treatment programs" here. Some programs operate over a period of one to several months, a period of time somewhere between "acute" and "long-term," and are included in the discussion of the "acute" group of programs because they share most similarities in terms of staffing and daily programming with that group of programs.

Treatment models also differ among these programs. Some treatment programs are based on a psychoeducational model in which youngsters learn the skills to manage themselves in the outside world (Frensch and Cameron 2002). Others are based on a psychodynamic and/or relational model that emphasizes the program environment, or *milieu*, as a treatment theater in which the adolescent "reenacts" difficulties with staff (Abramovitz and Bloom 2003; Kennard 2004; Redl 1966). Most programs are a blend between these and other models that combine the teaching of objective information with the difficult-to-define set of clinical interactions that occur during the provision of any mental health treatment.

This broad group of "residential services," with elastic time parameters and flexible theoretical and clinical orientations, is offered to more or less homogeneous groups of children, depending on the program mission. Some programs are highly homogeneous, developed for the treatment of adolescents with, for example, eating disorders, obsessive-compulsive disorder, or substance abuse disorders. Other programs are designed for more heterogeneous groups of children running the gambit from disruptive behavior disorders to psychotic disorders.

The cost of residential treatment is substantial (Dickey et al. 2001; Lyons et al. 1998; Sheidow et al. 2004). School systems, state social services and mental health budgets, and private insurance plans pay the largest portion of these programs costs, with private insurance paying the majority of the dollars spent on acute residential treatment and public funding paying for the majority of the costs of long-term residential treatment (Dickey et al. 2001; Hirshberg et al. 1997; Whittaker 2004). A mix of private and public insurance and private payment pays for interim-range programs. In some instances a family undertakes to pay privately for residential treatment because they feel a major intervention needs to occur for their child to recover and there is no alternative source of payment.

Linking residential services to other community-based treatment resources is crucial, because the gains made in residential treatment dissipate quickly if they are not capitalized on in the transition back into the community. Family therapy has become an increasingly emphasized aspect of most treatment models because children and families must continually try to resolve the problems that led to the need for out-of-home placement (Hirshberg et al. 1997; Landsman et al. 2001). The child or adolescent is typically placed as close to his or her community as possible to facilitate family contact.

Residential treatment offers options in the broader continuum of care when intensive services become necessary for children and adolescents who fail less restrictive options. As of 2003, almost 66,000 youth were living in long-term residential treatment centers in the United States, and these numbers are on the rise (Leichtman 2006). In addition, tens of thousands of children and adolescents are served each year in acute residential treatment settings.

History

Residential treatment centers existed in the eighteenth and nineteenth centuries in the form of or-

phanages and reform schools (Zimmerman 2004). These original sites were not structured around a self-consciously designed "therapeutic environment" but were the product of acts of social and religious charity as well as social pragmatism that deemed it wise to isolate youth identified as social misfits (Cohler and Friedman 2004). The children in these programs received basic necessities such as food and shelter. The "treatment" often consisted of punitive measures taken against antisocial behavior. The goal was not community reintegration but community insulation (Zimmerman 2004).

Many trends in the United States over the past several decades led to the shift in residential treatment toward a more therapeutic approach. First, the number of orphans in this country declined dramatically (Cohler and Friedman 2004). This was due to both the increase in life expectancy of adults and a major decrease in the number of immigrants coming to the United States. Second, as the public became more aware of the number of incidents of child abuse in orphanages, the government wanted to ensure that children would be safe from these traumatizing experiences (Cohler and Friedman 2004; Hylton 1964). In response to these societal shifts, the variety and quality of services for children with emotional or behavioral problems began to increase.

Initially, there were no standards for the type of care being offered to children in residential placements. Other than providing a safe environment, there was no consensus as to what model "succeeded" with children and adolescents (Zimmerman 2004). Early centers that included "treatment" used a psychoanalytic model that emphasized the importance of the 1-hour therapy session. The other 23 hours of care were initially deemed unimportant to the rehabilitation of the individual, but soon psychoanalysts discovered the additive value of the time spent on the ward (Davids 1975; Redl 1966). They proposed that a therapeutic milieu could allow children to relearn how to manage their world in more adaptive ways (Davids 1975; Kennard 2004; Redl 1966).

Milieu therapy was subsequently incorporated into more child residential programs. One key principle of milieu therapy, termed *marginal interviewing* or *the life space interview*, encompassed the techniques of intervening with a child or adolescent in the moment of difficulty rather than relying on scheduled therapeutic hours (Redl 1966).

Referrals for out-of-home care in the United States numbered more than 500,000 by the mid-1970s (Cohler and Friedman 2004). The amount of money allotted for these services became significant. Children were spending years in residential facilities, and many were not then able to transition smoothly back into their communities (Zimmerman 2004). Child advocates and public policy makers questioned the efficacy of these institutions. Did so many children need to be away from their families? Could some be served as well in the community?

The Adoption Assistance and Child Welfare Act (P.L. 96-272) was passed in 1980. This law stated:

> No child will be removed from a home unless he or she was shown to be at imminent risk of harm; that authorities must at all times make "reasonable efforts" to assure safety and maintain the child in the home whenever possible; and that if a child is removed from home, subsequent placement must be in the "least restrictive environment" (closest to home, closest to community).

This legislation helped promote the concept of a continuum of care, with mental health intervention ranging from less restrictive community-based treatments to out-of-home placements for those with repeated failures at lower care intensity levels.

Short-Term Residential Treatment

Child and Adolescent Characteristics

Community-based interventions are successful for many children and adolescents (Hoagwood et al. 1996; Kazdin and Whitley 2006). Outpatient therapy and psychotropic medication are enough for these children to maintain an acceptable amount of success in school and at home. However, some children at some times cannot be safely or successfully treated in the home environment.

The children and adolescents who cannot be treated in the community typically are those who have more than one current psychiatric diagnosis (Pottick et al. 2005). Children with these complex clinical presentations are more likely to engage in unpredictable and unsafe behaviors and more likely have medication-resistant illness (Connor et al. 1997). For example, substance abuse, criminal and disruptive behaviors, and posttraumatic stress disorder are more prevalent in residential treatment programs than in outpatient treatment (Hussey and Guo 2002). Residential treatment centers have an inflated population of children and adolescents raised in chaotic, abusive, or neglectful environments. Divorce, poverty, and drug abuse among the parents of the children and adolescents are more common in residential treatment centers than in outpatient treatment settings (Landsman et al. 2001).

Entry Points and Patient Selection

Common entry points into an acute residential program include emergency departments and inpatient units. Staff in emergency departments might assess a child or adolescent as needing to be out of his or her current environment, without requiring the full intensity of an inpatient unit. An inpatient unit might assess the child or adolescent as no longer requiring inpatient services but still requiring intensive work on coping skills, illness management, or family systems issues prior to being able to manage in a community setting. The term *level of care* is a way to define and designate medical necessity criteria that are requisite to treat children and adolescents in out-of-home placements (Sowers et al. 2003). If the child does not meet the requirements for an inpatient stay, he or she may meet the criteria for a short-term residential facility. Alternatively, if safety is an acute concern, the child or adolescent may be placed in a locked inpatient unit and then "stepped down" to a residential facility prior to returning to the community.

Intake staff members at short-term residential facilities assess the "fit" between the treatment center and the referred youth. "Fit" has to do with the youth's characteristics and treatment goals. Different residential centers have different exclusionary criteria for their program. At the McLean Hospital Acute Residential Treatment Center, for example, adolescents with moderate to severe mental retardation do not tend to tolerate the focus on group interactions and require more individualized treatment than the program is designed to offer. Youth with sexual offending behaviors tend to have extremely low impulse control and frustration tolerance, and their behavioral responses pose unmanageable risks to themselves and others in the treatment setting.

Admissions Process

After a child is deemed an appropriate fit by the intake staff, his or her guardian must sign the admission forms. The standard forms required in this process provide physical, contact, and insurance information along with authorization for the program to treat the child, contact outside providers, and bill for services. Families also are routinely provided education at the point of intake regarding the Health Insurance Portability and Accountability Act regulations.

In a short-term residential model, the child is seen by a licensed clinician, either a social worker or a psychologist, and by a psychiatrist within 24 hours of admission (Hirshberg et al. 1997), versus the "within a few hours" protocol for an inpatient hospitalization. Case conceptualization and a plan for discharge are developed rapidly. There is frequent communication with the insurance company. Many programs employ an insurance reviewer whose job is to communicate focused treatment plans for the child's initial and ongoing stay in the facility. Coverage is authorized in units of days at a time to encourage a quickened tempo to the clinical work and discharge planning (Hirshberg et al. 1997). Interventions must be brief and focused. Once focal problems are addressed, the child or adolescent can be transitioned to the community for the treatment of more chronic or underlying issues (Curry 1991; Leichtman et al. 2001; Mikkelson et al. 1993).

It is imperative that acute treatment centers have the ability to quickly identify and address these focal treatment goals because commercial insurance companies manage residential mental health benefits tightly. When benefits are not authorized, children who do not meet criteria for Medicaid cannot access these services unless parents or guardians can cover the cost (Federation of Families for Children's Mental Health 2003). In order to access Medicaid services, parents may have the option of sharing custody of their child with the state. This option is anxiety-producing for all families and unacceptable for many. Many family rights agencies have been pursuing legislation that would change current practices and allow children the access to the mental health services they need without the issue of custody being introduced (Federation of Families for Children's Mental Health 2003).

Clinical Course

In the short-term model, a child and his or her family work with a treatment team that includes a case manager, who usually provides individual and family therapy as well as helps coordinate transition to the community. This person can be a licensed mental health counselor or a master's-level clinician (Hirshberg et al. 1997). Often the case manager is a psychologist or social worker by training. A psychiatrist supports the case manager, manages medication during the stay, and communicates with community medical personnel such as psychiatrists and pediatricians. In a short-term residential program, the psychiatrist meets with the resident a few times per week, whereas in a long-term residential program the psychiatrist may see the

resident only on a monthly basis (Leichtman 2006). The clinical educator is often a third treatment team member. The educator has primary responsibility for the program's psychoeducation and skills teaching curriculum, because most children and adolescents have ongoing academic objectives that need to be maintained within the residential context.

The short-term residential model emphasizes and reinforces prosocial behaviors often implemented via a point or level system (Mohr and Pumariega 2004). "Respect and responsibility" is a theme that speaks to the core ethic communicated to children and adolescents in these programs. When the child demonstrates identified positive behaviors, such as completion of a treatment module or sustained nondisruptive behavior, the staff provide increased privileges and freedoms to the patient (Mohr and Pumariega 2004). The child or adolescent is seen as "working toward discharge" with these behaviors. This ability to show cooperation and motivation in treatment is a key indicator of functioning within the parameters of the treatment program, and it is seen as indicative of the resident's ability to move toward discharge and a decreased intensity of clinical services.

Family passes and visits off-site of the program are important measures of success in short-term programs. These passes, which can last from 1 hour to the entire day, provide a litmus test as to the child's or adolescent's ability to translate his or her functioning in the program back to the home and community setting.

Treatment Outcomes

Children are discharged from short-term residential programs with the idea that they have become better able to manage in the community. Many studies have shown the effectiveness of short-term residential treatment. Leichtman et al. (2001) found that short-term residential treatment was effective for youngsters who had not responded well to outpatient therapy and brief psychiatric hospitalizations. This study found a decrease in both internalizing (anxiety/depression) and externalizing (disruptive/conduct disordered) behaviors up to a year after discharge. The subjects showed both an increase in their functional capacities and a decrease in their symptoms. Hirshberg et al. (1997) found that their short-term residential program was able to contain and stabilize 90% of their population. They also found that families whose child had spent time in a short-term unit overwhelmingly reported improved family relations and improved behavior of the child. Mikkelson et al. (1993) found that children who were admitted to a short-term residential treatment facility were less likely to have future hospitalizations.

Although promising, the results lack the rigor of true experimental design. More sophisticated research needs to further validate this treatment modality. Efficacy studies for residential treatment tend to have a within-group design without a true control. Also, no studies have shown which populations respond best to acute residential intervention or whether certain treatment models better help the child prepare for a successful discharge. Although more sophisticated studies are necessary, the studies available provide persuasive evidence as to the efficacy of acute residential treatment as a needed intervention in a continuum of care.

Although these studies tend to lack the rigor of experimental research in terms of scientific methodology, there is nonetheless clear evidence for the effectiveness of the short-term residential treatment approach. When children cannot succeed in the community, a brief problem-focused out-of-home placement can allow the patient and the family to solve the acute problems contributing to the child's functional difficulties and set up supports that will allow the child to better manage after discharge.

Long-Term Residential Treatment

Child and Adolescent Characteristics

The vast majority of children and adolescents with mental illness respond to outpatient or intensive short-term interventions. However, some do not. The child's or adolescent's problems may be so impairing that long-term behavioral work and full removal from a community setting are necessary. The pathology may lie in the family and not with the child, and foster care options may not be available. Families who have children in long-term residential treatment tend to have high rates of parental alcohol use, violence, and physical or sexual abuse (Connor et al. 2004; Hussey and Guo 2002).

Because long-term residential care represents the most structured, intensive, and costly form of treatment for a child or adolescent, it is a treatment of last resort (Frensch and Cameron 2002). The process of a long-term care referral is lengthy and complicated.

Entry Points and Child Selection

Long-term care for severely emotionally disturbed children or adolescents may be initiated and paid for by their families (Smollar and Condelli 1990). This se-

lects for affluent families, as the cost of this treatment is great. This particular group is more likely to be demonstrating behaviors such as drug use and truancy that the parents cannot control (Smollar and Condelli 1990). A majority of children and adolescents, however, are referred through the child welfare system (Andrews et al. 1986). These youth tend to come from dysfunctional homes and from a low socioeconomic class (Connor et al. 2004). Their placement in a facility may be due to the maladaptive behaviors they developed as a result of their chaotic development or simply because there is nowhere else these children can go. A third group of children and adolescents are referred through the Department of Mental Health because the severity of their psychiatric illnesses requires prolonged and intensive services (Teplin et al. 2005).

Child welfare agencies are always seeking alternatives to residential placement because it is expensive and tends to have a negative psychological effect on the family (Andrews et al. 1986). Many parents perceive the placement into out-of-home care as a repudiation of their ability as caretakers. Although attempts have been made to come up with a standardized way to determine the necessity of placement, such as linking specific behaviors with a need for the service (Andrews et al. 1986), to date there remain complex and subjective aspects to admission into these programs.

Admissions Process

The costs of long-term residential care can exceed $100,000 per year (Lyons et al. 1998). Due to the Individuals With Disabilities Education Act, the child's school district is required to pay for the academic portion of the residential facility if it is determined that the least restrictive place for the child to receive an education is in a long-term treatment center. Schools, especially those with limited funds, can be profoundly burdened by these costs. At times, the school system can find creative, less restrictive alternatives that work for the psychiatrically ill child or adolescent. At other times, financial matters present obstacles for necessary service provision. The nonschool "residential" portion of the cost is most often paid for by public funding, channeled through the social services agency involved with the child and family.

A major objective of this long intake process, with multiple diversion points to less restrictive treatment built in, is that when a child or adolescent is ultimately placed in a long-term facility, the need for this placement is clear. This type of placement is often a highly intrusive intervention because it takes a child or adolescent away from his or her family and community for a substantial length of time. During this time, the facility attempts to teach the child more adaptive behaviors, repair the family, and have the child be able to generalize these newly learned behaviors and modes of coping in a community setting.

Clinical Course

Many children and adolescents who reach a long-term treatment center have been subjected to significant trauma and abuse (Hussey and Guo 2002). These childhood experiences, along with a high rate of genetic loading for a major mental illness in this patient population, leave the long-term residential group of patients with severe impairments in managing emotions, coping with frustration, and succeeding in relationships. It is the goal of the long-term program to establish and offer a therapeutic milieu to shape new behaviors that are more prosocial and adaptive (Redl 1966).

The therapeutic milieu is based on the idea that the troubled child or adolescent will reexperience and reenact the difficulties he or she has had in relationships with others while he or she is at the program (Abramovitz and Bloom 2003; Kennard 2004; Redl 1966). As these difficulties arise, it is the job of the child care staff to help the child learn better ways to function emotionally, cognitively, and behaviorally in the given situation (Bonier 1982; Hylton 1964; Youngren 1991). Appropriate behavior is modeled, taught, and reinforced. If the child makes a bad decision, the staff members attempt to not react emotionally or aggressively, as might have been the case within the family or community environment. A consequence may be given, but it is done with an attempt at neutrality of emotion and predictability of the consequence (Kennard 2004). This predictable and muted response by authority is probably the opposite of what the child is used to and can allow the child to feel incrementally more safe and contained. Over time, the goal for the child or adolescent is to experience relationships with the staff based on trust and respect and to experience a personal sense of agency and mastery over feelings, thoughts, relationships, and the environment. The importance of this relational aspect to longer-term residential care is exemplified by the finding that the ability to make strong therapeutic relationships is one of the most important nonspecific predictors of success in residential treatment (Bickman et al. 2004; Pfeiffer and Strzelecki 1990).

Due to this finding, there has been an effort to limit seclusion and restraint use in residential programs, because such interventions can be hurtful to the development of these important relationships (Donovan et al. 2003). The use of seclusion and restraint techniques is most likely to occur when a child fails to comply with the expectation made by direct care staff (Ryan et al. 2004). The manner in which the expectation is communicated influences the need for this intervention. De-escalation models aiming to limit the use of restraints and physical interventions have increased greatly.

Each resident in long-term care typically has a case manager and psychiatrist. Compared with time in short-term programs, the time spent with these individuals is much less (Hirshberg et al. 1997). There is not the immediate need to reintegrate the child back into the community, and therefore individual therapy can happen less frequently, medication changes can take place more gradually, and there are more opportunities for behavioral observation. Most of a resident's time is spent with milieu staff whose training and experience are variable (Myers et al. 2004).

There are alternatives to this therapeutic milieu model. There has been growing popularity of more military-style "boot camp" programs whose goal is to provide a structured and demanding environment that teaches "responsibility and respect" through more punitive means (Weis and Whitemarsh 2005). These programs offer strict monitoring, goal-directed activities, and alternative education environments geared toward individuals with histories of chronic truancy, substance abuse, and antisocial behavior. Although this model is not as supportive as that of more traditional residential programs, past participants in these programs maintain favorable perceptions of the program model, specifically citing how much care and concern were shown by staff as well as the fairness of practices (Deschenes and Greenwood 1998). For children with more disruptive externalizing behaviors and without a clear psychiatric mood or thought disorder, these behavior-oriented programs may be desirable.

Treatment Outcomes

It has been very hard for long-term residential treatment to demonstrate clinical effectiveness as a treatment model. Although individual agencies may do well at monitoring how their own populations improve as a result of treatment, no agency or group can provide rigorous studies with large samples (Leichtman 2006). Thus although much research has been done showing that some programs have positive results for their residents, there is no empirical study that truly substantiates the use of this intensive and costly form of care.

There is some information on who tends to be more successfully treated in long-term programs. Lyons et al. (2001) used a sophisticated growth modeling technique to determine the rates of change of symptoms during a residential stay. They found tremendous variability in which symptoms improved and which did not. The results showed that residential treatment was effective at reducing risky behaviors and improving depressive symptoms. On the other hand, hyperactivity and anxiety increased over the course of the treatment stay.

The work of Conner et al. (2002) supported this finding. They found that higher internalizing scores were predictive of favorable treatment gains. They also found that the higher a child is functioning upon admission, the more likely he or she will show improvement at the end of treatment.

Studies are beginning to focus on gender differences when trying to determine who may be successful in residential treatment. Gender has been overlooked in the past as a potential treatment variable (Blotcky et al. 1984). Recently, however, studies have shown that residentially placed females demonstrate more behavioral and emotional problems than males in their age group (Handwerk et al. 2006). This finding may be due to the fact that females are more likely to have been physically and sexually abused than males. Also, because girls are not as overtly aggressive as boys, their problems may go unnoticed and unchecked for longer periods of time before any treatment interventions are begun (Handwerk et al. 2006).

Research relating to the success of residential treatment has shown that, as with shorter-term residential treatment, an important variable in long-term residential treatment is the amount of contact and involvement the family has with the child (Joshi and Rosenberg 1997; Landsman et al. 2001; Leichtman 2006; Whittaker 2000). Children in out-of-home care who do not have the support of their parents tend to do poorly in comparison with youth whose parents are involved in care. The goal of residential treatment to transition the child to a less restrictive setting is helped tremendously by family work done with motivated and eager parents or guardians. As a result of this research, residential centers are pushing to make family therapy and contact a more integral part of their treatment model (Hirshberg et al. 1997).

Special Populations

Although many residential centers serve individuals with a variety of needs, some serve populations requiring a more homogeneous and specialized environment. Adolescents with eating disorders, for example, face both medical and psychological problems related to their illness (Steiner and Lock 1998). They require more medical staff on the premises than most long-term centers have available. In addition, the behavior planning around meals and food intake is more codified than can be effectively administered in a general care setting. This section explores residential treatment for adolescents with eating disorders as well as other specific patient populations that benefit by specialized programming: substance abuse, sexual offending, emerging personality disorder, and obsessive-compulsive disorder patient populations.

Residential treatment for eating disorders is becoming more common (Frisch et al. 2006). Inpatient hospitalizations occur for patients when their weight drops to life-threatening levels. The goal is to bring the adolescent to a more normal weight and nutritional/hemodynamic status. Once this is done, there is value in continued acute work to address underlying causes of the illness and behaviors that are likely to lead to rapid weight loss and rehospitalization if not addressed (Wiseman et al. 2001). Non-hospital-based residential programs offer a site for this "subacute" work.

In response to increased demand for this service, residential programs focused on eating disorders have more than tripled in recent years. Therapies tend to be eclectic, ranging from cognitive therapy to spiritual and experiential models (Frisch et al. 2006). Along with the difference in philosophy, there is also a great difference in cost. Program costs range from $500 to $1,500 dollars per day. The variation in service provision along with the dearth of scientific research to substantiate what is effective has been a major shortcoming of these services (Frisch et al. 2006). Although there is clearly a need for residential eating disorders programs due to decreases in inpatient stays, this burgeoning industry will become more standardized as programs are called on to provide indices for their effectiveness.

Alcohol and drug use is currently a major health problem for children and adolescents. Many adolescents with substance use disorders have comorbid mental illness. Among individuals in substance abuse programs, 25%–61% have a comorbid affective illness. The use of substances has also been linked to increased risk of suicidal and criminal behaviors (Weiner et al. 2001). This group of patients tends to be highly treatment resistant. There are high rates of recidivism and dropout rates from treatment (Wise et al. 2001).

Two residential treatment models have shown the most promising results with this population. The first, the Minnesota Model, is based on the 12-Step approach to substance abuse treatment. In this model, chemical dependency is treated as a primary disease in which the only treatment regimen that works is abstinence. The typical length of stay in a program is 1 month, and during this time the patient attends group and individual therapy, Alcoholics Anonymous lectures, and family counseling (Winters et al. 2000). The second model is termed the *therapeutic community approach.* This program emphasizes mutual self-help, behavioral consequences, and a shared set of values concerning "right living" (Jainchill 1997; Morral et al. 2004). Instead of viewing substance abuse as the primary disease, this model views dependence as a symptom of larger personality or psychiatric problems. The goal of the therapeutic community is to treat the personality problems with the hope that substance use will decrease (Morral et al. 2004).

Both program models report modest gains (Morral et al. 2004). However, adolescents with comorbid disruptive disorders do particularly poorly in these settings (Wise et al. 2001). Ironically, increases in referrals to these programs are coming overwhelmingly from the juvenile justice system (Teplin et al. 2005). Wise et al. (2001) found that only 20% of patients who had a comorbid disruptive disorder were successful treatment participants.

Sexual offenders are a very complex population with many unique issues. Although they are likely to get referred for treatment through the criminal justice system, they have different treatment needs than nonsexualized conduct disorder patients (Letourneau et al. 2004). Sexual offenders tend to have more internalizing symptoms, are more likely to have a history of significant sexual abuse, and are more susceptible to the negative effects of congregating with conduct disordered individuals (Mager et al. 2005). As a group, they tend to respond well to intensive family-based treatment options. Interestingly, the variable most highly correlated with treatment success is the amount of caregiver involvement (Letourneau et al. 2004). Other aspects of the work with sexual offenders involve medication for attention-deficit/hyperactivity disorder and dysthymia (M. Kafka, M.D., personal communication, May 3, 2007), and cognitive-behavioral therapy approaches to enable the patients to identify and disrupt their "abuse cycle" of behaviors.

The treatment of adolescents with "emerging" personality disorders in long-term residential centers has been increasing (Walsh 2004). These programs gener-ally employ modified dialectical behavior therapy, an outpatient therapy for the treatment of parasuicidal and suicidal behaviors, within the context of a residential unit in order to help the adolescent better manage his or her emotions, curb self-mutilation behaviors, and interact more effectively in social situations with peers and family (Linehan 1993). Research has shown that the use of this approach reduces suicidal behavior, dropout from treatment, future psychiatric hospitalizations, substance abuse, and overall interpersonal difficulties (Walsh 2004).

Obsessive-compulsive disorder has a long history of health care providers utilizing a behavioral approach to treatment. The same exposure therapies that are used in outpatient care settings have become the primary means of care offered to patients in adolescent residential care facilities for this disorder. Because behavioral techniques require consistent reinforcement in order to extinguish the relationship between obsession and compulsion, it is often very important that this diagnostic group receive intensive residential services. Currently, research efforts at the Menninger Clinic and at Rogers Memorial Hospital in Wisconsin have both shown promise in the intense exposure and behavioral work that can be done with this population of adolescents in a residential treatment setting (Björgvinsson et al. 2007; B. Reiman, personal communication, 2007).

Community-Based Alternatives: Multisystemic Therapy

The pressure to provide least-restrictive, cost-effective services has led to community-based treatments that manage some high-risk adolescents in the community, thereby avoiding out-of-home placement (Halliday-Boykins and Henggeler 2004).

Multisystemic therapy is a leading choice in a growing continuum of less restrictive services available in the community (Henggeler et al. 1999; Huey et al. 2005; Schoenwald et al. 2000; Sheidow et al. 2004). The program model revolves around the idea of creating the structure and intensity of services necessary to stabilize an acute crisis but doing so without removing the patient from the home. By embedding interventions in the home environment, this treatment approach is aimed at altering the social system of the child or adolescent (Schoenwald et al. 2000). As in the acute residential model, each child or adolescent in community-based treatment has a psychiatrist and a case manager. The child or adolescent also typically has two bachelor's degree–level crisis caseworkers who are trained in the multisystemic therapy philosophy (Henggeler et al. 1999). With the frequent help and multidisciplinary aspects of staff support the child and family receive, multisystemic therapy is bringing very intensive structure and expertise right into the home.

In an effort to clearly distinguish itself from residential treatment, multisystemic therapy has prided itself on stringent standardization of care and scientifically rigorous research methods (Henggeler et al. 1999). Treatment studies are highly organized, with a control group and random assignment of youth to either a residential or multisystemic treatment condition. Also, professionals practicing multisystemic therapy are consistently monitored so as to determine how rigidly they are following the treatment model and philosophy (Henggeler et al. 1999).

Structured studies have reliably shown the ability of multisystemic therapy to keep children and adolescents at home while stabilizing crises. Henggeler et al. (1999) found that this therapy effectively prevented psychiatric hospitalization in 75% of the youth it served. It was also able to lower the use of psychiatric hospitalizations well after the 4 months of treatment were completed. This research is important because not only is multisystemic therapy keeping children and adolescents within their home and community, but it also is much more cost-effective than either residential placement or inpatient hospitalization.

Future Needs

Many factors have created a real need for major change in the practices of residential treatment. First, there is great pressure to keep the child or adolescent in the community as much as possible (Dickey et al. 2001). This has led to much shorter lengths of stay and an increased focus on family work and reunification efforts (Terling 1999). Second, the targeted clinical population has changed. Residential facilities are being asked to manage much more difficult clinical situations because of the shortened length of inpatient stays (Hirshberg et al. 1997). This patient population provides great challenges and a need for specialized, sophisticated, and standardized treatment models. Last, there is pressure from third-party payers to hold treatment centers more accountable for the work they do (Boyd et al. 2007; Curry 2004; Hirshberg et al. 1997; Lieberman 2004). This has led to a need for these organizations to study their own programs to determine what works and what does not.

One clear direction for residential facilities is to increase connections between themselves and community interventions (Lieberman 2004). Residential services have been shown to be most effective for many populations when the family is intensively involved. Because the goal is reunification with the community, there needs to be as much contact with the community as possible during the child's residential stay (Leichtman 2006). There must be outreach so that the skills and behaviors learned in the center can be easily generalized at home, which includes an increased focus on family work. It is imperative that parents or guardians be a part of the process, both within therapy and in the planning of stepdown, wraparound services and other community supports.

Residential treatment programs must also respond to the calls for increased accountability. As discussed earlier, "residential treatment" is a nebulous term; there is very little that unifies these wide-ranging services into a cohesive whole. There must be more effort put into standardization of care. When a child or adolescent is referred for long-term out-of-home placement, payers, family members, and school personnel must have the knowledge of which program and what length of stay are most likely to work for that child or adolescent. With these adaptations, intensive mental health services such as residential treatment can be a leader in the development of a connected and supportive continuum of care for adolescents and youth.

References

Abramovitz MD, Bloom SL: Creating sanctuary in residential treatment for youth: from the "well-ordered asylum" to the "living-learning environment." Psychiatr Q 74:119–135, 2003

Adoption Assistance and Child Welfare Act of 1980, P.L. 96-272 (94 Stat. 500)

Andrews DA, Robinson D, Balla M: Risk principle of case classification and the prevention of residential placements: an outcome evaluation of the share the parenting program. J Consult Clin Psychol 54:203–207, 1986

Bickman L, Vides de Andrade AR, Lambert EW, et al: Youth therapeutic alliance in intensive treatment settings. J Behav Health Serv Res 31:134–148, 2004

Björgvinsson T, Wetterneck CT, Webb SA, et al: Treatment outcome for adolescent OCD in an inpatient setting. Poster presented at the 27th Annual Meeting of the Anxiety Disorders Association of America, St. Louis, MO, March–April 2007

Blotcky MJ, Dimperio TL, Gossett JT: Follow-up of children treated in psychiatric hospitals: a review of studies. Am J Psychiatry 141:1499–1507, 1984

Bonier RJ: Staff countertransference in an adolescent milieu treatment setting. Adolesc Psychiatry 10:382–390, 1982

Boyd AS, Einbinder SD, Rauktis ME, et al: Building research capacity in residential treatment centers: an approach for empirical studies. Child Youth Care Forum 36:43–58, 2007

Cohler BJ, Friedman DH: Psychoanalysis and the early beginnings of residential treatment for troubled youth. Child Adolesc Psychiatr Clin N Am 13:237–255, 2004

Connor DF, Ozbayrak KR, Kusiak KA, et al: Combined pharmacotherapy in children and adolescent in a residential treatment center. J Am Acad Child Adolesc Psychiatry 36:248–254, 1997

Connor DF, Miller KP, Cunningham JA, et al: What does getting better mean? Child improvement and measure of outcome in residential treatment. Am J Orthopsychiatry 72:110–117, 2002

Connor DF, Doerfler LA, Toscano PF, et al: Characteristics of children and adolescents admitted to a residential treatment center. J Child Fam Stud 13:497–510, 2004

Curry JF: Outcome research on residential treatment: implications and suggested directions. Am J Orthopsychiatry 61:348–357, 1991

Curry JF: Future directions in residential treatment outcome research. Child Adolesc Psychiatr Clin N Am 13:429–441, 2004

Davids A: Therapeutic approaches to children in residential treatment. Am Psychol 30:809–814, 1975

Deschenes EP, Greenwood PW: Alternative placements for juvenile offenders: results from the evaluation of the Nokomis Challenge Program. Journal of Research in Crime and Delinquency 35:267–294, 1998

Dickey B, Normand SL, Norton EC, et al: Managed care and children's behavioral health services in Massachusetts. Psychiatr Serv 52:183–188, 2001

Donovan A, Plant B, Peller A: Two-year trends in the use of seclusion and restraint among psychiatrically hospitalized youths. Psychiatr Serv 54:987–993, 2003

Federation of Families for Children's Mental Health: Relinquishing Custody for Mental Health Services. Rockville, MD, Federation of Families for Children's Mental Health, 2003

Frensch KM, Cameron G: Treatment of choice or a last resort? A review of residential mental health placements for children and youth. Child Youth Care Forum 31:307–349, 2002

Frisch MJ, Herzog DB, Franko DL: Residential treatment of eating disorders. Int J Eat Disord 39:434–442, 2006

Halliday-Boykins C, Henggeler SW: Heterogeneity in youth symptom trajectories following psychiatric crisis: predictors and placement outcomes. J Consult Clin Psychol 72:993–1003, 2004

Handwerk ML, Huefner JC, Smith G, et al: Gender differences in adolescents in residential treatment. Am J Orthopsychiatry 76:312–324, 2006

Henggeler SW, Rowland MD, Randall J, et al: Home-based multisystemic therapy as an alternative to the hospitalization of youth in psychiatric crisis: clinical outcomes. J Am Acad Child Adolesc Psychiatry 38:1331–1339, 1999

Hirshberg DL, Horgan A, Douglass D: Acute residential treatment: adapting our expertise for managed care. Residential Treatment for Children and Youth 15:51–72, 1997

Hoagwood K, Jensen P, Petti T, et al: Outcomes of mental health care for children and adolescents: a comprehensive conceptual model. J Am Acad Child Adolesc Psychiatry 35:1055–1063, 1996

Huey SJ, Henggeler SW, Rowland MD, et al: Predictors of treatment response for suicidal youth referred for emergency psychiatric hospitalization. J Clin Child Adolesc Psychol 34:582–589, 2005

Hussey D, Guo S: Profile characteristics and behavioral change trajectories of young residential children. J Child Fam Stud 11:401–410, 2002

Hylton LF: The Residential Treatment Center: Children, Programs and Costs. New York, Child Welfare League of America, 1964

Jainchill N: Therapeutic communities for adolescents: the same and not the same, in Community as Method: Therapeutic Communities for Special Populations and Special Settings. Edited by De Leon G. Westport, CT, Praeger, 1997, pp 161–177

Joshi P, Rosenberg LA: Children's behavioral response to residential treatment. J Clin Psychol 53:567–573, 1997

Kazdin AE, Whitley MK: Comorbidity, case complexity, and effects of evidence-based treatment for children referred for disruptive behavior. J Consult Clin Psychol 74:455–467, 2006

Kennard D: The therapeutic community as an adaptable treatment modality across different settings. Psychiatr Q 75:295–307, 2004

Landsman MJ, Groza V, Tyler M, et al: Outcomes of family centered residential treatment. Child Welfare League of America 30:351–379, 2001

Leichtman M: Residential treatment of children and adolescents: past, present, and future. Am J Orthopsychiatry 76:285–294, 2006

Leichtman M, Leichtman ML, Barber CC, et al: Effectiveness of intensive short term residential treatment with severely disturbed adolescents. Am J Orthopsychiatry 71:227–235, 2001

Letourneau EJ, Schoenwald SK, Sheidow AJ: Children and adolescents with sexual behavior problems. Child Maltreat 9:49–61, 2004

Lieberman RE: Future directions in residential treatment. Child Adolesc Psychiatr Clin N Am 13:279–295, 2004

Linehan M: Cognitive Behavioral Treatment of Borderline Personality Disorder. New York, Guilford, 1993

Lyons JS, Libman-Mintzer LN, Kisiel CL, et al: Understanding the mental health needs of children and adolescents in residential treatment. Prof Psychol Res Pr 29:582–287, 1998

Lyons JS, Terry P, Martinovich Z, et al: Outcome trajectories for adolescents in residential treatment: a statewide evaluation. J Child Fam Stud 10:333–345, 2001

Mager W, Milich R, Harris MJ, et al: Intervention groups for adolescents with conduct problems: is aggregation harmful or helpful? J Abnorm Child Psychol 33:349–362, 2005

Mikkelson EJ, Bereika GM, McKenzie JC: Short-term family based residential treatment: an alternative to psychiatric hospitalization for children. Am J Orthopsychiatry 63:28–32, 1993

Mohr WK, Pumariega AJ: Level systems: inpatient programming whose time has passed. J Child Adolesc Psychiatr Nurs 17:113–125, 2004

Morral AR, McCaffrey DF, Ridgeway G: Effectiveness of community based treatment for substance abusing adolescents: 12 month outcomes of youths entering Phoenix Academy or alternative probation dispositions. Psychol Addict Behav 18:257–268, 2004

Myers PG, Bibbs T, Orozco C: Staff supervision in residential care. Child Adolesc Psychiatr Clin N Am 13:309–327, 2004

Pfeiffer SI, Strzelecki SC: Inpatient psychiatric treatment of children and adolescents: a review of outcome studies. J Am Acad Child Adolesc Psychiatry 29:847–853, 1990

Pottick KJ, Warner LA, Yoder KA: Youths living away from families in the US mental health system: opportunities for targeted intervention. J Behav Health Serv Res 32:264–281, 2005

Redl F: When We Deal With Children. New York, Free Press, 1966

Ryan EP, Hart VS, Messick DL, et al: A prospective study of assault against staff by youths in a state psychiatric hospital. Psychiatr Serv 55:665–670, 2004

Schoenwald SK, Ward DM, Henggeler SW, et al: Multi-systemic therapy versus hospitalization for crisis stabilization of youth: placement outcomes four months post-referral. Ment Health Serv Res 2:3–12, 2000

Sheidow AJ, Bradford DW, Henggeler SW, et al: Treatment costs for youths receiving multi-systemic therapy or hospitalization after a psychiatric crisis. Psychiatr Serv 55:548–554, 2004

Smollar J, Condelli L: Residential placement of youth: pathways, alternatives, and unresolved issues. Child Today 19:2–8, 1990

Sowers W, Pumariega AJ, Huffine C, et al: Level of care decision making in behavioral health services: the LOCUS and the CALOCUS. Psychiatr Serv 54:1461–1463, 2003

Steiner H, Lock J: Anorexia nervosa and bulimia nervosa in children and adolescents: a review of the past 10 years. J Am Acad Child Adolesc Psychiatry 37:352–359, 1998

Teplin LA, Abram KM, McClelland GM, et al: Detecting mental disorders in juvenile detainees: who receives services. Am J Public Health 95:1773–1780, 2005

Terling T: The efficacy of family reunification practices: reentry rates and correlates of re-entry for abused and neglected children reunited with their families. Child Abuse Negl 23:1359–1370, 1999

Walsh B: Using dialectical behavior therapy to help troubled adolescents return safely to their families and communities. Psychiatr Serv 55:1168–1170, 2004

Weiner DA, Abraham ME, Lyons J: Clinical characteristics of youths with substance use problems and implications for residential treatment. Psychiatr Serv 52:793–799, 2001

Weis R, Whitemarsh SM: Military style residential treatment for disruptive adolescents: effective for some girls, all girls, when, and why? Psychol Serv 2:692–705, 2005

Whittaker JK: The future of residential group care. Child Welfare League of America 29:59–74, 2000

Whittaker JK: The re-invention of residential treatment: an agenda for research and practice. Child Adolesc Psychiatr Clin N Am 13:267–279, 2004

Winters KC, Stinchfield RD, Opland E, et al: The effectiveness of the Minnesota Model approach in the treatment of adolescent drug abusers. Addiction 95:601–612, 2000

Wise BK, Cuffe SP, Fischer T: Dual diagnosis and successful participation of adolescents in substance abuse treatment. J Subst Abuse Treat 21:161–165, 2001

Wiseman CV, Sunday SR, Klapper F, et al: Changing patterns of hospitalization in eating disorder patients. Int J Eat Disord 30:69–74, 2001

Youngren VR: Opportunity's hard knocks: clinical training in adolescent milieu therapy. Psychotherapy 28:298–302, 1991

Zimmerman DP: Psychotherapy in residential treatment: historical development and critical issues. Child Adolesc Psychiatr Clin N Am 13:347–363, 2004

CHAPTER 23

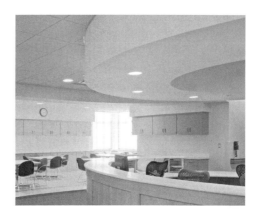

HOSPITAL-BASED PSYCHIATRIC EMERGENCY SERVICES

Glenn W. Currier, M.D., M.P.H.

The Psychiatric Emergency Service as the Canary of the Mental Health Coal Mine

Over the past four decades, psychiatric emergency services (PESs) emerged and matured largely in response to external changes in the public mental health treatment system. The widespread deinstitutionalization or closure of state psychiatric beds was coupled with poorly planned and executed community alternatives. Money that accrued from state bed closure did not follow patients into the community, and with notable exceptions, most community mental health centers did not consider emergency interventions within their scope of business. With the advent of managed care, private psychiatric beds disappeared in the wake of hospital closures and network consolidations. Between 1960 and 1994, the number of U.S. psychiatric beds per capita decreased by about two-thirds, from 4 per 1,000 to 1.3 per 1,000, with a correlative increase in deaths due to mental illness (Currier 2000). More

recently, the widespread availability of cheap smokable cocaine and other powerful drugs of abuse made disabled patients with a reliable source of public income easy targets for drug dealers, often destabilizing their underlying psychiatric conditions and touching off a "revolving door" of frequent PES presentations and discharges. Public intolerance of visible homeless people and involuntary commitment laws predicated solely upon dangerousness led to a funneling effect, with increasingly disturbed, volatile individuals channeled to general hospital–based emergency departments.

In response to these and other factors, the number and organizational complexity of PESs have risen substantially. Patients with primary psychiatric disturbances now compose at least 8% of all emergency department visits (Larkin et al. 2005). Additionally, although many perceive this to be a uniquely urban phenomenon, mental health presentations to rural "critical access" hospital emergency departments show similarly troubling trends (Hartley et al. 2007).

Despite the growing—and, some would say, alarming—increase in demand for emergency psychi-

311

atric services, mention of PESs is virtually absent in both the President's New Freedom Commission on Mental Health (2003; Unutzer et al. 2006) and the more recent Institute of Medicine report on U.S. emergency departments (Institute of Medicine 2006). This is both troubling and baffling. Unlike other care venues, emergency departments cannot refuse to treat patients for any reason, and this open access provides an excellent snapshot of the level of functionality of the mental health treatment system as a whole. For example, the numbers of presentations of children and adolescents seeking care at one large urban PES in Rochester, New York, have increased substantially, presumably in response to school districts' "zero tolerance" policies for violence and suicidal behavior in the wake of the Columbine incident and others. PESs serve as the leading edge for recognizing the changing need for psychiatric services among specific subpopulations.

The Psychiatric Emergency Service as Black Box

In spite of the escalating quantity of PES visits over time, the evidence base testing clinical practice in this setting is almost nonexistent. Few descriptive studies exist of PES protocols and procedures, and even fewer high-quality randomized, controlled trials exist to test the efficacy of treatments rendered in that environment. The scope, quantity, and quality of PES services remain poorly characterized and highly variable across regions, institutions, and providers. In a survey by Allen and Currier (2003, 2004) of PES directors, several findings helped shed some light on these issues. The most common reasons for presentation included mood disorders, psychotic-spectrum disorders, and substance abuse or dependence. A majority of patients were not subsequently admitted to psychiatric inpatient beds from the PES, and approximately two-thirds were discharged from the PES either with no aftercare or with referrals to outpatient treatments of some type. In some centers, the PES can be a volatile place. Use of restraints (chemical or physical) is common, as is assault of staff by patients. Unfortunately, data are not routinely collected in a uniform fashion across settings, and comparing outcomes is hampered accordingly. As the leading edge of treatment for many patients, the PES is in the unique position of detecting changes in types of populations served and the after-effects of changes in other parts of the mental health service delivery system.

Conceptual Models of Psychiatric Emergency Service Care: *Primum Non Nocere* (First, Do No Harm)

In 1980, Gerson and Bassuk first articulated a "triage model" of PES care in which the main function of embattled and underresourced services was to decide who got access to scarce inpatient beds. Diagnostic precision was downplayed, and dangerousness was the key determinant. Two decades later, Allen (1999) described a "treatment model" whereby advances in medications and community programming allowed for initiation of definitive treatment within the PES. This approach hinges on more rigorous diagnostic precision so that condition-specific treatments can be initiated. Treatment initiation was also fostered by the development of 48- or 72-hour extended observation units, allowing for ongoing assessment of many patients who ultimately were found not to require inpatient care but were too unstable to discharge within the first 24 hours. Strategies such as "Depakote loading" and initiation of selective serotonin reuptake inhibitors were possible to consider within this time frame. Mobile crisis teams and other hospital diversion strategies were developed with varying degrees of success. Although the treatment model was a major step forward in emergency care, the task of ameliorating acute symptoms of mental illness within a few days remains an elusive goal. In spite of many advances, the primary focus of PES clinicians for the majority of patients remained the decision to admit or discharge. Unfortunately, many patients with behavioral complaints who are treated in overwhelmed emergency services find the experience so off-putting that trust in the mental health delivery system can actually be damaged, hindering willingness to follow through with prescribed care (Cerel et al. 2006). Meaningful communication with outpatient providers was all too often an afterthought, and patients who required assistance navigating a complex treatment system were often left to their own devices to follow up with prescribed aftercare.

Now, another decade later, it seems possible to imagine another model of PES care that prioritizes the interface between the PES and outpatient treatment referral sources. In this "staging model," emphasis would be placed on actively engaging and educating clients and their families about the value of following through with appropriate prescribed care. Based on an assessment of readiness to change and use of psychotherapeutic techniques such as motivational interviewing (Miller and Rollnick 2002), clinicians may not only refer patients to appropriate community-based care but also increase treatment adherence and improve treatment outcome (Sheldon et al. 2003). We have recently reported results of a randomized trial using a PES-based mobile crisis team to meet with discharged suicidal patients in the community and engage them in further services. This intervention was successful in 60% of cases, versus 20% for usual care (referral to an outpatient psychiatric appointment within 5 business days). Novel models that capitalize on the provider–patient relationship developed in the PES offer promise. Other models that allow representatives of community mental health centers, substance abuse treatment providers, and others to meet with the patients before they leave the PES also hold promise. However, widespread development of such bridging strategies will require adaptations of payment rules, because currently ambulatory providers are unable to bill for services while patients are registered in the PES. Further research to demonstrate the clinical utility and cost-effectiveness of new approaches is clearly desirable.

A Road Map for Psychiatric Emergency Service Evaluation

For the practicing clinician, treating the sometimes overwhelming volume of patients supersedes any consideration of national trends in health care delivery. Clinicians are charged with making rapid decisions based on imperfect and incomplete information. Should things go wrong, the stakes can be high for both service providers and service recipients. Nonetheless, at its core, the goals of the PES evaluation are fairly straightforward. Clinicians must first decide if a patient belongs in the PES and route those who do not to more appropriate venues. Examples of patients who do not belong in a PES include individuals who are acutely medically compromised (e.g., overdoses disclosed after the triage process) and patients whose behavior is grounded in criminality rather than mental illness. For patients who do have a mental illness that warrants immediate voluntary or involuntary intervention, the next order of business is to decide if definitive care can be initiated within the PES or if the time frame for effective treatment is likely to be so long as to require inpatient hospitalization. Then the search for a bed begins. However, it is the gray zone of patients who describe or manifest signs of mental illness, but who may or may not meet a severity thresh-

old or who are estimated to be likely to improve rapidly, who linger in the PES. What follows is a suggested logical framework for dealing humanely and judiciously with such individuals.

Emergency Assessment Steps

It cannot be emphasized enough how important it is that all patients coming into the PES are searched and that an arch or at least a wand metal detector is employed at triage. Contraband weapons represent a real risk to staff and other patients. Likewise, to maximize safety for all involved, protocols should be worked out with local law enforcement departments to make gun lockers available so that officers can remove their weapons prior to entering the PES.

Once patients are safely through the door, hospital-based emergency assessments are composed of a few steps that are largely consistent across most institutions: 1) triage, 2) medical assessment, 3) psychiatric assessment, and 4) disposition. Each step may be straightforward or not, depending on the complexity of the case, but at the end of the day, each of these four steps needs to be not only performed but also articulated in the medical record.

Triage

Triage simply means "to sort." The first clinician most patients encounter in an emergency department is a triage nurse whose major function is to route patients to either medical, surgical, or psychiatric care tracks. Most often, these are medical-surgical nurses with limited specialty mental health training. As discussed in the next section, in many institutions a cursory physical examination and *pro forma* set of orders for laboratory tests may begrudgingly precede a transfer to psychiatry, but from the medical/surgical perspective, the goal is to "clear" patients as quickly as possible for transfer.

Triage can also be thought of as the process by which PES clinicians get an initial impression of case severity as patients roll through the door. As opposed to treating patients sequentially based on time of admission, it makes sense to establish a two-stage assessment process for prioritization of potentially volatile and violent cases. In other instances, if it appears on initial screening that a person clearly does *not* belong in the PES, a clinician may decide to see such patients more rapidly to decompress the PES. Finally, an internal triage can establish quickly who should and should not be allowed to leave the PES without a full assessment, regardless of whether the person presented voluntarily or involuntarily.

There are several triage algorithms and tools available (Lewis and Roberts 2001). However, one of the oldest, best established, and most clinically useful is the Crisis Triage Rating Scale (Bengelsdorf et al. 1984; Figure 23–1). This scale is designed specifically to aid in making admission decisions by rating patients on three domains: support system, dangerousness, and ability to cooperate. Each domain has a Likert-type scale scored from 1 (most severe) to 5 (least severe). Patients who score 8 or below warrant serious consideration for admission. Isolated low scores on any one of these particular domains also suggest an intervention strategy while the patient is in the PES to maximize chances for a safe discharge. For example, many patients present with suicidal thoughts without clear intent and are clearly motivated to seek treatment. For such patients, involving friends and family to shore up the social support network may make discharge a realistic option. Operationalizing this assessment through the use of this or other standardized rating tools can be enormously beneficial.

Medical Assessment

PES patients present with a large number of concurrent psychiatric, social, and medical needs. "Proper" assessment of the latter is a debatable issue and is often a point of conflict between busy PES and medical emergency department staff. As such, there is wide variation across and within emergency services in terms of the extent of medical screening and interventions undertaken. Certainly, the "baton" model of care, in which blanket "medical clearance" is granted by emergency physicians and the patient is irrevocably passed on to the PES, is outmoded. However, efforts to design more appropriate treatment algorithms are hampered by lack of consensus on the type, scope, and duration of adequate assessment. This is worrisome in light of the enormous medical morbidity in PES patients. As early as 1980, Carlson et al. (1981) documented medical issues as the sole reason for PES presentation in 7% of patients seen. By the mid-1990s, Olshaker et al. (1997) found serious medical issues requiring urgent intervention in 19% of psychiatric patients presenting to a medical emergency department. More recently, data from the Clinical Antipsychotic Trials of Intervention Effectiveness study indicated that metabolic syndrome was present in 36% of male and 52% of female subjects at enrollment, respectively (McEvoy et al. 2005). In the same cohort, 30% of people who entered the study with diabetes were not re-

---

Instructions: score 1 to 5 in each category using descriptive statements as guidelines.

A. Support system (circle number)

1. No family, friends or others. Agencies cannot provide immediate support needed.

2. Some support might be mobilized, but its effectiveness will be limited.

3. Support system potentially available but significant difficulties exist in mobilizing it.

4. Interested family, friends, or others but some question exists of willingness of availability to help.

5. Interested family, friends, or others able and willing to provide support needed.

B. Dangerousness (circle number)

1. Expresses or hallucinates suicidal/homicidal ideas or has made serious attempt in present illness. Unpredictably impulsive/violent.

2. Same as #1, but ideas or behavior are to some degree ego-dystonic or history of violent or impulsive behavior but no current signs.

3. Expresses suicidal/homicidal ideas with ambivalence or has made only ineffective gestures. Questionable impulse control.

4. Some suicidal/homicidal ideation or behavior, or history of same, but clearly wishes and is able to control behavior.

5. No suicidal/homicidal ideation or behavior. No history of violent or impulsive behavior.

C. Ability to cooperate (circle number)

1. Unable to cooperate or actively refuses.

2. Shows little interest in or comprehension of efforts to be made on his/her behalf.

3. Passively accepts intervention maneuvers.

4. Wants to get help but is ambivalent or motivation is not strong.

5. Actively seeks outpatient treatment, is willing and able to cooperate.

Total score: _____

Disposition

Referred for admission screening

Accepted as crisis patient

FIGURE 23–1.   Crisis Triage Rating Scale.

Source.   Reprinted from Bengelsdorf H, Levy LE, Emerson RL, et al: "A Crisis Triage Rating Scale: Brief Dispositional Assessment of Patients at Risk for Hospitalization." *Journal of Nervous and Mental Disease* 172:424–430, 1984. Copyright 1984, Lippincott Williams & Wilkins. Used with permission.

ceiving treatment, and 62.4% of subjects with hypertension were not receiving outpatient care (Nasrallah et al. 2006). Compared with the general population, individuals with mental illness are more often uninsured and more often unlinked to a primary care provider (Druss and Rosenheck 1998).

Given all that, the likelihood of untreated medical conditions being detected in the PES is very high. Lines of responsibility for addressing these issues are not so clear. The relationship between medical illness and psychiatric conditions can be causative, contributory, or incidental. Causative medical conditions are the reason that the aberrant behavior manifests and are the grounds for the emergency department visit. An example is urinary tract infections in elderly nursing home patients, with resulting delirium and agitation. Most prudent clinicians would agree that such cases usually belong on the medical side of the department, at least initially. However, even when the cause of psychiatric symptoms is clearly medical in nature, there will be times when a medical admission is not prudent. For example, a severely agitated patient's behavior may prove so disruptive to the functioning of a medical unit that psychiatric admission is nonetheless warranted, even if such behavior results from recent medical causes such as head trauma or encephalitis. Such patients will clearly require close medical follow-up, regardless of their inpatient location. On the other end of the spectrum are incidental illnesses, often chronic in nature, that may need "tuning up" but are well within the scope of practice of the PES psychiatrist in a tertiary care medical center. An example would be a known diabetic who stopped insulin treatment briefly and needs a sliding scale written to control blood sugars until her insulin doses can be verified. This is something any competent PES psychiatrist should be able to handle. The most confusing and largest category of patients is the gray zone of contributory conditions. These include patients with behavioral disturbances with unclear and unexplored thyroid disease, lupus, alcohol withdrawal, and so on. Each PES staff needs to work out a relationship with medical colleagues whereby these gray-zone patients can be handled on a case-by-case basis, and patients can flow back and forth between psychiatry and medicine as the clinical picture evolves.

Another contentious issue includes blanket laboratory screening. Henneman et al. (1994), writing in the *Annals of Emergency Medicine*, recommended a relatively extensive battery of laboratory tests, a head computed tomography scan, and potentially a lumber puncture for all patients with new-onset psychiatric illness. However, real-world constraints of time, cost, and patient resistance and a high likelihood of false-positive results argue for a more conservative approach. Blanket laboratory screenings for all PES patients are not recommended. However, rational and targeted testing grounded in a good history and physical examina-

tion is critical. Examples would be a thyroid-stimulating hormone level in a depressed patient with known thyroid disease, electrolyte levels in volume-depleted patients, lead levels in high-risk children, and a urinalysis in elderly patients with acute mental status changes. If patients tell you they are not experiencing current medical concerns, and they are walking and talking, available evidence suggests that you can believe them (Korn et al. 2000). A wasteful and lengthy battery of laboratory tests, drawn either in the PES or perhaps on the medical side as a way to forestall access to the PES, is not advised. However, a basic panel of screening studies (complete blood count, basic metabolic panel, urinalysis, and toxicology) and *pertinent* medication blood levels, radiological studies, electrocardiograms, and the like are usually necessary before PES patients will be accepted onto psychiatric units.

Psychiatric Assessment

Patients' time in the PES is generally measured in hours and sometimes, in spite of legal restrictions to the contrary, in days. Documentation of clinical history and assessments should not be static but rather should establish an initial set of relevant clinical data and build upon this in a linear and coherent narrative as the period of observation lengthens. The PES medical record should prompt a series of questions that form the basis for an informed (if provisional) diagnosis. Untoward behavior needs to be grounded in and arise from a treatable mental or medical disorder in order for psychiatric or medical hospitalization—as opposed to jail, shelter placement, or myriad other disposition alternatives—to make sense. However, because involuntary commitment laws in all U.S. states hinge on dangerousness to self or others, and not on a firmly established psychiatric diagnosis, a solid risk assessment for both violence and suicide is crucial. The evaluation should be internally consistent, with assessments by physicians, nurses, and other clinical staff cross-referenced and incorporated into the documentation left by each. Ultimately, the assessment should conclude with a well-reasoned and well-informed statement of the logic for the clinical course of action pursued.

Using a public health model of analysis (Table 23–1), there are only four outcomes possible from the PES intervention: patients can be appropriately or inappropriately discharged or admitted. Each outcome has potentially far-reaching consequences for patients, providers, and the health system as a whole.

True-positive cases represent persons who meet criteria for a treatable mental illness that can only be

TABLE 23–1.   Roman square for psychiatric admission decisions

	Admitted to Inpatient Bed	Not Admitted
Appropriate for admission	TRUE POSITIVE	FALSE NEGATIVE
Not appropriate for admission	FALSE POSITIVE	TRUE NEGATIVE

addressed in the highest level of services available, the inpatient psychiatric setting. Such patients may seek admission voluntarily, or if significant risk of harm to self or others is established, involuntary detainment laws (which vary from state to state) may be invoked if needed.

Patients who meet criteria for illness severity but who are discharged from the PES constitute *false-negative* cases. Inexperienced clinicians may fear the outcome of letting patients go based on the incomplete data set available in the PES and may be tempted to admit every patient they evaluate. Clinicians are not clairvoyant, and even in the best of services, some decisions are made that in hindsight appear ill advised. Good documentation of the rationale for discharge is the best defense should something untoward occur after discharge (Simon 2000; Simon and Shuman 2006). However, the risks of wrongful detainment are real, and psychiatric hospitalization has potentially catastrophic ramifications for patients in terms of stigma, financial burden, and erosion of trust in mental health providers.

False-positive cases represent persons admitted to psychiatric units who are more appropriate for detoxification units, criminal justice environments, medical services, or release to the community. A small minority of patients seeking secondary gains may make specious threats of suicide to force clinicians' hands. Clinicians in chronically busy treatment settings may start to believe that the vast majority of patients fall into this category. This is the *sine qua non* of staff burnout, and PES managers should be mindful of the potential for corrosive countertransference. Every effort should be made to work with outpatient providers to make informed admission decisions. False-positive cases can be an extreme drain on hospital resources, because most payers will not cover such admissions.

True-negative cases are people who do not need admission, probably do not want admission, and can be referred to ambulatory treatment settings in a safe and effective manner.

The Appendix shows an example of a clinical intake form currently in use at a large tertiary care medical center. This is offered simply as a model of a form that has stood up to regular use in a busy PES. Several

aspects of this examination warrant consideration. Data accrue over time, and documentation should reflect that fact. The parts of the assessment must be internally consistent, and information should be added as it is obtained. All staff who are responsible for direct patient care should provide written information on this form, although more detailed nursing notes may be documented in other parts of the chart. If physician staff notes are not congruent with the clinical impressions and observations of nurses, social workers, and so on, any discrepancies should be addressed directly in the notes.

In high-volume services, a two-stage evaluation process is the norm. Part 1 is usually completed by a registered nurse, social worker, psychiatric resident, or other clinical staff member. This is a history-gathering phase, and salient parts of the reasons for presentation, prior history of psychiatric conditions or substance use, acute medical concerns, social history, and family history are assessed and recorded. Most important, a standardized set of questions related to dangerousness to self or others must be included and filled out completely. Part 2 is completed by the attending psychiatrist or, in some states, by a nurse practitioner who has a collaborative agreement with that physician. To save time, a check-box statement that the physician has reviewed Part 1 and found no factual discrepancies is included. A multiaxial diagnosis is given, although often with provisional qualifiers. This note must again be dated and timed, because it usually represents the endpoint of the decision-making period.

Disposition

The assessment should culminate in a coherent summary statement, often incorporating a description of the main sources of clinical data, the clinician's level of trust in the veracity of those sources (including the patient), and a logical conclusion as to course of action taken, either admission or discharge. If discharge is selected, efforts to link patients with appropriate aftercare should be explained. Every effort should be made to inform the clinicians who will "inherit" the patients about the patients' PES visit(s). Changes in medications must be clearly articulated. The patient or family should be educated about steps to take if the clinical picture declines after discharge. If a patient is to be discharged under somewhat anxiety-provoking circumstances, it should be clear in the note that the circumstances did not allow for involuntary commitment and that the patient was offered and refused voluntary inpatient psychiatric treatment.

Clinical documentation around the decision to admit "true positive" cases may be appropriately rather brief, for example: "Patient still actively suicidal with plan and requires continuous monitoring to prevent suicide." However, writing a discharge note can be very tricky for recurrently "false positive" patients. Examples abound, for instance, patients who made an actual suicide attempt but did so while intoxicated, or self-injurious patients with borderline personality disorder who present for PES services weekly or sometimes daily. Clinicians may be reluctant to discharge these people, not wanting to be the last to carry the "hot potato."

In closing, a few examples of discharge notes are provided that cover the clinical and legal bases for these sorts of individuals.

1. The intoxicated mild overdose:

   > Mr. X. presented in the context of acute inebriation and the breakup of his relationship. This was an impulsive act. Now that he is sober and reunited with his fiancée, he denies any intention to harm himself or others. He has no prior history of self-injurious behavior and denies symptoms consistent with a treatable Axis I mood or psychotic disorder. He appears to be a reliable historian, and his story is verified by his fiancée and primary care physician. In my opinion, he is not at imminent risk of self-harm and therefore is no longer legally detainable. He declines voluntary admission or an outpatient counseling referral. Both he and his fiancée agree to call 911 or present voluntarily here if his condition worsens and SI [suicidal ideation] occurs.

2. The frequent PES habitué:

   > Ms. Y is well known to me from prior emergency department visits. Although she is at chronically elevated risk of self-harm, nothing in this recent episode suggests that risk has increased over this high baseline. In fact, the patient sought help by calling 911 in this current presentation. The patient is well connected with her outpatient therapist, who concurs with this assessment. This patient does not appear at imminent risk of self-harm and therefore is no longer legally detainable. Plan: discharge directly to dialectical behavior therapy skills group this afternoon; follow up with therapist tomorrow at 11 A.M. Patient agrees with plan.

Conclusion

PESs are a critical component of the U.S. mental health services delivery system. Policy makers are now paying increased attention to the importance of PESs in the efficient functioning of the entire emergency response system. They are forced to do so: Demand is clearly outpacing supply by a wide margin. Emergency medicine as a specific specialty only came into being over the past few decades. In a somewhat delayed but similar trajectory, emergency psychiatry is now clarifying and codifying the unique set of skills and training necessary to practice in this challenging environment. There is growing momentum to establish fellowship training to meet these needs. Certainly, as the portfolio of high-quality medical evidence grows (in the form of randomized trial data), clinical practice will come to be based on a more sure footing. In the meantime, clinicians must operate largely on the basis of caring, compassion, experience, and common sense to do their best by the multiply challenged people who seek care in the PES.

References

Allen MH: Level 1 psychiatric emergency services: the tools of the crisis sector. Psychiatr Clin North Am 22:713–734, 1999

Allen MH, Currier GW: Use of restraints and pharmacotherapy in academic psychiatric emergency services. Gen Hosp Psychiatry 26:42–49, 2004

Bengelsdorf H, Levy LE, Emerson RL, et al: A crisis triage rating scale: brief dispositional assessment of patients at risk for hospitalization. J Nerv Ment Dis 172:424–430, 1984

Carlson RJ, Nayar N, Suh M: Physical disorders among emergency psychiatric patients. Can J Psychiatry 26:65–67, 1981

Cerel J, Currier G, Conwell Y: Consumer and family experiences in the emergency department following a suicide attempt. J Psychiatr Pract 12:341–347, 2006

Currier GW: Psychiatric bed reductions and mortality among persons with mental disorders. Psychiatr Serv 51:851, 2000

Currier GW, Allen M: Organization and function of academic psychiatric emergency services. Gen Hosp Psychiatry 25:124–129, 2003

Druss BG, Rosenheck RA: Mental disorders and access to medical care in the United States. Am J Psychiatry 155:1775–1777, 1998

Gerson S, Bassuk E: Psychiatric emergencies: an overview. Am J Psychiatry 137:1, 1980

Hartley D, Ziller EC, Loux SL, et al: Use of critical access hospital emergency rooms by patients with mental health symptoms. J Rural Health 23:108–115, 2007

Henneman PL, Mendoza R, Lewis RJ: Prospective evaluation of emergency department medical clearance. Ann Emerg Med 24:672–677, 1994

Institute of Medicine: IOM report: the future of emergency care in the United States health system. Acad Emerg Med 13:1081–1085, 2006

Korn C, Currier G, Henderson S: Medical screening of psychiatric patients in a general emergency department. J Emerg Med 18:173–176, 2000

Larkin GL, Claassen CA, Emond JA, et al: Trends in US emergency department visits for mental health conditions, 1992 to 2001. Psychiatr Serv 56:671–677, 2005

Lewis S, Roberts AR: Crisis assessment tools: the good, the bad, and the available. Brief Treat Crisis Interv 1:17–28, 2001

McEvoy JP, Meyer JM, Goff DC, et al: Prevalence of the metabolic syndrome in patients with schizophrenia: baseline results from the Clinical Antipsychotic Trials of Intervention Effectiveness (CATIE) schizophrenia trial and comparison with national estimates from NHANES III. Schizophr Res 80:19–32, 2005

Miller WR, Rollnick S: Motivational Interviewing: Preparing People for Change, 2nd Edition. New York, Guilford, 2002

Nasrallah HA, Meyer JM, Goff DC, et al: Low rates of treatment for hypertension, dyslipidemia and diabetes in schizophrenia: data from the CATIE schizophrenia trial sample at baseline. Schizophr Res 86:15–22, 2006

Olshaker JS, Browne B, Jerrard DA, et al: Medical clearance and screening of psychiatric patients in the emergency department. Acad Emerg Med 4:124–128, 1997

President's New Freedom Commission on Mental Health: Achieving the Promise: Transforming Mental Health Care in America. Rockville, MD, U.S. Department of Health and Human Services, 2003

Sheldon KM, Joiner TEJ, Pettit JW, et al: Reconciling humanistic ideals and scientific clinical practice. Clin Psychol Sci Pract 10:302–315, 2003

Simon RI: Taking the "sue" out of suicide: a forensic psychiatrist's perspective. Psychiatr Ann 30:399–407, 2000

Simon R, Shuman DW: The standard of care in suicide risk assessment: an elusive concept. CNS Spectr 11:442–445, 2006

Unutzer J, Schoenbaum M, Druss BG, et al: Transforming mental health care at the interface with general medicine: report for the President's commission. Psychiatr Serv 57:37–47, 2006

APPENDIX

Sample "Comprehensive Psychiatric Emergency Program Evaluation" Form

The form presented here was developed at the Department of Psychiatry, University of Rochester Medical Center, Rochester, New York, and is not copyrighted. It is provided as a resource for the reader, as an example of an intake form that has stood up to regular use in a busy psychiatric emergency service.

STRONG 🜲 HEALTH

STRONG MEMORIAL HOSPITAL

SMH 873 MR – SAMPLE DOCUMENT
Strong Behavioral Health
Comprehensive Psychiatric Emergency Program Evaluation

Page 1 of 7

PSYCHIATRIC TRIAGE Date: _____ Time: _____ Legal Status On Arrival: ☐ Voluntary ☐ MHA ☐ Other (explain)

Accompanied By: Method of Travel to ED:

Print Name:	Signature:	Date:

INITIAL EVALUATION

Initial Evaluation Begun   DATE: _____   TIME: _____   Reason for presenting to ED (provide brief narrative)

SEVERAL BLANK LINES DELETED TO SAVE SPACE

History of Presenting Illness:

Symptoms contributing to today's presentation, if present	√	Please check box if there has been a change or identified problem in the following categories in the recent past. Describe/clarify *each* change or problem below with brief narrative.	Time Duration for change/problem
Depression			
No symptoms of Depression found			
Depressed Mood			
Decreased Energy			
Appetite Disturbance			
Sleep Disturbance			
Decreased Interest			
Suicidality			
Psychomotor Activity			
Concentration Disturbance			
Feelings of Hopelessness			
Mania			
No symptoms of Mania found			
Inflated Self-Esteem			
Decreased Need for Sleep			
Pressured Speech			
Racing Thoughts			
Easy Distractibility			
Goal-Directed Activity			
Excessive Involvement in Pleasurable Activities			
Print Name:		**Signature:**	**Date:**

Appendix.   Sample "Comprehensive Psychiatric Emergency Program Evaluation" Form

History of Presenting Illness – Continued			
Symptoms contributing to today's presentation if present	√	Please check box if there has been a change or identified problem in the following categories in the recent past. Describe/clarify *each* change or problem below.	Time Duration for change/problem
Psychosis:			
No symptoms of Psychosis found			
Delusions			
Hallucinations			
Disorganized Speech			
Disorganized or Catatonic Behavior			
Negative Symptoms		☐ Flat Affect ☐ Avolition/Apathy ☐ Poverty of Speech/Thought	
Social or Occupational Dysfunction			
Anxiety:			
No symptoms of Anxiety found			
Palpitations			
Sweating			
Trembling			
Shortness of Breath			
Feeling of Choking			
Chest Discomfort			
Nausea			
Dizziness			
Derealization or Depersonalization			
Feelings of Losing Control			
Fear of Dying			
Numbness/Tingling			
Chills/Hot Flashes			
Agoraphobia			
Obsessions			
Compulsions			
Specific Phobias			
Recurrent Thoughts of a Traumatic Event			
Avoidant Behavior			
Increased Arousal			
Excessive Anxiety/Worry			
Restlessness			
Print Name:		**Signature:**	**Date:**

Appendix.   **Sample "Comprehensive Psychiatric Emergency Program Evaluation" Form** *(continued)*

Addictive Behavior Assessment

☐ **No contributory Addictive Behaviors** | **WITHDRAWAL SYMPTOMS**

Substance	Method/Type of Use	Amount	Frequency	Last Use	CURRENT		PAST	
Alcohol					☐ No symptoms ☐ Tremors ☐ Nausea	☐ Sweating	☐ No symptoms ☐ Tremors ☐ Nausea	☐ Sweating ☐ Seizure ☐ Delirium Tremens
Benzodiazepines					☐ No symptoms ☐ Tremors ☐ Nausea	☐ Sweating	☐ No symptoms ☐ Tremors ☐ Nausea	☐ Sweating ☐ Seizure
Heroin/Opiate					☐ No symptoms ☐ Tremors ☐ Nausea	☐ Sweating	☐ No symptoms ☐ Tremors ☐ Nausea	☐ Sweating ☐ Seizure
Cocaine					☐ No symptoms ☐ Other–specify		☐ No symptoms ☐ Other–specify	
Marijuana					☐ No symptoms ☐ Other–specify		☐ No symptoms ☐ Other–specify	
Nicotine					☐ No symptoms ☐ Other–specify		☐ No symptoms ☐ Other–specify	
OTHER					☐ No symptoms ☐ Other–specify		☐ No symptoms ☐ Other–specify	
					☐ No symptoms ☐ Other–specify		☐ No symptoms ☐ Other–specify	
					☐ No symptoms ☐ Other–specify		☐ No symptoms ☐ Other–specify	

Prior Rehab/Detox Dates (Begin with Most Recent) ☐ None	Location	Length of Stay	Completed?	
			☐ Yes	☐ No
			☐ Yes	☐ No
			☐ Yes	☐ No

Print Name: **Signature:**   **Date:**

Appendix. Sample "Comprehensive Psychiatric Emergency Program Evaluation" Form *(continued)*

Social History

☐ Information covered in Social Work Risk/ Psychosocial Assessment – 1056PSY MR (Go to Next Section)

Resides: ☐ Alone ☐ With Family or Others	Marital Status:	Legal: ☐ No ☐ Yes (specify)
☐ Homeless ☐ In Facility/Group Home	Children:	

☐ History of abuse as victim (specify):

Psychiatric History

Previous Diagnoses: ☐ None	Family History: ☐ None

Current providers: ☐ None ☐ See SW Risk Assessment – 1056PSY MR ☐ Providers w/contact #'s listed immediately below

Prior Dates – Begin With Most Recent	Location	Length of Stay	Prior Dates – Begin With Most Recent	Location	Length of Stay
Psych ED Visits			Hospitalizations		
EOB Stays			Partial Hospital Prgrm		

Previous Medication Trials ☐ None

	Name of Rx	Start	End	Side effects	Benefit Y / N
1					
2					
3					
4					
5					
6					

Lethality Assessment

Danger to Self				Danger to Others			
Suicidal Thoughts	☐ No	☐ Yes–specify		Violent Thoughts	☐ No	☐ Yes–specify	
Current Attempt	☐ No	☐ Yes–specify		Current Violence	☐ No	☐ Yes–specify	
Past Attempts	☐ No	☐ Yes–specify		Past Violence	☐ No	☐ Yes–specify	
Current Plan	☐ No	☐ Yes–specify		Current Plan/Threat	☐ No	☐ Yes–specify	
Barriers to Suicide?				Barriers to Harming Others?			
Command Hallucinations To Self-Harm	☐ No	☐ Yes–specify		Command Hallucinations To Harm Others	☐ No	☐ Yes–specify	
Self-Injurious Behavior – Current	☐ No	☐ Yes–specify		Identified Target	☐ No	☐ Yes–specify	
Self-Injurious Behavior – Past	☐ No	☐ Yes–specify					

Print Name:	Signature:	Date:

Appendix. Sample "Comprehensive Psychiatric Emergency Program Evaluation" Form *(continued)*

Physical Assessment
–May be completed by Nursing and Physician Disciplines–

Medical History:	Medications	Dosage	Allergies	☐ NKA
			Latex: ☐ No ☐ Yes	
			Medications	Reaction
			Food/Environmental:	

Date/Time: _____

Pain Scale: *(if above 4, notify NP or MD)* Location: _____ Frequency: _____

0	1	2	3	4	5	6	7	8	9	10
No Pain										Severe

Weight in Kg:

☐ No intervention indicated

Medication Offered/Given: _____ Response: _____ Date/Time of Reassess: _____

Fall Risk Assessment:

Yes	No		Yes	No	
☐	☐	Impaired Mobility due to Unsteady Gait	☐	☐	Poor Standing or Sitting Ability
☐	☐	Unable or Unwilling to call for assistance appropriately	☐	☐	History of Syncopal Episodes
☐	☐	History of Incontinence	☐	☐	Use of Assistive Ambulatory Device

If Yes to any of the above, implement Fall Prevention Plan: Side rails up, call bell within reach, appropriate footwear; other: _____

Specify Device: _____

Safe to Use on Unit? **YES NO**

Fall Prevention Plan Implemented – Date: _____ Initials: _____

Advance Directive (AD): ☐ **None** ☐ <18yr ☐ AD placed on chart ☐ AD teaching info given

MOLST* Form filed with chart

Code Status: ☐ **Full Code** ☐ DNR filed with chart

(*Medical Orders for Life-Sustaining Treatment)

Review of symptoms patient is *currently* experiencing: ☐ **Patient is not reporting any physical complaints at this time**
(no documentation below required if box is checked)

HEENT:	Cardiac:
Neck:	Resp:
Abdomen:	Extremities:
Skin:	Vascular:
Endocrine:	Neuro:
Other:	Other:

Additional Evaluation Information: [Sign and Date Each Entry]

SEVERAL BLANK LINES DELETED TO SAVE SPACE

Physician/NP Physical Assessment: Diagnostic Tests/Findings/Interventions

☐ History, Physical Assessment, Vital Signs, Addictive Behavior Assessment, Lethality Assessment and Pain Scale [score of 4 or above requires intervention] have been reviewed and confirmed.

SEVERAL BLANK LINES DELETED TO SAVE SPACE

Printed Name with Credentials:	Signature:	Date:

Appendix. Sample "Comprehensive Psychiatric Emergency Program Evaluation" Form *(continued)*

Physician /NP Evaluation	*Brief statement of presenting problem *Prior Psychiatric history and other pertinent medical social and family history (reference previous documentation as appropriate) *Additional clinical observations * Formulation (organized summary of the patient's current situation based on data collected, differential diagnosis, rationale for medication strategy) * DSM-IV Diagnosis Axis I - Axis V *Treatment Plan **Please use progress note for additional documentation if needed.**

Date and Time Patient Seen by Physician/NP:

SEVERAL BLANK LINES DELETED TO SAVE SPACE

Mental Status Exam:	Muscle Strength and Tone:
General:	Abnormal Movements:
Speech:	Gait and Station:
Mood:	Affect:
Thought Process:	Thought Content: (SI/HI)
Memory:	Perceptions/Associations: (AH/VH)
Concentration:	Attention/Level of Consciousness:
Language:	Fund Of Knowledge:
Judgement:	Other:
Insight:	

Assessment and Plan:

SEVERAL BLANK LINES DELETED TO SAVE SPACE

Axis I:
Axis II:
Axis III:
Axis IV:
Axis V:

_____ _____ _____
Print Name   Physician Signature   Date

Patient search at CPEP Triage and Screening Intake	Searched By:	Time:

Method: ☐ Pocket/Purse ☐ Pat Down ☐ Metal Scan ☐ Other

Articles removed:

Articles Placed: ☐ Bag ☐ Cabinet ☐ Lock Box ☐ Family ☐ Other

Admit Note: ☐ Patient introduced to unit ☐ Patient brought to Waiting Room ☐ Patient brought to Rm _____

☐ Patient educated to evaluation process ☐ Q 15 minute checks maintained

Print Name: | **Signature:** | **Date:**

☐ Articles, as above, given to Inpatient Staff at Admission. **Receiving Staff Signature:** **Date:**

Collateral, Additional Interventions, Pertinent Triage & Screening Course of Events *Date, Time and Sign Each Entry

SEVERAL BLANK LINES DELETED TO SAVE SPACE

Appendix. **Sample "Comprehensive Psychiatric Emergency Program Evaluation" Form** *(continued)*

	✓	(Check all that apply)		✓	(Check all that apply)
Summary of Interventions (check all that apply)					
Patient Interview	☐	Psychiatric Technician (1)	Collateral Contacts	☐	Family Member (1)
	☐	RN Evaluation (2)		☐	Therapist (1)
	☐	NP Evaluation (2)		☐	Psychiatrist (1)
	☐	SW Evaluation (2)		☐	Primary Care Physician (1)
	☐	Resident Evaluation (2)		☐	Other: (1)
	☐	Attending Evaluation (3)			
Crisis Intervention	☐	Family Meeting (2)	Safety Plan	☐	Follow-up Appointment (1)
	☐	Psychoeducation regarding support services (ABW, CD, etc) (2)		☐	Lifeline Number Given (1)
				☐	Home with Family Member (1)
	☐	Intensive Staff Contact (1)		☐	Increased Supervision (1)
Discharge Referral To:	☐	Primary Therapist (1)	Diagnostic Tests	☐	Imaging (4)
	☐	Psychiatrist (1)		☐	Labs (4)
	☐	PCP (1)		☐	EKG (4)
	☐	COPS Appointment (1)		☐	Pulse Oximetry (2)
	☐	Other: (1)			
Social Work Risk Assessment	☐	Low (Risk Screen) (3)	Medication(s)	☐	General Meds (Tylenol, Advil, etc) (1)
				☐	Psychotropics PO (3)
	☐	High (Second Page Completed) (5)		☐	Psychotropics IM (5)
				☐	Prescription Given (3)
Lethality Assessment	☐	(2)	General Psychoeducation	☐	(4)
Physical Assessment	☐	(3)	Restraints	☐	Observation Log complete (764MR) (5)
				☐	Nursing Documentation (763A) (5)
				☐	Physician Documentation (763B) (5)
Addictive Behavior Assessment	☐	(2)	Medicaid Application	☐	(3)
Observation	☐	Q 15 minute checks (2)	Legal Status Explained and Rights Given	☐	(1)
	☐	Continuous (quiet rooms with monitor) (3)			
CIWAs	☐	(5)	Other	☐	( )
Other	☐	( )	Other	☐	( )
Printed Name with Credentials:			**Signature:**		**Date:**

Appendix. Sample "Comprehensive Psychiatric Emergency Program Evaluation" Form *(continued)*

CHAPTER 24

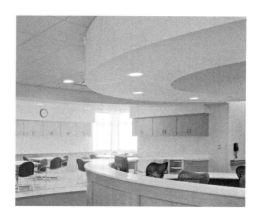

OUTPATIENT COMMUNITY MENTAL HEALTH SERVICES

Francine Cournos, M.D.
Stephanie LeMelle, M.D.

The locus of psychiatric treatment has progressively shifted from inpatient to outpatient care. In this chapter we describe this trend and some of the structures that have evolved to provide a continuum of care outside of the hospital. We illustrate the general approach to care by using our own program, a comprehensive service for people with severe and persistent mental illness (SPMI), as a model.

Deinstitutionalization and Community Care

To provide some context, it is helpful to review the history of the decline of long-term institutional care and the growth of community-based outpatient services. This trend began in the mid-1950s (Kiesler and Sibulkin 1987) and continues to evolve even in the present. In the early 1950s most seriously mentally ill people in the United States were treated in long-term

hospitals, and most outpatient services were offered by clinicians in private practice to people with less incapacitating disorders. This system is still in place in many developing countries that have not yet established community services.

In the United States the movement to reduce the use of hospital care for mentally ill people was driven by many factors, including the introduction of antipsychotic medications, an increasing bias against the use of large institutions (Goffman 1961), and a number of important legal decisions concerning the rights of patients (Bloche and Cournos 1990). The evidence suggests, however, that the most important impetus was the opportunity for state governments to shift patients from large state hospitals, where care was paid for by the states, to alternative sheltered care, where newly developed federal entitlement programs such as Medicare, Medicaid, and Social Security disability payments would pay most of the costs (Bloche and Cournos 1990; Foley and Sharfstein 1983; Kiesler and Sibulkin 1987).

The term *deinstitutionalization* is inaccurate in the sense that the use of institutional care changed but did not diminish. Rather, there was a depopulation of state hospitals while the population of other types of institutions grew (Bloche and Cournos 1990; Kiesler and Sibulkin 1987). According to the U.S. census, a consistent 1.05%–1.1% of the U.S. population resided in institutions between 1950 and 1980. However, in 1950, 40% of institutionalized people were in mental hospitals, and 20% were in homes for the aged and dependent. By 1980, however, only 10% of the institutionalized were in mental hospitals, and 57% were in homes for the aged and dependent. The degree to which this represented transferring those in need of supervision from one institution to another is not entirely clear, but certainly new types of institutions opened to house disabled elderly and people with developmental disabilities (Bloche and Cournos 1990). A criticism of deinstitutionalization has long been that despite the establishment in 1963 of a new federal funding stream to build community mental health centers, adequate resources did not follow patients with SPMI into the community (Bloche and Cournos 1990; Greer and Greer 1984).

By the 1980s three new and intertwined concerns about people with severe mental illness became prominent: substance use, homelessness, and the "criminalization" of mentally ill people. Jails and prisons became a more frequent site for the long-term institutional care of people behaving in a disorderly way as the result of mental illness (Hall et al. 2003; Quanbeck et al. 2003). In the face of these problems, some commentators lamented the loss of long-term hospital care. Yet although hospitalization had provided housing and supervisory functions that made these problems less likely, virtually every study that compared patients who remained in the hospital with those who lived in the community demonstrated that most patients functioned better once they left the hospital and reported an improved quality of life (Okin 1983; Segal and Aviram 1978). It became clear that there was no turning back, and the work of mental health advocates has largely focused on the development of more effective and comprehensive outpatient services and on parity between mental health care and general health care to provide the funding needed to expand community services. Although a detailed discussion of these developments is beyond the scope of this chapter, the primary outcome is that today hospital beds are used for increasingly shorter periods of time, and the long-term management of patients with major mental illnesses must be carried out in the community.

Principles of Community Treatment

The philosophies and goals of community outpatient services have gradually shifted from maintenance strategies to recovery-based models. Following the loss of state hospital beds, the primary goal of community outpatient care for people with severe mental illness was to stabilize patients' symptoms and prevent hospitalizations. These are still important goals, because it is difficult to work on longer-term strategies before patients achieve stability. A variety of strategies have been developed to promote stability that are largely focused on maintaining community housing and family ties; reducing patient exposure to criticism and hostility (often referred to as creating environments with low expressed emotion) (Anderson et al. 1986; Beels et al. 1984; Cournos 1987); and promoting adherence to treatment through continuity of care, outreach, and use of depot medications. Yet as the voices of patients and their families grew more powerful within the mental health system, it became clearer that stability by itself does not achieve a good quality of life and that patients' assets are often underestimated.

Today's recovery-oriented programs have more ambitious goals that include rehabilitation strategies to improve social, occupational, and recreational skills. Rehabilitation interventions include social skills training, supported employment, cognitive enhancement, and illness management strategies. The body of evidence for the effectiveness of rehabilitation interventions on role functioning is stronger for some interventions (e.g., supported employment; Anthony and Blanch 1987; Catty et al. 2008; Cook et al. 2005) than for others (e.g., cognitive enhancement; Hogarty et al. 2004).

It has also become clearer that many illnesses are best treated using medication and psychotherapy together. Many different therapies, including family and multiple family group therapy (McFarlane et al. 1996), interpersonal psychotherapy (Weissman 2007), cognitive-behavioral therapy (Weissman 2007), dialectical behavioral therapy (Lynch et al. 2006), motivational interviewing (Rüsch and Corrigan 2002), and psychodynamic therapies (Fonagy et al. 2005), have shown efficacy in the treatment of major mental illnesses, with or without pharmacological interventions.

Hospital-Based Outpatient Mental Health Care Programs

Community mental health outpatient services can be provided in a variety of settings. In this chapter we focus on outpatient mental health care that is delivered as part of the ambulatory services of a hospital. Hospital settings vary as to their mission and funding, depending on whether they are public, voluntary, or private and whether the hospital is a general medical facility or is a standalone psychiatric hospital. This chapter focuses broadly on outpatient care in a manner that is applicable to all of these settings.

Hospital-based outpatient psychiatric programs have unique structural, staffing, and patient care delivery advantages that include benefits for staff and for patients.

Structure

Hospitals are well-organized systems with structures in place for all of the basic activities needed to establish and run outpatient programs. This includes systems to hire and train staff, register and bill patients, provide fiscal and legal services, develop and maintain code-compliant space, and respond to the multiple requirements of regulatory agencies.

Staffing

Outpatient staff who are hired through a hospital have the advantages of the resources of a large institution. This can improve the types of benefit packages that staff can choose from and may allow staff access to unions and collective bargaining. Often licensed clinicians can be credentialed through the hospital, which allows them admitting privileges and the flexibility to work in both inpatient and outpatient settings. Hospitals can also provide staff with training and continuing education programs that are often too costly for freestanding clinics to provide. The common practice of affiliation with a university provides an academic environment for supervision of junior staff, the teaching of students, and research collaborations. These activities help stimulate senior clinicians and contribute to their staying up to date on current developments in psychiatry. Student programs can also be an importance source of recruitment to junior staff positions.

Patients

Hospital-based outpatient programs also benefit patients. One of the benefits is a continuum of psychiatric care from emergency services to inpatient care to outpatient treatment. In general hospitals, patients can also get their medical evaluations and care in the same organization, creating the optimal conditions for integrating medical and psychiatric treatment. Some medical evaluation and treatment is usually present in freestanding psychiatric hospitals as well.

Hospital emergency services afford patients priority access to the hospital's beds and other programs. Once patients are familiar with a hospital's services, they may be more willing to move from one level of care to another. Inpatient and outpatient staff can readily share information and consult with one another. As more programs adopt electronic medical records, there are unprecedented opportunities for the instantaneous exchange of information among a hospital's components of care.

Many general hospitals have outpatient or walk-in medical clinics that are open to the community. These are good settings for detecting mental disorders, because people with psychiatric illnesses often initially present to medical practitioners. In addition, patients with established psychiatric disorders can receive general medical health care in these settings. Having access to a general hospital for patients who are on medications that require blood level monitoring or regular blood work can greatly improve patient adherence to monitoring. This setup also provides opportunities for medical and psychiatric practitioners to collaborate. The psychiatry program can provide psychiatric assessments and recommendations for patients seen by medical staff, and the medical program can provide comprehensive medical care for psychiatric patients.

Challenges

Hospital-based outpatient services may also face some greater challenges than programs run by community-based organizations. These might include maintaining good community relations and responding to the unique cultural customs and languages of local populations. Some patients prefer being seen in more informal community-based settings that are not reminiscent of prior hospitalizations. These problems can be reduced by including members of the local community among program staff and on advisory groups and by locating some programs off site from the main hospital buildings. For example, we have located our outpatient programs in the local community and have systematically recruited bilingual and bicultural staff to meet the needs of the Latino population that we serve.

Often hospital-based staff earn higher salaries than staff working for smaller, not-for-profit organizations. These staff costs can be a barrier to creating those elements of a comprehensive program that are not well reimbursed. For example, in New York State, where our program is located, cost considerations result in the operation of most housing programs by organizations that pay lower salaries than are given to the hospital-based workforce. In general, the higher overhead incurred in hospital settings combined with the limitations of reimbursement for psychiatric disorders can make mental health outpatient services a challenge to sustain.

Another financial stress occurs because although private practitioners can attempt to collect fees from self-pay psychiatric patients for missed appointments, such visits cannot be billed to insurance companies, which are the primary source of revenue for most hospital-based services. Strategies to reduce missed appointments include scheduling appointments around patients' other obligations, making reminder telephone calls, arranging for patient transportation, offering on-site child care, and obtaining the assistance of family members where appropriate. Our program is large enough to designate on-call clinicians who leave their time free for a specific morning or afternoon during the week. This allows us to overschedule appointments on the assumption that if everyone shows up, the on-call clinician can help out. It also allows us to see patients who show up unexpectedly, which helps to retain patients in treatment. When on-call clinicians are not seeing patients they use the unscheduled time to catch up with required paperwork. Some programs offer financial incentives for patients to come to appointments, which is a matter of some controversy and not a practice that our program utilizes.

The Continuum of Care

Outpatient services exist on a continuum from the most intensive to the least intensive interventions. A comprehensive community mental health service allows patients to move from one level of care to another depending on current needs. High-intensity services include day programs, residential care with around-the-clock staffing, assertive community treatment, emergency department services, and crisis intervention. Intermediate-intensity services include intensive outpatient treatment and housing programs with more limited staff oversight. Routine outpatient treatment is most often a low-intensity service, as are peer-led programs such as support groups and clubhouses. Most hospital-based community mental health programs offer some but not all components of this continuum of care and collaborate with local providers for the elements that are not available through the hospital.

The continuum of services needed is in part determined by the types of patients the hospital serves. Hospitals routinely accept Medicare and Medicaid, which are the primary funding streams for people with SPMI, and many outpatient programs focus on this group of patients. Hospitals may also elect to establish specialized programs that focus on children or adults with particular illnesses such as attention-deficit disorders, autism spectrum disorders, mood disorders, anxiety disorders, eating disorders, and substance use problems. Hospitals that choose to target particular illnesses and populations often set up parallel inpatient and outpatient services.

The timing and settings in which services can be delivered most successfully may vary with patients' ages. For example, children may benefit from school-based programs, working adults from clinics with early morning or evening hours, and the elderly from outreach teams that serve the homebound. Providing labor-intensive services that are poorly reimbursed, such as geriatric outreach, often depends on the hospital securing state or local funding or charitable gifts to help cover the costs.

Patient Movement Through the Continuum of Services

In hospital-based outpatient programs, patients with acute and severe psychiatric illness are often seen initially in the emergency department, where they are screened, evaluated, and most commonly referred for inpatient hospitalization or crisis services. Some hospitals are in a position to take almost all of their emergency patients who require admission, whereas others may have to refer at least some patients to hospital beds outside of their system. Having a perspective on the long-term trajectory of a patient's needs and circumstances should contribute to the decision about where he or she is hospitalized.

Hospital-based programs should ideally have a direct line of communication between emergency department, inpatient, and outpatient staff. Patients with recurrent illness usually become familiar with staff in all three settings, which enhances the transfer of information and gives staff a historical perspective on what helps a particular patient. When patients are moved in and out of unaffiliated systems, their histories can be lost, and new treating staff may need to start from scratch each time. Acutely ill patients are often unable to report on important treatment and psychosocial facts that are crucial to their treatment and recovery. There is, therefore, a distinct advantage to keeping patients in one system of care that has continuity.

Once patients are hospitalized, there is a unique opportunity for input from outpatient staff regarding patients' progression toward their normal baselines. This input can occur through rounds and clinical case conferences that take place on the inpatient unit and involve the patient and the inpatient and outpatient treatment teams. This collaboration improves treatment planning and patient adherence. Collaboration also encourages respectful and trusting relationships, decreases workload, and reduces clinician burnout. Conversely, staff from the inpatient units can participate in case conferences in outpatient settings and have the opportunity to see how patients live and function when they are well in the community.

For people with SPMI, often their outpatient psychiatric treatment providers are their major and most frequent social contacts. The attachment between the patient and treating clinician can be intense and can foster an overly paternalistic and dependent relationship that can hinder the patient's recovery. Having multiple staff members treat a patient diminishes the intensity of the patient's relationship to a single provider. In our setting we assign patients to two staff members, a psychiatrist and a case manager. The case manager can be of any specialty (e.g., a nurse, social worker, or psychologist). The role of each clinician is determined by the patient's needs and by the comfort and/or training of the clinicians.

The psychiatrist can exclusively focus on medication management with some patients and provide additional therapies with others. Similarly, the case manager can help the patient obtain concrete services and/or act as the primary therapist. Patients often become familiar with other staff as well, for example, the nurse who provides depot medication injections, the receptionist who helps the patient with transportation reimbursement, or the other clinicians that patients meet during times of crises or therapists' vacations. This arrangement encourages the diffusion of the transference and allows the patient to benefit from a multidisciplinary treatment team. It also supports the development of a shared or collective risk among staff. Often, when treating high-risk patients with SPMI, there is the tendency for staff to "burn out" or for individual staff members to become overwhelmed with the fear of a patient's potential for violence or for suicide. The assignment of two staff members and the encouragement of transference to the whole program and its staff help to reduce these phenomena.

The type and intensity of treatment needed for a patient with SPMI will vary over time, and there are different models for providing flexible care. Here we use our own program to illustrate one possible model for providing a continuum of treatment.

The Washington Heights Community Service (WHCS) is a hospital-based program in northern Manhattan that focuses exclusively on SPMI patients. The program consists of two community-based outpatient clinics that follow approximately 1,000 patients and a 22-bed inpatient unit. The latter is one of three inpatient units housed at the New York State Psychiatric Institute, the major research institute for the New York State Office of Mental Health. WHCS is the only component of the institute that operates on clinical rather than research funds. Although WHCS's productivity and reimbursements are monitored by the Office of Mental Health, there is no doubt that state funding has been key to the program's stability. In addition, the New York State Psychiatric Institute has an affiliation with Columbia University that has aided in the recruitment and retention of WHCS's professional staff, many of whom seek and receive academic appointments and take advantage of teaching and/or research opportunities.

WHCS has a low turnover of both staff and patients. The low turnover of staff can be attributed to the philosophy of sharing risk, assigning manageable case loads, using community-based harm reduction approaches, having an academic affiliation, and maintaining a respectful and supportive environment. The low turnover of patients can be attributed to the unique continuum and multiple levels of care that are provided, under the authority of one program, to a population of patients with severe chronic illness requiring long-term care. The realities of funding and location will dictate the programming that most hospital-based programs can provide. New York State is known for its generous financial support of health care for disadvantaged citizens. WHCS is also in an urban area where there is a high density of health care professionals and readily available patient access to transportation, social services, and other supports. Our urban environment, however, has very limited housing opportunities, and the cost of living is high. Rural programs often have very different challenges. These are some of the variables that must be taken into consideration when a hospital establishes mental health outpatient services for a particular geographical region.

Continuing Day Treatment Program

To address the issue of the changing clinical needs of patients, WHCS offers two levels of outpatient care, a continuing day treatment program (CDTP) and an outpatient program. The CDTP, as the name implies, has clinical activities that run throughout the day, 5 days per week. Patients can participate in as many or as few activities as is recommended in their treatment plans and can stay in the program for any length of time deemed clinically appropriate. Patients have some autonomy to choose activities and the frequency of contact. The CDTP is often a better fit for people who have significant residual symptoms and who are more disorganized. The program allows for a more structured environment with a higher staff-to-patient ratio. The CDTP also allows for peer-to-peer interaction in safe, low-expressed-emotion settings.

CDTP programming is geared toward rehabilitation and recovery. The staff-to-patient ratio is higher than in the outpatient program, and the staff are a mix of licensed clinicians, mental health aides, and peer workers. A typical day in the CDTP might include a social skills group targeting free-time management, a medication management group that reviews the benefits and side effects of medications, a current events group to keep people oriented to news events, a vocational skills group geared toward future employment, and a healthy lifestyle group geared toward diet and exercise. These groups are designed to promote skills development and provide psychoeducation to help patients gain independence and progress toward recovery. The group settings also allow for peer interactions, modeling, skills practice, and feedback from both staff and peers. Specific therapeutic techniques can be used in this setting, including modified motivational interviewing, cognitive-behavioral therapies, multiple family groups, and many of the other evidence-based practices that have been developed for this population.

The rates of employment among people with severe mental illness are low, and many patients express a desire to engage in productive work and to earn money. A variety of program models have shown efficacy in helping patients obtain and maintain competitive employment, most often on a part-time basis (Cook et al. 2005). Many patients receive disability payments from the Social Security Administration, and if they earn too much income, they fear losing these benefits. There is no guarantee that patients whose disability benefits are discontinued as a result of full-time employment will have them reinstated if they cannot sustain their jobs.

We run a transitional employment program as part of our CDTP, although we also accept outpatient program participants. We help patients who would like to attempt full-time competitive employment to realistically assess the disability benefits issue, and we provide ongoing support throughout the pre-employment and employment process.

Patients participating in the CDTP program have the opportunity to meet with their psychiatrists or case managers as needed. Staff of the CDTP are familiar with all patients and their treatment plans, and they regularly participate in clinical rounds to ensure that these treatment plans are informed by all disciplines.

Outpatient Program

The outpatient program is geared to patients who are higher functioning and who would benefit from a less intense, less frequent therapeutic intervention. In the outpatient program, patients are also assigned both a case manager and a psychiatrist. Typically, the case manager acts as the primary therapist, and the psychiatrist provides medication management. Patients attend the program by appointment with either clinician. The frequency of visits is dependent on a patient's needs and can vary from twice per week for new or acute patients, to monthly, to every 3 months for stably maintained patients.

For many reasons, some clinical and some psychosocial, patients often have difficulties keeping their appointments. It is our program policy to see patients whenever they show up at the clinic. To accomplish this there is always a doctor and a case manager on call to see patients if they arrive unexpectedly and their assigned clinicians are unavailable. This strategy improves patient adherence and retention.

Patients in the outpatient program also tend to have community, vocational, and family obligations, so treatment is designed to accommodate each patient's lifestyle with minimal disruption. Ideally, the program should be able to provide treatment before and after regular working hours to improve accessibility for employed patients. Creating an atmosphere in which patients who are parents can comfortably bring their young children to the clinic also enhances adherence, as does such simple things as offering reading materials and access to snacks for waiting patients. The outpatient program is also sometimes used for more symptomatic patients who cannot tolerate the structured therapeutic atmosphere of the CDTP.

There is continuity of care between the CDTP and outpatient program, and patients can move between these two levels of care as their therapeutic and psychosocial needs change. Patients often start in the CDTP after an acute hospitalization, and as they recover and need a less structured or intense program, they can transfer to the outpatient program. Conversely, patients in the latter in need of a more structured environment can transfer to the CDTP.

There is community outreach in both programs, and staff attempt to understand and integrate the clinical care of a patient with the patient's life in the community. As staffing allows, outpatient programs can conduct home visits and help patients utilize other community resources. This can include escorting patients to benefit offices for the purpose of helping them with entitlement applications and linking patients to food pantries, day care, home health aides, and other services as needed. Because many of the patients we see in our own program are new immigrants from Spanish-speaking countries, we help patients access English language programs, pass citizenship tests, and obtain legal help for immigration issues as needed.

Community outreach can also involve escorting and advocating for patients in the medical health care system. Because members of the psychiatric treatment team often see patients with SPMI more frequently than their medical providers see them, psychiatric and nursing staff often provide some basic primary care services and help coordinate care across the medical and psychiatric systems, advocating for improved access as needed.

Collaborations Promoting Continuity of Care

Most ambulatory services do not have the mission, funding streams, or other resources to provide every element of comprehensive care. Although our program is part of a freestanding psychiatric hospital, we are on the same campus as a large general hospital (New York Presbyterian Hospital) with which we collaborate in the provision of most psychiatric emergency and crisis services as well as needed medical care. We do not have the capacity to run our own housing programs, so we collaborate with those providers who establish residential care in or near the neighborhood we serve. We also refer patients to consumer-run programs that might benefit them, such as clubhouses that offer evening and weekend activities or more sophisticated vocational services. These collaborations are essential and often take considerable effort to maintain.

Treating Comorbid Substance Abuse and Mental Illness

People with SPMI often have other co-occurring disorders. It is estimated that almost half of people with schizophrenia and other severe mental illnesses will have a lifetime diagnosis of an alcohol or other substance use disorder (Kessler 2004). The use of substances in the absence of a disorder can also be problematic. It is crucial, therefore, to create treatment programs that can address both mental illness and sub-

stance use. There are several models of dual diagnosis treatment that are often used in mental health settings. One is a traditional substance abuse treatment model that uses a peer-run, 12-Step design. This works well for patients who have a primary substance use disorder and a secondary psychiatric history. For SPMI patients who have secondary substance abuse or who self-medicate with substances, a harm reduction model (Magura et al. 2003) that involves more professional staff is often recommended. Both of these models can be adapted for use in a day treatment or outpatient psychiatric setting.

The model created by Drake et al. (1998) is another example of a program geared toward people with primary mental illness and secondary substance abuse. This integrated model employs a single program that provides both psychiatric and substance abuse treatment, using clinicians trained to treat both disorders.

Substance abuse treatment is tailored to patients who have severe mental illness and differs from many standard substance abuse treatments by focusing on anxiety reduction instead of denial; emphasizing trust and understanding instead of confrontation and criticism; using harm reduction approaches in place of abstinence; maintaining a long-term perspective instead of a focus on rapid withdrawal; providing clinical support beyond clinic hours; and utilizing neuroleptics and other pharmacotherapy as needed rather than excluding these medications. Programming includes motivational interventions, community outreach, intensive case management, family psychoeducation, and psychosocial rehabilitation in addition to medication management (Drake et al. 1998).

In addition to the models already noted, the National Institute on Drug Abuse offers manuals for a wide range of substance use interventions that, depending on the population served, may be usefully adapted.

Substance use problems are also associated with medical sequelae, and people who have substance use disorders combined with other mental illnesses have the highest risk of becoming infected with HIV (McKinnon et al. 1997). Other infections, including hepatitis B, hepatitis C, and a variety of other sexually or parenterally transmitted infections are considerably elevated in the dually diagnosed population when compared with the general population (Rosenberg et al. 2001).

Managing Co-Occurring Medical Disorders

People with SPMI are generally at increased risk for many other co-occurring medical disorders. People with schizophrenia have up to a 20% reduction in life span attributable to medical illness when compared with the general population (Marder et al. 2004). Metabolic and cardiovascular diseases are common, including hypertension, diabetes, emphysema, obesity, and coronary artery disease (Marder et al. 2004). Factors contributing to this increased risk include poverty, poor eating habits, decreased physical activity, alcohol and cigarette use, stigma on the part of medical providers, and more recently the side effects of atypical antipsychotics and other psychotropic medications. Often the task of monitoring and coordinating medical treatment falls to mental health staff.

SPMI patients taking psychotropic medications should have an annual physical examination with routine blood work. Outpatients on mood stabilizers and certain antipsychotics such as clozapine require more frequent blood work or other tests to monitor for therapeutic blood levels, bone marrow suppression, liver toxicity, renal disturbances, and/or hypothyroidism, depending on the medications being used. There is now a concerted effort to get baseline metabolic parameters and body measurements on all patients prior to starting psychiatric medications to help monitor, prevent, or reduce metabolic complications, especially among patients taking newer-generation antipsychotics. Testing patients for HIV and viral hepatitis is now also more common, and the U.S. Centers for Disease Control and Prevention now recommends routine opt-out HIV testing in all health care settings for all patients (Branson et al. 2006). Monitoring and coordination of medical care can be done through the psychiatric outpatient program. Our program staff make considerable efforts to be effective across institutional boundaries to provide coordinated medical and psychiatric care, sometimes with remarkable results (LeMelle and Entelis 2005).

Clinician Cultural Competence

When conducting assessments and selecting clinical interventions, the culture of both the clinician and the patient must be taken into consideration. Clinicians use their experiences and knowledge as tools to determine if a patient's response or behavior is reasonable or normal. This may pose a problem if the patient is from a different culture, and the clinician uses only his or her own experiences as a frame of reference. There are many examples of behaviors that can be misconstrued as pathological, including religious practices, spiritual experiences, and expression of intense affect. For example, if a male patient comes from a culture

where it is appropriate for men to cry in public, and the clinician is not from the same cultural background, the clinician may incorrectly assume the patient's crying is a symptom of depression. It is imperative that clinicians not make assumptions about what is normative behavior based solely on their own cultural background. The clinician must ask the patient or get collateral information regarding what is normal behavior for the patient's particular culture. There have been several studies that have shown that minorities in the United States are often misdiagnosed. This is partially due to culturally insensitive assessments that can lead to inappropriate diagnoses and treatment recommendations (Copeland et al. 2003; Neighbors et al. 1989; Primm et al. 2005).

It is obvious but worth stating that clinicians must be able to communicate effectively with patients. If the clinician is not fluent in a patient's language, a translator is required. Even within a shared culture there are often multiple dialects of the same language. When conducting a psychiatric assessment, there are subtle nuances in a patient's oral presentation that can aid in making a diagnosis. These can be missed if there is a language barrier, and the use of translators is second best to employing clinicians who are fluent in the languages that patients speak.

Our program is located in a largely Latino community. Seventy percent of our patients are Spanish speaking, and a substantial number of these are monolingual in Spanish. We therefore conduct all programming in English and in Spanish. The majority of our staff is also bilingual and bicultural. The physical environment of our clinics and our activities for patients reflect Latin culture, and we accept patients incorporating traditional practices into their self-management strategies. Culturally appropriate environments and programming contribute to patient adherence and retention and also improve the quality of care that patients receive. It is important, however, to understand that as the cultural makeup of the community changes, so should the culture of the mental health programming.

Residential Programs

Housing options for people with severe psychiatric disabilities have progressively expanded in most states, not only because they are important alternatives to long-term hospitalization but also because disabled patients usually live on small benefit checks that have not kept up with the growing cost of housing, thereby making shelter otherwise unaffordable (Ropers 1988).

The levels of supervision in these residential programs vary from intense, on-site, around-the-clock supervision to situations in which mental health organizations hold housing leases and provide only occasional staff visits to patients who are living relatively independently in the community. These more independent individuals often find that the major impediment to moving out into their own housing is lack of affordable opportunities (Goldfinger and Schutt 1996; Shern et al. 1997; Won and Solomon 2002). Housing programs have been shown to decrease hospitalization and homelessness, to increase quality of life, and to improve social and occupational functioning (Hawthorne et al. 1994; Okin et al. 1995). These programs can be run by various organizations, including hospitals.

Some residential programs specialize in the treatment of patients who are homeless, dually diagnosed, criminally involved, require a highly structured residential program, or are otherwise not eligible for other types of residential options. The terms *supported, supportive,* and *independent living* are among those used to describe a gradual decrease in the level of structure, supervision, and staffing of different housing programs. Programs also differ in their eligibility criteria, staffing patterns, and intended length of stay. They usually require that patients participate in some type of daily programming, and the programming is usually conducted outside of the housing setting. Patients are also usually required to sign a standard housing lease to participate in these residential programs.

Transitional housing is highly supervised, supported housing that is designed to allow patients to make a gradual transition from the inpatient setting to the outpatient setting. This type of housing is often used for patients who have a history of difficulty in residential programs, who have had long inpatient stays, and/or who need a transition to less structured housing programs. A stay in transitional housing can sometimes be required by other types of more permanent housing programs to allow patients time to establish a "positive track record" in an outpatient setting. Transitional housing is staffed with 24-hour on-site coverage. The staffing usually consists of a nurse, social workers, and mental health aides. Programming includes medication management and supervision of medication self-administration, social and recreational activities, links to the community, activities of daily living training, behavioral interventions for safety, and discharge planning and community linkage. The average length of stay can be up to 4 months. This is temporary housing, and the goal is to move patients as quickly as possible to permanent housing in the community.

Crisis residences are supported housing that can be used in one of two ways: to help patients who have "housing crises" and are on the verge of becoming homeless, or to help patients who have psychiatric crises that are related to their psychosocial environments and who need a short-term, higher level of care but do not qualify for inpatient hospitalization. In both cases, the stay is short, perhaps 2–4 months, and the staffing is similar to transitional housing, with 24-hour coverage by a nurse, social workers, and mental health aides. These programs are designed to make quick interventions to defuse crises and get patients into stable living environments in the community. All patients in this type of residential program are required to remain in some sort of outpatient treatment. The residential programming is geared toward psychosocial assessment and stabilization, benefits acquisition, and family/residential interventions.

Community residences are supportive housing programs that are freestanding in the community and are staffed by mental health aides. The intensity of supervision varies from 24 hours a day to occasional staff visits. The length of stay in this type of program can be months to years. Programs with lower levels of supervision are designed for higher-functioning patients who do not have significant impulse-control problems, who can manage and administer their medications independently, and who are able to perform all of their activities of daily living unassisted. This type of supportive program is often used for patients who are transitioning to independent housing. Patients are required to attend off-site programming, which may include continuing day programs, rehabilitation or vocational programs, competitive employment, community integration programs, or recreational programs. So-called low demand housing relaxes these daytime requirements and serves patients who do not tolerate the demands of more traditional programs, for example, those who have been chronically homeless and prefer to be left alone.

Independent living programs are scatter-site housing in the community that have no on-site supervision. There are staff who meet with patients on a regular basis at a frequency of once per week to once per month depending on the patients' needs. There is no required programming associated with this type of housing program, but there are social activities that patients can participate in voluntarily. Patients are expected to be engaged in some sort of outpatient treatment program. There is little to no daily monitoring of patient activity, and patients are allowed to have overnight visitors, smoke, and essentially do anything that is permissible within the usual tenant laws.

Family care programs are essentially adult foster care programs where foster families take in adult patients with mental illness. These families are screened and certified through the state and receive financial support. The families are trained and supported in the general and emergency care of people with mental illness. This type of housing is designed for patients who cannot tolerate living in large, communal settings such as a community residence and who need permanent housing in a structured and nurturing setting. This is more of a custodial care model where the family often acts as the representative payee or power of attorney for the patient. For many older patients, this is the ideal setting. The families are supported by the psychiatric staff and play an integral role in the patient's treatment and care.

Retaining Patients in Outpatient Treatment

In contrast to most inpatient care, outpatient settings struggle with patient adherence to treatment. A variety of techniques are available to address this problem. The most important of these is creating smooth and well-coordinated transitions from one level of care to another. Flexibility is crucial, so that if a patient misses a scheduled appointment but shows up at another time a staff member is available to at least briefly see the patient and schedule another visit. Other strategies that help enhance adherence are low staff turnover allowing for long-term therapeutic alliances between staff and patients; engaging with patients on their own goals for recovery; use of outreach techniques when patients fail to show for appointments; and the involvement of families in patients' treatment plans.

Monitoring patient adherence to psychotropic medication and the use of long-acting injectable medications for psychotic disorders are helpful in addressing nonadherence to drug regimens. Assertive community treatment (Dixon 2000), intensive case management, and outpatient commitment are among the strategies employed when seriously ill patients repeatedly fail to adhere to treatment and either present a danger to themselves or others or are heavy users of inpatient and emergency department care (Van Dorn et al. 2006). Small inducements may also help keep seriously ill patients in treatment. These include serving meals, offering transportation reimbursement, and engaging patients in pleasurable activities such as creative arts groups and recreation. Forensic patients may be subject to other forms of monitoring, such as parole, that track adherence to mandated care (Monahan et al. 2005).

Outpatient commitment laws vary from state to state. In New York State, an assisted outpatient treatment law, commonly referred to as Kendra's Law, was enacted in 1999. The intent of the law is to mandate treatment for people with severe mental illness who are nonadherent, primarily to medication, and who have a history of violence and/or multiple hospitalizations. This law was enacted in response to a tragic incident in which a young woman, Kendra Webdale, was pushed to her death in New York City's subway system by a man with mental illness (who incidentally was being turned away from treatment, not refusing it). The law requires that eligible adults be mandated to treatment that must include either an assertive community treatment team or an intensive case manager. The law also allows for disturbed people to be picked up and held for up to 72 hours for psychiatric evaluation. Assisted outpatient treatment provides a new process for identifying, investigating, and evaluating individuals with high need. It has improved accountability in local mental health service systems and enhanced access to services and coordination of treatment for these individuals. New York State allocated additional funding to support more assertive community treatment teams and intensive case manager programs, which helped to improve community services.

Initial outcomes of assisted outpatient treatment showed an increased participation in case management from 53% to 100%, in day programs from 15% to 22%, in substance abuse services from 24% to 40%, and in supported housing services from 19% to 31%. Most significantly, there was an increased adherence to prescribed medication from 34% to 69% in the first 6 months (Brennan 2005). This program, and its equivalent in other states, is one of several legal approaches that have been developed to assist in patient adherence to treatment and to decrease recidivism. Other programs operated by the legal system include mental health courts, specialty probation programs, and criminal diversion programs (Elbogen et al. 2003).

Patients may accept some types of treatment and reject others. For example, some patients accept psychiatric care but refuse placement in a residential setting because they object to living with others, to the rules and regulations of housing programs, or to the fact that most of their entitlement checks will be used for housing and thereby leave little spending money. Other patients are willing to talk about their problems but refuse to accept medication. In our program we work with patients where they are. Using techniques that are now often referred to as *harm reduction* and *motivational interviewing,* we help patients examine their own views about the advantages and disadvantages of the choices they make and try to help them adopt health-promoting behaviors. We reserve mandated treatment for patients who do not respond to a more collaborative approach.

Conclusion

The spectrum of psychiatric illness has not changed, but our understanding about treatment efficacy, recovery, and patients' quality of life has changed, and our systems of care need to reflect this new knowledge. As large, long-term state psychiatric hospitals have downsized, treatment and services for people with severe mental illness have shifted to the community. Many different models of community care have evolved. There are some distinct advantages for both patients and staff to having hospital-based outpatient programs, which we have enumerated in this chapter. Although varying somewhat by hospital, these advantages usually include well-developed administrative structures, a continuum of integrated patient services, the capacity to recruit and retain well-trained staff, and the ability to coordinate medical and psychiatric treatment.

References

Anderson CM, Reiss DJ, Hogarty GE: Schizophrenia and the Family: A Practitioner's Guide to Psychoeducation and Management. New York, Guilford, 1986

Anthony WA, Blanch A: Supported employment for persons who are psychiatrically disabled: a historical and conceptual perspective. Psychosocial Rehabilitation Journal 11:5–23, 1987

Beels CC, Gutwirth L, Berkeley J, et al: Measurements of social support in schizophrenia. Schizophr Bull 10:399–411, 1984

Bloche MG, Cournos F: Mental health policy for the 1990s: tinkering in the interstices. Journal of Health, Politics, Policy and Law 15: 387–411, 1990

Branson BM, Handsfield HH, Lampe MA, et al: Revised recommendations for HIV testing of adults, adolescents, and pregnant women in health-care settings. MMWR Recomm Rep 55:1–17, 2006

Brennan KJ: Appendix 2, in Kendra's Law: Final Report on the Status of Assisted Outpatient Treatment. New York, New York State Office of Mental Health, 2005

Catty J, Lissouba P, White S, et al: Predictors of employment for people with severe mental illness: results of an international six-centre randomised controlled trial. Br J Psychiatry 192:224–231, 2008

Cook JA, Leff HS, Blyler CR, et al: Results of a multisite randomized trial of supported employment interventions for individuals with severe mental illness. Arch Gen Psychiatry 62:505–512, 2005

Copeland LA, Zeber JE, Valenstein M, et al: Racial disparity in the use of atypical antipsychotic medications among veterans. Am J Psychiatry 160:1817–1822, 2003

Cournos F: The impact of environmental factors on outcome in residential programs. Hosp Community Psychiatry 38:848–852, 1987

Dixon L: Assertive community treatment: twenty-five years of gold. Psychiatr Serv 51:759–765, 2000

Drake RE, Mercer-McFadden C, Mueser KT, et al: Review of integrated mental health and substance abuse treatment for patients with dual disorders. Schizophr Bull 24:589–608, 1998

Elbogen E, Swanson J, Swartz M: Effects of legal mechanisms on perceived coercion and treatment adherence in persons with severe mental illness. J Nerv Ment Dis 191:629–637, 2003

Foley H, Sharfstein S: Madness and Government. Washington, DC, American Psychiatric Press, 1983

Fonagy P, Roth A, Higgitt A: Psychodynamic psychotherapies: evidence-based practice and clinical wisdom. Bull Menninger Clin 69:1–58, 2005

Goffman E: Asylums. New York, Doubleday Anchor, 1961

Goldfinger SM, Schutt RK: Comparison of clinicians' housing recommendations and preferences of homeless mentally ill persons. Psychiatr Serv 47:413–415, 1996

Greer S, Greer A: The continuity of moral reform: community mental health centers. Soc Sci Med 19:397–404, 1984

Hall LL, Graff AC, Fitzpatrick MJ, et al: Shattered Lives: Results of a National Survey of NAMI Members Living With Mental Illnesses and Their Families. Arlington, VA, National Alliance for the Mentally Ill, 2003

Hawthorne WB, Fals-Stewart W, Lohr JB: A treatment outcome study of community-based residential care. Hosp Community Psychiatry 45:152–155, 1994

Hogarty GE, Flesher S, Ulrich R, et al: Cognitive enhancement therapy for schizophrenia. Arch Gen Psychiatry 61:866–876, 2004

Kessler RC: The epidemiology of dual diagnosis. Biol Psychiatry 56:730–737, 2004

Kiesler C, Sibulkin A: Mental Hospitalization: Myths and Facts About a National Crisis. Newbury Park, CA, Sage, 1987

LeMelle SM, Entelis C: Heart transplant in young man with schizophrenia. Am J Psychiatry 162:453–457, 2005

Lynch TR, Chapman AL, Rosenthal MZ, et al: Mechanisms of change in dialectical behavior therapy: theoretical and empirical observations. J Clin Psychol 62:459–480, 2006

Magura S, Laudet AB, Mahmood D, et al: Role of self-help processes in achieving abstinence among dually diagnosed persons. Addict Behav 28:399–413, 2003

Marder SR, Essock SM, Miller AL, et al: Physical health monitoring of patients with schizophrenia. Am J Psychiatry 161:1334–1349, 2004

McFarlane WR, Dushay RA, Stastny R, et al: A comparison of two levels of family aided assertive community treatment. Psychiatr Serv 47:744–750, 1996

McKinnon K, Carey MP, Cournos F: Research on HIV, AIDS, and severe mental illness: recommendations from NIMH National Conference. Clin Psychol Rev 17:327–331, 1997

Monahan J, Redlich AD, Swanson J, et al: Use of leverage to improve adherence to psychiatric treatment in the community. Psychiatr Serv 56:37-44, 2005

Neighbors HW, Jackson JS, Campbell L, et al: The influence of race factors on psychiatric diagnosis: a review and suggestions for research. Community Ment Health J 25:301–311, 1989

Okin R: The future of state hospitals: should there be one? Am J Psychiatry 140:577–581, 1983

Okin RL, Borus JF, Baer L, et al: Long-term outcome of state hospital patients discharged into structured community residential settings. Psychiatr Serv 46:73–78, 1995

Primm AB, Osher FC, Gomez MB: Race and ethnicity, mental health services and cultural competence in the criminal justice system: are we ready to change? Community Ment Health J 41:557–569, 2005

Quanbeck C, Frye M, Altshuler L: Mania and the law in California: understanding the criminalization of the mentally ill. Am J Psychiatry 160:1245–1250, 2003

Ropers K: The Invisible Homeless. New York, Human Sciences Press, 1988

Rosenberg SD, Goodman LA, Osher FC, et al: Prevalence of HIV, hepatitis B, and hepatitis C in people with severe mental illness. Am J Public Health 91:31–37, 2001

Rüsch N, Corrigan PW: Motivational interviewing to improve insight and treatment adherence in schizophrenia. Psychiatric Rehabilitation Journal 26:23–32, 2002

Segal S, Aviram O: The Mentally Ill in Community-Based Sheltered Care: A Study of Community Care and Social Integration. New York, Wiley, 1978

Shern DL, Felton CJ, Hough RL, et al: Housing outcomes for homeless adults with mental illness: results from the second-round McKinney program. Psychiatr Serv 48:239–241, 1997

Van Dorn RA, Elbogen EB, Redlich AD, et al: The relationship between mandated community treatment and perceived barriers to care in persons with severe mental illness. Int J Law Psychiatry 29:495–506, 2006

Weissman M: Cognitive therapy and interpersonal psychotherapy: 30 years later: Am J Psychiatry 164:693–696, 2007

Won YL, Solomon PL: Community integration of persons with psychiatric disabilities in supportive independent housing: a conceptual model and methodological considerations. Ment Health Serv Res 4:13–28, 2002

CHAPTER 25

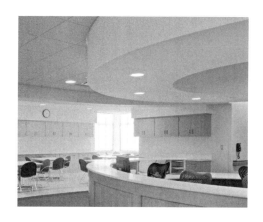

DAY HOSPITALIZATION AND INTENSIVE OUTPATIENT CARE

Donna T. Anthony, M.D., Ph.D.
Joan K. Feder, M.A., O.T.R./L., C.P.R.P.

In an era of brief inpatient hospitalizations, psychiatric intensive outpatient treatment has a number of important missions. Intensive outpatient services can prevent hospitalization or decrease inpatient length of stay. They allow for treatment in the least restrictive setting while still providing structure and support. In this chapter, the terms *intensive outpatient treatment* and *intensive outpatient services* refer to a range of programs, including the partial hospital program (PHP), continuing day treatment program (CDTP), and intensive outpatient program (IOP).

Mental illnesses affect functioning and quality of life. Intensive programs can help the participant resume functioning in roles that have been disrupted or facilitate development of new roles. Although intensive treatment can occur in a number of settings, hospital-based intensive outpatient programming provides an array of services to address the client's strengths, interests, and goals by integrating a range of therapeutic and rehabilitative interventions, focusing not only on symptom stabilization but also on community integra-

tion. Hospital-based programs provide a high staff-to-patient ratio with an array of clinical specialists ranging from psychiatrists to occupational therapists. Present-day programs aim to be client centered and rely on the patient's perception of his or her illness. Treatment depends on patients' active participation in choice of goals and volition for achieving them (Feder 1998). This working alliance propels the treatment forward, ensuring quality care and positive rehabilitation outcome. Treatment goals include symptom stabilization as well as restoration of meaningful life roles and functioning. Flexibility of treatment and adequate resources provide patients with a sense of control over life decisions and a feeling that their judgment is valued. The aim is to support the patient's goals while gently challenging vague or unrealistic expectations.

A range of potential intensive outpatient services exists. The terminology in the literature is often confusing and inconsistent. Different labels are being used for the same services, and to complicate matters further, services with the same label may actually be significantly different, depending on location, funding sources, and other factors. In this chapter, a PHP, at times referred to elsewhere as *day hospitalization*, is utilized to prevent inpatient admission or shorten the duration of an inpatient stay. A PHP provides up to several weeks of daily treatment, typically Monday through Friday. Studies have shown that up to 40% of people meeting criteria for a voluntary inpatient admission could be treated in a PHP setting, often with more rapid symptom relief and, in the short term, improved psychosocial functioning (Kallert et al. 2007; Schene 2004). A CDTP typically provides care over several months or more to enable individuals with psychiatric disorders to stabilize and function more independently in the community. In the European literature, CDTPs include day treatment programs for affective and personality disorders as well as day care centers for severe chronic mental illnesses such as schizophrenia (Marshall et al. 2001b). An IOP provides integrated individual and group treatments at a lesser frequency of up to three times per week. There is support in the literature for treating personality disorders (Gratz et al. 2006; Gunderson et al. 2005; G.W. Smith et al. 2001) and addictions (Avants et al. 1999; Gottheil et al. 1998; Kleber et al. 2007; Timko et al. 2003) in an IOP setting. Reviews of randomized, controlled trials provide evidence for more rapid symptom relief in PHP, CDTP, and IOP levels of care compared with inpatient treatment (Marshall et al. 2001a, 2001b). It has been more difficult to compare relapse rates, cost-effectiveness, and functional outcomes (Priebe et al. 2006).

Intensive outpatient services are part of a larger continuum of care in a hospital setting that includes the emergency department, inpatient setting, and clinic. A continuum of care facilitates communication and efficiency of referral to the intensive program. Another model is that of vertical integration of services, in which the same provider follows the client for continuity of care (T.E. Smith et al. 1999). There are also many types of community-based intensive programs. Regardless of the setting, all three forms of intensive outpatient services reviewed in this chapter provide assessment, stabilization, skill development, rehabilitation, and community integration to varying degrees.

History of Intensive Outpatient Treatment

Group-oriented and milieu-based treatment approaches were developed by T. F. Main in England based on experiences from treating combat-related posttraumatic stress disorder in World War II (Piper et al. 1996). Bion, Foulkes, and others also contributed to the development of group and milieu treatment. The first day hospital in North America was started in Montreal in 1946 at the Royal Victoria Hospital by Ewen Cameron. In 1971, based on experience with the Montreal program, H.F.A. Azim opened the Edmonton Day Treatment Program with a residential facility at the University of Alberta Hospital. Azim developed an 18-week treatment program for personality and affective disorders that incorporated services research. The Massachusetts Mental Health Center also had a tradition of intensive transitional services starting in 1946 and opened a day hospital in 1956 that accommodated patients admitted directly from the community to prevent hospitalization. In the United States, the Mental Retardation Facilities and Community Mental Health Centers Construction Act of 1963 mandated an expanded array of outpatient services to be provided by community mental health centers (Kraus and Stroup 2006). Financial issues have played a significant role in shaping outpatient services. Funding influences mental health policies, determining access to care and quality. There have been shifts in responsibilities for determining reimbursement and programming among local, state, and federal governments. The introduction of Medicare and Medicaid in the mid-1960s shifted financial responsibility from the state to federal sources (Gottlieb 1995). In recent years there has been a greater shift to managed Medicare and Medicaid, causing a reorganization of service delivery and limiting coverage for both inpatient days and outpatient services.

Treatment Outcomes in Intensive Outpatient Services

Acute episodes of mood disorders, including unipolar major depression and bipolar disorders, are often successfully managed in a PHP or IOP setting or a continuum of care from inpatient unit to PHP or IOP. Literature focusing on outcomes for affective disorders alone is generally positive but quite limited (Marshall et al. 2001a). Patients with more chronic mood disorders who have impairments in functioning can benefit from CDTP and IOP levels of care as well. Mood disorders complicated by personality disorders and/or substance abuse are more often described in studies on the efficacy of intensive outpatient services.

Severe episodes of major depression can often be treated in a PHP or IOP setting to avert hospitalization, providing that the patients are not acutely suicidal, have some supports in the community, and are able to maintain adequate self-care and medication compliance. PHP and IOP levels of care sometimes achieve the goals of inpatient treatment with less disruption to the patient's life and are perhaps more cost-effective (Goodwin and Jamison 2007b). Intensive outpatient services more commonly offer a stepdown for patients in a resolving manic episode after sufficient stabilization on the inpatient unit. Goodwin and Jamison (2007c) stressed that patients must have sufficient insight and commitment to maintain medication compliance out of the inpatient unit; for these individuals, an intensive service is helpful because symptoms might still fluctuate, and there is the risk of cycling into a depressive episode. Furthermore, patients with bipolar illness are at substantial risk for suicide in the first 6–12 months after discharge from the hospital, with the highest risk in the first week, regardless of polarity of the acute episode, warranting more intensive follow-up in a PHP or IOP (Goodwin and Jamison 2007a, 2007c). Rucci et al. (2002) found that an intensive treatment program that closely monitored treatment adherence significantly decreased suicide attempts in patients with bipolar illness recovering from an acute manic episode. Also, short-term therapies recommended for bipolar illness can be incorporated into PHP and IOP programming, including cognitive-behavioral therapy (CBT), interpersonal and social rhythm therapy, and family-focused treatment, among others (Goodwin and Jamison 2007d).

There is evidence that borderline personality disorder can be effectively treated at PHP, CDTP, and IOP levels of care (Gunderson et al. 2005). The goals of treatment are to decrease subjective distress, maladaptive behaviors, interpersonal problems, and self-injurious behaviors. An IOP level of care can effect improvements in social and interpersonal functioning (Bateman and Fonagy 1999, 2001; G.W. Smith et al. 2001). Bateman and Fonagy (1999) studied the treatment of borderline personality disorder in a longer-term psychoanalytic PHP and demonstrated fewer suicide attempts after 6 months, decrease in anxiety and depression in 9 months, and decrease in self-harm after 12 months, with consolidation of gains on follow-up. Patients in a borderline personality disorders program at McLean Hospital who transitioned from a PHP level of care to an IOP were followed up over 18 months (Gratz et al. 2006). Within the first few months there were improvements in emotional dysregulation and parasuicidality, followed by gradual improvement in functioning and quality of life. Treatment of a range of personality disorders was studied in a Norwegian treatment research network; individuals with borderline personality and Cluster C personality

disorders benefited more than those with Cluster A personality disorders, and an IOP was as effective as a more intensive day hospital (American Psychiatric Association 2000; Karterud et al. 2003; Vaglum et al. 1990). In general, evidence supports a time-limited day treatment program followed by an IOP for personality disorders (American Psychiatric Association 2001; Dazord et al. 1997; Wilberg et al. 1998).

Individuals with schizophrenia often have positive symptoms, negative symptoms, and cognitive impairment along with poor insight into the illness. Medication management and psychosocial therapies in a PHP or CDTP address positive symptoms and poor treatment adherence (Schwartz et al. 2006). Negative symptoms and impairments in social skills and cognition are more intractable and result in chronically impaired functioning (Muser et al. 2006). Schizophrenia and other psychotic disorders often start in early adulthood and adversely affect acquisition of independent living skills. Repeated episodes of psychosis disrupt educational and vocational pursuits as well as interpersonal relationships. Day treatment is effective at preventing relapse and repeated hospitalizations and improving independent living skills and vocational functioning (Lehman et al. 1998, 2004; Miller et al. 2006). Resnick et al. (2004) reviewed data from the Schizophrenia Patient Outcomes Research Team (PORT) survey and showed that participation in a CDTP had a significant positive association with knowledge of illness and services along with improvement in life satisfaction. Recently the efficacy of cognitive remediation has been studied in intensive outpatient treatment with promising outcomes (McGurk et al. 2007; Medalia and Lim 2004). Results have shown improvement in cognitive function, especially in areas of memory and attention. A 2-year follow-up also revealed a significant decrease in rehospitalization rates and overall success in achieving rehabilitation goals. Finally, CBT for psychosis, a new approach in the United States but a mainstay of treatment for patients with schizophrenia in the United Kingdom, is a potential adjunct to services already offered (Turkington et al. 2006).

Rehabilitation in Intensive Outpatient Services

Rehabilitation focuses on the patient's need for a sense of mastery or the ability to cope with symptomatology and demands of daily living. The biopsychosocial aspects of each individual are factored into efforts to encourage development of skills. This concept dates back to the foundation of psychosocial occupational therapy in 1917 and was supported by Adolf Meyer, who proposed a psychobiological approach to mental health. In 1922, while director of the Henry Phipps Psychiatric Clinic at Johns Hopkins Hospital, Meyer described mental illness as "problems of living" and not merely diseases of a "structural and toxic nature," and he proposed "habit training." At the time it was viewed as the most successful type of treatment program, providing "intensive care and re-education" (Schwartz 2005b). Today, occupational therapy is based on a patient-centered approach and focuses on functional skills essential to everyday tasks of living.

Psychiatric rehabilitation has been an emerging field over the past 15 years. There is a range of philosophical and technical differences within the field (Anthony and Liberman 1986; Anthony et al. 1978), but the common goal is to support recovery and restore ability for independent living and effective life management. The strongest value of psychiatric rehabilitation is that each individual has the right of self-determination and the capacity to learn and grow (Pratt et al. 2002). Both occupational therapy and psychiatric rehabilitation models promote development of an individualized map of recovery, helping clients acquire social and functional skills while developing the supports needed to adapt to their environment.

Partial Hospital Program

Admission Criteria

The PHP is a transition or diversion from inpatient level of care. Participants are acutely symptomatic but not at imminent risk of self-injurious or aggressive behaviors posing a threat to others, and they have adequate self-care and cognitive organization to live in a community setting. They are not actively abusing drugs or alcohol. The level of academic and intellectual functioning should be appropriate to the cognitive demands of the program. The preliminary diagnostic assessment determines whether the patient is experiencing the acuity and intensity of symptoms that would likely benefit from this level of care. Acute symptoms might include depression, anxiety, hypomania, and psychosis, among others. Patients with a range of diagnoses can benefit from a PHP. Because treatment is generally limited to several weeks or less, the clinician should identify target symptoms as a focus of treatment planning. Adequate community supports, housing, transportation, and benefits must be available. The patient needs a support system, especially during evenings and weekends. Medication compliance or direct supervision of medication administration is essential. The participant must be medically stable for monitoring of adjustments in the psychotropic regimen without inpatient supervision. The ability to tolerate four groups or activities per day within a structured program lasting several hours a day is a general expectation.

Psychiatric Assessment

The initial psychiatric assessment is completed by a multidisciplinary treatment team and actually applies to all levels of intensive outpatient care discussed in this chapter. Referral documents and collateral information are obtained with informed consent of the participant. A thorough history includes the elements outlined in the American Psychiatric Association's (2006) "Practice Guideline for the Psychiatric Evaluation of Adults." Basic areas addressed at intake include demographics, history of present illness and current symptoms, past psychiatric history, substance abuse, medical history, current medications and drug allergies, family history, and psychosocial history. A thorough assessment of risk factors for self-injurious behaviors and aggressive behaviors is conducted in the course of obtaining the history and mental status examination.

The treatment team identifies acute or persistent symptoms and maladaptive behaviors preventing optimal functioning at a lower level of care. The designated primary therapist, a team member who may be a nurse, social worker, or other clinician, elicits the patient's grasp of warning signs of decompensation. Commonly used rating scales could be utilized to assess and track symptoms and warning signs in a more systematic manner. Some of these rating scales are the Independent Living Skills Survey (Loeb 1996), Hamilton Rating Scale for Depression (Hamilton 1960), Beck Depression Inventory (Beck et al. 1961), Brief Psychiatric Rating Scale (Overall and Gorham 1988), and Positive and Negative Syndrome Scale (Kay et al. 1987). Data on symptoms and functioning from structured interviews are then integrated into the overall formulation.

Medical Assessment

Essential medical information includes a recent physical examination, laboratory tests, and an electrocardiogram. An intake assessment often includes weight, calculation of body mass index, abdominal girth, vital signs, and review of physical complaints or medication side effects. Programs often develop a health assessment form to be completed on day of admission by the patient. If a patient does not have a primary care provider, he or she is assisted with referrals. The assessment identifies the need for health maintenance services, in particular nutritional problems and conditions exacerbated by psychotropic medications.

Psychosocial Assessment

The initial comprehensive assessment explores psychosocial stressors precipitating the current episode. Stressors can be related to interpersonal issues, changes in living situation, or difficulties in school or a job, among others. The patient's life story, including current living situation, developmental milestones, family structure, friendships, relationships, educational background, work history, and leisure interests, should be explored. Premorbid and interepisode functioning both have significant bearing on expectations for treatment. In addition, history of emotional, physical, or sexual abuse and any other trauma is obtained. Support systems are identified, including family, friends, case managers, residential counselors, and others, with an expectation of further collaboration. The level of insight of family and friends is also explored, including understanding of the participant's illness. If there is a legal history, contact with probation officers or other agencies might be necessary. If the patient is a parent or caretaker, the therapist should explore issues around the safety of the dependents and provide links to community agencies.

Stabilization Phase

For direct admissions from the community, partial hospitalization provides rapid stabilization of acute symptoms with medication trials in a setting that allows for frequent assessment and medical monitoring. Referrals from an inpatient unit to PHP as a stepdown allow for consolidation of treatment effects. Some programs also offer electroconvulsive therapy on an acute or maintenance basis. For patients on mood stabilizers and certain antidepressants, blood levels are monitored. For patients on antipsychotics, monitoring of weight, abdominal girth, and laboratory tests helps follow risk factors for the metabolic syndrome. Examination for extrapyramidal side effects and periodic electrocardiograms, if indicated, should be conducted. Depot antipsychotics such as haloperidol decanoate (Haldol decanoate), fluphenazine decanoate (Prolixin decanoate), or risperidone (Risperdal Consta) could be administered in this setting for patients with a history of poor treatment adherence. Titration of the antipsychotic clozapine (Clozaril) also requires close medical monitoring that can be accomplished in a PHP.

The practitioner providing psychopharmacological management maintains contact with the primary care provider or other specialist if there are medical comorbidities. Nutritional counseling is ideally provided as part of medical management, with referrals initiated for better follow-up and maintenance. Education about short- and long-term risks for medications is important. A team approach to tracking symptoms and behavioral changes allows active adjustments in the medication regimen and formulation of other aspects of treatment.

Treatment Planning and Establishment of Goals

Effective stabilization and skill development procedures include the patient in setting goals and objectives. It is also highly desirable to involve the family and significant others in the establishment of the treatment plan. Goal setting should not be solely based on diagnosis or clinicians' expectations but rather should be founded on assessment of the patient's strengths, deficits, interests, needs, and supports. Table 25–1, developed by one of the authors (J.K.F.), provides a sampling of behaviorally written goals and objectives for partial hospital or continuing day treatment levels of care expressed in terms of the client's measurable functioning. Goals should be assessed and reevaluated regularly, engaging the patient as much as possible. The self-report chart shown in Figure 25–1 was developed for the CDTP at New York–Presbyterian Hospital, Payne Whitney Manhattan; it demonstrates how the client's perspective contributes to the treatment plan and determination of discharge readiness. In the PHP and CDTP, the client helps to steer the course of treatment and assess progress with the assistance of the multidisciplinary team. Estimated length of stay, which can be driven by reimbursement and institutional expectations, influences goal setting.

Program Structure

A PHP is often situated near the emergency department or inpatient services department. The programs meet Monday through Friday, generally offering 4 hours of group a day. Individual sessions with the primary therapist and psychiatrist or nurse practitioner are typically scheduled on a weekly basis but may occur more frequently. Some programs provide or assist with transportation. All groups, whether they are skills training or supportive therapy, rely on effective group leadership. The therapist must ensure that the group remains committed to its goals while responding to the evolving needs of the participants to keep the treatment active.

Psychoeducation is an important component of

TABLE 25–1. Sample goals and objectives in intensive outpatient services

Goals	Objectives
Improve attention and organization	1. Client will describe two strategies to help focus. 2. Client will utilize a daily planner. 3. Client will remain at task for 50% of the group. 4. Client will verbalize two strategies to better organize the environment.
Reduce self-injurious behavior	1. Client will contract for safety. 2. Client will utilize diary cards to increase insight into self-injurious behaviors. 3. Client will self-initiate skills coaching prior to engaging in self-injurious behavior.
Increase social activities	1. Client will initiate conversation once a day in a group. 2. Client will report satisfaction with increase in social contacts outside of program. 3. Client will develop three strategies to communicate needs more effectively.
Improve ability to manage anxiety	1. Client will identify three triggers to anxiety. 2. Client will describe two coping strategies for dealing with anxiety. 3. Client will utilize one stress reduction activity on a daily basis.
Maintain sobriety	1. Client will attend Alcoholics Anonymous meetings twice per week. 2. Client will discuss two effective coping strategies to deal with stress. 3. Client will develop a daily schedule.
Improve self-care	1. Client will develop a nutritional chart. 2. Client will exercise at least 20 minutes, three times a week. 3. Client will discuss weight management activities by attending a nutritional group on a weekly basis.
Increase work readiness	1. Client will identify vocational goals realistic to current situation. 2. Client will identify strengths in area of work. 3. Client will identify three possible internship sites.
Increase control of anger	1. Client will identify triggers to outburst. 2. Client will describe two anger management techniques. 3. Client will identify two alternative actions when experiencing an outburst.

the PHP accomplished in individual sessions and groups. The aim of psychoeducation is to teach symptom management as well as health and safety awareness. The patient learns to monitor and share information about symptoms and medications as an active participant in treatment. In addition to verbal discussion of the risks and benefits of treatments, patients are also directed to Internet sites providing beneficial information about their medication. A hospital is likely to have its own health education department for current literature.

Discharge Planning

Participants demonstrating resolution of the most acute symptoms but still experiencing persistent symptoms or functional impairment can be referred to a CDTP or an IOP. Those who demonstrate significant improvement are referred to an outpatient clinic

or individual provider for extended treatment issues and relapse prevention. Many of the patients in a PHP are able to return to their previous level of functioning, which may include parenting, work, and/or school. Not all patients require extensive rehabilitation, although some may benefit from a referral to a job coach or additional vocational training. Occasionally patients do not respond adequately to treatment at the PHP level of care and ultimately require inpatient care. Further decompensation of the presenting symptoms leading to self-injurious or other types of impulsive behaviors would require inpatient admission. Also, medication management that has led to the need for more intensive medical monitoring would warrant inpatient admission. Termination from the program may also be necessary when the patient is unable to tolerate the intensity of the program or is not committed to the treatment.

PLEASE COMPLETE THE FOLLOWING FORM	Yes	No
Benefits of treatment		
Did you complete any objectives (steps) on any of your goals?		
Were there any days in which your symptoms were less bothersome than usual?		
Were there any days on which you were able to keep symptoms from interfering with your activities?		
Considering your involvement in community life (outside of program), did you		
a. Get better at taking care of the place you live?		
b. Add any hours of work (volunteer or paid) or attend a class?		
c. Add any leisure activities or socialize with anyone in the community?		
Considering your life as a whole, were there days in which you		
a. Were particularly pleased with any of your activities?		
b. Were particularly pleased with any of your relationships?		
c. Felt healthier or more competent or skillful?		
Were there any days in which your symptoms were worse than usual?		
If day treatment services had not been available to you during this month, would this have made a difference in the following areas?		
a. Work you are doing on your goals?		
b. The amount of support you needed at home?		
c. Your involvement in school or work (volunteer or paid)?		
d. Your involvement with other people?		
e. Your involvement in leisure activities?		
Please describe how you will know if it is time to move on from the outpatient program.		

FIGURE 25–1. Sample client self-report monitor.

Continuing Day Treatment Program

A CDTP, for the purposes of this chapter, is a comprehensive, structured, and supportive program committed to sustaining individuals in the community and diminishing need for repeated hospitalizations. Intervention is both therapeutic and rehabilitative, focusing not only on symptom stabilization but also on graded cognitive and psychosocial rehabilitation strategies. The CDTP differs from the PHP in terms of duration of treatment, acuity of symptoms, chronicity of conditions, and baseline functioning. Length of stay depends on goal acquisition, regulatory demands, and program philosophy as well as insurance benefits. Historically, patients remained in programs for years, but in recent years there has been a gradual shift toward providing time-limited intensive treatment. Strong emphasis is placed on maximum community integration, requiring the program to create linkages with an array of community services including self-help groups, state-funded vocational programs, independent living centers, and supportive housing. Principles of psychiatric rehabilitation are incorporated into the program because they are based on the belief that rehabilitation can prevent further deterioration and help a person function better in the community.

Admission Criteria

CDTPs serve individuals with chronic mental illness and functional impairments affecting their ability to sustain themselves in the community. They may have difficulties adhering to a medication regimen. They should not be at imminent risk for suicide or aggressive behaviors. Participants need to verbalize personal goals and expect to benefit from this level of intensive services. Family involvement is highly desirable. Individuals with schizophrenia, schizoaffective disorder, and chronic major affective disorders make up the bulk of the population, with a core of special services for those diagnosed with borderline personality disorder, eating disorders, or substance abuse. Other specialized programs may be geared toward the adolescent or geriatric population.

Assessment Phase

The initial psychiatric and medical assessments include all of the elements outlined for the PHP. The psychosocial assessment is similar, although there is greater emphasis on assessing potential for skill development and rehabilitation. Functional assessments are often administered by occupational therapists who collect data through semistructured interviews, observation, and standardized tests. The evaluation includes the client's history and premorbid functioning in areas of self-care, education, work, and leisure. The present capabilities and problems contributing to functional deficits, such as inattention, inability to focus, poor planning, and organizing, are assessed (Allen 1985). Finally, contextual factors affecting the client's functional performance are reviewed in depth, including living environment, finances, and health status. A comprehensive functional assessment also explores the client's interests and values regarding roles and occupational expectations. The client's perception of his or her disability and ability to engage in a therapeutic alliance is important (Law et al. 1998). Ultimately a functional assessment will identify potential strengths and help develop realistic and applicable rehabilitation goals. The assessment tool can be used at the beginning of treatment and as an integral part of the program. Occupational therapists administer standardized assessments such as the Allen Cognitive Level (Allen 1985).

Liberman et al. (1995) reviewed the need to identify past and present skills to guide the rehabilitation process, allowing development of a comprehensive treatment plan. Psychiatric rehabilitation specialists stress the need to assess motivation and examine factors influencing rehabilitation readiness (Cohen et al. 1992). Areas considered include motivation and commitment to change, awareness of roles, and ability to establish a therapeutic alliance. Finally, goal setting is the most critical stage of functional assessment. It is a powerful tool that actively engages the client in developing an individualized service plan. This is an ongoing collaborative process designed to provide strategies for achieving patients' personal goals in settings of their own choice. The plan serves as a road map, prioritizing overall objectives and identifying strengths, barriers, and time frames for monitoring the journey.

Treatment

A well-designed program offers a structured environment where treatment is individualized, with clear expectations and estimated duration. Programs are generally offered for the entire day from Monday through Friday but may have a more limited schedule tailored to the needs of some patients. The primary therapist oversees the treatment, providing individual therapy and case management. The psychiatrist evaluates the patient on admission and at least monthly but more often if necessary for active symptoms or medication changes. A treatment schedule is developed between the patient and therapist involving an array of groups ranging from skill development to psychoeducation around illness management to preparation for community living.

A CDTP provides an opportunity for more extensive medication trials. Medical issues that require monitoring include the metabolic syndrome and extrapyramidal syndromes, including tardive dyskinesia for patients on antipsychotics. Resources are generally available to administer depot medications and prescribe clozapine, with all of the necessary laboratory tests and medical monitoring. Random urine toxicology screenings might be indicated. Psychoeducation is aimed at symptom management; understanding risks, benefits, and potential side effects; and perhaps most importantly, compliance.

Skills training and activities therapy compose core components of CDTPs. Direct instruction and experiential learning of functional skills are of particular importance for acquisition of new skills and generalization. Emphasis is placed on interventions that facilitate basic skill acquisition (physical, cognitive, and social) without unduly challenging individual thresholds for stress and disorganization. Combining social skills training with maintenance of antipsychotic medication yields better social functioning while minimizing relapse (Liberman et al. 1995). In addition, services provided during recovery may include case management, family intervention, crisis intervention, and community linkage.

Group Programming

A wide range of group models is available to meet the therapeutic and educational needs of clients. Below is a sampling of groups offered in outpatient day treatment programs.

INDEPENDENT LIVING SKILLS

Independent living skills programs teach self-care skills such as meal preparation, nutrition, budgeting, and home maintenance. Basic foundation skills such as organization, problem solving, and decision making are reviewed in these groups to increase awareness of potential difficulties in the patient's environment. Skills are taught using a variety of strategies involving instruction and practice, such as preparing a meal and inviting the hospital nutritionist to review the food pyramid and special diets.

INTERPERSONAL SKILLS

Interpersonal skills groups teach social skills and communication. Clients learn to identify verbal and nonverbal communication behaviors and become more effective in starting a conversation and keeping it going. These groups involve a range of methods, including pencil-and-paper activities, role-playing, videotaping interactions, and modeling.

RECREATION/LEISURE PLANNING

Effective use of time includes exploration of leisure interests. Clients are provided with information and the opportunity to explore the benefits of recreational activities as a means to develop social skills and better management of unstructured time. In addition, providing a supportive community where interests can be pursued increases the likelihood that a client will further explore the activities in his or her own community. Clients support each other in the pursuit of activities, and it may not be uncommon to observe two clients spending time after the program pursuing a leisure activity.

COPING SKILLS

Coping skills groups focus on developing effective ways to manage stress and associated destabilization. Clients are taught a range of adaptive skills for coping with stressors and becoming more effective in crisis situations. Techniques to cope better with daily life demands are explored, with emphasis on developing problem-solving strategies and awareness of effective communication patterns. Topics can include relaxation, assertiveness skills, or review of the stress–vulnerability model.

PSYCHOEDUCATION

Psychoeducation groups provide explicit training to increase patients' awareness of their symptoms, vulnerability, and the environmental stressors that exacerbate the symptoms. Psychoeducational groups also focus on increasing the understanding of patients and families about the phases of the recovery process and development of resilient behaviors. Some CDTPs use specific modules such as the University of California–Los Angeles Social and Independent Living Skills Modules developed by Robert Liberman (Schwartz 2005a). For instance, a medication management group focuses on teaching patients to monitor their own medications by being aware of side effects and learning to talk with the health care provider. Another psychoeducation group focuses on symptom management skills to help patients identify warning signs of relapse and become more effective in coping with persistent symptoms. Many other modules are available that address additional community reentry skills, including a wide array of skills from self-care to job readiness.

SPECIALIZED GROUPS

Additional specialized groups may be provided in a CDTP, such as the following.

Dialectical behavior therapy. Dialectical behavior therapy (DBT) groups are most effective if they are reinforced by a DBT-certified therapist in the individual sessions and throughout the day. DBT groups are designed for patients with the diagnosis of borderline personality disorder who have severe emotional dysregulation and behavioral dyscontrol. The DBT skills training groups comprise four modules that address 1) emotion regulation, 2) interpersonal effectiveness, 3) surviving crises without engaging in maladaptive behaviors, and 4) developing a stable sense of self. Patients learn to replace maladaptive behavior with more adaptive skills. Groups involve specific skills teaching, consultation, and homework (Linehan 1993).

Cognitive-behavioral therapy for psychosis. CBT groups address the needs of patients with persistent positive symptoms of psychosis and, in some cases, negative symptoms. The groups aim to reduce distress by challenging the patients' beliefs about their symptoms. They teach how to identify and correct cognitive biases, evaluate beliefs, and assess whether the beliefs can be changed. Specific cognitive and behavioral strategies are developed to cope more effectively with the symptoms. CBT for psychosis has been utilized effectively as a treatment modality in the United Kingdom (Garety et al. 2000; Turkington et al. 2006), although it has limited dissemination in the United States.

Cognitive remediation. Cognitive remediation groups, not offered in most routine clinical settings, are designed to treat cognitive deficits that commonly occur in psychiatric conditions (McGurk et al. 2007; Medalia and Richardson 2005). Groups provide cognitive training by the use of either computer or cognitive-related activities. Some of the groups have been combined with a focus on the relationship with daily function and vocational training.

Substance abuse relapse prevention. Groups for substance abuse relapse prevention are specifically designed for those patients with a history of substance abuse, and the focus is on assessing the need for lifestyle adjustments from drug use to healthy habits of daily living and meaningful occupations. Integration of cognitive-behavioral interventions helps clients use varying coping skills in place of substances to help them avoid relapse and return to meaningful roles (Comerford 1999). Topics include identification of triggers, development of healthy habits, and effective management of nonusing activities (Precin 1999). Clients may also be introduced to the 12-Step model and encouraged to affiliate with a community-based Alcoholics Anonymous group.

Work readiness. In work readiness groups, clients are provided with the opportunity to explore their future roles as students and/or workers in supportive recovery-oriented groups. These groups help clients acquire the skills, resources, and supports necessary to pursue their chosen work or educational goals. Underlying skills are assessed, and a rehabilitation plan is developed with the goal of establishing real work or educational experiences. In some settings clients can be placed in internships or attend a course while receiving treatment in the program. Ultimately, success for community integration relies on programs having an explicit focus on supporting work integration and developing relationships in the community that will support this mission. Research has shown that clients who were discharged from day treatment to supported employment improved their vocational outcome without experiencing any increased risk of relapse (Bailey et al. 1998). Supported employment has expanded in recent years and is considered to be an evidence-based mental health practice, providing clients with the opportunity to obtain employment based on skills and experience while providing professional help they may need to sustain it (Salyers et al. 2004).

Family Interventions

Psychoeducation and consultation with the families of patients are important elements in a CDTP. The definition of *family* may extend to other support systems based on the needs of the patients. Permission is required prior to contact but may be a stated expectation of the program. Most family interventions are educationally oriented, with the goals of helping family members cope more effectively with the patient's illness and maximizing their ability to support the patient's recovery. Families are taught the stress–vulnerability model and encouraged to create a low-stress environment for the patient, with improvement in effective communication and decreases in arguments and use of substances. In addition, families may be asked to help with medication compliance and provide emotional and, at times, financial support. Multifamily groups provide a forum to disseminate recent information and develop a supportive network among families and patients (McFarlane et al. 2002).

Community Integration and Discharge Planning

Ideally, timing of discharge is linked to completion of goals established in treatment planning. At a minimum, the individual should be stabilized to the point that relapse is unlikely. Safety assessments indicate there is minimal risk of self-injurious or aggressive behaviors and that self-care and other activities of daily living can take place with less structure. Patients should be able to identify warning signs and have acquired skills to manage persistent symptoms. Appropriate aftercare should be established for ongoing medication monitoring, relapse prevention, and psychotherapy. It is hoped that the rehabilitation phase has enabled patients to pursue a work or educational goal that may include holding a volunteer job and/or resuming education or paid employment.

Intensive Outpatient Program

An IOP is intended for individuals who require more intensive treatment than routine outpatient care but less intensive treatment than a PHP. On the average, participation is up to 3 hours a day for at least 3 days a week over a period of a few weeks, although some programs offer individual and group therapy on a more extended basis. Often patients begin treatment in the PHP and then step down to an IOP. However, sometimes the selection of the IOP is driven by the patient's insurance benefits. In general, the patients are less acutely symptomatic than patients enrolled in a PHP or CDTP level of care, have some structured activities outside of the IOP, and do not require supervision. IOPs have been successful for treatment of some personality and affective disorders (Gratz et al. 2006; Gunderson et al. 2005; G.W. Smith et al. 2001). They allow individuals to engage in educational and vocational pursuits while pursuing intensive treatment. In some cases, insurance benefits do not support PHP or CDTP levels of care, but IOP provides some structure and intensive therapy. Many of the skills and psychoeducation groups described earlier for CDTPs or partial hospitalization could be adapted for an IOP format. The patient is also assigned an individual psychiatrist and therapist.

Administrative Issues

Management practices and policies in outpatient psychiatric services have moved toward standardization and accountability in service delivery to increase cost-effectiveness of care and ensure quality services. Guidelines started to be developed in the early 1990s, with performance indicators for evaluating care appearing in the mid-1990s. Mental health monitors have proliferated in recent years, although there is a scarcity of data on the prevalence of these practices in intensive outpatient treatment (Timko et al. 2003). Programming is influenced by many factors, including staffing patterns, the milieu, emergency services, documentation requirements, reimbursement, and regulatory agencies. In particular, reimbursement issues often dictate the range of services provided and have an influence on staffing patterns and overall accessibility of services. Following is a brief discussion of administrative issues that must be considered when developing intensive outpatient services.

Staffing

Intensive outpatient services employ providers with at least a master's-level degree in a counseling or related profession. A psychiatric attending physician prescribes medications or supervises residents in a teaching hospital. Medication management may also be provided by a nurse practitioner with oversight from a psychiatrist. Social workers, psychologists, and nurse practitioners are often the primary therapists, but other mental health providers may be involved in the case management. The rehabilitation counselors are usually occupational therapists, certified rehabilitation counselors, and/or psychiatric rehabilitation therapists. In addition, mental health workers, creative art therapists, and substance abuse specialists may also work in intensive outpatient services. Staff members need to have experience working with persons with chronic mental illness and an ability to work in a multidisciplinary team with a focus on rehabilitation. Volunteers with specific expertise such as yoga, writing, and art sometimes provide services. Staff members lead groups for symptom stabilization and skill development and provide treatment coordination and family counseling. Occupational therapists or other rehabilitation therapists provide treatment geared toward activities of daily living, work, and/or education. The treatment team interacts with residential settings, case managers, social clubs, vocational programs, peer counseling, and advocacy organizations.

Milieu

The therapeutic nature of the milieu plays a significant role in the rehabilitation of the patient. The design of the milieu involves a wide array of variables, including site location, architecture and design, channels of communication, organizational structure, and administration. Ultimately, the rhythm and pace of treatment all play a role in the milieu (Nosphpitz 1984). Today an effective outpatient milieu incorporates the patient in all levels of programming, from patient government to patient satisfaction surveys. As a result of increasingly client-centered treatment, there is a high level of expectation that patients play an active role in the program and take personal responsibility for their recovery. At the same time hospitals are being challenged to personalize the health care experience and encourage collaboration among patient, family members, and providers.

Emergency Services

Clear guidelines should be established about managing crises outside of program hours. At all levels of outpatient care, the patients should be aware of resources available in an emergency to help maintain their safety. Emergencies requiring immediate care should be referred to an emergency department or hospital evaluation center. If crisis team services are available, therapists, families, residential programs, and patients should know how to access them. If possible, the psychiatrist, therapist, or program administrator should be available to consult with an emergency department provider or crisis team. In some programs the treatment team is accessible to the patients after hours, but this is not always the case, and expectations about using community resources should be clear.

Documentation

Expectations for documentation are governed by state and federal regulations and, most importantly, the hospital or program agency. A treatment chart generally includes the referral documents, initial evaluation, individual and group progress notes, treatment plans, laboratory and medical reports, and any structured assessments or patient self-evaluations. Documentation also includes written consents from the patient for contacts with previous providers, community supports, and discharge planning. At the start of treatment, the patient is informed of his or her rights as a patient in the program and provided with the institution's policy on confidentiality regulations.

Reimbursement

The structure of insurance benefits for various levels of care varies from state to state. There is a risk that intensive treatment will not be supported due to limitations in spending for health care in state and national budgets. Private insurance generally pays for very limited duration of participation in a PHP or an IOP. Limits are set on the number of days per year covered, and such benefits often get subtracted from the number of inpatient or outpatient benefits remaining. Standards for Medicaid payments are set on the state level, and Medicaid reimbursement is subjected to the constraints of managed care in many areas. Medicare currently limits billing for therapeutic activities and vocational rehabilitation. Therefore, assignment to a level of care is driven by insurance benefits in addition to clinical considerations. Hospitals and community health care organizations have had to make decisions about which programs to maintain based on financial considerations, and the issue of reimbursement for levels of care has become one of the main considerations.

Regulatory Agencies

The Joint Commission, the arbiter of hospital accreditation, has developed reporting criteria focusing on outcome. A mandate was implemented in 1998 to integrate performance measures into the accreditation process (Babiss 2002). In 2001 hospitals started to collect data on 15 measures of outcome, which are then submitted to the commission. Assessments of whether patients have resumed roles in their lives, improved socialization, and sustained sobriety are just a few outcome measures identified. In addition, continuum of care from one level of service to another is closely assessed by reviewers, in regard to both appropriateness of the level of care and ease of transitioning from one level to the next. Programs are additionally monitored by the Centers for Medicare and Medicaid Services but often are deferred to the state department of health or office of mental health. Community- and hospital-based programs might utilize other agencies for accreditation and quality assurance, including the Commission on Accreditation of Rehabilitation Facilities. The National Committee for Quality Assurance provides oversight for managed behavioral health organizations.

Conclusion

Intensive outpatient services such as PHP, CDTP, and IOP offer care to individuals with acute exacerbations of symptoms or persistent symptoms who do not require inpatient level of care. They provide intensive diagnostic assessments, medication trials, and a range of therapeutic modalities aimed at stabilization and skill development to prevent future relapses and help the individual engage in further rehabilitation. A PHP provides acute stabilization for referral to a less intensive level of care. It can offer a diversion from inpatient admission or a stepdown from an inpatient service. A CDTP provides more extensive skills training and rehabilitation in a structured setting with some amount of daily supervision. An IOP offers stabilization in integrated individual and group therapy. The goals of these programs are to provide symptom relief, decrease maladaptive behaviors, and provide improved quality of life through enhanced interpersonal skills and functional and vocational rehabilitation. Intensive services provide a setting for education of trainees. They are also ideal sites for clinical research protocols in psychopharmacology, therapeutic modalities, programming, and services research.

These programs are cost intensive. Although remarkable benefits are apparent in many cases, qualitative input that defines outcome in a subjective manner requires further research, and more objective quantitative measures need to be developed (Babiss 2002). Multidimensional outcome measurements are needed to establish cost-effectiveness and to provide longitudinal data on quality of life and community reintegration. Research on outcomes could preserve and even expand funding for intensive outpatient services while informing the design of evidence-based treatment. Simultaneously, the voices of patients must never be forgotten. They provide a unique perspective on treatment and the recovery process, a perspective eloquently expressed by a former CDTP patient, Chaya, in her poem "Free Dove" (Figure 25–2).

Free Dove

We walked through these doors

Blindly

Mindless

Unaware

Of our surroundings.

Daily we walked through these doors,

We cried

We struggled

We fell

And pulled each other up.

And as we continued to walk through these doors,

All pride and shame left

We exposed our souls and secrets

Our fears yet to be conquered

We learned to believe.

Daily we walk through these doors,

Time has strengthened us

Bonded our hearts

Strong links,

Of which we have never known.

Now that I walk out these doors,

I want to thank you

And love you

For you have made me a better person

Now I bid you farewell with gratitude

You released me from my cage

And you're letting me fly....

FIGURE 25–2. **Poem written by Chaya upon discharge from a continuing day treatment program.**

References

Allen C: Measurement and Management of Cognitive Disabilities. Boston, MA, Little, Brown, 1985

American Psychiatric Association: Diagnostic and Statistical Manual of Mental Disorders, 4th Edition, Text Revision. Washington, DC, American Psychiatric Association, 2000

American Psychiatric Association: Practice guideline for the treatment of patients with borderline personality disorder. Am J Psychiatry 158 (suppl):1–52, 2001

American Psychiatric Association: Practice guideline for the psychiatric evaluation of adults, 2nd edition. Am J Psychiatry 163 (suppl):3–36, 2006

Anthony WA, Liberman RP: The practice of psychiatric rehabilitation: historical, conceptual and research base. Schizophr Bull 12:542–559, 1986

Anthony WA, Cohen MR, Vitalo R: The measurement of rehabilitation outcome. Schizophr Bull 4:365–383, 1978

Avants SK, Margolin A, Sindelar JL, et al: Day treatment versus enhanced standard methadone services for opioid-dependent patients: a comparison of clinical efficacy and cost. Am J Psychiatry 156:27–33, 1999

Babiss F: An Ethnographic Study of Mental Health Treatment and Outcomes: Doing What Works. Binghamton, NY, Haworth Press, 2002

Bailey EL, Ricketts SK, Becker DR, et al: Do long-term day treatment clients benefit from supported employment? Psychiatric Rehabilitation Journal 22:22–29, 1998

Bateman A, Fonagy P: Effectiveness of partial hospitalization in the treatment of borderline personality disorder: a randomized controlled trial. Am J Psychiatry 156:1563–1569, 1999

Bateman A, Fonagy P: Treatment of borderline personality disorder with psychoanalytically oriented partial hospitalization. Am J Psychiatry 158:36–42, 2001

Beck AT, Ward CH, Mendelson M, et al: An inventory of measuring depression. Arch Gen Psychiatry 4:53–63, 1961

Cohen MR, Farkas MD, Cohen B: Training Technology: Assessing Readiness for Rehabilitation. Boston, MA, Boston Center for Psychiatric Rehabilitation, 1992

Comerford AW: Addiction and vocational intervention. J Subst Abuse Treat 16:247–253, 1999

Dazord A, Gerin P, Seulin C, et al: Day-treatment evaluation: therapeutic outcome after a treatment in a psychiatry day-treatment center. Another look at the "Outcome Equivalence Paradox." Psychother Res 7:57–69, 1997

Feder J: Bridging the gap: integration of consumer needs into a psychiatric rehabilitation program, in New Frontiers in Psychosocial Occupational Therapy, Vol 14. Edited by Scott A. Binghamton, NY, Haworth Press, 1998, pp 89–95

Garety PA, Fowler D, Kuiper SE: Cognitive-behavioral therapy for medication-resistant symptoms. Schizophr Bull 26:73–86, 2000

Goodwin FK, Jamison KR: Clinical management of suicide risk, in Manic-Depressive Illness, 2nd Edition. New York, Oxford University Press, 2007a, pp 953–980

Goodwin FK, Jamison KR: Medical treatment of depression, in Manic-Depressive Illness, 2nd Edition. New York, Oxford University Press, 2007b, pp 747–796

Goodwin FK, Jamison KR: Medical treatment of hypomania, mania, and mixed states, in Manic-Depressive Illness, 2nd Edition. New York, Oxford University Press, 2007c, pp 721–746

Goodwin FK, Jamison KR: Psychotherapy of bipolar illness, in Manic-Depressive Illness, 2nd Edition. New York, Oxford University Press, 2007d, pp 869–905

Gottheil E, Weinstein SP, Sterling RC, et al: A randomized controlled study of the effectiveness of intensive outpatient treatment for cocaine dependence. Psychiatr Serv 49:782–787, 1998

Gottlieb GL: Financial issues, in Comprehensive Textbook of Psychiatry. Edited by Kaplan HI, Sadock BJ. Baltimore, MD, Williams & Wilkins, 1995, pp 2656–2657

Gratz KL, LaCroce DM, Gunderson JG: Measuring changes in symptoms relevant to borderline personality disorders following short-term treatment across partial hospital and intensive outpatient levels of care. J Psychiatr Pract 12:153–159, 2006

Gunderson JG, Gratz KL, Newhaus EC, et al: Levels of care in treatment, in The American Psychiatric Publishing Textbook of Personality Disorders. Edited by Oldham JM, Skodol AE, Bender DS. Washington, DC, American Psychiatric Publishing, 2005, pp 239–255

Hamilton M: A rating scale for depression. J Neurol Neurosurg Psychiatry 23:56–62, 1960

Kallert TW, Priebe S, McCabe R, et al: Are day hospitals effective for acutely ill psychiatric patients? A European multicenter randomized controlled trial. J Clin Psychiatry 68:278–287, 2007

Karterud S, Pederson G, Bjordal E, et al: Day treatment of patients with personality disorders: experiences from a Norwegian treatment research network. J Personal Disord 17:243–262, 2003

Kay SR, Fiszbein A, Opler LA: The Positive and Negative Syndrome Scale (PANSS) for schizophrenia. Schizophr Bull 13:261–276, 1987

Kleber HD, Weiss RD, Anton RF Jr, et al: Practice guideline for the treatment of patients with substance use disorders, 2nd edition. Am J Psychiatry 164 (suppl):5–123, 2007

Kraus JE, Stroup TS: Treatment of schizophrenia in the public sector, in The American Psychiatric Publishing Textbook of Schizophrenia. Edited by Lieberman JA, Stroup TS, Perkins DO. Washington, DC, American Psychiatric Publishing, 2006, pp 395–405

Law M, Baptiste S, Carswell A, et al: Canadian Occupational Performance Measure (COPM), 3rd Edition. Thorofare, NJ, Slack, 1998

Lehman AF, Steinwachs DM, Survey Co-Investigators of the PORT Project: Patterns of usual care for schizophrenia: initial results from the schizophrenia patient outcomes research team (PORT) client survey. Schizophr Bull 24:11–20, 1998

Lehman AF, Lieberman JA, Dixon LB, et al: Practice guideline for the treatments of patients with schizophrenia, 2nd edition. Am J Psychiatry 161 (suppl):1–56, 2004

Liberman RP, Voccaro JV, Carrigan PW: Psychiatric rehabilitation, in Comprehensive Textbook of Psychiatry. Edited by Kaplan HI, Sadock BJ. Baltimore, MD, Williams & Wilkins, 1995, pp 2696–2717

Linehan M: Cognitive Behavioral Treatment of Borderline Personality Disorder. New York, Guilford, 1993

Loeb PA: Independent Living Skills Survey Manual. San Antonio, TX, Harcourt Brace, 1996

Marshall M, Crowther R, Almaraz-Serrano AM, et al: Day hospital versus outpatient care for psychiatric disorders. Cochrane Database Syst Rev (3):CD003240, 2001a

Marshall M, Crowther R, Almaraz-Serrano AM: Systematic reviews of the effectiveness of day care for people with severe mental disorders: (1) acute day hospital versus admission; (2) vocational rehabilitation; (3) day hospital versus outpatient care. Health Technol Assess 5:1–75, 2001b

McFarlane WR, Gingerich S, Deakins SM, et al: Problem solving in multifamily groups, in Multifamily Groups. New York, Guilford, 2002, pp 142–171

McGurk SR, Twamley EW, Sitzer DI, et al: A meta-analysis of cognitive remediation in schizophrenia. Am J Psychiatry 164:1791–1802, 2007

Medalia A, Lim R: Treatment of cognitive dysfunction in psychiatric disorders. J Psychiatr Pract 10:17–25, 2004

Medalia A, Richardson R: What predicts a good response to cognitive remediation interventions? Schizophr Bull 31:942–952, 2005

Miller AL, McEvoy JP, Jeste DV, et al: Treatment of chronic schizophrenia, in The American Psychiatric Publishing Textbook of Schizophrenia. Edited by Lieberman JA, Stroup JS, Perkins DO. Washington, DC, American Psychiatric Publishing, 2006, pp 365–381

Muser KT, Glynn SM, McGurk SR: Social and vocational impairments, in The American Psychiatric Publishing Textbook of Schizophrenia. Edited by Lieberman JA, Stroup TS, Perkins DO. Washington, DC, American Psychiatric Publishing, 2006, pp 275–288

Nosphpitz JD: Milieu therapy, in the American Psychiatric Association Commission on Psychiatric Therapies. Edited by Karasu TB. Washington, DC, American Psychiatric Press, 1984, pp 619–665

Overall JE, Gorham DR: The Brief Psychiatric Rating Scale (BPRS): recent developments in ascertainment and scaling. Psychopharmacol Bull 24:97–99, 1988

Piper WE, Rosie JS, Joyce AS, et al: Historical evolution of day treatment, in Time-Limited Day Treatment for Personality Disorders: Integration of Research and Practice in a Group Program. Washington, DC, American Psychological Association, 1996, pp 11–34

Pratt CW, Gill KJ, Barrett N, et al: Goals, values and guiding principles of psychiatric rehabilitation, in Psychiatric Rehabilitation. San Diego, CA, Academic Press, 2002, pp 137–160

Precin P: Living Skills Recovery Workbook. Woburn, MA, Butterworth-Heinemann, 1999

Priebe S, Jones G, McCabe R, et al: Effectiveness and costs of acute day hospital treatment compared with conventional in-patient care. Br J Psychiatry 188:243–249, 2006

Resnick SG, Rosenheck RA, Lehman AF: An exploratory analysis of correlates of recovery. Psychiatr Serv 55:540–547, 2004

Rucci P, Frank E, Kostelnik B, et al: Suicide attempts in patients with bipolar I disorder during acute and maintenance phases of intensive treatment with pharmacotherapy and adjunctive psychotherapy. Am J Psychiatry 159:1160–1164, 2002

Salyers MP, Becker DR, Drake RE, et al: A ten-year follow-up of a supported employment program. Psychiatr Serv 55:302–308, 2004

Schene AH: The effectiveness of psychiatric hospitalization and day care. Curr Opin Psychiatry 17:303–309, 2004

Schwartz KB: Groups, in Psychosocial Occupational Therapy. Edited by Cara E, MacRae A. Clifton Park, NY, Thomson Delmar Learning, 2005a, pp 529–564

Schwartz KB: The history and philosophy of psychosocial occupational therapy, in Psychosocial Occupational Therapy. Edited by Cara E, MacRae A. Clifton Park, NY, Thomson Delmar Learning, 2005b, pp 58–79

Schwartz MS, Lauriello J, Drake RE: Psychosocial therapies, in The American Psychiatric Publishing Textbook of Schizophrenia. Edited by Lieberman JA, Stroup TS, Perkins DO. Washington, DC, American Psychiatric Publishing, 2006, pp 327–340

Smith GW, Ruiz-Sancho A, Gunderson JG: An intensive outpatient program for patients with borderline personality disorder. Psychiatr Serv 52:532–533, 2001

Smith TE, Hull JW, Hedayat-Harris A, et al: Development of a vertically integrated program of services for persons with schizophrenia. Psychiatr Serv 50:931–936, 1999

Timko C, Sempel JM, Moos RH: Models of standard and intensive outpatient care in substance abuse and psychiatric treatment. Admin Policy Ment Health 30:417–436, 2003

Turkington D, Kingdon D, Weiden PJ: Cognitive behavior therapy for schizophrenia. Am J Psychiatry 163:365–373, 2006

Vaglum P, Friis S, Irion T, et al: Treatment response of severe and nonsevere personality disorders in a therapeutic community day unit. J Personal Disord 4:161–172, 1990

Wilberg T, Karterud S, Urnes O, et al: Outcomes of poorly functioning patients with personality disorders in a day treatment program. Psychiatr Serv 49:1462–1467, 1998

Part IV
STRUCTURE AND INFRASTRUCTURE

CHAPTER 26

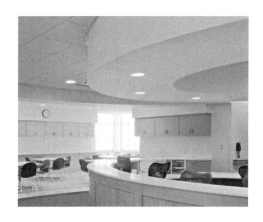

ADMINISTRATION AND LEADERSHIP

Harold I. Schwartz, M.D.
Steven S. Sharfstein, M.D., M.P.A.

It has been said that hospitals are among the most complex of organizations. Although the narrower focus of psychiatric hospitals, as a subset of the whole, might seem to diminish the complexity somewhat, the reach of organizational, systems, business, legal, regulatory, ethical, policy, clinical, professional, and academic concerns central to the administration of the psychiatric hospital today raises the bar for leadership to heights previously unknown. The complexity of this task is suggested by the degree to which the term *psychiatric hospital* fails to capture the depth and breadth of the enterprise. Although the word *hospital* has traditionally suggested inpatient care, psychiatric hospitals have evolved into continuums of services of which inpatient care may be only the briefest component; and, increasingly, into systems of care that are themselves components of integrated delivery networks (Sharfstein et al. 2001). These organizational changes reflect a shift—driven by financial pressures, policy, and, to a degree, the consumer/recovery move-

ment—away from the hospital as the central locus of treatment to the hospital as only one of the many levels of service necessary on the road to recovery from severe mental illness (Mechanic et al. 1995; Schreter et al. 1997). For the administrator/leader, the term *hospital* suggests a far narrower scope of responsibility and degree of challenge than actually exists for today's psychiatric health system leader.

The complexity of the psychiatric hospital system is reflected in the organizational forms these institutions have taken. Whereas the 1980s marked a huge expansion in the number of (mostly for-profit) psychiatric hospitals, fueled by changing demographics, attitudes toward mental health treatment, and the generous availability of insurance coverage (Geller 2006; Sharfstein 1995), by the early 1990s a number of important trends had converged that would force a radical rethinking and reorganization of the roles of psychiatric hospitals. The first, and clearly the most important, of these was the emergence of managed care, which drove the utilization of inpatient services down dramatically through techniques such as precertification and utilization review, encouraged the growth of less intensive levels of care, and revolutionized hospital business practices through the shift from fee-for-service to at-risk methods of payment (Mechanic et al. 1995; Schreter 1993). The emergence of modern psychopharmacology had earlier provided the therapeutic basis for fewer hospitalizations and lower lengths of stay, while the nascent recovery movement provided an additional rationale (Davidson et al. 2006; President's New Freedom Commission on Mental Health 2003), as did the establishment of an evidence base for shorter hospitalization for many patients (Glick and Hargreaves 1979; Glick et al. 1984). The result was a dramatic shift in the psychiatric hospital industry that left both the for-profit and the not-for-profit hospitals in search of survival strategies. The progressive and systematic underfunding of psychiatric services throughout America in recent years (Appelbaum 2003) has created a relentless pressure either to downsize and rationalize programs and services or to reinvent business and clinical practices to make them sustainable. Although the circumstances of individual markets may influence the survival strategy greatly (Schlesinger et al. 1997), the administrative and leadership challenges have been great everywhere.

This chapter uses case studies and vignettes to illustrate the leadership challenges and the changes in hospital organization, business practice, and clinical models central to the evolution of psychiatric hospitals over the past generation. We select our illustrations from the recent histories of America's earliest asylums, the eight private, not-for-profit hospitals that constitute the informal "Ivy League" of psychiatric hospitals. These prototypical not-for-profit psychiatric hospitals, whose efforts to remain viable into the twenty-first century contain important lessons in hospital administration and leadership, include the Institute of Pennsylvania Hospital, Friends Hospital, the Institute of Living, Sheppard and Enoch Pratt Hospital, Butler Hospital, the Westchester Division of New York Presbyterian Medical Center, McLean Hospital, and the Brattleboro Retreat. As McCue and Clement (1993) predicted in their comparison of private for-profit and not-for-profit hospitals, the not-for-profits toward the end of the twentieth century were disadvantaged by the burden of older facilities, higher costs, the absence of ready capital, and a not-for-profit–inspired sense of mission. Rapid change, with the emulation of for-profit business practices, would be required, with the risk of closure for those who could not adapt.

Modern Adaptations of the Early Asylums

At one extreme—the closure of a hospital in substance and in name—lies the Institute of Pennsylvania Hospital. The Pennsylvania Hospital, established in 1751, was chartered to treat the "sick poor and insane" in the same facility. In 1841 a separate facility, the Pennsylvania Hospital for the Insane, was established. It was renamed the Institute of Pennsylvania Hospital in 1959 and continued to operate as such until 1997. In that year, under the relentless pressure of diminishing revenue from insurance providers, the institute was closed, the facility sold, and psychiatric services downsized and returned to the Pennsylvania Hospital (Sudak 2007). Other well-known hospitals were either closing or radically reorganizing at the time. These included Chestnut Lodge, which was bankrupt and closed its doors in 2001, and Taylor Manor, which sold its license to operate inpatient beds to the Sheppard Pratt Health System in 2002 (Geller 2006).

The Institute of Living

Established as the Hartford Retreat for the Insane in 1822, the Institute of Living was the third asylum established in America and the first hospital of any kind in Connecticut (Goodheart 2003). The name change in 1939 reflected the vision of then Psychiatrist-in-Chief C. Charles Burlingame to fashion an institution that was "a combined hospital, country club and university campus" (Clouette and Deslandes 1997, p. 526). The institute flourished for a time in this model, although by the 1970s it had moved into the medical mainstream, treating the great variety of patients made available by the emergence and growth of commercial insurance and Medicare. All was to change with the emergence of managed care. In 1988 the institute operated 420 inpatient beds with an average daily census of 368 and an average length of stay of 33 days. By 1992 it had undergone nine consecutive downsizings and was operating only 150 beds with an average daily census of 119 and an average length of stay of 13 days (Institute of Living 1993). The downsizings and other increasingly frantic efforts to meet the requirements of managed care payers were not enough to ensure survival. Revenues did not meet expenses, and reserves in the form of endowments would not last forever. By 1992 the institute had either to be merged, sold to a for-profit chain, or closed. The solution most consistent with the institute's long history of moral treatment (antecedent to the biopsychosocial model) was a merger in 1994 with Hartford Hospital, a large, voluntary, not-for-profit general hospital that was physically contiguous.

In the process of merging with a large and successful general hospital, the Institute of Living gave up its private psychiatric hospital license and proceeded to operate as the department of psychiatry of a general hospital. All of the programs and services of the Hartford Hospital psychiatry department were merged with those of the institute, using a best practices analysis to determine the program features, site, and staffing of the surviving programs. The medical staff of the institute joined the medical staff of Hartford Hospital. All infrastructure departments of the institute were either absorbed into those of Hartford Hospital or eliminated.

Although the boards of directors of the merging institutions had committed themselves to "maintaining the mission, tradition and identity" of the Institute of Living, it was clear that, going forward, the Institute of Living was now the department of psychiatry of Hartford Hospital, doing business as (and looking for all the world to be) a private psychiatric hospital. The confusion of identity was heightened by the decision to maintain a board of directors for the institute with limited responsibilities while the Hartford Hospital board assumed the traditional governance role. For several years the tension between the charge to maintain the identity of the Institute of Living and the requirement to fully merge into the general hospital produced "us and them" tensions. Active and creative leadership interventions were necessary to strike a workable balance.

Early challenges included the organization of administration and leadership. In the first years postmerger, the Institute of Living shed its president and several vice presidents. Harold I. Schwartz, M.D., the Director of Psychiatry of Hartford Hospital, ultimately became the psychiatrist-in-chief of the merged entity and, in recognition of the size and complexity of this service for the parent organization, the vice president of Behavioral Health for Hartford Hospital. Because the Institute of Living joined the hospital as a self-contained entity, it seemed appropriate to transition the operation of the merged Institute of Living as Hartford Hospital's first product line division. The very nature of the merger, with the shift to Hartford Hospital support departments, meant that the organization would have to find its way through a matrix of product line functioning and integration with the central organization. This has been challenging in an organization not otherwise committed to a product or service line organization. The establishment of a "collaborative management team" consisting of medical and nursing directors and a director of operations, along with the psychiatrist-

in-chief, ultimately provided the degree of support necessary for a modified product line management.

Operating as a component of a general hospital had several immediate and significant financial ramifications. First, and perhaps most important, was termination of the hospital's exclusion as an institution for mental disease (the so-called IMD [Institution for Mental Disease] exclusion) from the Medicaid program for adults. The ability to hospitalize Medicaid patients created a new revenue source and marked an expansion of the Institute of Living's mission to the community; however, (managed) Medicaid reimbursement in Connecticut does not meet the cost of providing care, which would come to be a serious drawback. The Institute of Living also had to give up its established TEFRA (Tax Equity and Fiscal Responsibility Act) rate for Medicare patients, accepting the somewhat lower rate established for Hartford Hospital. The transition from traditional fee-for-service billing to all-inclusive contracting was also accelerated by the merger. Prior to the merger, the Hartford Hospital department had one inpatient unit staffed largely by private practitioners in fee-for-service billing arrangements. The Institute of Living, in contrast, had transitioned to all-inclusive contracts staffed by contract to psychiatrists in a related professional corporation. With the merger, payers were unwilling to proceed with dual billing procedures. The growth of managed care argued strongly for transition, and the Hartford Hospital unit was moved to the institute's inpatient building and transitioned to all-inclusive billing. This allowed for standardization of business and clinical practices, facilitated a hospitalist model for inpatient care, and alienated the private practitioners who felt unable to adapt their traditional practice to this new arrangement.

The postmerger managerial and leadership challenges faced by the Institute of Living emerged in three stages. In the first, the integration of the institute into Hartford Hospital provided a secure base of operation from which it could focus its attention on adapting its continuum of programs and services to better meet the challenges of the behavioral health marketplace. This period of stability provided an environment that allowed the institute's research and teaching programs to flourish and adapt to changing circumstances. These adaptations included the reconfiguration of research initiatives into translational research centers that aligned closely with the institute's core mission and clinical programs. In each of these examples, the closer alignment of research and clinical programs produced synergies of benefit to the Institute of Living and its patients. For example, the institute's Braceland Center for Mental Health and Aging had focused for many years on geriatric health services–related research. Typical studies examined issues related to Medicaid funding of geriatric mental health treatment in nursing homes or Medicare funding of such in the community. Although important, such studies were distant from the core mission of the psychiatric hospital and its programs. The center was gradually transitioned to one that focused on clinical dementia studies, and with the establishment of a Memory Disorders Center, research initiatives were integrated into an important clinical program that provides clinical assessment of individuals in the early stages of dementing illness. The center became a study site in the federally funded Alzheimer's Disease Neuroimaging Initiative (Thal et al. 2006), marking the transition to a fully relevant state-of-the-art research/clinical program working in an area of central relevance to the hospital's patient base.

At the same time, a "schizophrenia initiative," supported philanthropically, led to the establishment of the Olin Neuropsychiatry Research Center, a functional and structural magnetic resonance neuroimaging research center with Connecticut's first 3-Tesla magnet. Research on cognitive rehabilitation in schizophrenia led to the establishment of a partial hospital program specializing in this computer-based rehabilitation approach. Most recently, a genetic screening research program has been added to the mix, leading to pharmacogenetic approaches to the treatment of mood disorders and schizophrenia. The Institute of Living's reestablishment of its own independently sponsored (by Hartford Hospital) adult and child and adolescent residencies has added still another important element to the synergy created by the mix of academic and clinical programs.

The second stage of postmerger activities involved the establishment, by Hartford Hospital's parent corporation, of a behavioral health (partially) integrated delivery system, the Behavioral Health Network, consisting (in addition to the institute) of another psychiatric hospital (as a corporate subsidiary), a substance abuse treatment system, the psychiatry department of a subsidiary general hospital, and a community mental health center. The network established its own behavioral health managed care organization that ultimately outlived its purpose and was merged with another not-for-profit but for a time helped to stabilize the environment for the network partners during a period of chaotic managed care growth and consolidation in Connecticut. The network has been most effective in negotiation of its carve-out managed care contracts, reflecting the enhanced regional clout of the combined entities.

In the third and current stage, the Institute of Living finds itself still challenged to rationalize its services and programs in an era of rising costs and limited revenues. Although the huge inefficiencies of a private psychiatric hospital struggling alone in an inhospitable environment were shed by the merger, they have been replaced by the equally huge and growing overhead costs of the general hospital. Network contracting has been successful at generating enhanced revenue from commercial payers, but Medicaid reimbursement remains inadequate to match the demands of mission to the community. Teaching and research programs have flourished, along with a regional reputation for excellence in clinical care, yet the translation of these into entities of financial survival value remains very much a work in progress.

Sheppard Pratt: From Asylum to Comprehensive System of Care

On his death in 1857, Moses Sheppard, a prominent Quaker philanthropist from Baltimore, left $571,000 to found the Sheppard Asylum. Inspired by Dorothea Dix 5 years earlier, Sheppard decided to put his entire fortune into building an institution in the image of York Retreat in England and Friends Hospital in Philadelphia. He admonished the trustees to "meet a need that not otherwise would be met" and to "do everything for the comfort of the patient." He also said, "lead the way." Insisting that only the interest of his gift and not the principal be used in the building of the asylum, it took more than 30 years for the original buildings, designed by Calvert Vaux, to be built. The first patient was admitted in 1891. The trustees then solicited a second gift from another prominent Baltimore philanthropist, Enoch Pratt. After Pratt's death in 1896, the Sheppard Asylum was renamed The Sheppard and Enoch Pratt Hospital (Forbush 1971; Gollaher 1995).

Sheppard's Quaker heritage, with its emphasis on moral treatment (Digby 1985), evolved into a long-term inpatient hospital for those who could afford to pay the fees. When psychoanalysis came to America, Sheppard Pratt was an ideal place to practice the art of this treatment and to research its efficacy. Harry Stack Sullivan was a psychiatrist in residence from 1922 to 1930 and established an all-male schizophrenia research unit on the grounds. He published papers on his findings and established the field of social psychiatry. William Rush Dunton, another staff psychiatrist, invented occupational therapy while at Sheppard Pratt to enrich the experience of long-term hospitalization. Originally consisting of 200 beds, Sheppard Pratt rapidly expanded to a high of 322 beds by the mid-1980s. The average stay in 1970 was 140 days. Even with 90% of revenue coming from long-term hospitalization, the winds of change began with the advent of private health insurance and the community mental health center movement.

Sheppard Pratt was the first private psychiatric hospital to establish and sponsor a community mental health center with a catchment area in Baltimore County in 1972. Dr. Robert Gibson, the fourth medical director of Sheppard Pratt, had the vision to anticipate that this mode of community practice would be the wave of the future. Although this was a small part of Sheppard Pratt, by the early 1990s it proved to be a model for change and growth. Day hospital programs were established, and the early efforts toward rehabilitation, supervised housing, and supportive employment all came into place during this era.

In 1986 Dr. Steven Sharfstein was named vice president and medical director. At that time, the average length of stay at Sheppard Pratt was 80 days for adults, 125 days for children and adolescents. There were 322 beds, which were almost always full, with 1,000 admissions per year to fill those beds. From 1990 to 1993, with the advent of managed care and a broad consensus by the payers not to continue paying for long-term hospitalization, length of stay decreased dramatically (Feldman 1992). By 1992, as Dr. Sharfstein became the fifth president of Sheppard Pratt, the length of stay had decreased to 30 days. By the year 2000, it decreased even further, to 10 days. In 2006, with an average stay of less than 10 days, there were 7,000 admissions to fill 220 beds (100 fewer beds than 20 years prior), but Sheppard Pratt was fundamentally different in a variety of other ways.

With the handwriting visible on the wall, Sheppard Pratt began a process of reinvention, initially through reorganizing of the hospital into a health system (including a reduction in force) and then by embarking on a growth strategy that led to Sheppard Pratt becoming the largest provider of psychiatric, behavioral, addiction, and special education services in Maryland. In reorganizing of the traditional hospital structure of departments into "service lines," the priority became growing the continuum of care (Schreter et al. 1997) with the establishment of day programs, outpatient clinics, residential care, and other initiatives in communities across the state. The trustees decided to reinvest in Sheppard Pratt by first building a 50-bed residential school in western Maryland and then developing programs in general hospitals throughout the state. Sheppard Pratt currently manages 10 general

hospital psychiatric units, emergency departments, and outpatient programs throughout the state of Maryland. Utilizing the community mental health center model of the 1970s, Sheppard Pratt began to establish and acquire nonprofit community agencies across the state. These comprehensive mental health centers included supervised living, supportive employment, and other rehabilitation programs and served as the major community resource for patients being discharged from increasingly short-term settings, either from Sheppard Pratt or from general hospital units. In 2003 Sheppard Pratt acquired another private psychiatric hospital, adding an additional 40 beds, and began to plan for the building of a new 192-bed tertiary psychiatric facility at the original historic site in Towson, Maryland.

The $100 million building and renovation project began in 2003 and was completed in 2005 (only 2 years this time around!). Sheppard Pratt is the largest regional resource for behavioral health care, with acute adult crisis stabilization services and highly specialized units for children (ages 3–12) and adolescents, geriatric patients with and without dementia, patients with eating disorders, severe posttraumatic stress, dually diagnosed substance abuse and mental illness, and dually diagnosed mental retardation and mental illness.

Sheppard Pratt, which sponsored its own residency program for years, affiliated with the University of Maryland in 1996; the combined residency in child, adult, and geriatric psychiatry continues to prosper. As one of the largest residency programs in the country, with more than 70 trainees in a variety of undergraduate and postgraduate programs, this academic partnership has been a major success. Research on long-term outcomes of patients with schizophrenia and clinical trials research grew as well.

From the early 1990s to today, three private psychiatric hospitals in Maryland went bankrupt and closed their doors. By surviving in a radically changed marketplace, Sheppard Pratt was able to grow and develop services in those areas that needed them the most. Approximately two-thirds of Sheppard Pratt's revenue comes from public dollars (including Medicare and Medicaid) and public education dollars; the rest is private funding. Sheppard Pratt is the largest provider of special education throughout the state—that is, education for severely emotionally disturbed children and adolescents, including those with autism, with 11 special education schools. The revenue from the education component of Sheppard Pratt Health System is approximately 30% of the overall revenue stream. The hospital itself represents about 40% of the revenue, and the other 30% comes from the other special programs of Sheppard Pratt, including its community-based services and general hospital programs.

Not everything worked, however. In the early 1990s, Sheppard Pratt put together its own managed care program called the Sheppard Pratt Health Plan. This program was sold in the late 1990s. It was not successful because it could not compete with the large managed care corporations. The latter managed costs, whereas the Sheppard Pratt plan was more focused on providing care. Outpatient services sponsored by the hospital similarly were downsized and shifted to community-based programs because of the inefficiencies and cost issues related to outpatient care.

The leadership at Sheppard Pratt adopted the philosophy that we were "not for profit but also not for loss" early in this process of reinvention. Thus, new services and programs that were added on and off campus had to meet this test. Schools that were begun in various areas that did not meet this test were closed after an 18-month to 2-year trial; outpatient services were particularly vulnerable to this test. Additional acquisitions and mergers allowed some outpatient services to continue to grow, however. An important partner to this process has been the public mental health system, which contracted with the Sheppard Pratt Health System in 2004 for care for the uninsured.

Much of this has occurred in a regulatory environment in Maryland that is highly proscriptive. Hospital rates are regulated, and there is a strong Certificate of Need law. These regulatory issues have helped keep for-profit medicine out of Maryland, and this has been a benefit to the growth of the not-for-profit Sheppard Pratt.

Although it is hard to summarize the role of leadership in this process, it is important to note that the recruitment of top clinicians as well as administrative leaders has been a key aspect of success. Clinical leaders are especially critical. The Sheppard Pratt Practice Association has developed attractive compensation models as well as academic appointments at the University of Maryland, which has led to the recruitment of some outstanding leaders in the treatment of schizophrenia, bipolar illness, geriatric illnesses, trauma disorders, eating disorders, and child and adolescent disorders. Although Maryland is the primary focus of activity and 85% of patients come from this state, there is a strong regional and national pull for a variety of our tertiary care programs. In 2004, The Retreat at Sheppard Pratt was established as a concierge-level program, initially composed of 6 beds but now 16 beds, for those who can afford to pay out of pocket. It does not accept insurance, is licensed as an assisted living facility, and has been a success in a marketplace in which the wealthy look for extra amenities as well as attention from top psychiatric clinicians.

In summary, the success of Sheppard Pratt, an independent, not-for-profit foundation and health system, has occurred due to a reinvention of the hospital into a health system, reorganization of the staff, focus on the development of diverse services in various communities throughout the state, an economic model that was not for profit but also not for loss, high volume care, and the recruitment and retention of the top clinicians in the field. Luck also played a role through the tax-exempt bond financing that helped finance the new hospital in 2003—$60 million was borrowed at the all-time low in long-term interest rates. The success of the markets in the 1990s led to an important growth in the Sheppard Pratt endowment (the original gifts of Moses Sheppard and Enoch Pratt), which helped establish the good health of the balance sheet of Sheppard Pratt to borrow money cheaply and to build a new hospital. With luck and leadership, Sheppard Pratt looks to the twenty-first century with optimism and high expectations.

Core Components of Psychiatric Hospital Administration

As our case studies suggest, the domain of concerns that constitute hospital administration is extensive and ranges from public policy, to business practice, to the professional concerns of multiple mental health professions. These concerns play out in the marketplace as well as the community, in which the demands of mission add still greater complexity. For in-depth treatments of these many areas, the reader may turn to more extensive resources (Reid and Silver 2003; Talbott and Hales 2001). For the purposes of this chapter, we will profile the most compelling elements of administration highlighted in our case studies, with emphasis on the challenges currently presented to hospital leadership.

Organizational Structure and Governance

Organizational structure has been defined as "the people, positions, functional groups, and lines of authority and accountability designed to accomplish the organization's mission, goals and objectives" (Veenhuis 2003, p. 107). Although structure does indeed reflect the mission and goals of an organization, overly rigid structure may come to constrain and even dictate goals and objectives. Organizational structure occurs at multiple levels. The psychiatric hospital may function as a subsidiary of a larger parent organization with governance (the board of directors) at the health system level. Other hospitals are governed directly by their boards, having integrated horizontally with a variety of owned or affiliated services. Two of our examples, the Institute of Living and the Westchester Division of the New York Presbyterian Hospital, are organized as components of large general hospitals but do business as psychiatric hospitals.

The hospital leader (generally the chief executive officer) operates the organization by virtue of the authority conferred by the governing body (board of directors) (Joint Commission 2007). In those instances in which the hospital is a component of another entity, the hospital director, psychiatrist-in-chief, or other leadership position may report to a general hospital or system chief executive who, in turn, reports to the board. In either case, beyond these constants, the organization of the hospital may vary widely, with senior leadership organized around professional discipline, program and service lines, or (usually) some combination of both.

Governing boards generally play a critical administrative role in times of crises. Our case study of the Institute of Living provides a very clear example of the powerful role that decisive board leadership may play in times of administrative crises for psychiatric hospitals. In 1992, the board of directors of the Institute of Living was faced with the inability of the institute to remain viable as a self-sustaining organization. Among the available choices—closure, merger or sale to a for-profit—only one was consistent with a sense of mission that could be traced to the earliest days of the moral treatment movement: integration into a large general hospital that, by virtue of allowing Medicaid reimbursement for adult patients, actually allowed for an expansion of mission to the community. Another compelling example of the role of decisive board leadership is to be found in the story of Friends Hospital.

Friends Hospital

The Friends Asylum was established by the Philadelphia Society of Friends in 1817. As such it is the only of the "Ivy League" hospitals to have been established by a religious order. It was modeled after the York Retreat in York, England, and was instrumental in establishing the moral treatment movement in America (Deutsch 1949). By the turn of the twenty-first century, the asylum had become Friends Hospital, a 192-bed acute care psychiatric hospital with a 26-bed adult residential program located in northeastern Philadelphia, and was struggling with inadequate revenues in the face of a long-established and religiously driven commitment to provide care to those in need. A number of programmatic joint ventures and explored affiliations all failed to produce a plan that could ensure fiscal viability. Between 2000 and 2004 the hospital experienced a $20 million loss from operations and the nearly total expenditure of unrestricted reserves (Carol Ashton-Hergenhan, personal communication, March 2007).

The executive committee of the hospital board explored all options, including closing the hospital. In what may be one of the most creative reconfigurations of a hospital in this era, the board determined that it could both "partner for profit" and maintain its Quaker-driven commitment to the community. The board's solution was to form a for-profit joint venture with Horizon Health Corporation, a large for-profit hospital chain. Friends Hospital sold an 80% interest in the buildings and assets to the joint venture in return for $16 million received by the newly established Thomas Scattergood Foundation, established to continue the Friends mission by providing education, advocacy, and access to care. The Scattergood Foundation (which retains a Quaker board) has significant representation on both the board of the joint venture that operates the hospital and the board of the hospital itself (including the chairmanship in the latter case), leaving the foundation with a far larger role in governance than might be suggested by its 20% ownership position. A number of other contractual commitments are intended to ensure that Friends will continue to be operated in a manner consistent with its Quaker mission. For example, the joint venture must continue to operate the hospital in a manner consistent with the former Friends Hospital charity care policy. In addition, the organizational entity that was the former Friends Hospital will continue as the (not-for-profit) Thomas Scattergood Foundation, committed to a grant program that provides access to care in the Philadelphia area and to reestablishing "the Quaker heritage of being thought leaders in mental health" (Carol Ashton-Hergenhan, personal communication, March 2007).

Integration and Product or Service Line Organization

The concept of integration has come to play an increasingly important role in modern hospital administration. Virtually all successful hospitals have integrated to some degree. In its most fundamental sense, integration reflects the degree to which psychiatric care has transitioned from inpatient to a continuum of ambulatory levels of care requiring virtually all psychiatric hospitals to either create such services or ally themselves with organizations capable of providing them. Integration can be thought of in its horizontal and vertical dimensions (Santiago 2001). It occurs horizontally through the coordination between organizations, programs, and clinicians at a single level of care, and vertically in systems that focus on the development of continuums of care that may reach from the hospital emergency department to supportive housing. The development of an integrated system may require alliances, mergers, joint ventures, and other creative business developments as well as the information systems and other business tools necessary to manage a broad horizontal and vertical domain. The extent of integration flows from the goals and objectives of administration. In the Institute of Living case study, the parent organization acquired additional mental health organizations that were geographically distant enough to limit clinical program collaboration. However, the capacity to contract jointly as subsidiaries of the same parent corporation has proved an effective strategy.

Our Sheppard Pratt case study reflects an organization that has employed extensive horizontal and vertical integration. Through a program of acquisitions, mergers, and contractual relationships and by establishing the business capacity to manage extensive at-risk reimbursement arrangements, Sheppard has increasingly fashioned itself into an organized delivery system providing a continuum of services, with clinical and fiscal accountability to defined populations (Shortell et al. 1994). At the same time, both the Institute of Living and Sheppard Pratt attempted to extend their integrated delivery systems to include managed behavioral care organizations but ultimately withdrew from these business lines.

The Westchester Division and the Behavioral Health Service Line of New York Presbyterian Hospital

We briefly review the organization of psychiatric services in the New York Presbyterian Hospital system to highlight the complexity of product line integration in a hospital system with extensive vertical and horizontal integration. Opened in 1792, New York Hospital, like its predecessor, the Pennsylvania Hospital in Phil-

adelphia, admitted mental patients. The New York Lunatic Asylum was established nearby in 1808 as demand grew, and moved uptown in 1821 to become the enlarged Bloomingdale Asylum (Ozarin 2006). The Bloomingdale Asylum moved to White Plains, New York, in 1895. The name was changed to New York Hospital Westchester Division in 1936. The Westchester Division, operating under the general hospital license of New York Hospital (rather than as a private psychiatric hospital), together with the Payne Whitney Psychiatric Clinic at New York Hospital's New York City location, constituted the psychiatric services of New York Hospital and the department of psychiatry of the Cornell University School of Medicine (later the Weill Cornell School of Medicine).

In 1998 New York Hospital and Columbia Presbyterian Hospital announced a full-asset merger, one of the largest of its kind, creating the largest hospital in New York City, with more than 13,000 employees and 2,200 beds (NewYork–Presbyterian Hospital 2007). At the time of the merger, Presbyterian Hospital had its own full-service psychiatry department, including two inpatient pavilions, a continuum of ambulatory services, and an integral relationship with the New York State Psychiatric Institute, New York State's flagship psychiatric research hospital. These services constituted the clinical base of the department of psychiatry of the Columbia University College of Physicians and Surgeons. Each hospital had its own academic department and very significant educational and research enterprises in addition to these clinical services.

The complexity of the administrative and leadership tasks necessary to bring these behemoth institutions into an effective single entity is almost unimaginable. A "service line" organization for key clinical departments was one of the first business and quality initiatives of the merged hospital system. The purpose of the service line initiative was to inform senior leadership on strategic direction, quality issues, and business planning for the clinical areas (Gail Ryder, personal communication, March 2007). A planning and operational committee was established, consisting of the two department chairs, the medical director from each site, and the service line executive. The goals of the committee included planning for and rationalizing services and programs, establishing uniform contracting, and enhancing quality by establishing uniform policies and procedures and quality indicators throughout the system. Much has been achieved to date despite the retention of separate medical school affiliations and distinctive physician incentive systems (and physician hospital organizations) at the two sites.

The establishment of the New York Presbyterian Health System, consisting of 42 medical institutions (27 hospitals) with 18,500 physicians, has added another level of complexity to the behavioral health service line with the sharing of policies, quality initiatives, and contracting within the larger systems.

Indeed, integration appears to have been an important part of the strategy for almost all of the Ivy League hospitals as they have reorganized and reengineered themselves in the face of the fiscal constraints and changing business practices of the past few decades. McLean Hospital in Belmont, Massachusetts, Harvard Medical School's largest psychiatric site, joined Partners Healthcare, an integrated health system consisting of six Boston area hospitals (three teaching affiliates of Harvard Medical School), community health centers, a physician network, home health, and long-term care services (http://www.partners.org). Likewise, Butler Hospital in Providence, Rhode Island, the flagship psychiatric service for the Brown University Medical School's department of psychiatry, became a founding member of Care New England Health System, consisting of three hospitals, wellness centers, and home health and hospice services (http://www.carenewengland.org).

Core Business Domains

Our case studies and vignettes have illustrated a number of intra- and extraorganizational relationships and the core business functions necessary to lead the administration of a successful psychiatric hospital. All psychiatric hospitals (and hospital systems) have important relationships with funding, policy, and regulatory organizations. Meeting the requirements of each will be critical to success (Hester 2003). The requirement to remain in regulatory compliance with the Joint Commission (formerly the Joint Commission on the Accreditation of Healthcare Organizations), the Centers for Medicare and Medicaid Services, and state and local authorities becomes a critical component of strategies to expand (through integration or new program development) or contract services. The requirements of regulators and payers for the demonstration of quality and safety has led to an intensive focus on quality measurement, outcome studies (Docherty and Dewan 1995; Sederer and Dickey 1996), and satisfaction surveys that will only continue as "pay for performance" is introduced into hospital reimbursement (Pelonero and Johnson 2007). Efforts to continuously improve the quality of psychiatric inpatient (and outpatient) care are expensive (Rosenau and Linder 2003), and the translation of these efforts into improved financial performance is, at best, indirect.

Relationships with funders are another issue critical to psychiatric hospital survival. For those hospitals that operate under a general hospital license (and therefore are not subject to the IMD exclusion), Medicaid has had an enormous influence on financial outcome. Because Medicaid is administered by individual states with support of and regulation by the federal government (Silver 2003b), rates vary by state. Higher Medicaid rates in New York have contributed significantly to the revenues of the Westchester Division of the New York Presbyterian Hospital, whereas lower rates in Connecticut have had the opposite effect for the Institute of Living. The establishment of Medicaid 1115 (Research and Demonstration) and Medicaid 1915(b) (Medicaid Managed Care) waivers has led to innovations in the administration of Medicaid that have allowed the participation of some psychiatric hospitals in managed Medicaid programs (Dixon et al. 2001). Participation in such programs increases the requirement for participation in integrated systems of care, often requiring public–private partnerships to ensure adequate care and fiscal viability.

The transition of the Medicare program to a prospective payment system for psychiatric units in 2006 (Centers for Medicare and Medicaid Services 2006) illustrates another challenge created by the funder. The complicated formula that replaced the prior exemption from the diagnosis-related-group reimbursement methodology promised revenue enhancements to some hospitals and reductions to others. The ethical challenges to health care providers of prospective payment systems have been the subject of much discussion (Dougherty 1989). In anticipation of this change, the Institute of Living reduced its length of stay on one geriatric inpatient unit by 4 days within 6 months through a variety of steps that ensured that treatment goals were rapidly established and pursued, that treatment intensity continued through weekends, and that care was constantly reviewed by the medical director.

Although it is beyond the scope of this chapter to review, our case studies suggest the importance of expertise in core business functions. We mention some of the most compelling. In our examples, strategic planning at the level of senior administration and governance has been critical to the successes achieved. Strategic plans are implemented through the financial analysis that creates business plans and the financial management at all levels of the organization that implements them (Silver 2003a). None of this can happen in today's world without an emphasis on the management of information. The business systems necessary to create integrated hospital systems, electronic medical records with algorithm-driven order entry systems, and systemwide outcome studies (to cite just a few examples) suggest that no hospital or hospital system can succeed in the future without significant attention to and investments in information technology (Trabin 1996; World Health Organization 2005). Attention must be paid to human resources issues, especially to relations with the medical staff strained by the challenge to sustain professional satisfaction as resources and professional autonomy are diminished.

An often overlooked function of hospital leadership is the development of philanthropy (fund development) initiatives for the organization. These may take many forms, including annual fund drives, capital campaigns, planned giving, or major gift development (Fitzpatrick and Deller 2000). For older, well-established hospitals such as those in the "Ivy League," it is often the case that a community of donors can be accessed if this function is sufficiently addressed. Yet even newer hospitals can tap into the enthusiasm of the community in annual fund drives that can fund capital improvements, new program development, enhancement of existing programs, research activities, and other initiatives that may greatly enhance quality but would otherwise go unfunded. At the Institute of Living, a major fund drive supported a "schizophrenia initiative" that funded, in part, a new neuropsychiatric research institute, a day program focusing on cognitive rehabilitation for individuals with schizophrenia, and a family resource center.

Closely related to issues of fund development is stewardship of the endowments and related resources that a hospital may be fortunate enough to possess. Several of the hospitals discussed in this chapter have been fortunate in their geographic locations. Butler Hospital, McLean, and Sheppard Pratt, all established initially in areas that would have been considered rural, now find themselves in expensive suburbs with the opportunity to engage in real estate development ventures that already have or will in the future contribute significantly to the future fiscal viability of these hospitals. The Brattleboro Retreat in Brattleboro, Vermont, although still rural, has sold its dairy farm and is considering further real estate transactions (Greg Miller, personal communication, April 2007). In contrast, Friends Hospital was established initially in a rural area that ultimately became northeastern Philadelphia, an economically deprived area. Despite a sizable land holding, Friends was not able to rely on real estate development to compensate for its downward revenue spiral.

Qualities of Leadership

The literature on organizational leadership has become an industry unto itself, focusing on management skills (Edershein 2006) and the qualities that facilitate organizational effectiveness, learning (Senge 1990), and change (Kotter 1996). Numerous reviews of theories and styles of leadership are available (Dubrin 2001; Norhouse 1974), including a focus on leadership within mental health administration (Levin et al. 2003; Shore and Vanelli 2001). What will constitute appropriate training for mental health leaders of the future remains an important question (Harrison and Gray 2003; Yu-Chin 2002), as is the question of the leadership role for psychiatrists (Greiner 2006).

A common denominator in most theories of leadership is the distinction between management, the oversight of (and sometimes day-to-day guidance through) ongoing organizational processes, and visionary or inspirational leadership that strategizes, focuses resources and ideas into achievable goals and incentives, and empowers the people and processes that lead to productive growth and change. Most good leaders attend to both tasks.

A compelling example of the importance of leadership style flows from efforts to move mental health professionals and services toward evidence-based practice (Aarons 2006). The transition in ways of knowing from subjective understanding to algorithmic pathways remains a difficult one for many psychiatrists (Donald 2001). Mental health clinicians' attitudes toward the adoption of evidence-based practice varies according to individual differences such as education and experience and organizational ones such as structure and policies (Aarons 2004, 2005; Young et al. 2006). Aarons (2006) studied the impact of transformational and transactional leadership styles on the acceptance of evidence-based practices by mental health clinicians in 49 programs providing mental health services to children and adolescents. These are well-characterized leadership styles that reflect the core distinctions central to most leadership paradigms: transformational leadership is visionary and inspirational (Howell and Frost 1989), whereas transactional leadership focuses on practical matters such as goal setting and rewards through performance review (Jung 2001). Aarons (2006) predicted that "transformational leadership would influence attitudes by inspiring acceptance of innovation through the development of enthusiasm, trust and openness, whereas transactional leadership would lead to acceptance of innovation through reinforcement and reward" (p. 1163). Indeed, both leadership styles were positively associated with the adoption of positive attitudes toward adopting evidence-based medicine. There is an important lesson here for the leadership of psychiatric hospitals as we struggle constantly to adapt our institutions (and the people who constitute them) to the technological, organizational, scientific, and professional changes that are guaranteed to dominate the psychiatric hospital industry throughout our lives. The most effective leaders for the future must embrace a broad set of qualities that range from effective frontline management, to strategic planning, to the capacity to envision and inspire.

The Challenges Ahead

The challenges faced by psychiatric hospital leadership over the past generation are only likely to intensify. The corporatization and commercialization of health care leaves entities such as psychiatric hospitals often seeming primarily like businesses delivering a commodity with professional components rather than vehicles for the primary purpose of delivering a social good through professional psychiatric services (Tischler and Astrachan 1996). Increasingly competitive and market driven, psychiatric hospital systems will be challenged to reduce cost without reducing quality (Rosenau and Linder 2003) and, conversely, to increase quality and safety without increasing cost. Efforts to reduce the use of restraint and seclusion is but one example of a hospital practice that raises vital safety and quality concerns with economic implications. Although intuition might suggest that managing extreme behavior without seclusion and restraint would increase staff costs, research findings suggest that the reduced use of restraint and seclusion yields the additional benefit of reduced cost (LeBel et al. 2005; Phillips et al. 1993), aligning the goals of quality, safety, and cost efficiency. Systems will be challenged to diversify and expand to meet market demands while simultaneously contracting and streamlining to remain efficient and competitive. They will have to stay several steps ahead of evolving information technologies and adapt to an ever-changing field of potential public and private partners, business relationships, and reimbursement methodologies. The one predictable constant will be the relentless pressure to do more with

less (Schreter 2004). They will have to accomplish all of this while evolving technologies of diagnosis (e.g., genetics and neuroimaging) and treatment (e.g., pharmacogenetics, vagal nerve stimulation, deep brain stimulation, transcranial magnetic stimulation) are reshaping our conceptions of illness and treatment. Indeed, the moral and ethical dilemmas that sit at the interface of market-driven forces, professional values, commitments to the sense of "mission," and evolving definitions of illness and treatment may be the quintessential challenge facing the leaders of psychiatric hospital systems in the early twenty-first century.

References

Aarons GA: Mental health providers attitudes toward adoption of evidence-based practice: the Evidence-Based Attitude Scale (EBPAS). Ment Health Serv Res 6:61–74, 2004

Aarons GA: Measuring provider attitudes toward evidence based practice: organizational context and individual differences. Child Adolesc Clin N Am 14:255–271, 2005

Aarons GA: Transformational and transactional leadership: association with attitudes toward evidence based practice. Psychiatr Serv 57:1162–1169, 2006

Appelbaum PS: The "quiet" crisis in mental health services: adequate reimbursement to providers of mental health services is the key to sustaining a viable care system. Commentary Sept/Oct:110–116, 2003

Centers for Medicare and Medicaid Services: Inpatient Psychiatric Facility PPS: Overview. Baltimore, MD, Centers for Medicare and Medicaid Services, 2006. Available at: http://www.cms.hhs.gov/InpatientPsychFacilPPS. Accessed March 2007.

Clouette B, Deslandes P: The Hartford Retreat for the Insane: an early example of the use of moral treatment in America. Conn Med 61:521–527, 1997

Davidson L, O'Connell M, Tondora J, et al: The top ten concerns about recovery encountered in mental health systems transformation. Psychiatr Serv 57:640–645, 2006

Deutsch A: The Mentally Ill in America. New York, Columbia University Press, 1949

Digby A: Madness, Morality and Medicine: A Study of the York Retreat, 1796–1914. New York, Cambridge University Press, 1985

Dixon L, Ridgely S, Goldman H: The evolving behavioral health system: the public sector, in Textbook of Administrative Psychiatry: New Concepts for a Changing Behavioral Health System, 2nd Edition. Edited by Talbott JA, Hales RE. Washington, DC, American Psychiatric Press, 2001, pp 17–26

Docherty J, Dewan N: Outcomes Assessment Monograph. Washington, DC, National Association of Psychiatric Health Systems, 1995

Donald A: The Wal-Marting of American psychiatry: an ethnography of psychiatric practice in the late 20th century. Cult Med Psychiatry 25:437–439, 2001

Dougherty CJ: Cost containment, DRGs and the ethics of health care: ethical perspective on prospective payment. Hastings Cent Rep 19:5–11, 1989

Dubrin AJ: Leadership: Research Findings, Practice and Skills. Boston, MA, Houghton Mifflin, 2001

Edershein E: The Definitive Drucker: Final Advice from the Father of Modern Management. New York, McGraw-Hill, 2006

Feldman S: Managed Mental Health Services. Springfield, IL, Charles C Thomas, 1992

Fitzpatrick JJ, Deller SS: Fundraising Skills for Healthcare Executives. New York, Springer, 2000

Forbush B: The Sheppard and Enoch Pratt Hospital, 1853–1970: A History. Philadelphia, PA, JB Lippincott, 1971

Geller JL: A history of private psychiatric hospitals in the USA: from start to almost finished. Psychiatr Q 77:1–40, 2006

Glick ID, Hargreaves WA: Psychiatric Hospital Treatment for the 1980s: A Controlled Study of Short Versus Long Hospitalization. Lexington, MA, Lexington Books, 1979

Glick ID, Klar HM, Braff DL: Guidelines for hospitalization of chronic psychiatric patients. Psychiatr Serv 35:934–936, 1984

Gollaher D: Voice for the Mad: The Life of Dorothea Dix. New York, Free Press, 1995

Goodheart LB: Mad Yankees: The Hartford Retreat for the Insane and Nineteenth Century Psychiatry. Amherst, MA, University of Massachusetts Press, 2003

Greiner CB: Leadership for psychiatrists. Acad Psychiatry 30:283–288, 2006

Harrison T, Gray AJ: Leadership, complexity and the mental health professional: a report on some approaches to leadership training. J Ment Health (UK) 12:153–159, 2003

Hester T: Extraorganizational relationships, in Handbook of Mental Health Administration and Management. Edited by Reid WH, Silver SB. New York, Brunner-Routledge, 2003, pp 240–260

Howell JM, Frost PJ: A laboratory study of charismatic leadership. Organ Behav Hum Decis Process 43:243–269, 1989

Institute of Living: 1992–1993 Annual Report. Hartford, CT, Institute of Living, 1993

Joint Commission: 2006–2007 Comprehensive Accreditation Manual for Behavioral Health Care (CAMBHC). Oakbrook Terrace, IL, The Joint Commission, 2007

Jung DI: Transformational and transactional leadership and their effects on creativity in groups. Creativity Research Journal 13:185–195, 2001

Kotter J: Leading Change. Cambridge, MA, Harvard Business School, 1996

LeBel J, Goldstein R: The economic cost of using restraint and the value added by restraint reduction or elimination. Psychiatr Serv 56:1109–1114, 2005

Levin BL, Hanson A, Kuppin SA: Leadership and training in mental health, in Handbook of Mental Health Administration and Management. Edited by Reid WH, Silver SB. New York, Brunner-Routledge, 2003, pp 22–40

McCue MJ, Clement JP: Relative performance of for-profit psychiatric hospitals in investor-owned systems and nonprofit psychiatric hospitals. Am J Psychiatry 150:77–82, 1993

Mechanic D, Schlesinger M, McAlpine DD: Management of mental health and substance abuse services: state of the art and early results. Milbank Q 73:19–55, 1995

New York–Presbyterian Hospital: History. New York, New-York–Presbyterian Hospital, 2007. Available at: http://www.nyp.org/about/history.html. Accessed April 2007.

Norhouse PG: Leadership: Theory and Practice. Thousand Oaks, CA, Sage, 1974

Ozarin L: From N.Y. Lunatic Asylum to New York Hospital's Westchester Division. Psychiatric News, July 21, 2006, p 29

Pelonero AL, Johnson RL: A pay-for-performance program for behavioral health practitioners. Psychiatr Serv 58:442–444, 2007

Phillips CD, Hawes C, Fries BE: Reducing the use of physical restraints in nursing homes: will it increase the costs? Am J Public Health 83:342–348, 1993

President's New Freedom Commission on Mental Health: Achieving the Promise: Transforming Mental Health Care in America. Final Report (DHHS Publ No SMA-03-3832). Rockville, MD, U.S. Department of Health and Human Services, 2003

Reid WH, Silver SB (eds): Handbook of Mental Health Administration and Management. New York, Brunner-Routledge, 2003

Rosenau PV, Linder SH: A comparison of the performance of for-profit and nonprofit US psychiatric inpatient care providers since 1980. Psychiatr Serv 54:183–187, 2003

Santiago JM: How selected behavioral health systems are changing: toward integrated systems: introduction to section v, in Textbook of Administrative Psychiatry: New Concepts for a Changing Behavioral Health System, 2nd Edition. Edited by Talbott JA, Hales RE. Washington, DC, American Psychiatric Press, 2001, pp 221–226

Schlesinger M, Dorwart R, Hoover C, et al: Competition, ownership and access to hospital services: evidence from psychiatric hospitals. Med Care 34:974–992, 1997

Schreter R: Ten trends in managed care and their impact on the biopsychosocial model. Hosp Community Psychiatry 44:325–327, 1993

Schreter R: Making do with less: the latest challenge for psychiatry. Psychiatr Serv 55:761–763, 2004

Schreter RK, Sharfstein SS, Schreter CA (eds): Managing Care, Not Dollars: The Continuum of Mental Health Services. Washington, DC, American Psychiatric Press, 1997

Sederer LJ, Dickey B (eds): Outcomes Assessment in Clinical Practice. Baltimore, MD, Williams & Wilkins, 1996

Senge PM: The Fifth Discipline: The Art and Practice of the Learning Organization. New York, Currency Doubleday, 1990

Sharfstein S: The role of private insurance in financing treatment for depression. Soc Psychiatry Psychiatr Epidemiol 30:236–239, 1995

Sharfstein S, Stoline A, Spizak C: Private psychiatric hospitals, in Textbook of Administrative Psychiatry: New Concepts for a Changing Behavioral Health System, 2nd Edition. Edited by Talbott JA, Hales RE. Washington, DC, American Psychiatric Press, 2001, pp 227–237

Shore MF, Vanelli M: Leadership, in Textbook of Administrative Psychiatry: New Concepts for a Changing Behavioral Health System, 2nd Edition. Edited by Talbott JA, Hales RE. Washington, DC, American Psychiatric Press, 2001, pp 43–51

Shortell SM, Gillies PR, Anderson DA: The new world of managed care: creating organized delivery systems. Health Aff (Millwood) 13:46–64, 1994

Silver SB: Financial analysis and management, in Handbook of Mental Health Administration and Management. Edited by Reid WH, Silver SB. New York, Brunner-Routledge, 2003a, pp 310–319

Silver SB: Payers and players, in Handbook of Mental Health Administration and Management. Edited by Reid WH, Silver SB. New York, Brunner-Routledge, 2003b, pp 324–335

Sudak H: A Remarkable Legacy: The Pennsylvania Hospital's Influence on the Field of Psychiatry. Philadelphia, University of Pennsylvania Health System, 2007. Available at: http://www.uphs.upenn.edu/paharc/features/psych.html. Accessed April 25, 2007.

Talbott JA, Hales RE (eds): Textbook of Administrative Psychiatry: New Concepts for a Changing Behavioral Health System, 2nd Edition. Washington, DC, American Psychiatric Press, 2001

Thal LJ, Kantarci K, Reiman EM, et al: The role of biomarkers in clinical trials for Alzheimer's Disease. Alzheimer Dis Assoc Disord 20:6–15, 2006

Tischler GL, Astrachan BM: A funny thing happened on the way to reform. Arch Gen Psychiatry 53:959–963, 1996

Trabin T: The Computerization of Behavioral Healthcare: How to Enhance Clinical Practice, Management and Communications. San Francisco, CA, Jossey-Bass, 1996

Veenhuis PE. Essential management functions, in Handbook of Mental Health Administration and Management. Edited by Reid WH, Silver SB. New York, Brunner-Routledge, 2003, pp 101–110

World Health Organization: Mental Health Information Systems. Geneva, Switzerland, World Health Organization, 2005. Available at: http://www.who.int/mental_health/policy/mnh_info_sys.pdf. Accessed April 2007.

Young GJ, Mohr DC, Meterko M, et al: Psychiatrists' self-reported adherence to evidence-based prescribing practices in the treatment of schizophrenia. Psychiatr Serv 57:130–132, 2006

Yu-Chin R: Teaching administration and management within psychiatric residency training. Acad Psychiatry 26:245–252, 2002

CHAPTER 27

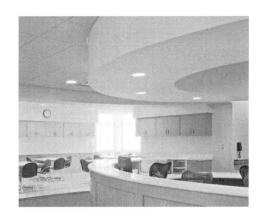

PSYCHIATRISTS AND PSYCHOLOGISTS

Robert P. Roca, M.D., M.P.H., M.B.A.
Barbara Roberts Magid, M.B.A.

In this chapter we discuss the patterns of practice and modes of compensation of psychiatrists and psychologists in current psychiatric hospital settings.

Patterns of Psychiatrist Practice

Hospitals use various employment and contractual options to ensure that their programs are staffed appropriately and that their patients are receiving the psychiatric services they require. The relationship between hospital and psychiatrist can range from an exclusive employment arrangement to a private attending model. In the latter model, the community-based private psychiatrist or psychologist admits and treats his or her own hospitalized patients. The psychiatrist may also provide contracted administrative services on a part-time basis to augment other sources of practice income.

The Community-Based Private Attending Psychiatrist

At one end of the continuum of hospital relationships with its professional staff is the community-based private attending psychiatrist (PAP) model. In this model, the community-based PAP has hospital privileges, admits and treats his or her own patients, and bills independently. Psychiatrists in this model may also participate in an on-call rotation for off-hours coverage. The advantage of this model is continuity of care; the psychiatrist with the greatest knowledge of the patient is providing care. The main disadvantage is that it is often inefficient both for the individual practitioner and for the hospital. The PAP must find a way to see the hospitalized patient daily and participate in multidisciplinary team meetings at which treatment is planned and reviewed; this is very difficult to fit into a busy day of outpatients or other clinical work and may produce conflict with hospital staff who are mandated to conduct the team meetings with all disciplines present. Furthermore, the community-based PAP may lack familiarity with hospital policies and procedures, documentation formats, managed care doctor-to-doctor review practices, and other activities that are particular to inpatient settings. Finally, in many environments all-inclusive managed care contracts preclude separate billing for professional services, rendering it financially impractical for independent community-based clinicians to provide hospital services.

For these reasons, it is increasingly common for hospital services to be provided by psychiatrists employed expressly for that purpose.

The Employed "Hospitalist" Psychiatrist

In general medicine, there is a growing trend toward the use of hospital-based physicians ("hospitalists") in the care of inpatients. There is evidence that the use of such physicians is associated with shorter lengths of stay, greater profitability (Wachter and Goldman 2002), and possibly better performance on measures of quality (Auerbach et al. 2002).

Although there has been very little study of the application of this practice model to inpatient psychiatric care, such care is increasingly being provided by employed hospital-based psychiatrists. A number of employment arrangements are possible. The psychiatrist may be employed by the hospital or by a closely associated or hospital-owned practice association on a full- or part-time basis. The contract with the psychiatrist may be exclusive, prohibiting practice outside the hospital contract, or it may permit or even encourage after-hours private practice or other professional activities. Hospitals may prefer an exclusive arrangement because it aligns the incentives of the hospital and the psychiatrist, ensuring that the clinician's professional effort is entirely devoted to meeting the needs of the hospital and its programs. However, this can be an expensive model because the hospital is forced to provide the entirety of the psychiatrist's income, which may be substantial in some geographical areas where psychiatrists have the option of lucrative outpatient practices treating a cash-paying clientele.

Roles of Psychiatrists and Psychologists

The Attending Psychiatrist as Clinician

The psychiatrist working with hospitalized patients takes a psychiatric history, performs a mental status examination, performs or reviews a general physical and neurological examination, and reviews the results of diagnostic tests. Ideally the psychiatrist also makes contact with other informants, including the family and the referring psychiatrist or other pertinent clinician, in order to obtain history, particularly the details of current or recent pharmacological treatment. At the end of this process, the psychiatrist makes a narrative formulation of the case and arrives at a working multiaxial diagnosis. Psychiatrists working with hospitalized patients provide treatment in teams that may include nurses, social workers, activities therapists (e.g., occupational, physical, and art therapists), mental health technicians, and utilization review specialists. These teams assemble soon after admission to identify—in collaboration with the patient—the reason(s) for admission, the objectives of the hospitalization, the means by which those objectives will be realized, the individuals responsible for those interventions, and the criteria by which it will be determined that discharge should occur. This discussion is documented in the "master treatment plan," the map that guides the therapeutic efforts of every member of the team. The team meets on a regular basis to share information and evaluate the effectiveness of the plan.

Generally the psychiatrist meets individually with the patient regularly to evaluate the patient's progress toward achieving the goals of treatment and serves as the attending clinician. Minimally, the psychiatrist assesses the extent to which the patient is benefiting from and tolerating pharmacological treatment. The attending psychiatrist may also obtain appropriate consultations from medical specialists and implement their recommendations. Routine visits usually include obtaining additional history, coordinating care, and providing advice and counsel. Sometimes formal psychotherapy is provided as well. More than one visit per day may be necessary if the patient is suicidal, aggressive, or otherwise in crisis.

Because many payers require concurrent review of the need for hospitalization, the psychiatrist may need to speak personally with a representative of the organization responsible for managing the patient's insurance benefit in order to make the case for continuing hospital care.

The Psychiatrist as Unit Medical Director

Most inpatient units have a designated medical director who receives an administrative stipend to provide essential administrative services for the unit and for the hospital. This is usually a part-time role played by an interested and capable inpatient attending psychiatrist. The unit medical director is generally expected to work closely with unit leadership (e.g., program director, nurse leader) and hospital entities (e.g., Medical Executive Committee, the Medical Staff Office) to develop practices and protocols (e.g., admissions criteria, clinical pathways) and serve on hospital committees requiring the participation of medical staff leaders (e.g., Medical Staff Credentialing Committee). It is also often the responsibility of the medical director to recruit, supervise, and evaluate the psychiatric medical staff, organize the on-call schedule, and help screen prospective admissions. In many settings the medical director also personally provides direct patient care.

Other Roles of the Psychiatrist in the Hospital Setting

Psychiatrists with hospital privileges have obligations not only to their individual patients but also to the hospital and their colleagues on the medical staff. These obligations and expectations may flow from regulations and standards set by such certifying and accrediting bodies as the Centers for Medicare and Medicaid Services and the Joint Commission (formerly the Joint Commission for Accreditation of Health Care Organizations). These responsibilities may also flow from the deliberations of the Medical Executive Committee, the governing body of the organized medical staff. These responsibilities are generally assembled into documents referred to as the "medical staff bylaws" and "departmental rules and regulations" and are distributed to new members of the medical staff at the time of orientation and available to all clinicians with privileges at the hospital.

At a minimum, medical staff members are expected to meet medical staff and hospital standards in terms of documentation requirements, on-call availability, collegiality, relationships with other hospital staff members, and other aspects of professional practice and conduct. In a world marked by increasing pressure to measure performance quantitatively, medical staff members are also expected to cooperate with efforts to measure aspects of their hospital-based practice (e.g., readmission rates, length of stay, satisfaction with services by patients and families) and to accept feedback about their performance on the measured dimensions.

In addition, medical staff members are expected to participate in a collaborative and constructive review of each other's work on a routine basis. Most often this involves reading and providing feedback about each other's medical record documentation. Occasionally peer review may be undertaken "for cause," such as when concerns have been raised about the practice of a particular clinician or when there is a need to review an adverse outcome. Depending on the provisions of the medical staff bylaws at the hospital, such review may be conducted by a specially selected senior clinician or by a committee appointed for this purpose.

Psychiatrists who are interested in playing an active role in the life of the hospital and/or the department of psychiatry may seek membership on medical staff (e.g., Pharmacy and Therapeutics, Credentialing) or hospital (e.g., Quality Improvement) committees. In some settings there is compensation for these activities, but in many hospitals such participation is considered part of the rights and responsibilities of medical staff "citizenship" and performed on a volunteer basis.

In psychiatric inpatient environments with an academic mission, psychiatrists may be involved in teaching medical students, psychiatric residents, and other trainees as well as conducting clinical research.

Roles of the Psychologist in the Hospital Setting

Psychologists who have hospital privileges may also serve on medical staff committees and participate in the governance of the hospital. Currently 37 states allow psychologists to serve on hospital medical staffs; however, this allowed status for psychologists is not implemented or utilized in many psychiatric hospital settings (Bailey 2006). When psychologists are credentialed to work in the inpatient setting, their roles are highly varied. The psychologist may serve in the role of attending clinician, although this is the exception rather than the rule. The psychologist may also perform psychotherapy with inpatients or may direct milieu-wide psychotherapeutic or behavioral programs on the inpatient unit. The psychologist may also evaluate inpatients with psychological tests to address specific clinical questions in response to a referral from the attending psychiatrist. In addition, psychologists may serve in managerial or administrative roles in the hospital organization (American Psychological Association Practice Directorate 1998). Like the psychiatrist who provides inpatient care, the psychologist is typically part of a treatment team and provides services in collaboration with other professionals, including nurses, social workers, and mental health technicians.

Models of Compensation for Employed Clinicians

Professionals employed by hospitals may be compensated by straight salary (e.g., $150,000 annually regardless of volume), per diem payments (e.g., $600 per day, regardless of volume), and/or productivity-based compensation systems (e.g., percentage-of-collections, fee schedule, or "relative value units"). Each of these models has advantages and disadvantages. In the decades between 1988 and 2008, Sheppard Pratt Health System, a freestanding not-for-profit mental health system, utilized and evaluated each of these approaches in an effort to accomplish three principal goals: 1) to change the mode of practice in response to a changing marketplace, 2) to align compensation with reimbursement, and 3) to recruit, retain, and motivate clinicians. What follows is a description of the Sheppard Pratt experience and the hybrid compensation system that emerged from it.

A Case Study: Professional Compensation at Sheppard Pratt

In 1988 Sheppard Pratt Hospital had 322 beds, an average length of stay of 180 days, and an average occupancy of more than 90%. The professional staff of psychiatrists, psychologists, and social workers were paid salaries that were significantly below market. Clinicians had private practices, and for a small "tax" paid to Sheppard Pratt, they could see their private patients in their hospital offices. There were no productivity requirements. Clinical assignments for all professionals were mostly on inpatient units, and the average caseload for psychiatrists and psychologists was between seven and nine inpatients. Clinicians had full benefits and vacation and sick leave accruals, and there were only limited expectations of providing weekend or evening services.

As the length of stay decreased with the advent of managed care, evolving changes in the nature of hospital work called upon staff to handle more admissions, meet with and evaluate patients daily, and discharge them more quickly. Weekend and vacation coverage became more demanding, and it became more difficult to attract psychiatrists to perform these functions. At the same time, the hospital census—once steady at 322—rose and fell, causing hospital revenues to fluctuate while professional staffing costs remained fixed. It became clear that the existing salaried arrangement was not providing psychiatrists and psychologists with incentives to adapt to the new mode of practice.

In this context, Sheppard Pratt's first volume- or productivity-based model of compensation—a system based on relative value units (RVUs)—was designed and adopted in 1991 (Schreter et al. 1997). The development of this system, which did not use the RVUs developed for the Medicare program, depended critically on the work of a committee that established an RVU for each clinical service provided in the hospital setting. RVU "targets" were set for every clinician, and annual compensation was based on the achievement of those targets. As the compensation system evolved, clinicians who exceeded 100% of contracted RVUs were eligible for additional compensation, which could be substantial.

The RVU system changed the corporate culture, increased productivity, and expanded the opportunity for clinicians to increase annual income by providing more services. Clinicians became engaged in discussing the merits of providing clinical care in a manner that was not only effective but efficient. Because the system directly rewarded the generation of billable services, it became easier to obtain coverage for clinicians on vacation and to staff new programs. The system was largely self-policing; if any clinician was below target in terms of generating a sufficient volume of RVUs, he or she usually made certain that the deficit was eliminated before the end of the contract year. Perhaps most importantly, the system demonstrated to the administration that it was possible to develop, implement, and manage a complex compensation system with the support and assistance of the clinical staff.

The RVU system also had weaknesses. Creating the system was very time-consuming and labor-intensive and diverted attention from other important activities. Some clinicians objected to having their professional services reduced to "widgets" and protested that the system negatively affected morale. However, the single greatest weakness of the RVU system was that the clinician was still to some extent insulated from the realities of the marketplace. By the mid-1990s—as reimbursement rates fell and the administrative hurdles required to receive payment became more unwieldy—levels of "bad debt" increased, and professional compensation was requiring unacceptable levels of subsidization from the rest of the health care system.

For this reason, a fundamental reexamination of the compensation system was undertaken in 1997. The result was a decision to adopt a system that would compensate clinicians on a percentage-of-collections basis, thereby putting clinicians much more closely in touch with the realities of the marketplace. The first hurdle to tackle in developing this system was to determine how to divide the collections, that is, what percentage to allocate for clinician compensation and what percentage to allocate for benefits and overhead. Because psychiatrists generated significantly more collections in a year than the other disciplines, the cost of their benefits and associated practice expenses represented a smaller percentage of their collections; therefore it was determined that psychiatrists would receive 65% of collections and psychologists would receive 50%. Several years later, the compensation paid to psychologists was increased to 65% so that all doctoral-level clinicians received the same compensation; this was in recognition of the time intensity of services delivered by psychologists and the more limited opportunities for psychologists to generate practice income.

A related challenge was creating a methodology for paying clinicians for the care of uninsured and indigent patients from whom no collections were expected. To address this issue, "floor payments"—Current Procedural Terminology (CPT) code–specific minimum compensation rates funded by Sheppard Pratt—were established for each service. These payments were set at levels that eliminated financial disincentives to the care of indigent patients while not creating an onerous subsidy burden on the organization.

It was also essential to deal with the time lag between the performance of the service and the receipt of collections. To address this time lag and the ups and downs of the collections process, Sheppard Pratt extended an interest-free advance, or "draw," to all employed psychiatrists and psychologists. The draw is a uniform sum paid 26 times each contract year without regard to actual monthly collections. The draw is a strong positive element because it means that paycheck amounts remain at a constant level even as collections ebb and flow during the contract term. A special challenge was developing a method for predicting the collections of individual clinicians over the course of a year so that the level of the draw could be adjusted accordingly. To accomplish this, administrators created productivity models based on the anticipated receipt of collections, taking into account the professional discipline, the clinical program and setting, the specific services delivered (e.g., distribution of CPT codes), anticipated service volume (e.g., patients per day), and the number of weeks the clinician expects to work during the contract year. By combining these variables, it was possible to arrive at an estimate of annual compensation.

Some clinicians, particularly those who are newly graduated from residency programs, are uncomfortable with pure productivity models. As a result, clinicians new to Sheppard Pratt have the option of a low guaranteed minimum salary with the opportunity to earn additional income in the event that 65% of the collections amount exceeds the minimum salary. This enables Sheppard Pratt to hire clinicians who are somewhat risk averse and still provide an incentive for high productivity.

Clinicians who teach residents or provide administrative services are paid stipends for these activities. These stipends are calculated on an hourly basis at rates that have been standardized to ensure that individuals performing the same administrative duties are being paid comparably. The duties, hours, and rates are specified in the employment contract, and the stipends are included in clinicians' biweekly paychecks over the course of the year.

The percentage-of-collections system has worked well in terms of keeping bad debt in check, increasing levels of productivity, and aligning the mode of practice with the demands of the market. A major positive consequence of the percentage-of-collections system has been greater clinician interest in billing and collections and in other aspects of financial oversight. Clinicians have come to understand the importance of the "charge ticket" (paper or electronic) as the direct accounting link between the clinical service and payment. Clinicians regularly review reports detailing such information as charges entered, collections in progress, accrued compensation, and productivity targets; they examine and analyze their reports and on a number of occasions have detected irregularities that led to the discovery of systematic errors that otherwise might have gone uncorrected.

The percentage-of-collections system has had its problematic aspects as well. Private practice had been prohibited for benefited employees with the advent of the percentage-of-collections system. Some long-tenured and highly respected psychiatrists and psychologists resigned because they were unwilling to give up highly remunerative and long-standing outpatient private practices. In the early years of the system, we lost some potential recruits who wanted the security of a salary without the pressure of productivity expectations. Some of those concerns of have been addressed with our salary option, although we do include a description of the volume of services needed to support the guaranteed salary in an addendum of the employment agreement.

Conclusion

The modern psychiatric hospital must continuously study the framework within which patient care services are provided in order to stay responsive to patients, families, and referrers. This chapter explores three critical questions with regard to the hospital's relationship with the psychiatrists and psychologists providing patient care services: 1) Should the hospital employ "psychiatric hospitalists," rely on private attending psychiatrists based in the community, or use a hybrid model? 2) What are the clinical and administrative roles of the psychiatrist and psychologist in the modern psychiatric hospital? and 3) Is it possible to develop systems of compensation that meet the needs of the clinicians, align the incentives of clinicians and the hospital, and fit within the budget? All three components are critical to the attainment of the hospital's goal of providing effective, responsive, and cost-efficient services. In an ever-changing marketplace, these three components must be evaluated as a unit and individually with the recognition that each component interacts with the others. Change must be carefully staged, with the active participation of key clinical and administrative staff. The goal is to create an environment in which patients receive safe and effective treatment and clinicians experience their work as appreciated and rewarding.

References

American Psychological Association Practice Directorate: Practicing Psychology in Hospitals and Other Health Care Facilities. Washington, DC, American Psychological Association, 1998

Auerbach AD, Qwachter RM, Katz P, et al: Implementation of a voluntary hospitalist service at a community teaching hospital: improved clinical efficiency and patient outcomes. Ann Intern Med 137:859–865, 2002

Bailey D: Psychologists' hospital privileges benefit patients. Monitor on Psychology, Vol 37, May 6, 2006. Available at: http://www.apa.org/monitor/may06/privileges.html. Accessed July 6, 2007.

Schreter RK, Sharfstein SS, Schreter CA (eds): Managing Care, Not Dollars: The Continuum of Mental Health Services. Washington, DC, American Psychiatric Press, 1997

Wachter RM, Goldman L: The hospitalist movement 5 years later. JAMA 287:487–494, 2002

CHAPTER 28

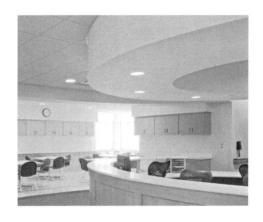

SOCIAL WORK AND REHABILITATION THERAPIES

Diana L. Ramsay, M.P.P., O.T.R., F.A.O.T.A.
Judith S. Gonyea, O.T.D., M.S.Ed., O.T.R./L.
Marlene I. Shapiro, M.S.W., L.C.S.W.–C.

Rehabilitation specialists and social workers play key roles in the therapeutic process within the acute care environment. Roles vary from site to site to reflect the needs of the region or community. Funding structures can affect the breadth and mix of services. Restructuring and cost-saving initiatives sometimes affect the roles of social work and rehabilitation.

One of the significant changes in hospital care has been a drastic decline in a patient's length of stay. Between 1990 and 2000, the total number of inpatient days fell by approximately one-half. Median length of stay declined 63% over the decade from 12.2 days to 4.5 days for most diagnostic categories and across types of patients and hospital settings (Case 2007). Admission, evaluation, intervention, and discharge phases of a stay are now compacted into a much briefer time frame. Stringent limits on the length of inpatient stays result in a critical need for step-down and community-based services. When individuals are not ready to step down to outpatient care, partial hospitals and crisis bed facilities may provide the bridge to community-based services.

Federal, state, and regional regulatory guidelines further influence service standards and delivery, as do professional credentialing requirements for clinicians within each jurisdiction. Worker shortages can have an impact on the availability of various types of professionals. Agencies may employ clinicians from several disciplines or may contract for specific services. Contractual providers may be available on a routine or as-needed basis, which may affect availability and roles within the team structure (Joint Commission Resources 2006). Sometimes these services are performed on a contractual basis; in other instances they are not part of the treatment package.

The acute care team typically includes psychiatrists, nurses, social workers, psychologists, various rehabilitative therapists (occupational, recreation, and psychiatric technicians), and, perhaps, a discharge coordinator. In these inpatient settings, tasks may be shared. Hence, it is important to differentiate which individual or discipline will take the lead for each respective task or process. As noted by Rosen and Callaly (2005, p. 239), "effective interdisciplinary teamwork in mental health services involves both retaining differentiated disciplinary roles and developing shared core tasks." There must be effective leadership and explicit mechanisms in place to resolve role conflicts and ensure safe practices. The team learns to operate quickly and efficiently. In order to continue providing services and oversight, team members rely increasingly on systems and agencies outside of the hospital, such as individual practitioners, outpatient community mental health centers, child or adult protective services, the forensic system, residential programs, psychiatric rehabilitation programs, assisted-living settings, peer support groups, and advocacy groups. In the wake of deinstitutionalization, "hospitals are recognizing that interdisciplinary [teamwork]…is an essential element of both effective patient care and organizational survival. The interdisciplinary team model, long cherished in psychiatry, remains the most efficacious model for carrying out the necessary tasks in acute psychiatric settings" (Rosen and Callaly (2005, p. 238); these tasks include admission, diagnosis, treatment planning, treatment, and, finally, discharge planning. Although team structures may vary, effective communication and understanding of roles are vital to efficient team process. Professionals within the acute care setting must also facilitate better links with the community in order to develop more integrated mental health services.

This chapter provides a general overview of the roles of social workers and the rehabilitation team within the acute care treatment setting.

Admission and Diagnostic Process

The first person a patient meets in the hospital may not be a psychiatrist but instead may be an intake coordinator, a nurse, a social worker, or a psychiatric technician. Figure 28–1 provides an overview of the acute care process from this point. In many acute care settings, individuals are evaluated upon admission by a cohort of professionals trained in various disciplines. The evaluation process often begins with structured diagnostic interviews and/or evaluations in which the patient, his or her family, and/or other community supports participate. Details of the patient's history,

community and family involvement, and current functional status are explored with a focus on the individual's current needs and desired outcomes. Psychiatric, nursing, psychological, social work, rehabilitation, and any other individualized assessments the team deems necessary will typically follow. These may include the following assessments: forensic, cognitive skills, motor skills, and/or a more intensive family evaluation.

Assessments may occur in one-to-one or group settings, depending on the hospital's admission protocol. They must be completed in a limited time frame and therefore require completion by staff members whose presence is guaranteed on a routine basis. Specialized assessments may be ordered by referral and may include (depending on the individual's presenting problems, insurance authorization, and/or the availability of services) psychological testing, a family consultation by the social worker, a neuropsychiatric exam, specialized occupational therapy testing, a substance abuse evaluation, and a forensic consultation. The goal of these assessments is to obtain a more detailed view of the individual's goals and specific strengths and challenges and to provide extra guidance and information for treatment planning.

After the information gathering is complete, the team collaborates with the patient to produce a workable, meaningful, and relevant treatment and discharge plan. Coordinated interdisciplinary discharge planning results in improved continuity of care, better functional status, decreased length of stay, less duplication of services, and improved education (Hansen et al. 1998).

When a patient is represented by a legal guardian, foster family, advocate, or others, it is necessary to confirm legal authorization in order to share with and receive information from those who speak on behalf of the patient. The Health Insurance Portability and Accountability Act of 1996 (U.S. Department of Health and Human Services 2003) provides specific guidelines and restrictions regarding protected health information that must be considered during any health care interaction. This can create a complex scenario for individuals who have been in multiple placements or who may be accompanied by someone other than their primary guardian at admission.

The Therapeutic Relationship

The therapeutic relationship remains the key element in acute care assessment, treatment, and outcome. Although inpatient stays are shorter than they were in

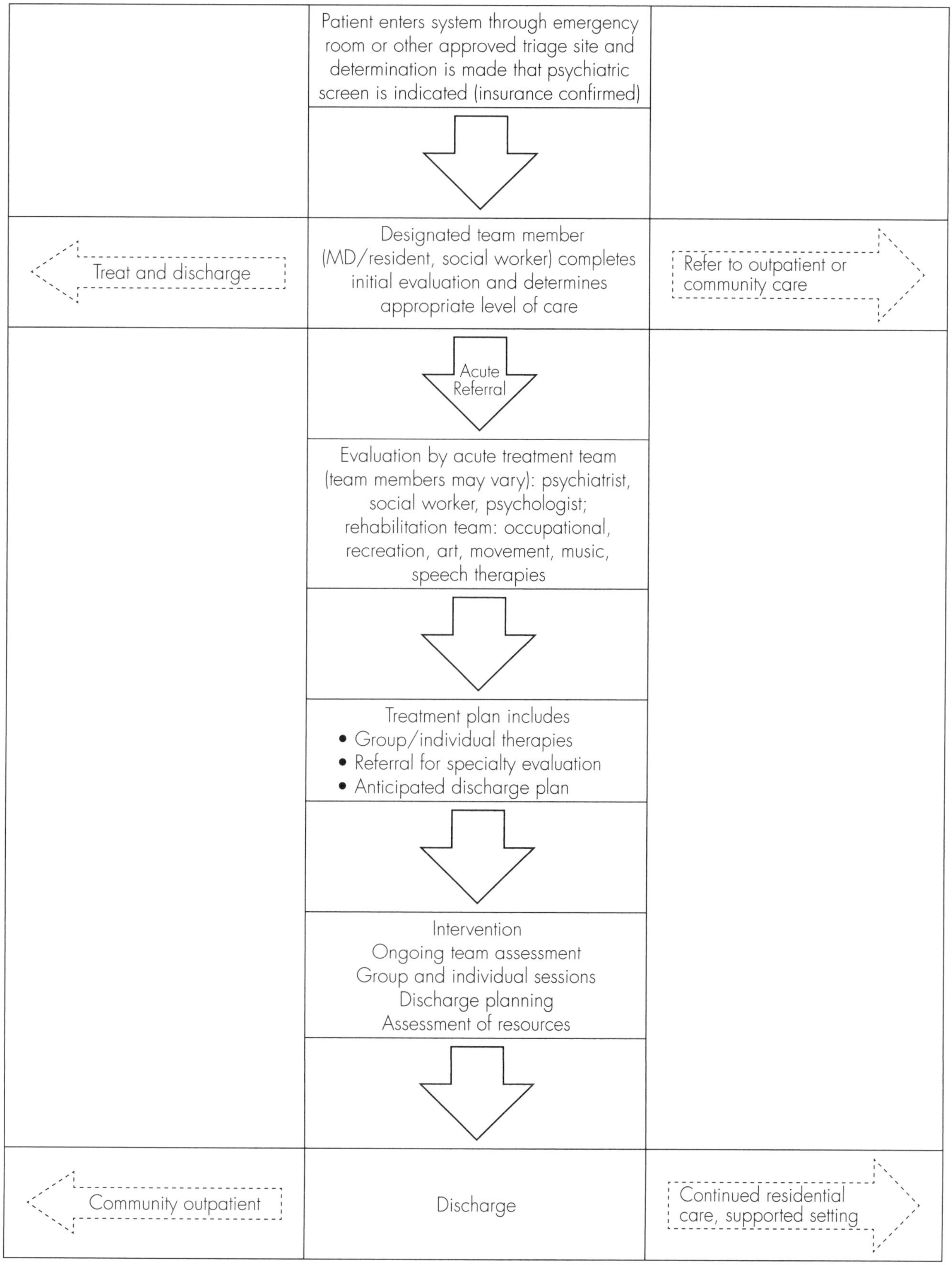

	Patient enters system through emergency room or other approved triage site and determination is made that psychiatric screen is indicated (insurance confirmed)	
⟵ Treat and discharge	Designated team member (MD/resident, social worker) completes initial evaluation and determines appropriate level of care	Refer to outpatient or community care ⟶
	Acute Referral	
	Evaluation by acute treatment team (team members may vary): psychiatrist, social worker, psychologist; rehabilitation team: occupational, recreation, art, movement, music, speech therapies	
	Treatment plan includes • Group/individual therapies • Referral for specialty evaluation • Anticipated discharge plan	
	Intervention Ongoing team assessment Group and individual sessions Discharge planning Assessment of resources	
⟵ Community outpatient	Discharge	Continued residential care, supported setting ⟶

FIGURE 28–1. Acute care system.

the past, the results of recently developed, briefer forms of therapies indicate that a significant and workable therapeutic relationship can be established within a short period of time. Team members typically become well versed in developing rapport with the patient. In addition, the patient on a unit is exposed to many professionals trained in various disciplines, and he or she has the opportunity to interact with more than one team member (Safran and Muran 1998).

Social Workers

Social workers have academic degrees (bachelor's degree or bachelor of social work; master's degree or master of social work) and are licensed at various levels. There are also social workers with doctoral degrees. Licensure and its requirements vary from state to state. The National Association of Social Workers (NASW) is the organization that establishes the ethics and practice guidelines for social workers. The Council of Social Work Education regulates social work education. Schools of social work must be accredited in order for their graduates to be licensed and call themselves social workers. Each state has a board that, along with national organizations, decides the parameters of social work practice. Social workers are required to maintain their qualifications for licensure with continuing education and/or postgraduate work (Hoon et al. 1978).

Social workers play a central role in the mental health system (Aviram 2002). They work in myriad public and private agencies, general hospitals, day hospitals, outpatient clinics, mobile treatment teams, shelters, and emergency departments. Some social workers function as part of an interdisciplinary team, whereas others may lead the team or direct a program; many work in private practice. In many states, depending on the level of licensure, social workers can conduct independent practices in which they diagnose as well as treat patients with mental illness. Their duties may include but are not limited to admission, evaluation and diagnosis, treatment planning, direct treatment, psychoeducation, family work, advocacy work, case management, and discharge planning. According to the NASW Standards for Social Work Practice in Health Care Settings (National Association of Social Workers 2005), "The basic values of social work, from promoting an individual's right to self-determination to having an attitude of empathy for the individual, are the foundation of social work practice. When confronting dilemmas or needs in health

care, social workers can use the principle of client self-determination in matters where clients or their proxies are faced with such issues" (National Association of Social Workers 2005, p. 8).

According to the NASW Standards for Social Work Practice in Health Care Settings National Association of Social Workers 2005), "professional social workers are well-equipped to practice in the health care field because of their broad perspective on the range of physical, emotional, and environmental factors that have an effect on the well-being of individuals and communities" (p. 6). The focus of social work is the transaction between the individual and his or her environment. Typically, if asked how to begin a patient assessment and plan for discharge, the social worker will probably respond, "I start from where the person is." The social worker assesses the interaction between the individual and the environmental systems that may affect the person's treatment. Some of these systems include the family; educational, outpatient, vocational, and cultural support; church or spiritual support; and social services systems. "Social workers have special skills in cultural awareness; it is a core value of the profession to respectfully respond to and affirm the worth and dignity of people of all cultures, languages, classes, ethnic backgrounds, abilities, religions, sexual orientations, and other diverse features found among humans" (National Association of Social Workers 2005, p. 6). In the hospital setting, the goals of the social worker are to assess the relevant systems, modify a system if needed (and if the individual and the system are able to do so) in order to optimize the individual's chances of success after discharge, and provide liaison between the inpatient setting and the outside systems.

In the era of short hospital stays, social workers and other members of the treatment team are accustomed to functioning with efficiency and precision in a short-term setting and to using the psychosocial assessment in a focused manner to formulate effective interventions. The emphasis has shifted to planning for an individual's transition to home or another level of care.

Social workers engage with the patient's family, however that may be defined, and are involved in all steps of the inpatient process: orienting the family to the hospital, providing psychoeducation for the family and the patient, and informing them of every step in the treatment. They provide individual, group, and family therapy and, with the treatment team, assist in formulating the discharge plan. Social workers often act as advocates in managing the hospital and community systems the patient may encounter. "Their role is to give information and to give hope" (R. Guth, personal communication, February 8, 2007).

No matter what the setting, social work has proven to be very flexible in fitting into the current framework of acute psychiatric care. Values of the social work profession such as negotiation, flexibility, and the right to exercise autonomy are useful on the interdisciplinary treatment team (Globerman 1995).

The psychosocial evaluation (PSE) is the basic operating document of the social worker. It is usually completed within 24 to 72 hours of admission. Given the fast pace of the setting, the social worker must be able to quickly establish a therapeutic relationship with the patient and, often, the family. "Social workers look at all of the influences and aspects of a person's life to complete a thorough assessment and treatment plan with the client, the family, and other health care professionals" (National Association of Social Workers 2005, p. 19).

The PSE is almost always conducted in an individual interview. It usually reflects the guiding philosophy of many social workers: "to start with where the person is." The PSE is a comprehensive document covering the following facts: basic demographic information; contact persons; plan for family involvement; information about the outpatient treatment team; notification contacts in case of seclusion or restraint; financial information; queries concerning advance directives, guardianships, or powers of attorney; history of harm to self or others; legal information; pertinent spiritual and cultural factors; and living arrangements. The PSE is also used to assess reasons for referral, prior psychiatric history, medication history, relevant stressors, substance abuse history, family composition and history, growth and developmental history (including trauma, medical problems, and abuse history), management of daily activity and interpersonal relationships (or other support networks), and education and employment history.

The last part of the assessment typically includes a clinical evaluation of a patient's strengths and challenges, suggestions regarding how the social system can be strengthened or modified to improve biopsychosocial functioning, participation by family and significant others, and social work treatment goals in discharge planning for the individual. The social work perspective draws from the strengths and abilities of the patient: "[A]wareness and use of the client's strengths form part of the foundation of social work theory and practice.... The strengths perspective helps patients use their past successful choices and behav-

iors, skills, and insights to resolve...a current crisis" (National Association of Social Workers 2005, p. 10).

Occupational and Rehabilitation Therapists

Credentialing and licensure for each rehabilitative discipline vary among states. For instance, occupational therapists enter the field at the master's or doctoral level. Occupational therapy assistants enter the field at the associate degree level. Supervised fieldwork is required at each level, and evidence of specialized education or training is required for some areas of practice. Licensure requirements vary across states, but most states do require successful initial certification by the National Board for Certification in Occupational Therapy (2003; see http://www.nbcot.org/web articles/anmviewer.asp?a=110&z=17).

Occupational and rehabilitative therapists work in tandem with other treatment team members to develop a profile of the patient's needs. Team members from each discipline incorporate their specialized view of the patient's needs, both within the acute care environment and upon discharge or transition to another treatment setting.

Occupational therapy practice guidelines ensure that "practitioners provide services to improve the ability of the individual or population to fulfill role obligations, to improve performance in occupations and activities, and resolve or compensate for impairments" (Moyers and Dale 2007, p. 15). The Occupational Therapy Practice Framework outlines the criteria for development of an Occupational Profile (American Occupational Therapy Association 2002). This profile may be developed using a variety of assessment instruments, both formal and informal. It is designed to identify individuals' unique characteristics, including how they perceive themselves, why they are in need of or are seeking services, the context from which they have come and/or to which they plan to return, their perceived roles and routines, their supports and liabilities, and, most importantly, what occupations or life skills are most significant to them (Cara and MacRae 2005).

The occupational profile will drive the course of occupational therapy treatment and may indicate areas where further evaluation is needed. Additional evaluation may address safety in areas of general mobility, personal care and care of others, cognitive processing ability (especially as it relates to performance skills), and sensory processing in relation to the individual's personal and environmental demands (Cara and MacRae 2005; Ikiugu 2007).

For occupational or other rehabilitative therapies, cognitive and motivational strategies may be critical in short-term treatment scenarios, especially those in which substance use is a relevant patient factor. A review of approaches by Stoffel and Moyers (2004) indicated that motivational interviewing as part of a brief intervention may encourage patients toward change. Their review revealed that it is not enough that an individual be motivated to begin treatment; his or her motivation must also be sustained and reenergized throughout the course of treatment.

Participation is another concept that is critical to both the occupational therapist's view of the patient and his or her assessment of the patient's needs. Simply knowing that an individual engages in or disengages from a particular behavior or task tells us nothing about that individual's strengths and needs. The therapist must also consider the context of the individual in his or her community, the roles he or she is expected to fulfill, and whether those roles are congruent with the individual's own perceived strengths and needs. As noted by Christiansen and Townsend (2004, p. 198), "it is not sufficient to understand that a person or a community is doing something. Rather, it is the exploration of what they are doing, why they are doing it, and what it brings to their lives individually or collectively that adds to our understanding of human behavior. A distinction needs to be made between occupations that [individuals or groups] *want* to do versus those that they *need* to do." For example, an individual who has engaged in high-risk behaviors for an extended period of time, such as substance abuse or sexual promiscuity, may have a difficult time replacing those behaviors with the safer behaviors that are deemed desirable by the treatment team or significant others. However, those high-risk behaviors may directly relate to that individual's sense of community and identified roles. Part of the occupational therapist's role may be to help refocus the patient's strengths or find community resources such as peer support groups that can enable the individual to feel motivated toward and supported in making behavioral alterations. To facilitate the desired occupational changes, the occupational therapist may need to work with the discharge planner to select the most supportive environment and services.

Occupational therapy places great emphasis on understanding a patient's habits and routines, which reflect the patterns of an individual's life. In some cases, these habits or routines may be reflective of an unhealthy lifestyle or physical or emotional challenges. Successful hospital discharge or life planning must take into account the individual's ability to sustain habits and routines that promote wellness while at the same time diminishing habits and routines that interfere with successful transition (Christiansen and Townsend 2004).

Occupational therapists have long been aware that underlying sensory, motor, and processing deficits may contribute to an individual's challenges. These challenges may include unusual ways in which the individual sees, feels, smells, hears, interprets, or interacts with his or her environment. Sensory integration was identified as a primary developmental concern in the field of occupational therapy in the 1960s. Later, King's (1974) work on the sensory-motor challenges faced by individuals with nonparanoid schizophrenia further exemplified the significant link between sensory-motor processing and functional participation. Although research continues in this area, some hospitals are already implementing sensory strategies or using sensory rooms (calming or exciting) within the milieu design. Champagne (2006) has warned that such strategies must be collaborative and well-thought-out and -designed in order for them to provide an effective alternative to other management approaches, specifically seclusion and restraint.

For example, an adolescent admitted to an acute care unit for stabilization following repeated high-risk behaviors may have a history that suggests poor environmental or sensory awareness. In this case, the adolescent could be referred to an occupational therapist for a sensory-integration or sensory-processing evaluation (Ikiugu 2007). The occupational therapist will select an evaluative approach that is consistent with the age and context of the client. Such an approach could include completion of an Adolescent/Adult Sensory Profile (Brown and Dunn 2002), clinical observation, chart review, or a variety of other sensory-referenced evaluations and interviews. Results of these focused assessments would typically indicate how well the individual is processing sensory information, whether the individual is seeking more or less sensory information than do typical individuals, and what effect the individual's sensory processing is having on his or her ability to interact with the environment and other people. Upon completion of the evaluation, the occupational therapist, in conjunction with the individual and treatment team, would establish sensory strategies that could be employed during and possibly after hospitalization.

In the case of a withdrawn suicidal patient, a referral to an art, music, or other expressive therapist may provide the best opportunity for insight into underlying issues or conflicts if the hospital stay is long enough for this type of assessment. In art therapy, the diagnostic workup usually includes a series of drawings that are foundational to the evaluation. They provide a view of the individual's sensory, spatial, and fine-motor processing; affect and emotion; sense of control; symbolic references; and other global areas of insight. Drawings completed in group also lend themselves to interpretation of the individual's responses to others and the group as a whole. In the case of forensic patients, the use of symbolism (cult, gang) or themes (death, hopelessness, violence) may provide further evidence of risky affiliations or aspirations (P. Prugh, personal communication, February 13, 2007).

Recreation therapy provides the patient with a focused opportunity to engage in and/or explore recreational pursuits within the milieu and for future needs. Recreational therapy interventions include structured activity focused on symptom reduction; education on social skills, stress management, and health maintenance; community functioning and integration activities; adventure/challenge activities; and family interventions (American Therapeutic Recreation Association 2004).

The Consumer Connection

Mental health consumers have found a voice within and outside the acute care environment. Consumer advocates help other consumers, and in this way, patients find a voice for their needs and concerns. They may also enable staff to see the patient's perspective more clearly through their ability to build trust with a client who may be intimidated by the system and its rules and restrictions. Advocates also provide a concrete link to community resources. It is important for clinicians working in these fast-paced short-term settings to appreciate the long-term challenges faced by the patient. Clinical partnerships with consumer advocates can lead to positive transitional plans across levels of care.

Models of care are becoming more patient/client-centered, and many treatment settings employ new approaches toward development of the individual's wellness plan. One model being applied in many settings is the Recovery Model (National Alliance on Mental Illness 1996), which places the individual in a position of control, focusing on the patient's need to understand and manage his or her own mental health care. Another approach is the Wellness Recovery Action Plan (WRAP), which can be introduced to patients as part of their overall treatment plan development. This approach was developed by Mary Ellen Copeland in response to her own challenges within the mental health system (Copeland Center for Wellness and Recovery 1995–2007; see http://www.copelandcenter.com/whatiswrap.html).

The Master Treatment Plan

The master treatment plan (MTP) is developed by the team on the acute care unit and becomes the guiding document for treatment during an individual's stay. The team leader for the development of the plan may be a psychiatrist or other psychiatric health professional. It is essential to have as much information as possible from all disciplines prior to creating the MTP. All team members have access to every evaluation completed, and this collection of data is used by the team, with the patient's consent and input, to develop treatment and discharge plans. An MTP typically consists of the following information: a diagnosis on Axis I through V, a list of current symptoms, a list of relevant problems, current prescribed medications, patient strengths and challenges, a plan for treatment with proposed interventions by staff, a measure to quantify patient improvement, and an initial discharge plan. After the MTP is completed, and depending on the custom of the hospital unit, the patient meets with the entire team or the case manager to review the MTP. Members of the team and the patient or patient advocate sign the document to affirm the treatment plan.

Therapies (or Who Does What)

Many types of therapies, both group and individual, in a variety of modalities are offered on an acute care unit. These may include occupational, activity, recreational, art, music, and other expressive therapies, depending on the patient's length of stay and the resources available. In some hospitals, one might find psychoeducational groups for patients and/or families. Less commonly, one might find support groups run by peers from advocacy organizations based in the local community. The leadership of various therapeutic activities depends on the hospital unit's organization, its theoretical preferences, its budget, and the availability of professionals within the hospital setting. Thus, one might find psychiatrists, social workers, occupational therapists, and others conducting similar groups across different hospital settings.

Milieu Management

Milieu management refers to the regulation of physical behaviors and personal interactions within the treatment environment. No matter what theoretical methodology is followed, the success of all teams depends on clear and effective communication among disciplines (Abramson and Mizrahi 1996). On a well-organized hospital unit where there is effective communication, the treatment team meets on a regular basis to discuss the practical elements of operating the unit, the unit organization, and any changes occurring on the unit (among the staff or in the institution) that might have an impact its operation. Problems in the milieu can affect the individual's experience and response to treatment and the staff's satisfaction with their work on the unit. The focus of clear communication should be on open and frank discussion, problem solving, and conflict management among the staff members and with individual patients and their families (Hansen et al. 1998).

All professionals should be trained to assist in the management of behavior on an acute care unit using nonconfrontational and least restrictive methods of control. Treatment team members may recommend modifications of the physical environment to reduce the incidence of aggressive or self-injurious behavior. Strategies may enable the patient to calm or control his or her response to "triggers," such as specific sights or sounds within the environment (Ikiugu 2007). However, some patients may not respond to typical calming or cognitive strategies. A history of trauma or neuropsychiatric problems may create a hypersensitivity that predisposes the patient to respond with extreme behavior. The patient may display aggression, withdrawal, hypersexuality, and other responses, which may be intended to be self-protective. Helping the patient to identify the personal triggers for these responses and/or the feelings associated with these triggers may enable him or her to develop strategies to preempt these extreme responses. The treatment team can then work together with the patient toward the development of more effective strategies, which can also continue to be used after discharge.

Discharge Planning and Length of Stay

At the time of discharge, individuals will have a detailed discharge plan, written in easily understood lay-person's language, that should include the following elements: a diagnosis; a clearly written list of medications; follow-up appointments for psychiatric care and/or other medical appointments; plans for housing, rehabilitation, and socialization; a number to call in an emergency; and any other referrals or recommendations related to continued care. The major goal of the plan is that the patient achieves the highest quality of life possible in the least restrictive environment (Tuzman and Cohen 1992).

Because a patient's length of stay is typically very short, discharge planning on an acute care unit must begin at the time of admission. At the same time, discharge planning has to be a fluid process due to the ongoing collection of evaluations, observations, and other data. The extent and type of family and other support of the patient are major considerations. A study on clinical decision making for discharge planning revealed that "the art of good discharge planning also involves the need to engage the patient, family, and care systems within briefer time frames" (Tuzman and Cohen 1992, p. 300).

Length of hospital stay is a significant consideration in both treatment and discharge planning. The length of stay is determined not only by insurance constraints but also by other factors, including the complexity of the patient's presenting problems, the preferences of the team and patient, and the availability of resources within the community for postdischarge care. It is important to note that evidence has shown that the presence of significant psychosocial problems is predictive of a longer length of stay (Keefler et al. 2001; Lechman and Duder 2006) and that this should be a significant consideration when planning a course of treatment for a particular patient (Keefler et al. 2001).

The entire treatment team is responsible for the development of the discharge plan. Table 28–1 lists the many considerations and preparation needed for each potential discharge setting. Because average hospital stays are so short, the team has to consider that the majority of an individual's treatment will occur after discharge from the acute setting. Thus, knowledge of resources is vital to discharge planning. It is critical that the team have a collective awareness of the benefits and risks of individual placement options and strive to create the best match for each person. Therefore, even though the entire team contributes, members representing specific disciplines may provide more precise input: the social worker may be instrumental in providing information about public entitlements such as Social Security, disability, or medical

TABLE 28–1. Discharge settings/services and considerations

Setting	Considerations	Preparation
Home	• Will individual need continuing care, and if so, what type? • What community resources exist in location where this individual will be discharged? • What personal resources are available to this individual (e.g., family or friends)?	• Check insurance coverage. • Check availability of funded services. • Check transportation options if needed. • Check individual's safety potential for home and community environments.
Outpatient/ day hospital	• Does this individual have the ability to follow up or have others who can remind him/her to do so? • Does the outpatient program provide an appropriate level of care for this individual? • Is the context/setting of outpatient program appropriate (e.g., age, community, culture)?	• Check insurance coverage. • Check transportation options if needed. • Check individual's safety potential for home and community environments.
Psychiatric residential treatment center	• Does the individual's diagnosis or current status require this level of care according to guidelines? • Are there beds available for this type of individual (e.g., age cohort, treatment needs)? • Can the anticipated plan of care be carried out in this setting?	• Check insurance coverage. • If individual is a child or adolescent, check educational program needs and availability.
Group home	• Does the individual possess the skills necessary for this type of setting (e.g., social, personal management)? • Are there beds available for this type of individual (e.g., age cohort, treatment needs)? • Can the anticipated plan of care be carried out in this setting?	• Check insurance coverage • Check individual's safety potential for home and community environments. • Check potential restrictions based on background, gender, etc. • Check vocational or work expectations and assess skills accordingly.
Supportive living	• Does the individual possess the skills (e.g., social, personal management, domestic) necessary for this type of setting? • Are there beds available for this type of individual (e.g., age cohort, treatment needs)? • Can the anticipated plan of care be carried out in this setting?	• Check insurance coverage. • Check individual's safety potential for home and community environments. • Check potential restrictions based on background, gender, etc. • Check vocational or work expectations and assess skills accordingly. • Check community resources (e.g., advocacy, peer support, transportation).

assistance; the occupational therapist may address safety skills; and the recreation therapist may find leisure resources within the community to promote a patient's engagement in the community.

Conclusion

Positive outcomes should be achievable for the individual in an acute care setting if, in addition to effective treatment, health care professionals focus on preventing conflict and aggression, positively affecting the patient's potential to improve performance in occupations and activities, and successfully transitioning the patient to placement in the community.

There are major differences in the roles and composition of social work and rehabilitation professionals across acute care settings. Careful consideration must be given to each profession's philosophical framework and approaches. In an environment where there are scarce resources as well as brief acute care stays, the need to achieve the best outcomes calls on leaders to identify the most effective staffing composition and role delineation for social workers, rehabilitation staff, and other health care professionals. Staff composition and role delineation should be determined by an assessment of the approaches offered by the respective professions in order to optimize accomplishment of the desired objectives.

In the course of treatment, staff members help patients cope, build strengths, and face life's challenges. In most acute care settings, the social worker plays a clearly defined and primary role in helping the patient, family, or primary support group. Occupational therapy, recreational therapy, and the expressive therapies also perform key roles and bring unique expertise to the treatment process. Acute care staff must be willing to share decision-making authority and information with families, guardians, and other community supports so that they all have a primary role in the care of the individual.

During the admission, evaluation, and treatment planning processes, staff form links with providers and resources to the communities to which the patient plans to return. The social worker plays a primary role in this linkage. The occupational therapist provides the individual, family, and team additional information about the qualities of the community environment. This professional also offers the supports necessary to improve the potential of the patient to fulfill role obligations, to improve performance in occupations and activities, and to resolve or compensate

for challenges. From the point of admission to the point of discharge, the entire team's focus is on the most functional, least restrictive outcome for patients and their significant others.

References

Abramson JS, Mizrahi T: When social workers and physicians collaborate: positive and negative interdisciplinary experiences. Soc Work 41:270–281, 1996

American Occupational Therapy Association: Occupational Therapy Practice Framework: Domain and Process. Bethesda, MD, AOTA Press, 2002

American Therapeutic Recreation Association: Summary of Health Outcomes in Recreation Therapy, 2004. Available at: http://www.atra-tr.org/benefitshealthoutcomes.htm. Accessed April 30, 2007.

Aviram U: The changing role of the social worker in the mental health system. Soc Work Health Care 35:615–632, 2002

Brown C, Dunn W: The Adolescent/Adult Sensory Profile Manual. San Antonio, TX, Psychological Corporation, 2002

Cara E, MacRae A: Psychosocial Occupational Therapy: A Clinical Practice, 2nd Edition. Clifton Park, NY, Delmar, 2005

Case BG, Olfson M, Marcus SC, et al: Trends in the inpatient mental health treatment of children and adolescents in US community hospitals between 1990 and 2000. Arch Gen Psychiatry 64:89–96, 2007

Champagne C: Creating sensory rooms: environmental enhancements for acute inpatient mental health settings. American Occupational Therapy Association: Mental Health Special Interest Section Quarterly 29:1–4, 2006

Christiansen CH, Townsend EA (eds): Introduction to Occupation: The Art and Science of Living. Upper Saddle River, NJ, Prentice Hall, 2004

Copeland Center for Wellness and Recovery: What is WRAP? Copyright 1995–2007, Mary Ellen Copeland, Ph.D. Available at: http://www.copelandcenter.com/whatiswrap.html. Accessed April 30, 2007.

Globerman J, Bogo M: Social work and the new integrative hospital. Soc Work Health Care 21:1–21; discussion 23–27, 1995

Hansen HE, Bull MJ, Gross CR: Interdisciplinary collaboration and discharge planning communication for elders. J Nurs Adm 28:37–46,1998

Hoon RA, Benedetti D, Cheng L, et al: Who does what? Role definition in a psychiatric hospital. Med J Aust 2:526–531, 1978

Ikiugu MN: Psychosocial Conceptual Practical Models in Occupational Therapy: Building Adaptive Capability. St. Louis, MO, CV Mosby, 2007

Joint Commission Resources: Comprehensive Accreditation Manual for Hospitals: The Official Handbook: CAMH Refreshed Core: Management of Human Resources: Standards, Rationales, Elements of Performance and Scoring, 2006. Oakbrook Terrace, IL, Joint Commission Resources, 2006, pp HR–3

Keefler J, Duder S, Lechman C: Predicting length of stay in an acute care hospital: the role of psychosocial problems. Soc Work Health Care 33:1–16, 2001

King LJ: A sensory integrative approach to schizophrenia. American Journal of Occupational Therapy 28:529–536, 1974

Lechman C, Duder S: Psychosocial severity, length of stay and the role of social work services. Soc Work Health Care 43:1–13, 2006

Moyers PA, Dale LM: The Guide to Occupational Therapy Practice, 2nd Edition. Bethesda, MD, American Occupational Therapy Association Press, 2007

National Alliance on Mental Illness: About Recovery. Arlington, VA, National Alliance on Mental Illness, 1996. Available at: http://www.nami.org/Template.cfm?Section= About_Recovery&Template=/TaggedPage/TaggedPage- Display.cfm&TPLID=23&ContentID=19107&lstid= 330. Accessed April 30, 2007.

National Association of Social Workers: NASW Standards for Social Work Practice in Health Care Settings. Washington, DC, National Association of Social Workers, 2005. Available at: http://www.socialworkers.org/practice/standards/NASWHealthCareStandards.pdf. Accessed March 1, 2008.

National Board for Certification in Occupational Therapy: Frequently Asked Questions, posted October 2003. Available at: http://www.nbcot.org/webarticles/anm-viewer.asp?a=110&z=17. Accessed March 1, 2008.

Rosen A, Callaly T: Interdisciplinary teamwork and leadership: issues for psychiatrists. Australas Psychiatry 13:234–240, 2005

Safran JD, Muran JC: The Therapeutic Alliance in Brief Psychotherapy. Washington, DC, American Psychological Association, 1998

Stoffel VC, Moyers PA: An evidence-based and occupational perspective of interventions for persons with substance-use disorders. Am J Occup Ther 58:570–586, 2004

Tuzman L, Cohen A: Clinical decision making for discharge planning in a changing environment. Health Soc Work 17:299–307, 1992

U.S. Department of Health and Human Services: Office for Civil Rights (OCR) Privacy Brief: Summary of the HIPAA Privacy Rule. Washington, DC, U.S. Department of Health and Human Services, 2003 (last revised 05/03). Available at: http://www.hhs.gov/ocr/privacy summary.pdf. Accessed March 1, 2008.

CHAPTER 29

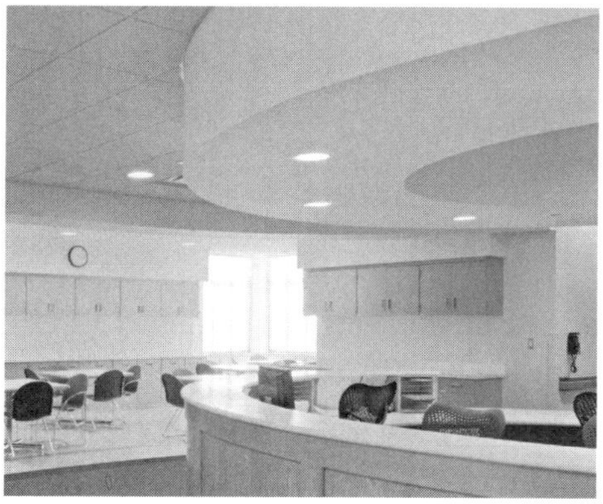

PSYCHIATRIC NURSING

Creating and Maintaining a Therapeutic Inpatient Environment

Kathleen R. Delaney, Ph.D., R.N., P.M.H.–N.P.
Suzanne Perraud, Ph.D., R.N.
Mary E. Johnson, Ph.D., R.N.

Psychiatric nurses are the largest professional workforce on inpatient psychiatric units; recent data counts indicate 78,500 nurses work in inpatient care (Manderscheid et al. 2004). Psychiatric nurses hold 24-hour accountability for the integrity of the inpatient treatment environment. They are responsible for maintaining the processes that ensure the physical and psychological *safety* of patients. Nursing also sustains the appropriate *structure* for the patient population, which provides expectancy and routine for those in acute crisis. At its heart, inpatient psychiatric nursing is a human endeavor. An essential element of the work is providing *support* to patients and ensuring they experience their needs being recognized, responded to, and understood (Barker et al. 1999; Raingruber 2003). Finally, persons who are hospitalized may be dealing with a chronic mental illness and are engaged with their own recovery. They may be coping with a recent exacerbation of their disease, and they may be trying to regain a sense of control over their illness (Delaney 1984). Nursing must create an environment that integrates *self-management* strategies that support recovery, coping, self-efficacy, and resiliency. Herein lies the work of nursing—work that, when it is going well, often goes unnoticed. Although nurses understand what maintaining a milieu requires, it is poorly understood outside the staff group. This chapter details how the everyday work of the nursing staff[1] creates and maintains the core therapeutic elements of the unit.

Much of this chapter will focus on the actual work of nursing in the milieu. Inpatient nurses also assume other responsibilities, particularly in their work with the interdisciplinary treatment team. In this vein, their efforts parallel the broad goals of hospitalization and the work of the interdisciplinary team: crisis resolution, instituting an aggressive treatment regimen; helping patients regain a sense of control and reestablish movement toward recovery; and aligning services so that the individual moves seamlessly along the continuum of care (Delaney et al. 2000; Glick et al. 2003). Accomplishing these goals usually involves pharmacological intervention, which may often include adding to or subtracting from the patient's current medication regimen. Because they monitor positive effects and any negative reactions to medication changes, inpatient nurses are essential to this effort (Volavka et al. 2005). Nurses have significant contact with patients at all times and are thus able to gather data on how patients' behaviors change with varying degrees of stimulation or stress. Their ongoing assessment of unit behavior is useful in clarifying diagnostic issues, particularly with children and adolescents (Delaney 2006b).

The Four-S Model

Gunderson (1978) determined that milieu operations could be conceptualized according to five therapeutic variables: containment, structure, support, involvement, and validation. During the 15 years that the authors have been working with the Gunderson model, we have changed the category labels and updated how they are operationalized during inpatient care (Delaney 1992; Delaney et al. 1995, 2000). Using these updated variables, this chapter organizes what nurses do in inpatient milieus by grouping their efforts into the following four categories (which we have termed the *Four-S model*): safety, structure, support, and self-management.

Safety

More than any other element in the milieu, safety is imperative. Criteria for hospitalization on an inpatient

unit stipulate that prior to admission, a person has displayed behaviors that have been deemed dangerous to self or others or have reached an acuity level that is interfering with the person's ability to function. This is not to imply that a patient is or should be viewed as dangerous but rather that the person's illness has reached a point where he or she may be experiencing extreme moods that are leading toward self-harm. An individual could, for example, be having a thought disturbance that significantly alters how he or she processes information or be undergoing periods of emotional dysregulation that disrupt functioning. Given the current short length of stay on inpatient units (National Association of Psychiatric Health Systems 2004), it is likely that at any one time several patients are in the acute phase of their illnesses. This creates high acuity and a milieu atmosphere that quickly changes, depending on admissions and discharges. In the face of such rapidly shifting milieu conditions, the safety of patients and staff must be maintained. If the basic safety of a unit is breached, no other treatments can proceed until it is restored (Bowers et al. 2005).

PRESCRIBED PRECAUTIONS AND MONITORING

On the most obvious level, the safety of an individual is maintained by a unit's system of precautions, such as implementing close watch or monitoring suicide risk. A precautions system sets out the frequency of monitoring commensurate with estimated risk (Temkin 2004). Monitoring suicide risk is a core duty of inpatient nurses and, as a component of keeping patients safe, is a basic function of an inpatient unit. Yet, close observation is not without controversy (O'Brien and Cole 2003). Patient accounts of being on close watch indicate that they may feel protected but at the same time also experience it as an intrusive measure that robs them of all privacy (Pitula and Cardell 1996). Recently, the Joint Commission (2007) placed identification of safety risks as its fifteenth National Safety Patient Goal. The new standards establish more explicit expectations for monitoring suicide risk and documenting suicide risk assessments, thus placing greater demands on the nurses and the interdisciplinary team for this extremely important, albeit time-intensive, responsibility.

Safety is also maintained by proactive control of the atmosphere of the milieu. This is accomplished by the way staff attend to the movement of patients, the

---

[1] Throughout this chapter, the term *nursing staff* is meant to denote the group of nurses and mental health workers who together create the therapeutic nursing elements of the milieu.

current at-risk behaviors of any particular patient, and any shifts in the pace and noise level of the milieu. At the most basic level, proactive control is accomplished by how staff members position themselves around the unit and thus maintain awareness of milieu action (Delaney and Johnson 2006). For instance, as they sit in the day room, staff members may notice two patients who exchange brief angry looks each time they pass by each other. As they observe such interactions, staff assess patients' behaviors in the context of what they know about the patients and their violence histories (Delaney and Johnson 2006). Anticipation is key to safety; it allows staff members to intervene early and to calmly interrupt a behavior that appears to be heading toward a volatile end (Delaney 2006c).

This does not mean that every patient on the unit needs intense monitoring. However, given the responsibility nurses hold for the welfare of both patients and fellow staff, and given the unpredictable nature of particular types of inpatient violence (Johnson 2004; Johnson and Delaney 2007), ongoing assessment of the milieu and patients is essential to safety. In other specialties, nurses use sophisticated machines to monitor patients during the acute phases of their illnesses. Psychiatric nurses must use the constant presence of staff. Intense monitoring can be interpreted or used as authoritarian control (Goffman 1961). This is particularly risky on units with low involvement, where, for example, nurses have not explained to patients the therapeutic context of routines and reasons behind different forms of monitoring (Alexander 2006). Keeping units safe in a humane way demands striking a balance; any restrictions on patient behaviors are enacted and explained within the therapeutic goal of keeping every patient physically and psychologically safe (Alexander 2006).

INGRAINED ROLE BEHAVIORS OF STAFF

Safety of the unit depends not only on how staff visually monitor space and assess behaviors but also on their ingrained role behaviors—actions that become second nature to inpatient staff. For instance, on any psychiatric unit a visitor may notice that when staff hear a loud noise, they will immediately stop what they are doing and (depending on whether they can safely leave the area) move toward the disruption. This is a seemingly simple response but is one that must occur almost automatically and with absolute consistency, given that it is key to reorganizing the staff group in the face of a possible emergency.

Staff members need to know each other's whereabouts at all times. Again, subtle role behaviors contribute to this aspect of safety. For example, nurses and mental health workers are in the habit of telling each other when they leave a common area of the unit. This is important for two reasons: first, it raises awareness that a staff member may be going to an unobserved area of the unit; second, it ensures that staff members know each other's whereabouts moment to moment, which allows for a rapid organization of the staff group in case of an emergency. Often, these role behaviors and assessment skills are acquired over time, usually by novice staff members as they work alongside more experienced peers (Hanneman 1996).

KEEPING THE UNIT SAFE: A STUDY

Although ingrained role behaviors represent one level of the safety net, most nursing interventions are not just reflexive but involve clinical judgment and reasoned action. Recently, two of the authors (M.J., K.D.) completed a study that entailed observing staff and patient interactions on two inpatient psychiatric units. We watched nurses interact with patients for 600 hours, over the course of 9 months, observing how staff members and patients moved about the milieu (Delaney and Johnson 2006; Johnson and Delaney 2006). Interviews were conducted with both staff and patients. We queried staff members on how they maintained safety and why they responded as they did to particular incidents. We also asked patients how they perceived the actions of staff as useful to helping them regain control. Study results detailed how staff kept the unit safe through actions that involved a complex set of four interconnected factors: ideology, people, space, and time.

The first dimension of safety, *ideology*, influences many aspects of unit life but was made especially evident by how the staff responded to patients' behavior. For example, a staff member who believed that a particular behavior was a function of the patient's paranoid thoughts would respond differently than a staff member who believed that the same behavior was a sign of the patient's "manipulations." Staff members who believed that patients were in control of their behavior would respond differently than those who believed that patients, because of the nature of their psychiatric illness, were not in control of their behavior. The important point was not that one set of beliefs was necessarily right or wrong but rather that the set of beliefs staff adopted about particular behaviors influenced how they responded to patients.

Likewise, the core values on the unit influenced how the staff responded to patients. Throughout our study, we were struck by how staff held respect as an important value. On one of the units in particular, the importance of respect was overtly communicated to patients. In community meetings and in day-to-day interactions, patients were told to "respect themselves, respect the staff, and respect the property." Additionally, respect was communicated more subtly through staff actions toward patients. Although the patients often exhibited strange behavior while in the acute phase of their illness, staff members were careful not to comment on this behavior in any way that could be interpreted as demeaning or pejorative. Rather, when necessary, the staff set limits on bizarre and inappropriate behavior using a kind and respectful tone of voice.

People on the unit—the patients and staff—are also critical variables in the complete framework of keeping the unit safe (Johnson and Delaney 2006). On each of the units, there was a kind of patient that was "typical." These patients might have seemed typical because of repeated hospitalizations, or they might have been patients whose diagnosis or behavior was customary for the unit. Staff knew how to respond to these patients because they had developed expertise working with certain types of behavior. On one of the units, at any given time, several patients paced up and down a long hallway. Usually, patients passed by each other without incident. However, on some days, due to the particular composition of the patient group, these pass-by pacers would seem to be muttering to each other, or there seemed to be a certain strain in the air. Staff took particular note of friction mounting between patients; often this behavior occurred between patients who knew each other from the streets and brought outside conflicts into the hospital (Delaney and Johnson 2006). By maintaining awareness of these individuals and their relationships, staff intervened quickly at the first signs of mounting tension. In doing so, they maintained the safety of the unit.

Space is an extremely important factor in keeping a unit safe; it has both objective and subjective properties. Objectively, the size of a space can be measured; the space in the unit we studied was large enough to give patients room to move around. One salient concept with relation to space was visibility. Larger units with more hallways or more bends and turns in the hallways were more difficult to keep safe than small units with only one hallway. Overall, the size and shape influenced how the staff positioned themselves so that most parts of the open space were visible to someone on staff. The configuration of the unit also helped determine how many staff members would be needed to attend to the safety of patients and their needs.

The final factor in this scheme is *time*. There was a core group of individuals who had worked on each unit for 5 or more years. These staff members tended to be the leaders and the culture bearers for the unit. Because of their longevity on the unit, the staff also knew patients who came into the hospital repeatedly. Knowing each patient meant that staff understood the patient's typical patterns of behavior and knew which strategies were effective with the patient. For example, during one of the investigator's observation periods, a man well known to the staff began to slam his door repeatedly in anger, yet the staff member in the hallway did not move. When asked about this behavior, the staff member assured the researcher that this gentleman often acted in such a way the first few days of hospitalization, and knowing the gentleman well, the staff member was certain that the anger would dissipate, which it did (Delaney and Johnson 2006).

For patients, time was a factor in the pattern of their illness trajectories. The patients who were newly admitted were more acutely symptomatic. If those patients were unfamiliar to the staff, it took the staff time to get a feel for the patient. However, getting to know the patient helped the staff get a sense of how the patient's trajectories of behavior might unfold. Illness trajectories were variable. Sometimes, patients who were anticipating discharge were also more symptomatic, especially in the time between knowing they were leaving and actually leaving. Thus, we found that, for the staff, the most hectic days were those in which many patients were admitted and discharged. Maintaining safety and stability in the milieu became more of a challenge on those days.

SAFETY AND THE USE OF SECLUSION AND RESTRAINT

Seclusion and physical restraint are emergency measures, only to be used when patients are exhibiting behaviors deemed dangerous to themselves or others. In the past decade, inpatient staff members have been engaged in scrutinizing practices that center on the use of seclusion and restraint (Goren and Curtis 1996; Mohr et al. 1998; Muir-Cochrane 1996; Wynn 2003). Tremendous effort is currently being expended in the psychiatric community on strategies that could produce restraint-free environments (Delaney 2006a; Huckshorn 2004; LeBel et al. 2004). Much of the federal focus has been on staff training and culture change (Substance Abuse and Mental Health Services Administration 2005a). What has not received sufficient study is how administration policies, such as floating staff among varied units regardless of training, mandatory overtime, and use of agency/part-time nurses breed resentful, fatigued, or dissatisfied staff—a factor associated with the proclivity to use restraint and seclusion (Morrison 1998). As nurses strive to keep units safe, they must also devise strategies to address larger organizational policies that affect safety, often policies in which they have little voice or control.

Structure

Structure is a part of milieu operations that may at first appear deceptively simple. At the most basic level, it is about nurses' and adjunct professionals' work in implementing a schedule that organizes a patient's day. The daily schedule usually includes a mix of activities: group therapy, psychoeducation, recreational activities, occupational therapy groups, and expressive therapies such as art. Usually, the schedule of the day includes a community meeting at which staff orient new patients and keep the patient group apprised of the day's events. It is a meeting that demands little participation; thus, even very ill patients can attend and feel part of the process but not invaded or pressured to communicate (Klein and Brown 1987).

The rationale for imposing a structure of activities has traditionally been to provide a clear, unambiguous scaffold to the day to control stimulation and to help patients reexperience competency (Alexander and Bowers 2004; Schulman and Irwin 1982). This is particularly important for patients who may be working on difficulties with concentration, information processing, or response flexibility (McClure et al. 2005; Seidman et al. 1995). In these instances, it is assumed that an environment that is predictable and controls stimulation would enhance organization (Sederer 1991).

The difficulty in imposing structure centers on when to encourage participation and when expectations infringe on patients' autonomy. Patients may not want to be involved in the groups offered on the unit or, when they attend, may choose not to participate. Not all persons admitted to the unit believe they need such groups to regain control of their illness or move toward recovery. In a qualitative study conducted on a short-term unit, only a small percentage of patients saw themselves getting better through development of coping skills or self-understanding. Indeed, patients saw themselves using the hospital for a variety of reasons, including as a sanctuary from stress and a place to recover while the medications took effect (Delaney 1984).

The results of a more recent study of patients with schizophrenic disorders confirmed this finding. The patients on the study unit said that they were seeking protection from vulnerability (created by the exacerbation of their illness) and needed help in empowering themselves to better cope with the outside world (Koivisto et al. 2004). These patients' goals may or may not align with the material presented to them in groups. Thus, in maintaining structure, employees must be mindful that the content of a group must match how individuals define their use of the hospital for recovery. When patients choose not to participate, as many do, complicated issues of power and coercion may arise.

On adult units, staff's work with regard to this issue is complex and often involves how the personnel implement the unit's rules and expectations. Limit setting and enforcement of rules are sometimes viewed by patients as nothing more than nurses exerting their control—practices that can leave patients feeling dehumanized, powerless, humiliated, and isolated (Alexander 2006; Duxbury and Whittington 2005). In such instances, there is no collaboration on the patients' goals, and they become passive recipients of care (Latvala et al. 2000). This is when nurses must work within the interdependence of structure and self-management, which demands that staff members consider structure within the context of what the patient's goals are and how patients believe hospital resources, including various groups, contribute to their recovery.

On child and adolescent units, implementing ward rules without coercion demands that youth understand the purpose of unit expectations. Novice staff members may hold the belief that they need to "shape up" a child's behavior by imposing stringent expectations. Actually, the reverse is true. Although there must be some guidelines for behavior to nourish coping abilities, nurses must support children's autonomy by providing choices and rationales for ward rules (Skinner and Wellborn 1994). In the unit where one of the authors (K.D.) practices, an effort is made to consciously structure the environment to reduce stress. Thus, children are afforded choices; staff aim at setting coping demands that are within the children's reach and providing sensible interventions that elicit cooperation.

On the Child Assessment Unit of the Cambridge Hospital (Cambridge, Massachusetts), nurses employ a child- and family-centered care model. Here, a child's refusal to attend group is met with a sincere staff effort to understand the reasons for refusal (Regan et al. 2006). Children are not given consequences for refusal. Instead, such interactions are viewed as opportunities for problem solving and for helping children adopt more flexibility to events perceived as frustrating (Regan et al. 2006). This model has met with excellent outcomes, and it challenges the traditional view that the unit structure would unravel if child/adolescent staff took a flexible approach to group attendance.

Although respect for freedom and autonomy is critical, a balance must be struck to ensure the psychological safety of all patients and personnel. Frueh et al.'s (2005) study documents the experiences of 142 patients who had been hospitalized on inpatient units. Many patients reported incidents they perceived to be traumatic: physical assault (31%), sexual assault (8%), and witnessing of traumatic events (63%). In addition, 54% reported experiences of being around frightening or violent patients, which is a situation that erodes psychological safety. To maintain structure, staff are put to the task of balancing tolerance for behaviors—not overcontrolling the environment yet not allowing the structure to relax to the point that patients are frightened.

The way in which staff members approach decisions regarding participation, rules, and behaviors determines the unit culture; these norms then become commonly held assumptions about how persons hospitalized on the unit should be treated. The culture of the unit can be dictated by rules and efforts to enforce them, or it can be permeated by a flexible interpretation of what is needed to keep order on the unit. It is played out every day in moment-to-moment decisions and responses to patients' behaviors. Currently, there are inpatient ideologies whose guiding principles are healing and creating a healthy social structure in which this can be accomplished (Bloom et al. 2003; Regan et al. 2006). As these newer models proliferate, so will the need to differentiate how they fit in a variety of populations; it will become increasingly important to be more precise about how to change cultures effectively and to be mindful of how to use these flexible structures while keeping the unit safe.

Support

Support is an essential milieu quality that must be available to persons hospitalized on a psychiatric unit. In their narratives of the hospitalization experience, patients have recognized the need for support—for becoming active participants in care (Latvala et al. 2000) so that they might be empowered to restructure their lives (Koivisto et al. 2004). Most importantly, patients need the support from a human connection that makes them feel they are responded to and understood (Carlsson et al. 2006; Thomas et al. 2002). Support is

a broad concept that has been framed in psychiatry in the context of crisis and stress (Hoff 1995), in the social support literature in the context of its moderating effects on illness (Mittelmark 1999), and in the treatment literature in the area of supportive psychotherapy (Winston et al. 2004).

Psychiatric nurses view support as occurring within the interpersonal aspects of care, especially in the context of the nurse–patient relationship. In the United States, this platform was established by the theories of Peplau (1952), and now, 50 years later, the relationship continues as the critical vehicle for nurses to join with persons with mental illness and support their movement toward health (Raingruber 2003). In the Peplau framework, it is within this relationship that persons come to master barriers to mental health arising from biological processes, development, or personal events (Beeber 2000). Researchers in Great Britain and Canada have examined the nurse–patient relationship during hospitalization (Cameron et al. 2005; Forchuk et al. 1998, 2000; Welch 2005). Their research confirms that much of the work of nursing is bound within the relationship; within that context nurses help patients move toward greater well-being (Barker 2001; Graham 2000).

The nurse–patient relationship is built on nurses' understanding of the patients' experience. To develop such an understanding requires staff's concerted and focused efforts to apprehend the patient's intents, attributions, and perceptions of incidents that have occurred in the past or are occurring now on the unit (Lewis 1978). Staff come to know the patient by observing the patient's nonverbal behaviors, patterning this presentation with what they know about the person, and sometimes interpreting those cues and feeding their interpretation back to the patient (Graham 2000; Raingruber 1999). Via this understanding, the nurse moves into the person's meaning system and, in doing so, begins to explore the significance of the illness experience for the person's life and with attention to what the patient currently needs to feel safe or to begin to rebuild her or his life (Barker 2001; Czuchta and Johnson 1998; Koivisto et al. 2004). This field of understanding is built by using empathy (Reynolds and Scott 1999), listening carefully to the patient's experiences, being present for the patient (accessibility), collaborating with the patient on problems, advocating for the patient, sharing power, and manifesting authenticity (Berg and Hallberg 2000; Forchuk and Reynolds 2001; Forchuk et al. 2000; Welch 2005).

Caring and support are neither the same for all persons nor the same for one person at different stages of his or her illness experience (Barker 2001). Patients living through psychosis and its attendant experience of vulnerability have reported needing support in dealing with the distress from a loss of self (Koivisto et al. 2003). They also report the need to feel safe, to sense they are in a reliable environment with nurses who are aware of and monitoring their situation (Koivisto et al. 2004). Patients who were depressed said they valued interventions that helped them regain a sense of control over their lives or a sense of control over their illnesses (Delaney 1984). Persons with a history of abuse particularly require that staff understand their need for personal boundary protection and provide explanation for instances when unit events pose a violation (Geanellos 2003). In all cases, the basic idea remains consistent: staff need to know patients by attending to their experiences of illness and how they define their needs, symptoms, and events (Cameron et al. 2005).

Establishing a base of support through the relationship is not always straightforward. Several factors inherent in the structure of inpatient care and in the nature of nurses' work may impede development of a supportive relationship. First, the pace of a brief hospitalization unit can take up much staff time. Brief lengths of stay produce high acuity, and as a result, nurses are apt to direct their attention not to relationship building but to the most acute patient or situation (Cleary and Edwards 1999). Clinical tasks such as tending to admissions, discharges, medications, and medical issues can also interfere with relationship building (Cameron et al. 2005; Hummelvoll and Severinsson 2001; Whittington and McLaughlin 2000). Although such aspects of the role are important, nurses must learn to become balancing artists for competing demands.

Another barrier to the nurse–patient relationship is shaped by interpersonal distance, sometimes mutually created by patients and staff and sometimes created when nursing staff members withdraw from patients (Forchuk et al. 1998). In an ethnographic study of three inpatient units, Bray (1999) found that staff members distanced themselves from patients who were harsh and insulting to them, those who did not take any accountability for behavior, and patients whose stories of abuse had the potential to lead to a vicarious traumatization. At times, nurses distanced themselves from patients because they were unsure of what they should to do, lacking confidence in their ability to address a situation. Obviously, relationship building is hampered when nurses distance themselves from patients; therefore, such behaviors should be examined in staff supervision.

A final barrier that nursing staff must overcome in establishing a relationship is the divide between what nurses expect a relationship to be versus what patients state they need. Nursing staff may approach patients with the expectation that they will talk out problems and use self-observing functions to review events of the past and their behavior (Forchuk et al. 2000). If they use the quality and quantity of one-to-one interaction as their way of evaluating the relationship, nurses may not believe they are developing meaningful relationships. However, the nurse–patient relationship is perceived to be quite satisfying if it is judged, on a practical level, by instances of nurses assisting patients with problem solving or helping them address the everyday dilemmas of unit life (McElroy 1996; Warelow and Edward 2007). Thus, to ensure that relationship-building proceeds in line with patients' needs, staff expectations and role definitions should become another important topic for supervision.

CARING, CONCERN, AND COERCION

Within this supportive stance, nursing staff maintain responsibilities around unit structure and safety. This means that the same person who is forming a relationship based on caring may be the one who sets limits during an escalating situation. At times, one aspect of this role may become dominant. Indeed, the nursing profession has an image of toughness, promulgated in part by the media but also by nurses themselves (Morrison 1990). Of course, coercion should be eliminated, but the reality of inpatient nursing is that, owing to a unit's acuity or staff's expertise level, aggression can occur, and, we might add, patients and nurses might be injured in these incidents (Flannery and Walker 2003; Nijman et al. 2005; Ryan et al. 2004). Patients who are involved in control situations and/or those who experience being restrained during emergency circumstances describe feeling demoralized (Bonner et al. 2002; Duxbury 2002; Johnson 1998; Olofsson and Norberg 2001). Times of strain therefore require skilled staff who respect the freedom of the individual; draw on a nonauthoritarian attitude; deal with situations in a straightforward, authentic manner; and offer the patient a way to save face (Carlsson et al. 2006; Johnson and Hauser 2001; Lowe 1992).

Self-Management

The term *self-management* is used to reflect a patient's active participation in his or her own disease care and generally refers to the day-to-day activities a person undertakes to maintain health. Although self-management is most often applied in interaction with health care providers, the optimal situation occurs when patients are active, identifying wellness-oriented tasks and seeking to learn and practice wellness-promoting skills (Lorig and Holman 2003). Self-management in the context of disease management is not new to psychiatry. But despite the rapid development of illness management programs, the integration of self-management into our existing mental health system has been slow. Recently, in its transformation plan for the mental health system, the Substance Abuse and Mental Health Services Administration (2003, 2005b) endorsed the idea of self-management as the cornerstone of a patient's recovery plan. Coupled with the expectations of the Joint Commission on Accreditation of Healthcare Organizations (2006) regarding recovery-based inpatient care, one expects that this ideology will quickly become a component of psychiatric hospital policy.

For many inpatient nurses, recovery and self-management involve increasing patient involvement in their own care, teaching self-care skills, and providing opportunities to practice newfound skills (Forchuk et al. 2003; Repper 2000). Providing self-management support on inpatient psychiatric units means that staff go beyond patient teaching to activities that help patients build confidence in their own abilities to manage their health. An inpatient self-management program might include generic lifestyle issues such as nutrition, exercise, and coping skills; role management; or programs that help individuals manage depression and stress (Robert Wood Johnson Foundation and Center for the Advancement of Health 2001). Desired program activities should include providing self-management education and engaging in goal setting with patients to control symptoms and thus avoid rehospitalization (Bachman et al. 2006; Rogers et al. 1999). Much of this inpatient work will be focused on with the notion of self-efficacy.

Self-efficacy is a framework used by some of the most successful self-management support programs. It refers to the confidence that one has in his or her ability to do what is necessary to achieve positive outcomes, in this case, to manage one's mental illness (Perraud 2000; Perraud et al. 2006). Improving self-efficacy for therapeutic activities will promote perseverance in the performance of targeted behaviors (Bandura 1997) and, based on the outcomes of other self-efficacy-based programs, will provide the resources needed to improve outcomes (Farrell et al. 2004; Lorig et al. 2001a, 2001b; Ludman et al. 2003).

Self-efficacy theory supplies inpatient staff with the framework for how to engage patients in the enactment of and persistence in their specific desired behaviors. On inpatient units, this becomes a plan in progress, with staff assessing patients' confidence in engaging in the specified behaviors, thus gauging the probability of success of the plan under development (Lorig 2006). If confidence is low, then the plan is adjusted. For instance, staff may teach patients about the relationship between staying active and reducing depression. If patients are interested in receiving support for staying active, then an action plan is developed that begins with involvement in activities on the unit. Confidence for participating in the plan (attending specific groups) is measured. If confidence is low, then obstacles to being active are discussed and the plan is adjusted until the patient becomes confident in his or her ability to follow through. Successful enactment of the plan should motivate the patient; adjustment is then made to take activity to the next level. As discharge nears, plans are developed that the patient can follow after discharge, using assessment of confidence as a guide (Perraud 2000; Perraud et al. 2006).

Inpatient treatment is uniquely suited to the development of self-efficacy because inpatient environments are rich in potential sources of self-efficacy. According to Bandura (1997), there are four sources of self-efficacy (in descending order of influence): mastery performance, vicarious experience, social persuasion, and management of physiological and affective states. The most effective way of enhancing confidence in one's ability to do something is to do it successfully. Because of their sustained contact with patients, inpatient nurses are in an excellent position to help patients identify a desired outcome, teach the skills to reach that outcome, and routinely encourage practice of targeted and taught skills. The boost in confidence provided by successful enactment of skills provides some assurance that, when coupled with reasonable and collaborative action plans, the patient is likely to continue the behaviors at home.

Self-efficacy is also boosted through vicarious experience of the successful behavior performed by a role model. This happens on inpatient units in groups and other milieu activities as patients actively observe and interact with each other. Inpatient staff can help by seeking and pointing out successful models for desired behaviors. Social persuasion, the third source of self-efficacy enhancement, is ubiquitous in inpatient settings. On inpatient units, nurses, physicians, and adjunct staff exhort patients to action by convincing them that they have the capability to succeed. Persuading patients to try, or to persist when they believe that they cannot succeed, and pointing out successes are critical to helping patients develop confidence in their ability to function independently. Finally, as action plans are developed, managing anxiety and stress related to performance and helping patients realistically assess their performance in relation to their emotions should be routinely addressed.

In the course of action planning, staff should also point out or provide resources to patients that can be used at home. A plethora of tools are available to help people manage their health. Electronic reminders can be programmed into pillboxes or personal digital assistants to structure self-management activities throughout the day. Self-help materials such as relaxation tapes, pamphlets, and other written material can be provided to assist patients both in the hospital and at home. As patients seek such information on their own, they will undoubtedly browse the Internet. The Internet is an important self-management support; it extends access to expertise and may result in the development of active patient self-management skills (Zuckerman 2003). Finally, referrals to self-help and information and support groups in the community can be made so that patients have a place to learn and practice new self-management behaviors.

Inpatient nurses are central to the provision of self-management support for chronically ill patients (Repper 2000), and inpatient treatment provides continuous opportunities for the process. Ultimately, the responsibility to manage one's health, well or poorly, belongs to each individual. Nurses and the interdisciplinary team can help by collaborating with patients to remove barriers to optimum choices and by providing them with the information, skill, and confidence they need to make those choices. Seriously mentally ill patients with impairments in self-care ability are at higher risk for rehospitalization (Lyons et al. 1997). There is evidence to suggest that active self-managers of psychiatric disorders have fewer hospitalizations (George et al. 2002; Pollack 1996a, 1996b, 1996c). It is therefore imperative that staff attend to the information needs of patients and families as they manage their day-to-day health so that they have the confidence and the ability to become active self-managers (Cleary et al. 2006; Lorig and Holman 2003).

Self-management programs are fairly robust. Patients tell us coping with acute psychosis is exhausting (Koivisto et al. 2004). The multidisciplinary team will need to partner with patients as they reach the point where they have the psychic energy to focus outward and engage in specific self-management strategies

(Forchuk et al. 2003). The team will more than likely focus on helping patients through the crises of illness and assist with symptom management. When these same persons reach a point where they sense their illness has stabilized, they may then turn their attention to how they can return to a meaningful life in the community (Barker 2001). Staff must move fluidly in both areas of care. For patients to shift successfully to the next level of care, both processes (recovery and self-management) must be supported by the work of the inpatient staff.

Conclusion

For the multidisciplinary team to accomplish rapid stabilization of symptoms and initiation of an aggressive treatment plan, seriously ill patients must be cared for in a consciously structured environment. Owing to their 24-hour contact with patients, nursing staff are at the center of the effort to create a safe milieu, with a structure that facilitates healing and recovery and an interpersonal context that encourages authentic interaction. It is terribly important that the work of nursing be recognized and understood. As described in this chapter, the skill set for maintaining psychiatric milieus is largely unarticulated outside the nursing community. When the skills required to keep the milieu safe are not understood by managers and hospital administration, they may fail to staff units with a nursing skill level that matches patient acuity, a situation that breaches basic principles of patient safety.

Inpatient clinicians must find ways to collect data that make obvious when staffing patterns are no longer supporting the basic functions of the unit and the staff expertise is no longer matching the intensity of the patient group's needs (Ellila et al. 2005; Furlong and Ward 1997). In other nursing specialties, the number and quality of staff are clearly related to patient safety and prevention of complications (Aiken et al. 2002, 2003). Selected hospitals are currently involved in pilot-testing core measures—indicators that have been found to correlate with the overall quality of care in a hospital (Joint Commission 2008; Table 29–1). These measures will yield important data that can be useful in correlating staffing patterns and organizational characteristics with restraint use and safety. These correlations can ultimately demonstrate the value of experienced and educated staff in preventing errors and preserving safety.

TABLE 29–1.   Hospital-based inpatient psychiatric services (HBIPS) candidate core measure set

The core measures for inpatient psychiatric treatment are currently in pilot testing. Measures being tested include the following:

- Assessment of violence risk, substance use disorder, trauma, and patient strengths completed
- Hours of restraint use
- Hours of seclusion use
- Patients discharged on multiple antipsychotic medications
- Discharge assessment and aftercare recommendations are sent to next level of care providers upon discharge

Source.   Joint Commission 2008.

References

Aiken LH, Clarke SP, Sloane DM, et al: Hospital nurse staffing and patient mortality, nurse burnout and job dissatisfaction. JAMA 288:1987–1993, 2002

Aiken LH, Clarke SP, Cheung RB, et al: Educational levels of hospital nurses and surgical patient mortality. JAMA 290:1617–1623, 2003

Alexander J: Patients' feelings about ward nursing regimes and involvement in rule construction. J Psychiatr Ment Health Nurs 13:543–553, 2006

Alexander J, Bowers L: Acute psychiatric ward rules: a review of the literature. J Psychiatr Ment Health Nurs 11:623–631, 2004

Bachman J, Swenson S, Reardon ME, et al: Patient self-management in the primary care treatment of depression. Adm Policy Ment Health 33:76–85, 2006

Bandura A: Self-Efficacy: The Exercise of Control. New York, WH Freeman, 1997

Barker P: The tidal model: developing a person-centered approach to psychiatric and mental health nursing. Perspect Psychiatr Care 37:79–87, 2001

Barker P, Jackson S, Stevenson C: What are psychiatric nurses needed for? Developing a theory of essential nursing practice. J Psychiatr Ment Health Nurs 6:273–282, 1999

Beeber LS: Hildahood: taking the interpersonal theory of nursing to the neighborhood. J Am Psychiatr Nurses Assoc 6:49–55, 2000

Berg A, Hallberg IR: Psychiatric nurses' lived experiences of working with inpatient care on a general team psychiatric ward. J Psychiatr Ment Health Nurs 7:323–333, 2000

Bloom SL, Bennington-Davis M, Farragher B, et al: Multiple opportunities for creating sanctuary. Psychiatr Q 74:173–190, 2003

Bonner G, Lowe T, Rawcliff D, et al: Trauma for all: a pilot study of the subjective experience of physical restraint for mental health inpatients and staff in the UK. J Psychiatr Ment Health Nurs 9:465–473, 2002

Bowers L, Simpson A, Alexander J, et al: The nature and purpose of acute psychiatric wards: the Tompkins acute ward study. Journal of Mental Health 14:625–635, 2005

Bray J: An ethnographic study of psychiatric nursing. J Psychiatr Ment Health Nurs 6:297–305, 1999

Cameron D, Kapur R, Campbell P: Releasing the therapeutic potential of the psychiatric nurse: a human relations perspective on the nurse-patient relationship. J Psychiatr Ment Health Nurs 12:64–74, 2005

Carlsson G, Dahlberg K, Ekebergh M, et al: Patients longing for authentic personal care: a phenomenological study of violent encounters in psychiatric settings. Issues Ment Health Nurs 27:287–305, 2006

Cleary M, Edwards C: "Something always comes up": nurse-patient interaction in an acute psychiatric setting. J Psychiatr Ment Health Nurs 6:469–477, 1999

Cleary M, Hunt GE, Walter G, et al: The patient's view of need and caregiving consequences: a cross-sectional study of inpatients with severe mental illness. J Psychiatr Ment Health Nurs 13:506–514, 2006

Czuchta DM, Johnson BA: Reconstructing a sense of self in patients with chronic mental illness. Perspect Psychiatr Care 34:31–36, 1998

Delaney KR: Short-term hospitalization and the depressed patient, in Nursing Interventions in Depression. Edited by Rogers CA, Ulsafer-VanLanen J. Orlando, FL, Grune & Stratton, 1984, pp 39–52

Delaney KR: Nursing on child psychiatric milieus, part 1: what nurses do. J Child Adolesc Psychiatr Ment Health Nurs 5:10–14, 1992

Delaney KR: Evidence base for practice: reduction of restraint and seclusion use during child and adolescent psychiatric inpatient treatment. Worldviews Evid Based Nurs 3:9–30, 2006a

Delaney KR: Learning to observe in context: child and adolescent inpatient mental health assessment. J Child Adolesc Psychiatr Ment Health Nurs 19:170–174, 2006b

Delaney KR: Top ten milieu interventions for inpatient child/adolescent treatment. J Child Adolesc Ment Health Nurs 19:170–174, 2006c

Delaney KR, Johnson ME: Keeping the unit safe: mapping psychiatric nursing skills. J Am Psychiatr Nurses Assoc 12:198–207, 2006

Delaney K, Ulsater van Lanen J, Pitula CR, et al: Seven days and counting: how inpatient nurses might adjust their practice to brief hospitalization. J Psychosoc Nurs Ment Health Serv 33:36–40, 1995

Delaney KR, Pitula CR, Perraud S: Psychiatric hospitalization and process description: what will nursing add? J Psychosoc Nurs Ment Health Serv 38:7–13, 2000

Duxbury J: An evaluation of staff and patient views of and strategies employed to manage inpatient aggression and violence on one mental health unit: a pluralistic design. J Psychiatr Ment Health Nurs 9:325–337, 2002

Duxbury J, Whittington R: Causes and management of patient aggression and violence: staff and patient perspectives. J Adv Nurs 50:469–478, 2005

Ellila H, Sourander A, Valimaki M, et al: Characteristics and staff resources of child and adolescent psychiatric hospital wards in Finland. J Psychiatr Ment Health Nurs 12:209–214, 2005

Farrell K, Wicks MN, Martin JC: Chronic disease self-management improved with enhanced self-efficacy. Clin Nurs Res 13:289–308, 2004

Flannery RB, Walker AP: Safety skills of mental health workers: empirical evidence of a risk management strategy. Psychiatr Q 74:1–10, 2003

Forchuk C, Westwell J, Martin M, et al: Factors influencing the movement of chronic psychiatric patients from the orientation to the working phase of the nurse-client relationship on an inpatient unit. Perspect Psychiatr Care 34:36–44, 1998

Forchuk C, Westwell J, Martin M, et al: The developing nurse-client relationship: nurses' perspective. J Am Psychiatr Nurses Assoc 6:3–10, 2000

Forchuk C, Reynolds W: Clients' reflections on relationships with nurses: comparisons from Canada and Scotland. J Psychiatr Ment Health Nurs 8:45–51, 2001

Forchuk C, Jewell J, Tweedell D, et al: Role changes experienced by clinical staff in relation to clients' recovery from psychosis. J Psychiatr Ment Health Nurs 10:269–276, 2003

Frueh BC, Knapp RG, Cusack KJ, et al: Patients' reports of traumatic or harmful experiences within the psychiatric setting. Psychiatr Serv 56:1123–1133, 2005

Furlong S, Ward M: Assessing patient dependency and staff skill mix. Nurs Stand 11:33–38, 1997

Geanellos R: Understanding the need for personal space boundary restoration in women-client survivors of intrafamilial sexual abuse. Int J Ment Health Nurs 12:186–193, 2003

George L, Durbin J, Sheldon T, et al: Patient and contextual factors related to the decision to hospitalize patients from emergency psychiatric services. Psychiatr Serv 53:1586–1591, 2002

Glick ID, Carter WG, Tandon R: A paradigm for treatment of inpatient psychiatric disorders: from asylum to intensive care. J Psychiatr Pract 9:395–402, 2003

Goffman E: Asylums: Essays on the Social Situation of Mental Patients and Other Inmates. New York, Anchor Books, 1961

Goren S, Curtis W: Staff members' beliefs about seclusion and restraint in child psychiatric hospitals. J Child Adolesc Psychiatr Nurs 9:7–14, 1996

Graham IW: Reflective practice and its role in mental health nurses' practice development: a year-long study. J Psychiatr Ment Health Nurs 7:109–117, 2000

Gunderson JG: Defining the therapeutic process in psychiatric milieus. Psychiatry 41:327–335, 1978

Hanneman SK: Advancing nursing practice with a unit-based clinical expert. Image J Nurs Sch 28:331–337, 1996

Hoff LA: People in Crisis: Understanding and Helping, 4th Edition. San Francisco, CA, Jossey-Bass, 1995

Huckshorn KA: Reducing seclusion and restraint use in mental health settings. Core strategies for prevention. J Psychosoc Nurs Ment Health Serv 42:22–33, 2004

Hummelvoll JK, Severinsson EI: Imperative ideals and the strenuous reality: focusing on acute psychiatry. J Psychiatr Ment Health Nurs 8:17–24, 2001

Johnson ME: Being restrained: a study of power and powerlessness. Issues Ment Health Nurs 19:191–206, 1998

Johnson ME: Violence on inpatient psychiatric units: state of the science. J Am Psychiatr Nurses Assoc 10:113–121, 2004

Johnson ME, Delaney KR: Keeping the unit safe: a grounded theory study. J Am Psychiatr Nurses Assoc 12:198–207, 2006

Johnson ME, Delaney KR: Keeping the unit safe: the anatomy of escalation. J Am Psychiatr Nurses Assoc 13:42–52, 2007

Johnson ME, Hauser PM: The practices of expert psychiatric nurses: accompanying the patient to a calmer personal space. Issues Ment Health Nurs 22:651–668, 2001

Joint Commission: 2007 Hospital/Critical Access Hospital National Safety Patient Goals. Oakbrook Terrace, IL, The Joint Commission, 2007. Available at: http://www.jointcommission.org/PatientSafety/NationalPatientSafetyGoals/07_hap_cah_npsgs.htm. Accessed February 15, 2007.

Joint Commission: Performance Measurement Initiatives: Hospital-Based, Inpatient Psychiatric Services (HBIPS) Candidate Core Measure Set, last updated February 15, 2008. Oakbrook Terrace, IL, The Joint Commission, 2008. Available at: http://www.jointcommission.org/PerformanceMeasurement/PerformanceMeasurement/Hospital+Based+Inpatient+Psychiatric+Services.htm. Accessed March 1, 2008.

Joint Commission on Accreditation of Healthcare Organizations: Approved Standards Additions for Behavioral Health Services, May 2005. Oakbrook Terrace, IL, Joint Commission on Accreditation of Healthcare Organizations, 2006. Available at: http://www.jointcommission.org/NR/rdonlyres/09CDAFFB-D502-40C7-973C-A935DF05BC5C/0/bhc_recovery_oriented_stds.pdf. Accessed April 1, 2008.

Klein RH, Brown SL: Large-group processes and the patient-staff community meeting. Int J Group Psychother 37:219–237, 1987

Koivisto K, Janhonen S, Vaisanen L: Patients' experiences of psychosis in an inpatient setting. J Psychiatr Mental Health Nurs 10:221–229, 2003

Koivisto K, Janhonen S, Vaisanen L: Patients' experiences of being helped in an inpatient setting. J Psychiatr Mental Health Nurs 11:268–275, 2004

Latvala E, Janhonen S, Moring J: Passive patients: a challenge to psychiatric nurses. Perspect Psychiatr Care 36:24–32, 2000

LeBel J, Stromberg N, Duckworth K, et al: Child and adolescent inpatient restraint reduction: a state initiative to promote strength-based care. J Am Acad Child Adolesc Psychiatry 43:37–45, 2004

Lewis GK: Nurse-Patient Communication, 3rd Edition. Dubuque, IA, William C Brown, 1978

Lorig K: Action planning: a call to action. J Am Board Fam Med 19:324–325, 2006

Lorig KR, Holman HR: Self-management education: history, definition, outcomes, and mechanisms. Ann Behav Med 26:1–7, 2003

Lorig KR, Ritter P, Stewart AL, et al: Chronic disease self-management program: 2-year health status and health care utilization outcomes. Med Care 39:1217–1223, 2001a

Lorig KR, Sobel DS, Ritter PL, et al: Effect of a self-management program on patients with chronic disease. Eff Clin Pract 4:256–262, 2001b

Lowe T: Characteristics of effective nursing interventions in the management of challenging behaviour. J Adv Nurs 17:1226–1232, 1992

Ludman E, Katon W, Bush T, et al: Behavioural factors associated with symptom outcomes in a primary care-based depression prevention intervention trial. Psychol Med 33:1061–1070, 2003

Lyons JS, O'Mahoney MT, Miller SI, et al: Predicting readmission to the psychiatric hospital in a managed care environment: implications for quality indicators. Am J Psychiatry 154:337–340, 1997

Manderscheid RW, Atay JE, Male A, et al: Highlights of organized mental health services in 2000 and major national and state trends, in Mental Health United States, 2002 (DHHS Publ No SMA 04-3938). Edited by Manderscheid RW, Henderson MJ. Rockville, MD, Substance Abuse and Mental Health Services Administration, 2004, pp 243–279

McClure EB, Treland JE, Snow J, et al: Deficits in social cognition and response flexibility in pediatric bipolar disorder. Am J Psychiatry 162:1644–1651, 2005

McElroy EC: Uncovering clinical knowledge in expert psychiatric nursing practice. J Am Psychiatr Nurses Assoc 2:208–215, 1996

Mittelmark MB: Social ties and health promotion: suggestions for population-based research. Health Educ Res 14:447–451, 1999

Mohr W, Mahon MM, Noone MJ: A restraint on restraints: the need to reconsider the use of restrictive interventions. Arch Psychiatr Nurs 12:95–106,1998

Morrison EF: The tradition of toughness: a study of nonprofessional nursing care in psychiatric settings. Image J Nurs Sch 22:32–38, 1990

Morrison EF: The culture of caregiving and aggression in psychiatric settings. Arch Psychiatr Nurs 12:21–31, 1998

Muir-Cochrane E: An investigation into nurses' perceptions of secluding patients on closed psychiatric units. J Adv Nurs 23:555–563,1996

National Association of Psychiatric Health Systems: 2004 Annual Survey. Washington, DC, National Association of Psychiatric Health Systems, 2004

Nijman H, Bowers L, Oud N, et al: Psychiatric nurses experiences with inpatient aggression. Aggressive Behavior 31:217–227, 2005

O'Brien L, Cole R: Close-observation areas in acute psychiatric units: a literature review. Int J Ment Health Nurs 12:165–176, 2003

Olofsson B, Norberg A: Experiences of coercion in psychiatric care as narrated by patients, nurses and physicians. J Adv Nurs 33:89–97, 2001

Peplau HE: Interpersonal Relations in Nursing. New York, JP Putnam, 1952

Perraud S: Development of the Depression Coping Self-Efficacy Scale. Arch Psychiatr Nurs 14:276–284, 2000

Perraud S, Fogg L, Kopytko E, et al: Predictive validity of the Depression Coping Self-Efficacy Scale (DCSES). Res Nurs Health 29:147–160, 2006

Pitula C, Cardell R: Suicidal inpatients' experiences of constant observation. Psychiatr Serv 67:649–651, 1996

Pollack LE: Information seeking among people with manic-depressive illness. Image J Nurs Sch 28:259–265, 1996a

Pollack LE: Inpatient self-management of bipolar disorder. Appl Nurs Res 9:71–79, 1996b

Pollack LE: Inpatients with bipolar disorder: their quest to understand. J Psychosoc Nurs Ment Health Serv 34:19–24, 1996c

Raingruber BJ: Recognizing, understanding and responding to familiar responses: the importance of a relationship history for therapeutic effectiveness. Perspect Psychiatr Care 35:5–17, 1999

Raingruber B: Nurture: the fundamental significance of relationship as a paradigm for mental health nursing. Perspect Psychiatr Care 9:104–112, 132–135, 2003

Regan KM, Curtin C, Vorderer L: Paradigm shifts in inpatient psychiatric care of children: approaching child- and family-centered care. J Child Adolesc Psychiatr Nurs 19:29–40, 2006

Repper J: Adjusting the focus on mental health nursing: incorporating service users' experiences of recovery. J Ment Health 9:575–587, 2000

Reynolds WJ, Scott B: Empathy: a crucial component of helping relationships. J Psychiatr Ment Health Nurs 6:363–370, 1999

Robert Wood Johnson Foundation and Center for the Advancement of Health: Essential Elements of Self-Management Interventions. Washington, DC, Center for the Advancement of Health, December 2001. Available at: http://www.cfah.org/pdfs/Essential_Elements_Report.pdf. Accessed April 28, 2007.

Rogers A, Flowers J, Pencheon D: Improving access needs a whole systems approach. And will be important in averting crises in the millennium winter. BMJ 319:866–867, 1999

Ryan EP, Hart VS, Messick DL, et al: A prospective study of assault against staff by youths in a state psychiatric hospital. Psychiatr Serv 55:665–670, 2004

Schulman JL, Irwin M: Psychiatric Hospitalization of Children. Springfield, IL, Charles C Thomas, 1982

Sederer LI: Schizophrenic disorders, in Inpatient Psychiatry: Diagnosis and Treatment, 3rd Edition. Edited by Sederer LI. Baltimore, MD, Williams & Wilkins, 1991, pp 70–107

Seidman LJ, Oscar-Berman M, Kalinowski AG, et al: Experimental and clinical neuropsychological measures of prefrontal dysfunction in schizophrenia. Neuropsychology 9:481–490, 1995

Skinner EA, Wellborn J G: Coping during childhood and adolescence: a motivational perspective, in Life Span Development and Behavior, Vol 12. Edited by Lerner RD, Featherman D, Perlmutter M. Hillsdale, NJ, Lawrence Erlbaum, 1994, pp 91–123

Substance Abuse and Mental Health Services Administration (SAMHSA): Promoting recovery with proven solutions. SAMSHA News 11(2):4–8, 2003

Substance Abuse and Mental Health Services Administration (SAMHSA): Roadmap to Seclusion and Restraint Free Mental Health Services (DHHS Publ No SMA-05-4055). Rockville, MD, Center for Mental Health Services, Substance Abuse and Mental Health Services Administration, 2005a. Available at: http://mentalhealth.samhsa.gov/publications/allpubs/sma06-4055. Accessed September 1, 2006.

Substance Abuse and Mental Health Services Administration (SAMHSA): Transforming Mental Health Care in America. The Federal Action Agenda: First Steps. Rockville, MD, Substance Abuse and Mental Health Services Administration, 2005b. Available at: http://www.samhsa.gov/Federalactionagenda/NFC_intro.aspx. Accessed September 1, 2006.

Temkin T: Suicide and other risk monitoring in inpatient psychiatry. J Am Psychiatr Nurses Assoc 10:73–80, 2004

Thomas SP, Shattell M, Martin T: What's therapeutic about the therapeutic milieu? Arch Psychiatr Nurs 16:99–107, 2002

Volavka J, Nolan KA, Kline L, et al: Efficacy of clozapine, olanzapine, risperidone, and haloperidol in schizophrenia and schizoaffective disorder assessed with nurses observation scale for inpatient evaluations. Schizophr Res 76:127–129, 2005

Warelow P, Edward KL: Caring as a resilient practice in mental health nursing. Int J Ment Health Nurs 16:132–135, 2007

Welch M: Pivotal moments in the therapeutic relationship. Int J Ment Health Nurs14:161–165, 2005

Whittington D, McLaughlin C: Finding time for patients: an exploration of nurses' time allocation in an acute psychiatric setting. J Psychiatr Ment Health Nurs 7:259–268, 2000

Winston A, Rosenthal RN, Pinsker H: Introduction to Supportive Psychotherapy (Core Competencies in Psychotherapy series). Washington, DC, American Psychiatric Publishing, 2004

Wynn R: Staff's attitudes to the use of restraint and seclusion in a Norwegian university psychiatric hospital. Nord J Psychiatr 57:453–459, 2003

Zuckerman E: Finding, evaluating, and incorporating Internet self-help resources into psychotherapy practice. J Clin Psychol 59:217–225, 2003

CHAPTER 30

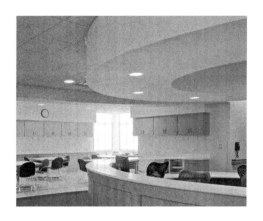

FINANCING OF CARE

Benjamin Liptzin, M.D.
Paul Summergrad, M.D.

The mechanisms used to finance inpatient psychiatric services have a major impact on the quantity, quality, and organization of care. The focus of this chapter is hospital psychiatry as it is practiced in the United States; therefore, financing mechanisms used in the United States will be emphasized. However, it is recognized that other countries may have very different ways to finance care, and much can be learned from the differences among systems of care in other countries.

History

In the eighteenth century, people with mental illness were labeled "insane" or "lunatics" and were generally cared for by their families or social groups. Those persons who could not be cared for by family were confined to jails if they were deemed to be dangerous or to poorhouses if they were unable to care for themselves. These institutions were funded by local governments, which encouraged communities to fund as little as possible so that poor persons would move from one community to another seeking shelter. According to Mora (1975), "the basic attitude of the general popula-

tion toward the mentally ill was uncharitable and punitive." In contrast, the Quakers in Philadelphia had a more humanitarian approach to the mentally ill. The provincial Assembly of Pennsylvania established the first general hospital in America in 1751 to be a "Hospital for the Relief of the Sick Poor of this Province and for the Reception and Cure of Lunaticks" (Mora 1975). When the Pennsylvania Hospital opened in 1756, mentally ill patients were admitted to the cellar. In 1796, a new wing was built just for the mental patients. The hospital was supported by public and private funds. In 1770, the colonial legislature of Virginia felt that poorhouses and jails were inadequate for the care of mentally ill persons and that it would be more equitable for the state, rather than local communities, to pay for their care. They established the first American asylum exclusively for the mentally ill, called "The Public Hospital for Persons of Insane and Disordered Minds," in Williamsburg. The facility, which opened in 1773, was designed to provide treatment for persons who had "curable mental illnesses" and who could ultimately be discharged to the community. Persons who were a threat to themselves or others as a result of their mental illness were also eligible for confinement.

Chronically mentally ill but harmless individuals were not thought to be appropriate for admission. The hospital had a physician on staff who was salaried, although the treatment mostly consisted of restraint use and unpleasant treatments designed to convince persons to change their behavior (William & Mary Crossroads Research Project 2001). "Treatments" included restraints, harsh drugs, cold plunge baths (via the ducking chair), bleeding, intimidation, cupping glasses, and blistering salves.

Early in the nineteenth century, a number of private institutions were established based on the experience of the York Retreat in England. Under the leadership of Samuel Tuke, the Quaker institution had an optimistic view of mental illness and provided a general atmosphere of kindness and sympathy that was referred to as "moral treatment." The Friends Asylum opened near Philadelphia in 1817. The McLean Asylum then opened in Charlestown, Massachusetts, in 1818 as part of the Massachusetts General Hospital. Like the Pennsylvania Hospital, the McLean Asylum saw the care of the sick and the insane as part of its charter. The Bloomingdale Asylum opened in New York under the auspices of the New York Hospital. The Hartford Retreat opened in 1824, the Brattleboro Retreat in 1836, and Butler Hospital in Providence opened in 1847. From 1825 to 1865, other states built public mental hospitals, including Georgia, Kentucky, New York, and South Carolina. For the next 100 years, patients with mental illness were treated in geographically separate institutions under the belief that "asylum" or refuge from the world would help heal their afflictions. Patients were cared for either in institutions funded by the state or in private institutions funded by their families or the generous contributions of philanthropic individuals. In the second half of the nineteenth century, state institutions admitted large numbers of immigrants judged to be mentally ill and in need of confinement. Given the pressures on state budgets, these institutions became overcrowded and were unable to deliver much in the way of treatment. Regardless of the exact form of financing, psychiatric hospital care became uniquely a state rather than a municipal or federal responsibility, a circumstance that has had important implications for the current organization of care.

Psychiatric Units in General Hospitals

In the 1930s, a few academic medical centers developed inpatient psychiatric services funded in part by grants from the Rockefeller Foundation (Summergrad and Hackett 1987). That development also recognized that some mentally ill patients had comorbid medical conditions that might require treatment and that medical or surgical patients treated at these institutions might require psychiatric inpatient care. At the time, there was no reliable source of funding for these units. When private health insurance was initiated in the mid-1930s, coverage for mental illness was generally excluded in the belief that these services were already provided by state mental institutions, which were funded by state tax dollars. The financing of psychiatric units in general hospitals changed dramatically with the enactment of Medicare and Medicaid in the 1960s. Medicare was developed as a federal program to provide universal health insurance coverage for persons older than 65 years but was later expanded to include younger persons who were disabled. Medicare paid for care in psychiatric units in general hospitals using the same cost-based reimbursement method used for other general hospital services. Medicaid was something of an afterthought, but it provided grants to states as a way of sharing in the cost of health care for poor people.

At the time Medicare and Medicaid were enacted, the inclusion of mental health coverage was considered progressive, given that many private health insurance plans continued to exclude such coverage. However, because of concerns that utilization would be difficult to control, both programs instituted special limitations on psychiatric coverage. Medicare limited care to 190 lifetime days in "mental hospitals," which included both state and private institutions but not general hospitals. Outpatient coverage for "nervous and mental conditions" was limited to $250 per year and was subject to a 50% copayment instead of the 20% copayment used for other medical conditions. Medicaid coverage to "institutions for mental disease" (IMD; i.e., hospitals in which more than 50% of discharges were psychiatric patients) was limited to persons younger than 22 and older than 64 years of age. Medicaid did not cover care for patients of all ages in general hospital psychiatric units.

Despite the funding's limitations, its availability led to a dramatic increase in the number of inpatient psychiatric beds in general hospitals. In 1970 there were 22,394 psychiatric beds in general hospitals with separate psychiatric services; by 1990 there were 53,479 (Center for Mental Health Services 2006). Annual admissions to these units increased as well, from 478,000 in 1969 to 959,893 in 1990. However, by 2002, the number of inpatient psychiatric beds in general hospitals had decreased to 40,202. The number of general hospitals providing psychiatric services also declined during this period, from 1,707 in 1998 to 1,285 in 2002 (Foley et al. 2006). Despite the recent reductions in psychiatric beds, the annual number of discharges with primary psychiatric diagnoses from general hospitals increased by approximately 35% between 1988 and 1994, from 1.4 to 1.9 million annual discharges. General hospitals increasingly replaced public mental hospitals as the primary institutions caring for publicly funded patients (Mechanic et al. 1998). This discharge trend continued between 1995 and 2002, especially in patients with serious mental illness, whose discharge rates from general hospitals increased by 34.7% during this time (Watanabe-Galloway and Zhang 2007). The number of beds in state and county mental hospitals declined dramatically over this 20-year period, from 413,066 in 1970 to 98,789 in 1990. The number of admissions declined as well, from 486,661 in 1969 to 276,231 in 1990. These trends toward deinstitutionalization had begun in the 1950s, as advocates criticized institutions for warehousing patients without providing treatment and state legislators saw an opportunity to reduce expenditures by discharging patients who no longer needed inpatient care. The development of psychotropic drugs to control or treat the symptoms of mental illness also facilitated the transfer of patients out of large state mental hospitals. Many of these patients showed up in the emergency rooms of their local community hospitals and were admitted there, either because they preferred those facilities or because they were unable to be readmitted to the state hospital that had discharged them.

Another trend that supported the development of units in general hospitals was the inclusion of psychiatric benefits in private health insurance coverage. By 1974, 95% of health insurance plans surveyed provided some coverage for hospital care of mental conditions (Reed 1975). This trend of increasing coverage under private health insurance led advocates in many states to successfully argue for "mandated coverage" of psychiatric care in all insurance plans regulated by the state.

Finally, general hospitals saw a marked reduction in the length of stay and, consequently, a decrease in bed utilization for medical and surgical patients as a result of the diagnosis-related group (DRG) payment system for Medicare and the use of a case rate by many private insurers for medical-surgical admissions. As a consequence, many community hospitals had empty beds, and opening a psychiatric unit was a way to fill some of those beds. Conversion to a psychiatric unit required little capital investment; given the increase in demand for those services, it made business sense for hospitals to do that. In addition, the expansion of insurance to the private sector and government programs brought increased numbers of patients into psychiatric care. Patients with mood disorders, comorbid medical and substance abuse illnesses, or dementing illnesses who might have never been cared for in the traditional state hospital system expanded the clinical range of patients treated in psychiatric units in general hospitals.

Private Psychiatric Hospitals

The increasing availability of coverage under public and private health insurance also led to increases in the number of beds and annual admissions to private psychiatric hospitals. In 1970 there were 14,295 beds; by 1990 this number had increased to 44,871. In 1969 there were 92,056 admissions to private psychiatric hospitals; in 1990 there were 406,522 such admissions (Center for Mental Health Services 2006). The enhanced availability of payment for these services encouraged the development of investor-owned psychiatric hospitals in addition to the small number of private nonprofit charitable institutions that had developed by the mid-nineteenth century.

Cost-Containment Pressures

Throughout the 1970s, overall expenditures under Medicare rose rapidly—faster than the original projections had predicted when the program was first enacted. As a result, Congress looked for ways to control the rise in expenditures. Public Law 98-21 mandated a new approach to hospital reimbursement using a pricing system linked to "diagnosis at discharge" (Iglehart 1982). On October 1, 1983, reimbursement was determined using a classification system that categorized diagnoses into 468 diagnosis-related groups. There was little or no previous experience using this approach for psychiatric care; therefore, Congress granted an exemption from this Prospective Payment System (PPS) for psychiatric hospitals and permitted psychiatric units in general hospitals to apply for an exemption. Congress asked the U.S. Department of Health and Human Services to report by the end of 1985 on the feasibility of including these facilities and specialty units in the Medicare PPS. Numerous studies were done, which concluded that available classification systems were poor predictors of resource use (Mitchell et al. 1987). Instead of including psychiatric patients in the DRG system, Medicare continued to reimburse psychiatric hospitals and exempt units in general hospitals under a system enacted by the Tax Equity and Fiscal Responsibility Act of 1982, which used complicated formulae and retrospective calculations to determine allowable costs and to set a target reimbursement rate per discharge irrespective of psychiatric diagnosis. This was in contradistinction to the DRG-based system for medical-surgical care, which, mirrored by the private insurance system, reduced payments for medical-surgical care, making psychiatric units and hospitals relatively more profitable and less competitive. The psychiatric cost-based reimbursement system remained in effect until the development of a PPS for psychiatric hospitals and exempt units mandated by the Balanced Budget Refinement Act of 1999, with phase-in of the new reimbursement rules starting January 1, 2005. The new PPS system has a base payment rate with adjusters for patient characteristics (e.g., age, psychiatric diagnosis, medical comorbidities) and facility characteristics (e.g., teaching status, presence of an emergency room, rural versus urban location). Despite Medicare data showing higher costs per case, often due to greater acuity and medical comorbidity in general hospital patients, the Medicare PPS for inpatient psychiatry is generally more favorable to freestanding hospitals (Centers for Medicare and Medicaid Services 2004). However, the new PPS does not fully account for costs of those patients cared for in general hospitals who have significant medical comorbidities or problems with activities of daily living (Drozd et al. 2006). While the initial version of the PPS system for psychiatry must, by statute, be budget-neutral overall, cost containment will depend on annual adjustments to the base rate and the behavior of providers. A rate adjustment below the increase in costs may save Medicare money but will disadvantage hospitals, whose operating margins will shrink as costs rise faster than reimbursement.

The Rise of Managed Behavioral Health Care

In contrast to Medicare's approach to cost containment, beginning in the 1980s private health insurance turned to specialized managed behavioral health companies subcontracted as so-called fourth-party payers

to manage their psychiatric benefits. These companies are often referred to as *carve-outs*. The growth of these companies occurred in response to rising expenditures as psychiatric care became less stigmatized and psychiatric benefits were included or improved in private health insurance as a result of consumer demand or state mandates. In addition, many primary private insurers did not have expertise in the management of psychiatric care. The carve-out companies responded to the complaints of insurance companies that reimbursed providers or the employers who purchased the insurance for their employees that psychiatric care was unstandardized and costs were growing rapidly. Just as experience with Medicare had taught people that psychiatric diagnosis did not predict resource use, purchasers were concerned that patients with similar diagnoses could remain in a hospital for stays that varied widely or could avoid hospitalization altogether. The carve-out companies developed programs of preadmission review and continued-care certification to control the utilization of psychiatric services, particularly on inpatient units. They developed review criteria (generally proprietary criteria that were kept secret from providers) and hired nonphysician reviewers to apply these criteria to approve or disallow inpatient admissions. Disallowals were supposed to involve a psychiatrist reviewer, and the provider was permitted to appeal an adverse determination. These review organizations avoided legal liability for any adverse outcomes that resulted from denied admissions or premature discharges by arguing that the clinician had the legal responsibility for admitting or discharging the patient, unlike the review organization, which was simply authorizing or denying payment. In addition to reviewing admissions and continued care, these carve-out companies negotiated rates with individual hospitals. Unlike Medicare, which had contracts with every hospital, often standardized by region, prevailing wage, and employment costs, these private for-profit companies could pick and choose what hospitals could have their contracts. As small carve-outs consolidated or were bought up by larger ones, these companies developed significant purchasing power. In many markets, their monopsony allowed them to dictate rates to hospitals. Hospitals frequently accepted rates below their costs, because not getting a contract would mean a loss of so much volume that the unit would have to be downsized or closed.

The effects of these carve-out companies on quality of care and patient outcomes has been difficult to measure. However, patient and provider dissatisfaction with these programs generated more complaints to state insurance regulators than any other area of health insurance. In part as a result of those complaints and because of uncertainty over the costs and benefits of these programs, many insurers began to bring the review of psychiatric care back into their core review activities rather than carving them out. Other considerations in this latter trend include the recognition of the high rates of medical and psychiatric comorbidity among patients with psychiatric illness. Patients with psychiatric illness often have undiagnosed or untreated medical illness and in severely ill populations die at higher rates from cardiovascular, pulmonary, and metabolic disorders than do age-matched controls (National Association of State Mental Health Program Directors 2006). In addition, substantial expenditures for psychopharmacological agents, often borne by the primary insurer rather than the carve-out payer, have led insurers to reclaim internal management of psychiatric services.

Medicaid

In the 1990s, state Medicaid programs also began to contract with these carve-out companies to manage their psychiatric benefits under special waivers from the U.S. Department of Health and Human Services. Medicaid rules define which services and hospitals are reimbursable (e.g., by nonallowance of payment in IMDs for patients ages 22–64 years). States can request modifications in traditional Medicaid payments (e.g., ability to admit patients of all ages to IMDs including private psychiatric hospitals, payments for residential or nonhospital emergency or community-based care). Waivers are quite variable among state programs, depending on the organization of the state mental health systems, and can be based on regional, county, or statewide programs. Because utilization of psychiatric services is generally significantly higher in the Medicaid population (especially in those considered disabled by their psychiatric illness) than in commercial populations, the organization of the Medicaid system has important implications for the overall system of care.

State Mental Health Systems

Because of the unique responsibilities that states bear for the direct provision of psychiatric services, the organization, budgeting, and interrelationship of state mental health systems with Medicaid and Medicare are unique components of hospital psychiatry. Prior to the 1930s, 96% of all psychiatric hospitalizations occurred in state or veterans hospitals. Large psychiatric hospitals, often set at some remove from major population centers, accounted for 25% of all hospital beds in the United States. Even as late as 1970, there were 413,066 psychiatric beds in state hospitals in the United States and 486,661 annual admissions (in 1969). By 2002, these figures had declined to 57,263 beds and 238,546 annual admissions.

State hospital systems vary greatly from state to state. In some states, state hospitals care only for those patients who require long-term care on transfer from general or private hospitals, in others, a county-based system provides acute psychiatric care in public hospitals. Some states run psychiatric emergency services in state facilities; other states have created mobile non-hospital-based emergency services. States have often modified their state-run systems in coordination with Medicaid waivers and have used state and federal funding streams from both Medicare and Medicaid programs to create more comprehensive systems of care.

Financial Effects of Changing Reimbursement

Partly as a result of the changes in reimbursement, the number of inpatient psychiatric beds has steadily declined since 1990. The number of beds in private psychiatric hospitals declined from 44,871 in 1990 to 25,095 in 2002. Beds on inpatient units in general hospitals were reduced from 53,479 in 1990 to 40,202 in 2002 (Center for Mental Health Services 2006). During the same time period, the number of available beds in state and county mental hospitals dwindled from 98,789 in 1990 to 57,263 in 2002. These changes may also reflect evolving approaches to treatment, as reliance has increased on outpatient, residential, or partial hospital services rather than inpatient programs and shorter lengths of stay for admitted patients. The shorter lengths of stay may have also led to more readmissions, because the total number of admissions increased in private psychiatric hospitals from 406,522 in 1990 to 477,395 in 2002, and in general hospital units from 959,893 in 1990 to 1,094,715 in 2002 (Center for Mental Health Services 2006).

As a result of the changes in reimbursement, operating margins for psychiatric hospitals and psychiatric units in general hospitals have been squeezed. Investor-owned psychiatric hospitals are no longer such attractive investments. Nonprofit psychiatric hospitals have struggled to stay in the black. As an example, McLean Hospital in Belmont, Massachusetts, has consistently been ranked as the best psychiatric hospital in the United States by the magazine *U.S. News & World Report*; yet it showed a loss from operations of $136,000 in 2001 and of $1,619,000 in 2003. It had surpluses of $190,000 in 2002, $282,000 in 2004, and $810,000 in 2005 (McLean Hospital Annual Reports [www.mclean.harvard.edu/about/annual/2002/operations.php]). Such results require substantial philanthropy to fund capital and keep the operations afloat.

Revenue Sources by Type of Hospital

An analysis of sources of revenue for different types of hospitals illuminates the financial challenges faced by these organizations. For private psychiatric hospitals the proportion of total revenue that came from patient fees, including private health insurance, decreased from 61.3% in 1990 to 42.7% in 2002. For general hospitals during this same time period, the decrease was from 36.5% to 31.5%. In contrast, for private psychiatric hospitals the proportion of total revenue from Medicaid increased dramatically, from 9.4% to 25.9%; the increase for Medicare revenue went from 10.8% to 18.2%. For general hospitals, Medicaid revenue was essentially unchanged from 1990 to 2002 (24.2% vs. 24.0%), but Medicare total revenue increased from 24.2% to 36.9%.

The Future Financial Viability of Inpatient Psychiatric Services

Given the trend of reimbursement increases that do not keep up with rising costs and a shift in revenue sources toward more publicly financed patients for whom reimbursement is typically less than for private patients, what can psychiatric services providers do to survive (Liptzin et al. 2007)? In strictly economic terms, there is likely to be a further reduction in the number of beds than has been the case since 1990. If reimbursement is not available to support the existing beds, more hospitals will be expected to close. At some point, the decrease in supply will fall below the demand for these services and reimbursement rates will

once again rise to encourage an expansion in the number of beds. Psychiatric units in general hospitals can be cross-subsidized by more profitable services in cardiology, oncology, or surgery. However, hospitals that need more beds for these profitable services may look to downsize, close, or move their inpatient psychiatric unit to an off-site location.

The American Hospital Association (2007) in a review of behavioral health care needs concluded: "As an important player in the continuum of care, hospitals that positively address behavioral health care needs will contribute to the more effective and efficient use of health care resources, while also helping to produce positive outcomes for patients and their communities." In contrast, investor-owned psychiatric hospitals will close if they do not generate the profits expected by their shareholders.

Psychiatric hospitals and services can also try to diversify into other lines of business that may be more profitable. However, historically, inpatient services generated the surpluses that allowed other less profitable services (e.g., emergency, consultation, and outpatient services) to survive. General hospitals may be able to use their contractual relationships with primary health insurers to negotiate better rates for their psychiatric services, especially as behavioral health carve-outs shrink. Psychiatric hospitals may then partner with general hospitals to divert less costly patients who do not need significant medical services away from general hospitals and thereby increase their volumes. Psychiatric services should participate in quality improvement programs that assure high quality to the process of care and excellent patient care outcomes (Institute of Medicine Committee on Crossing the Quality Chasm 2006). Pay For Performance systems could conceivably provide enhanced reimbursement to high-quality programs. Psychiatric services should also encourage patients who have benefited from psychiatric treatment, whether as inpatients or outpatients, to tell their stories publicly so that the stigma associated with psychiatric illness and its treatment can be reduced. Grateful patients should also be encouraged to provide philanthropic support to nonprofit psychiatric services.

References

American Hospital Association: Community hospitals: addressing behavioral health care needs. TrendWatch February 2007. Washington, DC, American Hospital Association, 2007

Centers for Medicare and Medicaid Services: 42 CFR Parts 412 and 413: Medicare program; prospective payment system for inpatient psychiatric facilities; final rule. Federal Register Vol 69, No 219. November 15, 2004

Center for Mental Health Services: Mental Health, United States, 2004 (DHHS Publ No. SMA-06-4195). Edited by Manderscheid RW, Berry JT. Rockville, MD, Substance Abuse and Mental Health Services Administration, 2006

Drozd EM, Cromwell J, Gage B, et al: Patient casemix classification for Medicare psychiatric prospective payment. Am J Psychiatry 163:724–732, 2006

Iglehart JK: Health policy report: the new era of prospective payment for hospitals. N Engl J Med 307:1288–1292, 1982

Institute of Medicine Committee on Crossing the Quality Chasm: Adaptation to Mental Health and Addictive Disorders: Improving the Quality of Health Care for Mental and Substance-Use Conditions. Washington, DC, National Academies Press, 2006

Liptzin B, Gottlieb GL, Summergrad P: The future of psychiatric services in general hospitals. Am J Psychiatry 164:1468–1472, 2007

Mechanic D, McAlpine DD, Olfson M: Changing patterns of psychiatric inpatient care in the United States, 1988–1994. Arch Gen Psychiatry 55:785–791, 1998

Mitchell JB, Dickey B, Liptzin B, et al: Bringing psychiatric patients into the Medicare prospective payment system: alternatives to DRGs. Am J Psychiatry 144:610–615, 1987

Mora G: Historical and theoretical trends in psychiatry, in Comprehensive Textbook of Psychiatry, 2nd Edition. Edited by Freedman A, Kaplan HI, Sadock BJ. Baltimore, MD, Williams & Wilkins, 1975, pp 1–75

National Association of State Mental Health Program Directors (NASMHPD) Medical Directors Council: Morbidity and Mortality in People With Serious Mental Illness. Alexandria, VA, National Association of State Mental Health Program Directors, 2006. Available at: http://www.nasmhpd.org/general_files/publications/med_directors_pubs/Technical%20Report%20on%20Morbidity%20and%20Mortaility%20-%20Final%2011-06.pdf. Accessed April 24, 2008.

Reed LS: Coverage and Utilization of Care for Mental Conditions Under Health Insurance–Various Studies, 1973–1974. Washington, DC, American Psychiatric Association, 1975

Summergrad P, Hackett TP: Alan Gregg and the rise of general hospital psychiatry. Gen Hosp Psychiatry 9:439–445, 1987

Watanabe-Galloway S, Zhang W: Analysis of US trends in discharges from general hospitals for episodes of serious mental illness, 1995–2002. Psychiatr Serv 58:496–502, 2007

William & Mary Crossroads Research Project: Brief History of Eastern State Hospital and the Treatment of Mental Illness in America. Available at: http://www.esh.dmh-mrsas.virginia.gov/crossroads/history.htm. Accessed April 24, 2008.

CHAPTER 31

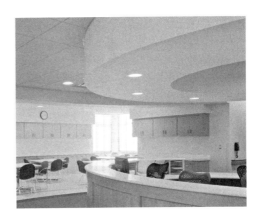

RISK MANAGEMENT

Marilyn Price, M.D.
Patricia R. Recupero, J.D., M.D.

Inpatient psychiatric facilities share risk management and patient safety concerns with general medical and surgical hospitals. When a patient is evaluated in the general emergency department or urgent care setting, clinicians seek to determine whether the patient's life is in immediate danger, whether the patient's illness poses any risk to others, and how the treatment team may help to improve the patient's condition. Similarly, in the psychiatric acute care setting, the clinical team must assess how the patient's safety can be ensured, whether the patient poses any danger to himself/herself or others, and how the patient can best be stabilized so that treatment may be effective. Many of the risk management concerns found in general hospitals are pertinent to hospital psychiatry including ensuring patient safety and quality improvement, preventing and managing adverse events, preventing staff misconduct toward patients, and complying with accreditation standards and the relevant laws.

However, there are areas that pose unique challenges for freestanding psychiatric hospitals and psychiatric units within general medical hospitals. These special issues for psychiatric facilities are manifest from the moment the patient is evaluated for admission. When a patient first presents for assessment, the team must determine whether the patient requires an inpatient level of care, and if so, whether the patient will be admitted on a voluntary or an involuntary basis. Involuntary civil commitment carries special implications for risk management. In general medical treatment, patients whose health status might pose a danger to others are typically identifiable through standardized tests for infectious diseases, and many notification procedures and precautions have become standardized. In contrast, in psychiatry, determining whether or not a particular patient poses a danger to himself or herself or others can be very difficult, but the duty to protect nonetheless still applies. In general medicine, if a patient elopes from the hospital or leaves against medical advice, the liability risk to the physician and hospital may be minimal. Psychiatric patients, however, may suffer from impaired judgment as a result of their mental illnesses, and an elopement or discharge against medical advice may not be a rational decision for which the patient bears the sole responsibility. Suicide, violence, and patients' legal

411

rights are significant concerns for risk reduction in hospital psychiatry. This chapter will discuss several prospective and retrospective risk management practices relevant to such scenarios.

Risk Management Techniques: A Culture of Patient Safety

Reducing risk to patients who are hospitalized in a psychiatric facility is best accomplished within a "culture of patient safety" (Murphy et al. 2007). This philosophy signifies that there is an institutional commitment to patient safety and quality improvement that encourages all members of the staff to become agents of change. It also implies that for questions of patient safety, the hierarchical environment is abandoned for one in which all members of the staff are encouraged to point out vulnerabilities in the system (Murphy et al. 2007). Achieving a culture of patient safety may require changing the guiding set of values of the organization in order to embrace this new approach. Otherwise, it becomes difficult to apply new policies, procedures, or practices that conflict with the existing organizational culture. Traditionally, physicians have considered risk management issues at the level of the care of an individual patient; they are concerned about suicide and violence risk assessment, medication side effects or errors, and accurate diagnosis. In contrast, hospitals have often approached risk management reactively, responding to a crisis by identifying the individual thought to be responsible, in what has been referred to as an *A-B-C* approach: "accuse, blame, and criticize."

Investigation of an incident should involve examination of the actions of the staff members involved, especially when the behavior has been willful, deliberate, or reckless or when an employee has violated well-established rules and regulations. However, this narrow focus on individual error precludes the assessment of organizational problems that could have contributed to the problem and which, if left unchecked, might lead to future incidents. Within a culture of safety, the focus turns to an examination of inherent weaknesses within the system that contributed to the medical error. The ultimate goal of the investigation is to implement modifications to prevent further injury. Although it is not exhaustive, the following list of issues could be considered: the behavioral or physical assessment process, patient observation procedures, the care planning process, the continuum of care, staffing levels, training programs for staff, and the competency of staff to perform assigned tasks (Joint Commission 2007a). One may also need to consider technology issues, the availability of information, the physical environment, and the security system. Problems in communication should be addressed, whether the difficulty rests in communication among staff members or communication with patients or family members. Some facilities have improved voluntary incident reporting through an intervention package that includes enhanced education, offering a range of reporting options and more feedback (Evans et al. 2007).

The organization must also respond proactively to safety concerns. The Joint Commission describes the process of risk management as "clinical and administrative activities undertaken to identify, evaluate, and reduce the risk of injury to patients, staff, and visitors and the risk of loss to the organization itself" (Joint Commission 2007a). Early indications of a problem within the system may come from analyses of incident reports, near misses, quality control data, occurrence trends, and patient complaints. Benchmarking with other institutions is another method of optimizing performance. In addition, implemented changes should be monitored on an ongoing basis and further modified, as appropriate (Martin and Federico 2007). The organization should appoint a patient safety officer to help oversee changes, paying special attention to issues that may affect the quality of care.

A culture of patient safety is enhanced by adherence to good clinical practices. These may include, but are not limited to, the following practices (Simon and Shuman 2007):

- Performing ongoing suicide risk assessments and violence risk assessments, including evaluating risk factors and protective factors
- Continually documenting all changes in a patient's clinical or risk status, as well as standardized communication of such changes to all staff members who will work with the patient
- Documenting treatment of modifiable risk factors
- Documenting communication among treatment team members about a patient's risk level
- Reviewing and documenting a patient's past history of hospital admissions
- Thoroughly documenting clinical reasoning, especially in regard to changes in observation or privilege status, detention for observation or safety, or changes in treatment regimen
- Involving family members in treatment (with the patient's permission) and building an alliance with the patient's family while remaining sensitive to protecting the patient's confidentiality

- Beginning discharge planning soon after admission
- Implementing strategies to decrease the risk of medication errors and adverse events
- Providing comprehensive and ongoing staff education, placing special emphasis on training for areas of increased risk (e.g., the proper use of de-escalation techniques, seclusion, and restraint; appropriate boundaries between staff and patients; addressing sentinel events and near misses)
- Improving communication and documentation at all levels of the organization, possibly through standardized communication methods (as discussed in this chapter)
- Modifying and enhancing discharge planning to address clinical risk and protective factors that affect discharge readiness (Simon and Shuman [2007] provide a very helpful table of discharge considerations for suicidal patients)

These practices represent, at best, a minimum of risk management practices that may help to reduce the risk of adverse events and improve patient safety.

The Institute of Medicine (IOM) Health Care Quality Initiative, begun in 1996, has brought nationwide attention to concerns about patient safety and quality in health care. The IOM's 1999 report *To Err Is Human: Building a Safer Health System* was a very influential review of medical errors and patient deaths resulting from preventable error in the health care system. The IOM issued another document in 2001, *Crossing the Quality Chasm,* which introduced suggestions for improving patient care. Following the publication of these reports and additional studies on patient safety and health care quality, there has been an increasingly stronger push toward standardized quality improvement, risk management, patient safety efforts, and evidence-based medicine throughout the health care system, including hospital psychiatry.

Reducing the incidence of medical errors is among the Joint Commission's national patient safety goals. Medication reconciliation and verification with outside pharmacies and other physicians involved in a patient's care are now essential functions of risk management in health care at all levels. Like other specialties, hospital psychiatry strives to avoid errors in dosing and administration of medicines to patients. Technological developments, such as automated electronic databases, promise to facilitate efforts to detect inappropriate dosages and drug–drug interactions, using either pharmacy management information technology or computerized physician order entry systems. The Joint Commission (2007a) calls for the use of two patient identifiers to improve the accuracy of patient identification; some hospitals may also use the more modern technology of radio frequency identification to avoid administering medication to the wrong patient. In hospital psychiatry settings, avoiding medical errors is especially pertinent when treating patients who are pregnant or have a compromised health status.

Coping With the Aftermath of a Sentinel Event

One of the most important aspects of risk management in hospitals is the manner in which the organization handles a *sentinel event* or a "near miss." Although changes should ideally be instituted before an adverse event occurs, in the aftermath of a sentinel event there is often an impetus to effect changes in the system. The Joint Commission defines a sentinel event as "an unexpected occurrence involving death or serious physical or psychological injury or the risk thereof. Serious injury specifically includes loss of limb or function. The phrase 'or risk thereof' includes any process variation for which a recurrence would carry a significant chance of a serious adverse outcome" (Joint Commission 2007b). The Joint Commission considers a patient suicide a sentinel event when the patient was housed around the clock, including suicide following elopement from such a setting. To demonstrate processes that are available to help identify areas of improvement following a sentinel event, the following fictional vignette is offered for illustrative purposes only:

> Mr. J, a 32-year-old married white male, was admitted for his first psychiatric hospitalization after presenting with depression and suicidal ideation and plan. Mr. J had recently separated from his wife and had been living with his brother. His brother was concerned because Mr. J had been drinking heavily and had missed several days at work. Mr. J's brother reported that Mr. J appeared depressed. He was not even showering or getting dressed most days. His brother brought Mr. J to the emergency room after he found a gun in the guest room. Mr. J admitted to his brother that he had purchased the gun 2 days prior to admission and had thoughts about killing himself. Mr. J revealed that he was spending most of his day thinking of suicide. He denied symptoms of psychosis. He agreed to hospitalization. Mr. J denied any previous psychiatric treatment or suicide attempts.
> Mr. J was started on an antidepressant. His family was very supportive, visiting daily, and Mr. J's brother and parents attended a family meeting. As

the hospitalization progressed, Mr. J reported to numerous staff members that he was feeling more hopeful. He stated that he could not consider suicide because of the effect that it would have on his family. He was very active and engaged in groups. Given the improvement in his clinical condition, the privilege level was advanced. A few hours later, a staff member performing checks found him trying to hang himself in the bathroom.

After Mr. J was discovered, his physical stabilization was the first priority. Fortunately, he did not sustain any permanent physical injury. However, in the event that Mr. J could not have been successfully resuscitated, staff members would have had to manage their own emotional responses to the patient's death while making difficult decisions. Family would have needed to be notified. Decisions would have had to be made about who should contact the family and what should be disclosed. Information about what happened would need to be gathered from staff and documented in the record (Leigh and Lagorio 2007). Administrators or directors of clinical units would have to be aware of any applicable mandates requiring reporting of adverse events. Additionally, Mr. J. may have indicated that he wished to have a family member or other significant other contacted in the event of an adverse event, such as any injury suffered during the attempt or as a result of other self-injury (e.g., cutting, head banging) or treatment.

It has been recommended that organizations develop a checklist to guide the response to such crises. The checklist may prove helpful to the clinical team members so that they may respond to the immediate needs of the family and staff members. The list allows for a systematic approach to information gathering, which can help identify the contributing factors that would need to be addressed immediately and the factors that could be studied further at a later date, using various risk management techniques (Leigh and Lagorio 2007). Risk management techniques like the checklist may be employed to improve patient safety even in "near miss" scenarios like the hypothetical vignette described above. Prudent risk management recognizes such near misses as opportunities to learn from problems and, if possible, to intervene before such problems lead to serious adverse events such as completed suicide.

An inpatient suicide, which would constitute a sentinel event, would require a comprehensive response. The checklist developed by Leigh and Lagorio (2007) is useful both for the early stages and for planning the organizational investigation. It directs staff to notify senior staff, management, and the critical response team and to ensure that documentation is complete before the medical record is secured. If equipment failure is a factor, the equipment is held and the chain of custody is maintained. Occurrence reports should be completed. The checklist also includes requirements for obtaining an accurate description of the occurrence and developing a detailed timeline, which would include response times. The names and positions of staff members who were present are gathered. Staff involved in the care of the patient would be interviewed.

The initial process includes assessing whether there were procedures in place to prevent the occurrence, and if so, why they failed in the instant case. The investigation would likely be performed under the auspices of a peer review committee. The initial analysis could indicate that immediate action must be taken. The checklist also offers suggestions for gathering information in anticipation of a *root cause analysis* (RCA; discussed below) and actions to be taken in determining whether there are system improvements that could mitigate risk.

One of the issues to be dealt with early in the process, if a serious adverse event has occurred, is its disclosure (Amori et al. 2003; Gallagher et al. 2003; Wojcieszak et al. 2006). Joint Commission Standard RI 2.90 requires that, when appropriate, patients and their families receive information about unanticipated outcomes. The National Quality Forum (NQF) has developed key elements of safe practices for disclosing unanticipated outcomes (NQF 2007). Appropriate information to disclose might include the facts of the event, a summary of the event analysis that allows informed decision making by the patient, an expression of regret and sympathy for the unanticipated outcome, and, when warranted, an apology if the outcome was the result of an error or systems failure (NQF 2007). The NQF directs institutions to integrate the disclosure process with patient safety and risk management activities. Institutions should establish background disclosure education and provide a system for disclosure coaching that should be available at all times. The institution should have a mechanism to provide emotional support for members of the community including administrators, health care workers, patients, and their families. The NQF also recommends developing performance tools to track and enhance disclosure (NQF 2007). In planning for a discussion with the patient or family after an adverse event, a decision must be reached about who would be involved and the timing, location, and extent of information that would be disclosed (Leigh and Lagorio 2007). Prior to making a disclosure, it may be appropriate to consult with legal counsel, insurance carriers, or risk management officers. Disclosures may not be warranted for near-miss scenarios.

There has been a growing endorsement by insurers and risk managers of the use of apology. Some states have taken action to mandate reporting of serious unanticipated outcomes. In 34 states, protection is now offered in the event of a malpractice suit through apology statutes that prevent introduction of the apology at trial. However, statutes differ as to the extent of information that is protected. Massachusetts, for example, narrowly defines what information is actually protected. In two-thirds of states, only the expression of regret is protected, while admissions of fault remain admissible at trial (Gallagher et al. 2007).

There is some empirical evidence foundation for the use of apology to mitigate risk of suit. Mazor et al. (2004) distributed eight questionnaires to study the effect of several variables affecting the patient response to disclosure. Patients had a more favorable response when physicians fully disclosed, accepted responsibility, and apologized rather than when information provided was vague or withheld. The severity of the outcome also influences the patient's response. However, none of the vignettes in their study resulted in patient death. Only in one scenario did full disclosure decrease the likelihood of seeking legal action. Kraman et al. (2002) found that a policy of full disclosure, including an apology and discussion of remedy and compensation, not only was the proper ethical response but also had financial ramifications. The authors noted that although the hospital they studied was in the top quarter of medical centers for number of torts claims filed, it was in the lowest quarter for malpractice payouts based on these claims.

The largest malpractice carrier in Colorado, COPIC, developed a program to facilitate disclosure. The *3Rs* program {(Recognize, Respond to, and Resolve patient injury)} includes linking disclosure to no-fault compensation for patients' out-of-pocket expenses up to $30,000. Because no fault is assigned, these disclosures are not reported to the National Practitioner Data Bank. The program provides disclosure training and coaching for physicians. There are exclusion criteria, such as death and clear negligence. The program is also not used when there has been a written demand or a complaint to a regulatory agency (Gallagher et al. 2007).

Research on the impact of disclosure to patients or family of unexpected outcomes is still in its infancy.

Some argue strongly for the use of apology (see, e.g., *Healing Words: The Power of Apology in Medicine*, 2nd Edition [Woods 2007]), whereas others suggest that there may be an increase in litigation as a result. Using conceptual modeling and statistical probability analyses, Studdert et al. (2007) found "the chances that disclosure [of medical error] would decrease either the frequency or cost of malpractice litigation to be remote. On the contrary, an increase in litigation volume and costs was highly likely." Regardless of the approach used, consultation with the appropriate insurance carrier immediately upon discovering a problem that may lead to litigation is essential.

Root Cause Analysis

General medical hospitals, as well as psychiatric facilities, are required to implement prospective and retrospective risk management techniques such as *root cause analysis* (RCA) and *failure modes and effects analysis* (FMEA; discussed below). Hospitals must have a sentinel event policy that allows a rapid response. After an occurrence such as the near-suicide of Mr. J. in the hypothetical vignette, the Joint Commission requires the hospital to undertake an analysis of the various systems that may have contributed to the event. The details of conducting an RCA are beyond the scope of this chapter; however, multiple resources are available at the Joint Commission Web site (www.jointcommission.org).

RCAs should be conducted after all events that have resulted in serious harm to a patient or that constitute a near miss of serious harm. The Joint Commission clearly states that not all sentinel events equate with medical error but, instead, that the process is designed to help identify problems that led to the event and to discover what changes *in process* may help to avoid repetitions of the event.

Each hospital is required to define a sentinel event in its own policies and procedures and to establish a procedure for conducting an RCA. Some of the events identified by the Joint Commission that may be applicable to a psychiatric hospital include the following:

> suicide of any patient receiving care, treatment and services in a staffed, around-the-clock care setting or within 72 hours of discharge; an abduction or elopement of any patient receiving care treatment services; a death in restraint; rape [any nonconsensual sexual conduct]; or surgery on the wrong patient or wrong body part [for example, electroconvulsive therapy on the wrong patient]. (Joint Commission 2007b)

There is currently no obligation to self-report a sentinel event. However, the Joint Commission requires that in accordance with the hospital's own policy, an RCA be conducted within 45 days of the event. Such a study is meant to focus on the underlying processes, not on individual actions; the outcome of an RCA is meant to be a systematic action plan to reduce the risk of similar events in the future. The plan must include "responsibility for implementation; oversight; pilot testing, as appropriate; time lines; and strategies for measuring the effectiveness of the actions" (Joint Commission 2007b). During a site visit, Joint Commission representatives may ask to review an RCA that has been conducted so that they may determine whether or not the analysis is acceptable. Acceptable analyses must include the following characteristics: a primary focus that is on systems and processes; an analysis that proceeds from special causes in clinical processes to more common causes and organizational processes; an attempt to "dig deeper" by asking "why" repeatedly; and identification of potential changes in the systems and processes that may avoid such events in the future.

The Joint Commission identifies multiple areas that must be investigated in order for an RCA to be considered credible:

- Behavioral assessment process
- Physical assessment process
- Patient identification process
- Patient observation procedures
- Care planning process
- Continuum of care
- Staffing levels
- Orientation and training of staff
- Competency assessment/credentialing
- Supervision of staff
- Communication with patient/family
- Communication among staff members
- Availability of information
- Adequacy of technological support
- Equipment maintenance/management
- Physical environment
- Security systems and processes
- Medication management

Not all of these processes will be relevant in every sentinel event; however, the institution is required to have a reasonable explanation for why analysis of a certain process is not relevant to the particular RCA being conducted. Any credible RCA must include a review of the literature and an analysis of how the literature applies to the case under consideration.

The Joint Commission also identifies 11 steps in the work plan for the completion of an RCA:

1. Organizing a team
2. Defining the problem
3. Studying the problem
4. Determining what happened and why
5. Identifying root causes
6. Designing and implementing an action plan for improvement
7. Designing improvements
8. Implementing the action plan
9. Measuring effectiveness of the action plan
10. Evaluating the implementation efforts
11. Communicating the results

Creating a checklist with benchmark dates and completion dates may be a useful tool in adhering to the 45-day timeline.

Although the patient (Mr. J) in the vignette described earlier did not sustain any permanent physical injury as a result of his attempted suicide, this event would be considered a sentinel event that justifies an RCA. In a 10-year summary of reported root causes of inpatient suicides, the Joint Commission identified environmental safety and security, patient assessment, orientation and training, and communication failures as the most common root causes (Joint Commission 2007b). Other areas identified as problematic include staffing, availability of information, continuum of care, care planning, leadership, procedural compliance, and, least likely, organizational culture. Although the vignette does not provide sufficient information to identify the root cause(s) of Mr. J's attempted hanging, one might speculate that in the interval after the family meeting, he had had an acrimonious telephone conversation with a family member and that the argument had heightened his feelings of hopelessness. If one staff member had been aware of this important event but failed to communicate it to other staff members, a systems issue or a training issue might well be identified. In addition, one must always evaluate the safety of the environment and whether or not the appropriate safety measures (e.g., breakaway bars in the bathroom) were in place. A review of the literature might reveal areas for potential improvement.

Failure Modes and Effects Analysis

While RCA approaches risk reduction by a thorough retrospective assessment of an adverse event, FMEA uses a prospective approach to eliminate or decrease risk (Battles et al. 2006). The goal of FMEA is to evaluate the vulnerabilities inherent in a process *before* an adverse outcome occurs and to implement modifications in order to decrease or eliminate potential injury to patients or staff (DeRosier et al. 2002). The Joint Commission requires that hospitals adopt prospective approaches such as FMEA when addressing patient safety concerns (Joint Commission on Accreditation of Health Care Organizations 2003).

FMEA was initially used as a strategy to anticipate and mitigate risk in manufacturing. In this model, a risk priority number was calculated through a three-variable equation in which each variable was assigned a score between 1 and 10. This process was used by medical device manufacturing firms to prevent problems or system failures (Cody 2006; DeRosier et al. 2002).

FMEA uses a systematic approach to identify failure modes, their frequency, and the associated probabilities of the consequences of the failure. The premise of FMEA is that individual failures within the process could be identified to prevent an adverse outcome. During FMEA, a process map and/or a table format is used to identify the contributing system components, to detect the ways that different elements in a system can fail, and to provide an estimate of how these failure points might affect the process and lead to a negative outcome (Battles et al. 2006).

Recent studies have demonstrated the positive benefits of implementing changes derived from FMEA in health care applications, such as protection of human subjects in research, improved safety of intravenous drug administration and trauma treatment, and safer administration of chemotherapy (Adachi and Lodolce 2005; Cody 2006; Day et al. 2006; Robinson et al. 2006; Sheridan-Leos et al. 2006; Spath 2003; Wetterneck et al. 2006; Woodhouse et al. 2004).

In an attempt to make the FMEA process more applicable to the health care setting, a hybrid model was developed by the Department of Veterans Affairs National Center for Patient Safety's Prospective Risk Analysis System and the Tenet HealthSystem (DeRosier et al. 2002). This new approach, which combines the features of FMEA, hazard analysis and critical control point, and RCA, has been termed *health care failure mode and effect analysis* (HFMEA) (DeRosier et al. 2002). As implemented by the Department of Veterans Affairs, the HFMEA process consists of five steps. Step 1 is selecting a high-risk or high-vulnerability area for study. Step 2 concerns the selection of a multidisciplinary team, including a subject-matter expert, an advisor, and a team leader. During Step 3, the team develops a process-flow diagram and adds the subprocesses.

If the process is complex, the team can decide to limit the scope to one aspect of the process. Step 4 involves conducting a hazard analysis. This includes identification of failure modes, assessment of the severity and probability of the potential failure mode, and the assignment of a Hazard Score on the Hazard Scoring Matrix. A decision tree is used to determine which of the failure modes merits further action. Consideration is given to criticality, absence of effective control measures, and lack of detectability. During Step 5, actions and outcome measures are planned (DeRosier et al. 2002). Several community hospitals have further refined HFMEA and have adopted what is termed *failure mode effects and criticality analysis* to reduce prospective risks (Coles et al. 2005).

Potential areas that FMEA might address within the psychiatric hospital include credentialing of physicians, de-escalation techniques, seclusion and restraint, participation in treatment plans by patients, prevention of medication errors, medication reconciliation, management of missed appointments, suicide prevention within the facility, prevention of patient self-injury, and elopement prevention. Choosing a process and examining it in advance may help to identify new best practices that can be implemented and, if possible, prevent or reduce risk to both patients and staff.

Prospective approaches such as FMEA offer a real opportunity to identify areas of vulnerability and institute changes that will decrease risk. In the hypothetical case example of Mr. J, the RCA might have revealed that information about a new stressor was not communicated to other members of the team so that the increased risk was not identified. The group may have concluded that barriers to effective communication needed to be studied further. In addition, FMEA could have identified other areas of vulnerability with regard to communication among staff members on the unit. There might have been a decision to implement standardized methods of communication, such as the *situation, background, assessment, and recommendation* method (SBAR; described below), to ensure that the appropriate information would be communicated in an effective and standardized manner.

Improved Patient Safety Through Communication

Communication problems in the health care setting contribute substantially to medical errors and associated legal risks. Among the strategies for quality improvement and error reduction set forth by the Institute of Medicine in its 2001 report *Crossing the Quality Chasm* are recommendations for improved communication between clinicians and patients, as well as improved communication among different clinical service providers.

Hospitals have begun implementing communication improvement strategies as part of efforts to improve patient safety and reduce medical errors. Improving communication among health care workers as well as between patients and staff are among the goals identified by the Joint Commission for improving patient safety (www.jointcommission.org); there is some evidence that approaches targeted at both forms of communication can enhance patient safety (Stebbing et al. 2007a). The Joint Commission lists communication as Goal 2 in its Patient Safety Goals for 2007; more specific recommendations are available through the Joint Commission Web site. Patient handoffs have been identified as one of the more problematic preventable medical errors, and the Joint Commission recommends standardizing the process for handoffs. One process that has shown some promise for improving handoff communication is appreciative inquiry, a strengths-based approach that emphasizes building on and learning from handoffs that have been effective in the past (Shendell-Falik et al. 2007).

Some health care organizations have adopted communication models or methods used in other high-risk settings, such as air and space travel, nuclear power plants, and the military; one such model gaining favor in medical settings, and specifically suggested by the Joint Commission, is the SBAR method of communication (Morin 2007). In the SBAR model, important communications must be conducted in a standardized format. First, one communicates the situation (e.g., vital signs and presenting complaint). Second, one provides information about the background (e.g., the patient's mental status, known medical conditions, and medications taken). Third, one expresses a preliminary assessment of the problem; if a particular diagnosis or syndrome is suspected, this should be expressed as part of the assessment. Finally, one posits a recommendation, such as suggested tests to be ordered and any emergency interventions or precautions that may be required.

In the psychiatric hospital setting, continued screening for suicide risk and communication about changes in suicide risk status or factors are crucial aspects of patient safety improvement. An initial suicide risk assessment must be conducted, with results com-

municated to all staff who will be involved in the care of a patient. Whenever the patient's status changes (e.g., immediately prior to discharge, after alterations in the observation level) or if other risks or precipitating factors change (e.g., death of a loved one), the patient's suicide risk should be reassessed and any changes in the level of risk should be communicated promptly to all staff members who will be working with the patient.

This discussion offers only several examples of the numerous methods and models for improving communication in the health care setting. Quality improvement efforts that target communication through systemwide administrative changes serve an important risk management function.

Boundaries and Staff Supervision

The study of boundary theory has evolved, in part, through attempts to reduce the incidence of therapist sexual misconduct toward patients. Gutheil and Gabbard (1993) defined a *boundary* as the "edge" of appropriate professional behavior. A "boundary violation" occurs when a clinician's behavior crosses the line into unacceptable conduct. Sexual contact between a clinician and a patient, which is proscribed by clinical ethics, constitutes a boundary violation. Boundary theory also attempts to identify behaviors that, while not constituting full boundary violations, may nonetheless be considered steps down a "slippery slope" toward more egregious boundary violations (Gutheil and Gabbard 1998). Boundary violations are among the most common reasons for malpractice suits against psychiatric treatment providers, second only to patient suicide (Norris et al. 2003). In the clinical setting, countertransference may lead staff to experience strong feelings of anger or affection toward patients. Helping staff to manage these feelings effectively, before they become boundary concerns, is an important step in managing risk on the unit. Uncontrolled anger may result in a staff assault against a patient, and feelings of attraction or affection may lead to staff sexual misconduct toward a patient. Patients have been harmed and treatment providers have been successfully sued as a result of both problems. Gutheil and Simon (2002) note that financial exploitation of patients may be more common than sexual misconduct; boundary training should address both sexual and nonsexual boundaries.

Helping staff to manage countertransference begins with staff education and training. Administrators should provide adequate training in what is and is not acceptable conduct toward patients, as well as tips on how to recognize the early warning signs of boundary problems (Epstein and Simon 1990). Keeping a record of staff training in human resources files will serve to document the training. Improving professionalism among direct care as well as support staff not only will help to lessen legal risks for the provider but also should result in improved patient care and a more positive treatment experience for the patient and his or her family.

Staff education should also address the symptoms and behaviors exhibited by patients with different psychiatric illnesses so that staff members will be able to recognize manifestations of each patient's illness and report back to the treating physician rather than reacting. For example, a manic patient may become hypersexual and flirtatious toward staff or other patients; staff members should be trained to recognize such behavior as a symptom of the patient's mania and should report this to the patient's psychiatrist when appropriate. Staff should also be trained in recognizing agitation and employing successful nonrestrictive de-escalation techniques. This will minimize the need for seclusion and restraint as well as reduce the risk of harm to the patient or to other patients or staff on the unit.

Staff selection and careful supervision are also important ways to reduce the risk of boundary or misconduct problems. Thorough background and reference checks are now required for employees or volunteers who will be working with patients or working on treatment units. Supervisors should be trained to recognize and address boundary violations as well as behavior that may lead to boundary violations. Staff should have a means by which to anonymously report known or suspected staff misconduct so that all potential boundary problems are recognized early and addressed before escalating into an assault or serious misconduct. The facility should have a policy in place for reporting and dealing with an assault or misconduct if such an incident does occur. This policy should be consistent with laws and regulations mandating reporting of adverse outcomes that govern the facility's operations. These rules may vary from one treatment center to another, and it may be necessary to seek assistance from a legal professional to ensure compliance with the relevant laws or rules.

Boundaries must be appropriately maintained even after the patient is discharged. Institutions have been sued for the misconduct of mental health technicians if there has been inappropriate contact between the technician and a former patient. One way to further reduce the risk of boundary-related problems, both during the inpatient stay and following discharge, is to provide education not only to staff but also to patients about sexual boundaries, dual relationships, and respect for nonsexual boundaries. Such training should be documented.

Civil Commitment

Hospitalization of psychiatric patients can occur on either a voluntary or involuntary basis. Voluntary admissions are further classified as either informal or conditional. A patient admitted on an informal voluntary basis retains the right to sign out at any time unless the criteria for commitment are met. A patient hospitalized under a conditional voluntary basis would need to provide notice of "an intent to leave," giving the hospital the opportunity to assess the need for involuntary commitment or to consider alternatives (Simon and Shuman 2007; Winick 2005). The issue of whether a psychiatric patient is competent to apply for a voluntary admission was addressed by the Supreme Court in *Zinermon v. Burch* (1990; Appelbaum 1990). The Court noted, "The very nature of mental illness makes it foreseeable that a person needing mental health care will be unable to understand any proffered explanation and disclosure of the subject matter." In addition, the Court recommended that the state establish a mechanism for assessing the competence of persons presenting for admission, explaining, "A person who is willing to sign forms but is incapable of making an informed decision is, by the same token, unlikely to benefit from the voluntary patient's statutory right to question discharge."

When a patient presents to the hospital in need of care, the hospital may obtain an emergency certification for a specified time period (usually 48–72 hours, but sometimes as long as a week, depending on the duration permitted by the state law) to help stabilize the patient. After the initial emergency period, a civil commitment may be initiated if it is determined that the patient will need continued care at the inpatient level. Unlike emergency certification, civil commitment requires court proceedings. The question of whether or not one can accept a health care proxy or an advance directive authorizing admission when the patient does not consent is a very unclear area of the law. States have varying rules regarding whether an appointed guardian can be authorized to consent to the patient's treatment or admission. Even more stringent rules may apply for specific forms of treatment, such as electroconvulsive therapy. If a question arises as to the legality of involuntary admission or treatment, it may be necessary to consult with legal counsel.

Civil commitment of a person who is mentally ill is a deprivation of freedom from detention. The justification for this deprivation is grounded in either the state's *parens patriae* authority or in its police power. The *parens patriae* right is derived from the state's interest in protecting citizens who are unable to care for themselves due to an infirmity such as a mental illness (Simon and Shuman 2007; Winick 2005). Police power allows the state to act to protect its citizens from harm; commitment is justified when a person who is mentally ill poses a danger to others (Simon and Shuman 2007; Winick 2005).

Involuntary hospitalization does not inherently allow involuntary treatment absent an emergency. Most states have their own procedures for substituted judgment in the event that a patient is deemed legally incompetent to consent to treatment. It is important to note that although a patient may, in a clinician's judgment, lack the capacity to make an informed decision, the patient may nonetheless retain the legal right to refuse treatment. The law draws a distinction between the clinical notion of *capacity* to consent and the legal status of *competence* to consent. Legal proceedings such as competency hearings are usually necessary in order to subject patients to involuntary treatment. Whenever possible, the clinician should allow the patient to fully participate in treatment decisions; when treatment is voluntary, the treatment alliance between the provider and the patient will help to facilitate better outcomes.

Although there is variability in the state statutes, there are common fundamental characteristics in the criteria and justification for commitment. Statutes require that commitment be based on the presence of a mental illness, which can be poorly defined. For example, in Ohio, mental illness is defined as a substantial disorder of thought, mood, or emotion that substantially impairs one's capacity for self-control, judgment, and discretion in the conduct of personal affairs and social relations (Ohio Rev. Code Ann. §5233.02[a] [b], 2003). The definition of mental illness in some states may also specifically exclude certain disorders. In Kansas, civil commitment for mental illness cannot be based solely on a diagnosis of "alcohol or chemical substance abuse; antisocial personality disorder; mental retardation; organic personality disorder; or organic mental disorder (Kan. Stat. Ann. §59–2946, 2003).

States also require that the impairment related to the mental illness result in one of the justifications for civil commitment. The typical criteria for commitment are *dangerousness to self or others* and *inability to provide for basic needs* (Simon and Shuman 2007). Some commitment statutes have specific criteria, such as *grave disability, refusing treatment and in need of hospitalization, destructive toward property,* and *lacking capacity to make rational treatment decisions* (Simon and Shuman 2007; Winick 2005). In most states, including Massachusetts, the commitment statutes introduce the concept of the "least restrictive alternative" (Mass. Gen. L. ch.123, §1, 2003). Winick (2005) has compiled a summary of the civil commitment statutes of all 50 states, which allows comparison of statutes. Some states have specialized commitment laws that govern involuntary treatment for alcohol or substance use disorders, treatment of minors with mental illness, and commitment of sexually violent predators. These issues are of limited applicability to general inpatient psychiatry. Likewise, the issue of outpatient commitment orders (e.g., Kendra's Law in New York State) is beyond the scope of this chapter, although information on this topic may be useful in discharge planning.

There are other consequences for patients involuntarily committed to a psychiatric facility rather than admitted on a voluntary basis. Many states now have statutes that restrict the access of persons with mental illness or substance abuse from possessing, purchasing, registering, or retaining a firearm or obtaining a firearm license. Some states have established a mental health database that is accessible to police. Norris et al. (2006) noted that as of 2005, 22 states had a mental health database, some maintained by departments of mental health and others by the state law enforcement agency. Some states require notification from the hospital when a person has been involuntarily committed, whereas other states obtain this information from court records of commitment proceedings (Norris et al. 2006). In Massachusetts, the names of persons committed to state psychiatric hospitals are recorded in a mental health database and are accessed during the firearm licensing process (Mass. Gen. L. ch.140, §129[b], 2004; et seq., 269–10). In the aftermath of the Virginia Tech tragedy, further limitations on access to firearms following mandated (or perhaps even voluntary) mental health treatment may be implemented. The passage of the National Instant Criminal Background Check Improvement Act was intended to expand reporting practices of states to the National Instant Criminal Background Check System (NICS) by providing significant financial incentives for releasing relevant records, including those contained in state mental health databases (Price and Norris 2008).

Seclusion, Restraint, and De-Escalation Techniques

The inappropriate use of manual restraint and seclusion in treatment settings has contributed to injuries, deaths, lawsuits, and negative public opinion toward the mental health profession. In the often-cited case *Youngberg v. Romeo* (1982), the mother of a mentally disabled man sued officials at the hospital where he was involuntarily committed, because the man had been subjected to prolonged periods of restraint as a result of his physically assaultive behavior. The Supreme Court ultimately ruled that reasonable clinical judgment should guide any decision to use seclusion and restraint but that patients should be afforded an opportunity to learn how to reduce the need for such restrictive interventions. In modern practice, patients are typically invited to identify in advance, as early in treatment as possible, their preferred methods for stabilizing or calming down. Alternative interventions, such as playing soothing music, sitting in a quiet room, and removing excessive sensory stimuli, should be offered to patients as first-line approaches to de-escalation, and patients should indicate which methods they prefer. Patient preferences for de-escalation interventions should be updated periodically by clinical unit staff, and a form documenting the patient's wishes should be included in the patient's chart. Following any incident of seclusion or restraint, the patient should be debriefed and afforded an opportunity to provide feedback to staff about the incident and what may be improved in the event of future incidents.

Joint Commission standards for seclusion and restraint call for specific policies and procedures to be followed, including mandatory debriefing after the use of either seclusion or restraint. Furthermore, hospitals are required to report to the Centers for Medicare and Medicaid Services any patient death occurring while a covered patient is in seclusion or restraint. Federal rules for seclusion and restraint may be found at 42 CFR 482.13(f). It bears noting that Joint Commission standards and federal guidelines may differ, and both are subject to ongoing and periodic changes. Hospitals are expected to remain up-to-date and informed with respect to the standards in place at any given time. Administrators should be aware that requirements may conflict; in such cases, seeking assistance from legal counsel or risk management officers may be appropriate.

Additional requirements may apply for the use of so-called chemical restraints. The use of psychotropic medicines to forcibly subdue a patient, independent of their therapeutic benefit, may be considered a type of restraint, as such use restricts the patient's freedom (see, e.g., Mossman 2002). On the other hand, the use of a neuroleptic to treat an individual's symptoms of psychosis may be considered a therapeutic use when used to treat psychosis rather than to control aggressive behavior. Documenting the rationale for the use of prn medications and monitoring patient response to chemical restraint are critical steps. Care must be taken to avoid the use of medication as a punitive measure, and all uses as a chemical restraint must meet appropriate evaluation, clinical, and documentation standards.

To reduce risk, psychiatric hospitals should endeavor to reduce the use of seclusion and restraint whenever possible and should consider implementing a program to continuously monitor and decrease the use of seclusion and restraint. Research has shown that effective de-escalation and behavioral management strategies can successfully reduce the incidence of violent behavior in treatment settings as well as improve relationships between staff and patients (Bisconer et al. 2006; Dean et al. 2007; Donat 2005; Hunter and Love 1996; Schreiner et al. 2004). Seclusion and restraint should be used only when required for legitimate safety concerns and when other de-escalation techniques have failed. The organization must follow the relevant rules and regulations for notifying family members or significant others about the use of seclusion and restraint, particularly in the treatment of children or adolescents. Adult patients may also indicate that they wish to have family members or others contacted in the event that seclusion or restraint becomes necessary; patients' wishes for such notification should be respected.

In 2003, the American Psychiatric Association, American Psychiatric Nurses Association, and National Association of Psychiatric Health Systems, with support from the American Hospital Association, published a resource guide on strategies for behavioral health care providers to reduce the use of seclusion and restraint in treatment settings, including tips for successful de-escalation (American Psychiatric Association 2003). The guide *Learning From Each Other: Success Stories and Ideas for Reducing Restraint/ Seclusion in Behavioral Health* is available online at the American Psychiatric Association's Web site (www.psych.org). The guide notes that change must be systemic and offers case studies from other organizations that have successfully implemented such changes. Included in the guide are suggestions for staff training, milieu improvement, risk assessments, individualized treatment plans, tips for documentation, and information about debriefing and improving de-escalation techniques. The appendix to the guide is a resource document with additional tips and tools, including examples of forms that may be useful for ensuring that documentation complies with Joint Commission and Centers for Medicare and Medicaid Services standards.

Tarasoff Duty

The *Tarasoff* duty to protect/warn third parties stems from the 1974 and 1976 California Supreme Court decisions in *Tarasoff v. Regents of the University of California* (1976). The well-publicized and frequently discussed case involved a lovesick young man who had disclosed to his treating psychologist an intention to kill an unnamed person identifiable as the young woman he had been pursuing, an intention he later carried out in what has since become a landmark case in mental health law. (For a detailed summary of the case and the court decisions, see, e.g., Mossman 2006.) The victim's parents sued the psychologist, the psychiatrists, and their employer for failing to detain the patient and failing to warn them of the danger.

In 1974, the California Supreme Court found that a mental health professional has a duty based on the special relationship between the patient and the psychotherapist: "When a doctor or a psychotherapist, in exercise of his professional skill and knowledge, determines or should determine, that a warning is essential to avert danger arising from the medical or psychological condition of his patient, he incurs a legal obligation to give that warning" (*Tarasoff I*). This decision, which came to be known as the *Tarasoff I* ruling, prompted the American Psychiatric Association to file an *amicus curiae* brief (summarized in *Tarasoff II*), arguing that psychotherapists cannot reliably predict future violence and that issuing a warning would be detrimental to the confidentiality that forms the cornerstone of the psychotherapist–patient relationship. The court reheard the case, and the 1976 *Tarasoff II* decision established a duty to protect, with a warning determined as one of the ways to satisfy this duty (Weinstock et al. 2006).

In response to the *Tarasoff* decisions and subsequent decisions expanding the *Tarasoff* duty, there was a move in California and in other states to more clearly define and limit the duty by statute. California Civil Code 43.92 served to confine the duty to the sit-

uations "where the patient has communicated to the psychotherapist a serious threat of physical violence against a reasonably identifiable victim or victims." It also provided that the "duty shall be discharged by the psychotherapist making reasonable efforts to communicate the threat to the victim or victims and to a law enforcement agency." Weinstock et al. (2006) recently reviewed these statutes, finding that 27 states have passed laws concerning the duty to protect third parties from harm by patients. These statutes are not uniform, and some allow for alternative actions other than warning. There are 9 states, along with the District of Columbia, that allow but do not mandate warning; 13 states lack a statute. The states of Virginia and Texas do not recognize a *Tarasoff* duty. In Minnesota and Ohio, the threat of harm need not be communicated by the patient himself or herself in order to trigger the duty to protect; such notice may come from collateral informants, such as the patient's family members (Weinstock et al. 2006).

Recent case law in California also suggests that the therapist's duty to protect may be triggered by information obtained from collateral informants. In two separate suits heard by the California Court of Appeals, the parents of a man murdered by a psychiatric patient sued the patient's therapist (*Ewing v. Goldstein* 2004) and the hospital that had discharged the patient a day prior to the murder (*Ewing v. Northridge Hospital Medical Center* 2004). The court ruled that a credible communication from the patient's father about his son's threat to kill the victim was sufficient to trigger the therapist's and the hospital's duty to warn the intended victim and law enforcement, and that the failure to communicate this warning could potentially be deemed negligence for which both the therapist and the hospital might be held liable.

In response to the *Ewing* decisions, there has been legislative action in California, an amendment to California Civil Code 43.92, AB 733, to clarify the duty as a duty to protect that can be discharged by warning, but that allows other measures to protect the potential victim. The reason for such legislation rests, in part, on the court's decision to impose an explicit requirement to *warn* on the therapist, who had sought to *protect* the victim by arranging for his patient's hospitalization. The amendment does not change the impact of the decision of the *Ewing* court with respect to credible threats communicated by collateral informants such as close relatives.

In duty-to-protect situations, Simon and Shuman (2007) recommend addressing three factors: 1) systematic assessment of the threat, 2) identification of the potential victim, and 3) implementation of preventive measures to decrease the risk. The systematic risk assessment would involve obtaining a history about past or present violence and inquiring about violence risk factors. Violence risk factors may be individual (e.g., threats against a specific person, previous history of violence, accessibility of the victim, motive); clinical (e.g., diagnosis, psychotic symptoms, ability to control anger, syntonic versus dystonic violent behavior, nonspecific threats, history of abuse, substance abuse, impulsivity); interpersonal (e.g., ongoing therapeutic alliance, strength and value attached to personal relationships, fear of control by others); situational (e.g., presence of a specific stressor; housing and employment stability; availability of lethal means, particularly firearms); and epidemiological (e.g., age, gender, base rates within the sociocultural group, violence base rates). Simon and Shuman (2007) provide a table to guide the identification of both risk and protective factors when determining an overall risk rating.

Although the duty to protect usually applies only to an identifiable victim, some courts have broadened the interpretation to a foreseeable risk of harm to the public at large or to threats to property rather than just person. The duty arises in the treatment of both inpatients and outpatients. Psychotherapists need to consider the specific statute within their state when considering the options for discharging the duty. Warning the victim and notifying the police are options, but there is also a responsibility to properly evaluate the patient for more intensive treatment. Hospitalization and treatment of the underlying disorder may be more effective measures, and there can be liability for a failure to hospitalize the patient when indicated. Simply warning the victim may be insufficient. In issuing a warning, a phone call is appropriate, especially when the patient is an outpatient or when the patient elopes from the unit and time is of the essence. The record should reflect that there has been a careful violence risk assessment and should provide the reasoning for breaching confidentiality, including the specific threats and the timing of the threats by the patient. The note should also document the timing of the warning and the content of the warning. If the potential victim cannot be reached, it may be necessary to contact persons who are close to the victim. When issuing a warning is necessary, the clinician should discuss with the patient the need to warn and may even invite the patient to be present during the warning (Simon and Shuman 2007). The clinician can help the patient to understand that in issuing the warning, the therapist is not merely protecting the potential victim but also helping to protect the patient by intervening before the patient's behavior escalates out of control, thereby reducing risks of adverse outcomes (e.g., incarceration, guilt) for the patient as well.

Elopement

An elopement from a psychiatric hospital can have dire consequences (Dickens and Campbell 2002; Hunt et al. 2007). Unlike discharges *against medical advice*, an elopement does not afford the treatment team sufficient time to assess whether the patient meets the criteria for commitment or to make a decision about discharge based on an evaluation of dangerousness to self and others. There is no opportunity to develop an aftercare plan, including medication and a safety plan, as appropriate. Furthermore, the patient who elopes usually leaves without arranging any follow-up. Because the elopement of an unstable patient can result in serious consequences, the matter has been addressed by regulatory agencies. One of the examples given by the Joint Commission of a reviewable sentinel event is "any elopement that is an unauthorized departure, of a patient from an around-the-clock setting resulting in a temporally related death (suicide, accidental death, or homicide) or major permanent loss of function" (Joint Commission 2007b).

Several studies have indicated that about 50% of patients elope primarily while off the unit on passes or walks (Kleis and Stout 1991; Richmond et al. 1991). Bowers et al. (1999a, 1999b, 1999c, 2000, 2003, 2005) performed a prospective study involving inpatients from 12 partially locked acute wards in five different hospitals in the United Kingdom. During the 5-month study period, 175 patients absconded (i.e., were absent from the unit without permission for a period of more than an hour) a total of 498 times. In contrast to earlier studies, 88% of the patients eloped directly from the unit. This may be due to the fact that the wards were generally left unlocked. Of the patients who eloped, 35% were confined to the unit. However, in only 1% of incidents was the unit door locked; in another 11%, a nurse was stationed at the door. For the remaining cases, the unit was unlocked at the time of the incident. Of those who eloped, 58% had expressed their intention to leave the unit within the previous 24 hours (Bowers et al. 1999a).

These patients differed from controls in exhibiting an increased frequency of noncompliant behaviors such as medication refusal and involvement in an officially reported ward incident within the previous week. They were more likely to be male, young, of minority ethnicity, and a member of a non-Christian religion and to have a diagnosis of schizophrenia. They also had a higher incidence of absconding during a past admission. There was no correlation with commitment status, level of ward security, or history of suicidal attempt or self-mutilation (Bowers et al. 1999c, 2000). Additional interviews with the patients who absconded (Bowers et al. 1999c, 2003) revealed that although psychiatric symptoms were related to the decision to elope, there were other reasons, such as boredom, fear of other patients, feeling trapped or confined, household responsibilities, feeling estranged from family and friends, and worries about the security of their income and property.

Bowers et al. (2003, 2005) implemented an *anti-absconding package*. This included the use of a log book for signing in and out of the ward, careful and supportive communication of bad news to patients, post-ward-incident debriefings, multidisciplinary review after repeated incidents, and identification of high-risk patients. High-risk patients were assigned daily nursing times to discuss concerns and staff-facilitated outside social contact. The rate of absconding was reduced by 25%. Other elopement-prevention measures such as the use of electronic wristbands and a triage protocol have been shown to be helpful as well (Macy and Johnston 2007).

Discharge Against Medical Advice

Significant numbers of patients who would benefit from hospitalization do not meet criteria for commitment and will not accept voluntary admission. Psychiatrists frequently encounter patients who wish to sign out *against medical advice* (AMA). Studies have revealed that 3%–51% of patients discharge themselves AMA, and the frequency of AMA discharges appears to have increased over time (Brook et al. 2006). Patients discharged AMA have been found to underutilize outpatient services, instead relying on expensive emergency care settings (Brook et al. 2006; Haupt and Erlich 1980). They are also more likely to be rehospitalized sooner than controls and with greater frequency (Brook et al. 2006; Dalrymple and Fata 1993; Dixon et al. 1997; Pages et al. 1998).

Seeking to identify risk factors for AMA discharges from inpatient facilities, Brook et al. (2006) synthesized data from 61 articles on the subject, excluding patients who had eloped. Patients who were at risk of

leaving AMA showed the following characteristics: young age; single; male gender; comorbid personality disorder or substance use disorder; pessimistic attitude toward treatment; antisocial, aggressive, or disruptive behavior; and history of multiple previous AMA discharges (Brook et al. 2006; Pages et al. 1998). AMA discharge was also predicted by the following facility/provider variables: failure to orient the patient to the unit; failure to establish a strong doctor–patient relationship; and time of day and time of year, with more AMA discharges being requested during evening and night shifts and during the spring and summer months (Brook et al. 2006; Dalrymple and Fata 1993; Jeffer 1993).

The majority of patients who signed out AMA from drug/alcohol treatment centers cited personal reasons, such as family illness or reconciliation with a spouse, or legal issues, such as a court date (Green et al. 2004). However, in a study by Blondell et al. (2006), 85% of patients admitted for drug and alcohol treatment who had all of the following risk factors left AMA: Latino ethnicity, detoxification from drugs, Friday or Saturday discharge, Medicaid or no insurance, and not being treated by one attending physician.

The case law concerning AMA discharges is limited. Devitt et al. (2000) were able to identify eight published court opinions involving AMA discharge, and only two involved patients in a psychiatric facility. Gerbasi and Simon (2003) found two other cases. In *Kelly v. United States* (1987) and *Solbrig v. United States* (1995), facilities were not held to be liable for negligence in AMA discharges preceding severe adverse outcomes (a stabbing and a patient suicide). Reviewing the potential legal ramifications of an AMA discharge, Gerbasi and Simon (2003) noted that voluntary admissions comprise 73% of admissions to psychiatric care facilities, with the majority of these patients being admitted on a conditional voluntary basis. Therefore, for a large pool of patients, AMA discharge is a possibility. The decision to allow a patient to sign out AMA is often made quickly, without a team meeting or a full assessment of the patient's capacity to understand the potential consequences of his or her actions.

There have been few studies of interventions designed to decrease the risk of AMA discharge. Targum et al. (1982) found that the rate decreased from 11.6% to 7.6% after a patient advocate system was started. Pages et al. (1998) recommend identifying high-risk patients early in the hospitalization and initiating an early-discharge plan. In addition to the foundation of patient safety efforts discussed earlier in this chapter, such as beginning discharge planning soon after admission, the following suggestions are offered from the literature (Gerbasi and Simon 2003):

1. Patients who are uncooperative with discharge discussions should, at a minimum, receive a referral list with options for follow-up outpatient care.
2. Even if an AMA discharge request is received in the evening, as is frequently the case, a contemporaneous evaluation for safety must be entered if the request is to be honored. If the request is denied, a similar assessment of the clinical purpose for retaining the patient should be documented. The assessment should evaluate the stability of the patient's psychiatric illness, as well as the patient's ability to attend to activities of daily living.
3. Endeavor to include the patient's family or significant others in the discharge process, and provide psychoeducation, as appropriate.
4. Provide an appropriate follow-up treatment plan and ensure reasonable access to medications, if indicated. Whether or not to provide the patient with discharge medications requires a separate risk–benefit analysis, but the mere fact that the discharge is against medical advice should not preclude provision of reasonable pharmacotherapy.

Gerbasi and Simon (2003) have offered several additional risk management strategies specific to AMA discharge concerns.

A patient's ability to understand the consequences of an AMA discharge or treatment refusal may be affected by the underlying mental illness. In such cases, one might consider pursuing authorization for continued hospitalization from a substitute decision maker as allowed by law. An advance directive for psychiatric care can also be helpful, although there may need to be further court intervention to enforce the directive. So-called Ulysses contracts (whereby a patient indicates her desire for future involuntary treatment should her condition worsen to the point that she would be deemed incompetent to consent to treatment) are not uniformly accepted in all jurisdictions, and subsequent court proceedings may be necessary even where such a "contract" exists. If the patient does not meet the criteria for involuntary commitment, the psychiatrist is obliged to inform the patient of the risks and consequences of an AMA discharge and to assess the patient's understanding of these risks (Gerbasi and Simon 2003).

Managed Care and Clinical Decision Making

There are times when the decision of a managed care company to deny further coverage of an inpatient stay may prompt the patient to request discharge. The attending psychiatrist and the facility are faced with a dilemma. The managed care company may deny reimbursement, but the responsibility for decisions about further management, including discharge, still rests with the attending psychiatrist and the hospital. In the event of a poor outcome, the physician may retain liability, particularly if there has been no appeal. In *Wickline v. State of California* (1986), the California Court of Appeals explained: "The physician who complies without protest with the limitations imposed by a third party payor when medical judgment dictates otherwise, cannot avoid his ultimate responsibility for the patient's care." However, liability may also be attached to managed care organizations in some circumstances in which the Employee Retirement Income Security Act does not bar suit. In *Wilson v. Blue Cross of Southern California* (1990), the court held that although the attending psychiatrist did not appeal the decision to discharge the patient after 10 days of hospitalization, this failure did not preclude action against the managed care company. In other cases, courts have found that managed care companies that actually supervise care or assert to subscribers that they direct care may incur liability for their decisions (Gerbasi and Simon 2003).

For risk management purposes, patients should never be discharged or otherwise denied clinically appropriate care merely because of restrictions imposed by managed care. The treating physician needs to be sure that the patient is safe for discharge. In cases when the patient's safety is at risk, the situation may require keeping the patient in the hospital, even when the managed care company denies reimbursement. The hospital and physician should continue to pursue any appeal rights that they have under the managed care contract. The documentation should reflect the patient's continued need for an inpatient level of care. Coverage issues may arise if, for example, the hospital is not part of the managed care network, the condition is not covered by the patient's policy, or the length of stay exceeds the authorized period. However, financial considerations are distinct from questions of clinical need. Patient safety and, if the patient is dangerous, the safety of others must guide clinical decision making.

Conclusion

Risk management must be continual in order to be successful. To achieve a culture of patient safety, systemwide changes to the organizational culture may be necessary. Even in a setting where sound risk management practices are in place, adverse events may occur, and the organization should address problems both retrospectively and prospectively. Standardized tools for risk reduction and management, such as RCA and FMEA, can help make investigations and troubleshooting less overwhelming. A crucial aspect of protecting patient safety is improving communication methods within the hospital—among staff members, as well as between staff and patients and staff and families. Staff orientation and training must be thorough, and any training program should address boundary theory and help staff to recognize countertransference reactions and the early warning signs of boundary problems. Improvements in communication and training should reduce the risk of malpractice lawsuits associated with negligence or misconduct.

Special care must be given to mandates and regulations concerning civil commitment or involuntary treatment, the use of seclusion or restraint, and the duty to warn or protect third parties from dangerous patients. Statutes often vary by jurisdiction, and there are additional regulatory considerations for accreditation or government agencies (e.g., the Joint Commission and the Centers for Medicare and Medicaid Services). For complicated legal and regulatory risk management, consultation with legal counsel, risk management officers, and insurance carriers may be necessary to ensure that rules are not overlooked.

Above all, patient safety and the safety of others should be first and foremost among the issues considered in clinical decision making. Elopement and AMA discharges are unfortunate occurrences, but patients' legal rights must be respected, and unduly coercive or restrictive treatment or confinement is not sound risk management. Because adverse outcomes may result when a patient elopes or discharges himself or herself against medical advice, advance planning and prospective risk reduction measures should be utilized to reduce the rate of treatment noncompliance. Finally, although reimbursement is a significant concern for medical care, staff should not allow managed care and financial considerations to trump clinical judgment. When a patient is hospitalized for psychiatric illness, the ultimate responsibility for the patient's safety rests with the treating psychiatrist and the hospital. Legal risk is a reality for hospital psychiatry in a litigious culture, but careful risk management can help to improve the safety and quality of patient care, thereby mitigating risks to the organization.

References

Adachi W, Lodolce AE: Use of failure mode and effects analysis in improving the safety of i.v. drug administration. Am J Health Syst Pharm 62:917–920, 2005

American Psychiatric Association, American Psychiatric Nurses Association, National Association of Psychiatric Health Systems: Learning From Each Other: Success Stories and Ideas for Reducing Restraint/Seclusion in Behavioral Health. Arlington, VA, American Psychiatric Association, 2003

Amori G, Kicklighter L, Kondis C, et al: Disclosure of Unanticipated Events: Creating an Effective Patient Communication Policy. Chicago, IL, American Society for Healthcare Risk Management, 2003

Appelbaum PS: Voluntary hospitalization and due process: the dilemma of Zinermon v Burch. Hosp Community Psychiatry 41:1059–1060, 1990

Battles JB, Dixon NM, Borotkanics RJ, et al: Sensemaking of patient safety risks and hazards. Health Serv Res 41:1555–1575, 2006

Bisconer SW, Green M, Mallon-Czajka J, et al: Managing aggression in a psychiatric hospital using a behaviour plan: a case study. J Psychiatr Ment Health Nurs 13:515–521, 2006

Blondell RD, Amadasu A, Servoss TJ, et al: Differences among those who complete and fail to complete inpatient detoxification. J Addict Dis 25:95–104, 2006

Bowers L, Jarrett M, Clark N, et al: Absconding: how and when patients leave the ward. J Psychiatr Ment Health Nurs 6:207–211, 1999a

Bowers L, Jarrett M, Clark N, et al: Absconding: outcome and risk. J Psychiatr Ment Health Nurs 6:213–218, 1999b

Bowers L, Jarrett M, Clark N, et al: Absconding: why patients leave. J Psychiatr Ment Health Nurs 6:199–206, 1999c

Bowers L, Jarrett M, Clark N, et al: Determinants of absconding by patients on acute psychiatric units. J Adv Nurs 32:644–649, 2000

Bowers L, Alexander J, Gaskell C: A trial of an anti-absconding intervention in acute psychiatric wards. J Psychiatr Ment Health Nurs 10:410–416, 2003

Bowers L, Simpson A, Alexander J: Real world application of an intervention to reduce absconding. J Psychiatr Ment Health Nurs 12:598–602, 2005

Brook M, Hilty DM, Liu W, et al: Discharge against medical advice from inpatient psychiatric treatment: a literature review. Psychiatr Serv 57:1192–1198, 2006

Cody RJ: Anticipating risk for human subjects participating in clinical research: application of failure mode and effects analysis. Cancer Invest 24:209–214, 2006

Coles G, Fuller B, Nordquist K, et al: Using failure mode effects and criticality analysis for high-risk processes at three community hospitals. Jt Comm J Qual Patient Saf 31:132–140, 2005

Dalrymple AJ, Fata M: Cross-validating factors associated with discharges against medical advice. Can J Psychiatry 38:285–289, 1993

Day S, Dalto J, Fox J, et al: Failure mode analysis as a performance improvement tool in trauma. J Trauma Nurs 13:111–117, 2006

Dean AJ, Duke SG, George M, et al: Behavioral management leads to reduction in aggression in a child and adolescent psychiatric inpatient unit. J Am Acad Child Adolesc Psychiatry 46:711–720, 2007

DeRosier J, Stalhandske E, Bagian JP, et al: Using health care failure analysis: the VA National Center for Patient Safety's prospective risk analysis system. Jt Comm J Qual Patient Saf 28:248–267, 2002

Devitt PJ, Devitt AC, Dewan M: An examination of whether discharging patients against medical advice protects physicians from malpractice claims. Psychiatr Serv 51:899–902, 2000

Dickens GL, Campbell J: Absconding of patients from an independent UK psychiatric hospital: a 3-year retrospective analysis of events and characteristics of absconders. J Psychiatr Ment Health Nurs 8:543–550, 2002

Dixon M, Robertson E, George M, et al: Risk factors for acute psychiatric readmission. Psychiatric Bulletin 21:600–603, 1997

Donat DC: Encouraging alternatives to seclusion, restraint, and reliance on PRN drugs in a public psychiatric hospital. Psychiatr Serv 56:1105–1108, 2005

Epstein RS, Simon RI: The exploitation index: an early warning indicator of boundary violations in psychotherapy. Bull Menninger Clin 54:450–465, 1990

Evans SM, Smith BJ, Esterman A, et al: Evaluation of an intervention aimed at improving voluntary incident reporting in hospitals. Qual Saf Health Care 16:169–175, 2007

Gallagher TH, Waterman AD, Ebers AG, et al: Patients' and physicians' attitudes regarding the disclosure of medical errors. JAMA 289:1001–1007, 2003

Gallagher TH, Studdert D, Levinson W: Disclosing harmful medical errors to patients. N Engl J Med 356:2713–2719, 2007

Gerbasi J, Simon RI: Patient's rights and psychiatrists' duties: discharging patients against medical advice. Harv Rev Psychiatry 11:333–343, 2003

Green P, Watts D, Poole S, et al: Why patients sign out against medical advice: factors motivating patients to sign out AMA. Am J Drug Alcohol Abuse 30:489–493, 2004

Gutheil TG, Gabbard GO: The concept of boundaries in clinical practice: theoretical and risk management dimensions. Am J Psychiatry 150:188–196, 1993

Gutheil TG, Gabbard GO: Misuses and misunderstandings of boundary theory in clinical and regulatory settings. Am J Psychiatry 155:409–414, 1998

Gutheil TG, Simon RI: Non-sexual boundary crossings and boundary violations: the ethical dimension. Psychiatr Clin North Am 25:585–592, 2002

Haupt DN, Erlich SM: The impact of a new state commitment on psychiatric patient careers. Hosp Community Psychiatry 31:745–751, 1980

Hunt IM, Kapur N, Webb R, et al: Suicide in current psychiatric in-patients: a case control study. Psychol Med 37:831–837, 2007

Hunter ME, Love CC: Total quality management and the reduction of inpatient violence and costs in a forensic psychiatric hospital. Psychiatr Serv 47:751–754, 1996

Institute of Medicine, Committee on Quality Health Care in America: Crossing the Quality Chasm: A New Health System for the 21st Century. Washington, DC, National Academies Press, 2001

Institute of Medicine, Committee on Quality Health Care in America: To Err Is Human: Building a Safer Health System.Washington, DC, National Academies Press, 1999

Jeffer EK: Against medical advice: a review of the literature. Mil Med 158:69–73, 1993

Joint Commission: 2007 National Patient Safety Goals. Oakbrook Terrace, IL, The Joint Commission, 2007a. Available at: http://www.jointcommission.org/PatientSafety/NationalPatientSafetyGoals/07_npsgs.htm. Accessed July 25, 2007.

Joint Commission: Sentinel Event Policy and Procedures, updated July 2007. Oakbrook Terrace, IL, The Joint Commission, 2007b. Available at: http://www.jointcommission.org/SentinelEvents/PolicyandProcedures/se_pp.htm. Accessed July 30, 2007.

Joint Commission on Accreditation of Healthcare Organizations (JCAHO): Comprehensive Accreditation Manual for Hospitals (Improving Organizational Performance, standard P13.1: "The organization collects data to monitor its performance"). Oakbrook Terrace, IL, JCAHO, 2003

Kleis LS, Stout CE: The high-risk patient: a profile of acute care psychiatric patients who leave without discharge. Psychiatr Hosp 22:153–159, 1991

Kraman SS, Cranfill L, Hamm G, et al: John M Eisenberg Patient Safety Awards. Advocacy: the Lexington Veterans Affairs Medical Center. Jt Comm J Qual Improv 28:646–650, 2002

Leigh J, Lagorio N: Clinical crisis management, in Risk Management Handbook for Health Care Organizations, Vol 2. Edited by Carroll R, Brown SM. Chicago, IL, Wiley, 2007, pp 37–51

Macy D, Johnston M: Using electronic wristbands and a triage protocol to protect mental health patients in the emergency department. J Nurs Care Qual 22:180–184, 2007

Martin PG, Federico M: Risk management's role in performance improvement, in Risk Management Handbook for Health Care Organizations, Vol 2. Edited by Carroll R, Brown SM. Chicago, IL, Wiley, 2007, pp 23–35

Mazor KM, Simon SR, Yood RA, et al: Health plan members' views about disclosure of medical errors. Ann Intern Med 140:409–418, 2004

Morin M: Patient safety efforts target communication at Rhode Island hospitals. Med Health R I 90:182–183, 2007

Mossman D: Unbuckling the "chemical straitjacket": the legal significance of recent advances in the pharmacological treatment of psychosis. San Diego Law Rev 39:1033–1164, 2002

Mossman D: Critique of pure risk assessment or Kant meets Tarasoff. U Cincinnati Law Rev 75:523–610, 2006

Murphy DM, Shannon K, Pugliese G: Patient safety and the risk management profession: new challenges and opportunities, in Risk Management Handbook for Health Care Organizations, Vol 2. Edited by Carroll R, Brown SM. Chicago, IL, Wiley, 2007, pp 1–21

National Quality Forum: Safe practices for better healthcare. Washington, DC, National Quality Forum, 2007. Available at: http:/www.qualityforum.org/projects/completed/ safe_practices/. Accessed July 1, 2007.

Norris DM, Gutheil TG, Strasburger LH: This couldn't happen to me: boundary problems and sexual misconduct in the psychotherapy relationship. Psychiatr Serv 54:517–522, 2003

Norris DM, Price M, Gutheil TG, et al: Firearm laws, patients, and the roles of psychiatrists. Am J Psychiatry 163:1392–1396, 2006

Pages KP, Russo JE, Wingerson DK, et al: Predictors and outcome of discharge against medical advice from the psychiatric units of a general hospital. Psychiatr Serv 49:1187–1192, 1998

Price M, Norris DM: National Instant Criminal Background Check Improvement Act: implications for persons with mental illness. J Am Acad Psychiatry Law 36:123–130, 2008

Robinson DL, Heigham M, Clark J: Using failure mode and effects analysis for safe administration of chemotherapy to hospitalized children with cancer. Jt Comm J Qual Patient Saf 32:161–166, 2006

Richmond I, Dandridge L, Jones K: Changing nursing practice to prevent elopement. J Nurs Care Qual 6:73–81, 1991

Schreiner GM, Crafton CG, Sevin JA: Decreasing the use of mechanical restraints and locked seclusion. Adm Policy Ment Health 31:449–463, 2004

Shendell-Falik N, Feinson M, Mohr BJ: Enhancing patient safety: improving the patient handoff process through appreciative inquiry. J Nurs Admin 37:95–104, 2007

Sheridan-Leos N, Schulmeister L, Hartranft S: Failure mode and effect analysis: a technique to prevent chemotherapy errors. Clin J Oncol Nurs 10:393–398, 2006

Simon RI, Shuman DW: Clinical Manual of Psychiatry and Law. Washington, DC, American Psychiatric Publishing, 2007

Spath PL: Using failure mode and effects analysis to improve patient safety. AORN J 78:16–37, 2003

Stebbing C, Wong ICK, Kaushal R, et al: The role of communication in pediatric drug safety. Arch Dis Child 92:440–445, 2007

Studdert DM, Mello MM, Gawande AA, et al: Disclosure of medical injury to patients: an improbable risk management strategy. Health Aff 26:215–226, 2007

Targum SD, Capodanno AE, Hoffman HA, et al: An intervention to reduce the rate of hospital discharges against medical advice. Am J Psychiatry 139:657–659, 1982

Weinstock R, Vari G, Leong GB, et al: Back to the past in California: a temporary retreat to a Tarasoff duty to warn. J Am Acad Psychiatry Law 34:523–528, 2006

Wetterneck TB, Skibinski KA, Roberts TL, et al: Using failure mode and effects analysis to plan implementation of smart i.v. pump technology. Am J Health Syst Pharm 63:1528–1538, 2006

Winick BJ: Civil Commitment: A Therapeutic Jurisprudence Model. Durham, NC, Carolina Academic Press, 2005

Wojcieszak D, Banja J, Houk C: The sorry works! Coalition: making the case for full disclosure. Jt Comm J Qual Patient Saf 32:344–350, 2006

Woodhouse S, Burney B, Costa K: To err is human: improving safety through failure mode and effect analysis. Clin Leadersh Manag Rev 18:32–36, 2004

Woods MS: Healing Words: The Power of Apology in Medicine, 2nd Edition. Oakbrook Terrace, IL, Joint Commission Resources, 2007

Legal Citations

42 CFR 482.13(f)

Cal. Civ. Code 43.92

Ewing v Goldstein, 15 Cal. Rptr.3d 864 Cal. Ct. App. (2004)

Ewing v Northridge Hospital Medical Center, 16 Cal.Rptr.3d 591 Cal. Ct. App. (2004)

Kan. Stat. Ann. §59–2946 (2003)

Kelly v the United States of America and John Doe, John Roe, & John Shoe. Civil Action 86-2864. U.S. Dist. LEXIS 2201 (1987)

Kelly v United States, No. 86-2864, 1987 U.S. Dist. LEXIS 2289 (E.D. Pa. 24 March 1987)

Mass. Gen. L., ch.123, §1 (2003)

Mass. Gen. L., ch. 140, §129(b) (2004) et seq., 269–10

Ohio Rev. Code Ann. §5233.02(a) (b) (2003)

Solbrig v United States, 1995 U.S. Dist. LEXIS 2201 (N.D. Ill. 23 February 1995)

Tarasoff v Regents of the University of California, 17 Cal.3d 425, 551 P.2d 334; 131 Cal. Rptr. 14 (1976)

Wickline v State of California, 192 Cal. App.3d 1630 (Cal. Ct. App. 1986)

Wilson v Blue Cross of Southern California, 222 Cal. App.3d 660 (Cal. Ct. App. 1990)

Youngberg v Romeo, 457 U.S. 307 (1982)

Zinermon v Burch, 494 U.S. 113 (1990)

CHAPTER 32

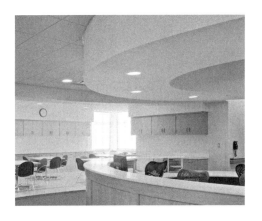

QUALITY INDICATORS

Marlin R. Mattson, M.D.

Quality of health care has assumed an increasingly prominent place in the issues confronting our nation, as we realize that problems regarding lack of quality care are hindering effective treatment and recovery of patients (Berwick et al. 1990; Institute of Medicine 2006b). The Institute of Medicine (2000, 2001) has played a major role in assessing how quality of care issues can be addressed. It has now extended the same thorough assessment to care for mental and substance use disorders by providing a detailed plan for addressing issues pertinent to these areas (Institute of Medicine 2006b).

Characterizing Quality

Quality of health care has been defined and characterized in many different ways. Donabedian (2003) was one of the earliest exponents of the various quality products that emerge from the application of the "science and technology of health care": efficacy, effectiveness, efficiency, optimality, acceptability, legitimacy, and equity. He defined these components of quality as follows:

1. *Efficacy:* ability of the science and technology of health care to bring about improvements in health when used under the most favorable circumstances
2. *Effectiveness:* degree to which attainable improvements in health are, in fact, attained
3. *Efficiency:* the ability to lower the cost of care without diminishing attainable improvements in health
4. *Optimality:* balancing of improvements in health against the costs of such improvements
5. *Acceptability:* conformity to the wishes, desires, and expectations of patients and their families
6. *Legitimacy:* conformity to social preferences as expressed in ethical principles, values, norms, mores, laws, and regulations
7. *Equity:* conformity to a principle that determines what is just and fair in the distribution of health care and its benefits among members of the population

The Institute of Medicine under the National Academy of Sciences has played a central role in the advancement of the health care improvement agenda for more than a decade. Its *Crossing the Quality Chasm* report made clear the consensus that had formed around the six aims of high-quality health care (Institute of Medicine 2001):

1. *Safe:* avoiding injuries to patients from the care that is intended to help them
2. *Effective:* providing services based on scientific knowledge to all who could benefit and refraining from providing services to those not likely to benefit (avoiding underuse and overuse, respectively)
3. *Patient-centered:* providing care that is respectful of and responsive to individual patient preferences, needs, and values and ensuring that patient values guide all clinical decisions
4. *Timely:* reducing waits and sometimes harmful delays for both those who receive and those who give care
5. *Efficient:* avoiding waste, including waste of equipment, supplies, ideas, and energy
6. *Equitable:* providing care that does not vary in quality because of personal characteristics such as gender, ethnicity, geographical location, and socioeconomic status

Many of the currently defined quality *indicators and measures* for mental disorders developed by national organizations initially focused on clinical therapies for depression, given its prevalence as a mental health condition. Substance abuse indicators and measures will follow (American Medical Association 2007). With time, many other opportunities beyond therapeutics will be developed as measures for improving the quality of psychiatric care (Greenberg et al. 2006). Some aims of quality health care have been more difficult to translate into meaningful mental or substance use disorder measures. The Institute of Medicine has called attention to the lack of national comprehensive measures for the domains of efficiency, equity, and patient-centered care. It recommended that "to measure quality better, the U.S. Department of Health and Human Services, in partnership with the private sector, should charge and financially support an entity similar to the National Quality Forum to convene government regulators, accrediting organizations, consumer representatives, providers, and purchasers exercising leadership in quality-based purchasing for the purpose of reaching consensus on and implementing a common, continuously improving set of mental/substance-use conditions health care quality measures for providers, organizations, and systems of care" (Institute of Medicine 2006b, p. 14).

The American Psychiatric Association Task Force on Quality Indicators has defined *quality indicator* as "a component of quality patient care" and *measure* as "a mechanism or instrument to quantify the indicator" (American Psychiatric Association 2002, 2007). They logically follow a *recommendation/goal*, defined as "an important clinical principle that reflects quality patient care."

In addition, exploration of variables that may lead to better results from quality measures continues to unfold. Examples include volume–quality interaction as well as disparities found in the National Committee for Quality Assurance Healthcare Effectiveness Data and Information Set results for mental health measures (Druss et al. 2002, 2004).

Central Role of Leadership

National leadership has been increasingly necessary for developing meaningful and feasible quality measures in mental and substance use disorder care (Hermann and Palmer 2002; Hermann and Rollins 2003). Quality indicators and measures in mental health have been and are being defined by many organizations, some of which are described below, as well as by hospitals and other health care systems. Although significant progress has been made, this area lags behind the development of quality measures in many other areas of medicine.

Several consensus organizations have taken an important leadership role in trying to draw all stakeholders together in developing core measures. Prominent among these organizations is the National Quality Forum, created "to develop and implement a national strategy for health care quality measurement and reporting" (see http://www.qualityforum.org/about) as well as to integrate behavioral health care performance measures into its strategy (see http://www.qualityforum.org/publications/reports/behavioral_health.asp).

Another consensus effort to identify and implement a set of core performance measures for hospital-based inpatient psychiatric services is currently under way (Joint Commission 2008). The set of core performance measures is being collaboratively developed by the Joint Commission, the National Association of Psychiatric Health Systems, and the National Association of State Mental Health Program Directors and its Research Institute, along with a broad-based advisory panel.

The Physician Consortium for Performance Improvement (organized by the American Medical Association) is developing evidence-based measures with links to health outcomes. Many specialty and state medical associations and other stakeholders are involved. Measures for major depressive disorder are included for both adult and child/adolescent psychiatry. Some measures are also available for problem drinking and tobacco use.

Hermann et al. (2004) brought together a panel of 12 stakeholders from national organizations to select core process quality measures for mental health care in seven domains (characteristics of quality) and review issues, including supporting research evidence, difficulties doing case-mix adjustment, and gathering the data. Through a consensus process, these researchers were able to characterize a core set of measures that they described as 1) meaningful, 2) feasible to diverse stakeholders, and 3) "broadly representative of the mental health care system." This stakeholder panel evaluated a total of 116 process measures and agreed on 28 related to treatment, safety, access, assessment, continuity, coordination, and prevention. It was hoped that this process and its results could inform the efforts of other groups, such as the National Quality Forum, involved in developing national standardized measures.

Other consensus organizations active in health care quality initiatives are the Hospital Quality Alliance and the AQA (formerly called the Ambulatory Care Quality Alliance). The Hospital Quality Alliance is developing a set of measures to be tracked and reported by all participating hospitals and accepted by a wide range of stakeholders. There currently are no quality measures for the care of mental and substance use disorders (Center for Medicare and Medicaid Services 2007c). The AQA, a public–private partnership representing an even larger group of stakeholders, is developing ambulatory care quality measures, many of which come from the American Medical Association Physician Consortium, the Centers for Medicare and Medicaid Services, and the National Committee for Quality Assurance (Institute of Medicine 2006c).

Customers for Quality Indicators and Measures

Users of quality indicators and measures can be viewed as internal or external to the hospital. Internally, there is a chain of accountability from staff to department/discipline to hospital to board of trustees. Increasingly, hospital executive leadership and their boards expect to be able to compare one hospital with another. Which hospitals run exemplary or benchmark programs, and how do other hospitals fare in comparison? Externally, accountability is linked to government and private purchasers of care, public re-porting programs, prospective patients, accrediting organizations, and incentive programs for providing data on quality measures for additional pay, among others.

Developing and Selecting Quality Indicators and Measures

To meet the expectations and demands of all potential customers, we need indicators and measures that are reliable, valid, and carried out accurately. However, the considerable variability in quality indicators and measures across facilities (Williams et al. 2007) indicates the need for consensus-building efforts to identify key core indicators and measures. Prioritizing areas of health care where attention needs to be focused is also required. Data can come from ever-expanding sources. They could include untoward occurrences such as medication errors and adverse drug reactions; safety rounds; application of current and past Joint Commission national safety goals; tracer methodologies; risk management (lawsuits and possible lawsuits); cases requiring reports to regulatory agencies; peer review of identified cases; complaint letters; team rounds/meetings; debriefing sessions following events such as seclusion or restraint use; hospitalwide concerns in provision of care; patient rounds; community meetings of patients and staff; findings from failure modes and effects analysis (FMEA) and external independent quality reviews; and data from Six Sigma studies. Six Sigma is "a systematic method for improving the output of the organization...by preventing error, solving problems, managing change, and monitoring long-term performance in quantitative terms" (Barry et al. 2002, p. 13). This is done through the definition of quality measures that address defects in the delivery of services (Barry et al. 2002). As described by Varkey et al. (2007, p. 737), Six Sigma is achieved through a series of steps: define, measure, analyze, improve, and control. A Six Sigma study from the Netherlands demonstrates the improved care processes and reduced costs (Van den Heuvel et al. 2006) that can result from such a methodology.

Measures are needed for health care areas in which errors are most likely to occur and carry the most severe consequences for patients. A patient-centered example could be transition care from one level of care to another or from one setting to another (Coleman 2006; Coleman et al. 2005). Here, discharge planning and ensuring continuity of care are the focus. Coleman (2006, p. 272) describes a "care transitions measure" of three questions for patients:

1. The hospital staff took my preferences and those of my family or caregiver into account in deciding what my health care needs would be when I left the hospital.
2. When I left the hospital, I had a good understanding of the things I was responsible for in managing my health.
3. When I left the hospital, I clearly understood the purpose for taking each of my medications.

Coleman et al. (2006) demonstrated that a care transitions intervention can reduce "serious quality deficiencies that occur...and may reduce the rate of subsequent readmissions." Their "coaching of chronically ill older patients and their caregivers" included medication self-management, a patient-centered medical record, participation in follow-up planning and activities, and knowledge of red flags and how to respond.

Among the six aims of high-quality health care identified by the Institute of Medicine, the domain or aim of *efficiency*, defined as "avoiding waste" (Institute of Medicine 2001, 2006a), can be difficult to evaluate. The goals of measuring "value-based health care" are to reduce underuse, overuse, and misuse of health care resources (Grazier 2006a). Another domain or aim of quality often not addressed effectively is *equity* (Institute of Medicine 2006a), which applies to areas where cultural, racial, language, age, gender, sexual orientation, or other disparities exist in the provision of care. Examples of such disparities include provision of mental health services to women in rural areas (Hillemeier et al. 2005) and standards for diabetes care in individuals with mental illness (Frayne et al. 2005).

Donabedian (2003) described three approaches to assessing health care quality: structure, process, and outcome. *Structural* measures are determined by how we set up our health care system—the environment, including the buildings, the staff, and their education and training. *Process* is illustrated by the specifics of how we carry out the provision of care. The process measure, however, has a connection to a desired outcome, thereby giving it validity (Charbonneau et al. 2004). *Outcome* measures are the gold standard. But because variables beyond the control of the hospital and its staff may influence outcomes, their use, at times, is limited. It is helpful to risk-adjust the results to make them more valid. Risk-adjustment issues for mental health services have been well described by Hendryx et al. (2001). Gender, race, and homelessness are important variables; and for readmission, length of previous hospitalization, therapy, or level of collaboration with outpatient providers may also predict outcome (Schacht and Hines 2003). Berghofer et al.

(2001) found that only first-time or long-term status was significantly associated with patient satisfaction. Long-term patients had a more positive impression of their care. Inpatient or outpatient setting was not related to satisfaction.

Practice guidelines can often provide appropriate quality indicators, although pitfalls in their use should be noted (Walter et al. 2004). Guidelines developed by the American Psychiatric Association or the American Academy of Child and Adolescent Psychiatry can contribute significantly to the development of specific quality indicators and measures, especially those that are evidence-based. In the American Psychiatric Association (2006) practice guidelines, each recommendation is coded according to the degree of clinical confidence with which it is made (I—recommended with substantial clinical confidence; II—recommended with moderate clinical confidence; III—may be recommended on the basis of individual circumstances).

Patient satisfaction surveys play an essential part in carrying out patient-centered aims in health care everywhere in the world. Examination of findings by gender, age group, or other characteristics (such as first-time admission vs. long-term patients or generic vs. psychiatric-specific questionnaire) can provide opportunities for improvement (Berghofer et al. 2001; Kuosmanen et al. 2006; Peytremann-Bridevaux et al. 2006).

A selection of other national organizations involved in quality measures is summarized below (the Institute of Medicine [2006c] has also provided such a summary):

- The Agency for Healthcare Research and Quality has a National Quality Measures Clearinghouse, which includes most current evidence-based quality measures available. However, there are currently no measures for mental health and substance use. This organization regularly presents reports on disparities in provision of health care (Agency for Healthcare Research and Quality 2007).
- The American Nurses Association's National Center for Nursing Quality manages a National Database of Nursing Quality Indicators, most of which are generic to nursing care. Several are pertinent to inpatient mental health services as well.
- The American Osteopathic Association provides a summary of quality and pay-for-performance initiatives in public and private sectors across the country, both nationally and state by state.
- The Centers for Medicare and Medicaid Services has an extensive history of efforts to improve quality in health care. One of its latest programs is the

Physician Quality Reporting Initiative (Centers for Medicare and Medicaid Services 2007), in which eligible clinicians may voluntarily report results from the application of specific Centers for Medicare and Medicaid Services–approved quality measures for a bonus payment (often referred to as pay-for-performance or pay-for-reporting). Several of the initial measures identified are pertinent to mental or substance use disorders. A Quality Measures Management Information System containing measures used in its quality initiatives is also offered (Centers for Medicare and Medicaid Services 2007; see https://www.qualitynet.org/qmis). One of the measures relates to the acute treatment phase of depression.

- The Center for Quality Assessment and Improvement in Mental Health provides a database that can be searched for quality measures (Center for Quality Assessment and Improvement in Mental Health 2007), a *Directory of Measure Sources*, and a valuable toolkit on using process measures (Hermann et al. 2002).
- The National Committee for Quality Assurance (http://www.ncqa.org), an independent nonprofit organization that accredits and certifies health plans and other entities, has refined over many years a quality measurement program called the Healthcare Effectiveness Data and Information Set (HEDIS).
- Originally launched by the Maryland Hospital Association, the Quality Indicator Project (http://www.qiproject.org) has developed numerous indicator sets, one of which covers mental health. Reports to the many participating hospitals are supplied with benchmarking percentiles.
- The Substance Abuse and Mental Health Services Administration (SAMHSA) is actively involved in establishing national outcome measures for the prevention and treatment of substance use and mental disorders. A program for developing benchmarking capabilities is to follow. SAMHSA funds the Evaluation Center at Human Services Research Institute, described below.

Data Collection Plans

A major component in planning to implement quality indicators and measures is whether there are consistent, reliable data available in the medical record, pharmacy database, or other locations. Government and other groups have encouraged hospitals to establish electronic medical record (EMR) systems. A component of such an effort has been electronic order entry. The Leapfrog Group (http://www.leapfroggroup.org) has made this one of its core measures. Electronic prescribing can eliminate many medication errors (Grazier 2006b). Key quality indicators and measures can be directly incorporated into the EMR. A close interface between a hospital's quality measurement effort and its development of the EMR can constitute an efficient use of resources (see Chapter 33, "The Electronic Medical Record," by Boronow). Medicare's Pay for Performance programs (originally called Physician Quality Reporting Initiatives) will stimulate the development of such integration. Many studies are beginning to demonstrate the feasibility of using the EMR to elicit needed quality measures data. Baker et al. (2007) have shown how the EMR can be used to assess quality of care, although their study also revealed that missing exclusion criteria remains an unsolved issue for medication-based measures. Goulet et al. (2007) also demonstrated that quality measures can be accurately elicited from the EMR. Opportunities and challenges associated with use of the EMR have been addressed in additional studies (Persell et al. 2006; Sequist 2007; Wahl et al. 2006).

Interpreting and Assessing Data

Determining what to do with measurement data in mental health care is an issue that is beginning to gain increased attention. Instead of data remaining available only in the hospital or department itself, there is increasing encouragement by boards of trustees for all measures to be reported and for as many as possible to have benchmarks.

The value of comparing measurement data with standards, norms, means, or averages (Hermann and Provost 2003) and of statistical benchmarking and risk (case-mix) adjustment (Hermann and Provost 2003; Schacht and Hines 2003) has been well demonstrated. Schacht and Hines (2003) defined risk adjustment as "a means of statistically controlling for group differences when comparing nonequivalent groups on the outcomes that are of interest" (p. 220). Factors such as age, gender, and legal status can have an impact on the measure results for which corrections can be made. Statistical benchmarking (Weissman et al. 1999) is defined as the performance achieved by the top 10% of providers after adjustment for the number of patients that each provider has. A recent key study by Hermann et al. (2006) provided substantial support for the use of statistical benchmarks to construct process measures of quality in mental health care. The study attempted to identify levels of high performance that were "potentially achievable." The authors noted that the benchmark results varied widely because "process measures differ not only in provider performance but also in the degree to which performance is under the provider's control" (Hermann et al. 2006, p. 1465). Kiefe et al. (2001) demonstrated the effectiveness of using achievable benchmarks when giving feedback to physicians on their performance regarding quality measures for diabetic patients.

The Institute of Medicine (2006b) report on mental and substance use conditions recommended "establishing models for the use of the quality measures for benchmarking." Examining the processes within the benchmark hospital to see what "best practices" contributed to the end result is also useful (Lefkovitz 2004).

Risk adjustments are also necessary because of the demand for hospitals to provide mental health quality measures for benchmarking with other similar facilities. Hendryx et al. (2001) have offered an overview of issues related to development and implementation of risk adjustment models in mental health care.

Sharing Data

The key objective of collecting and sharing data is to bring about change in performance. In a study that surveyed frontline providers about their views on various quality monitoring indicators and processes used in mental health services, Valenstein et al. (2004) found that whereas 65% felt that feedback would be "valuable in efforts to improve care," only 38% felt able to influence performance, and 41% indicated that the monitoring "did not assist them in improving care." Providers who had the most positive attitudes toward quality monitoring measures were those who believed that they had the power to influence these measures. Ultimately, however, provider engagement is predicated on accurate implementation of measures and a health-system context supportive of meaningful change in the face of identified shortfalls (Valenstein et al. 2004).

The most important challenge is how to share quality monitoring feedback in a productive and collegial way with clinical staff. Engagement of staff is more likely to be sustained if members are involved in the selection of performance measures from the outset. Formulating some questions to ask clinical staff may also be helpful—for example: "Will these results (on a specific measure) make any difference in how you interact/treat/care for patients?" "Did your work specifically affect this measure?" The goal is to motivate staff not just to hear the results but also to reflect on what the data may mean to them, their team members, and patients.

The "balanced scorecard"—a framework used in business for measuring a company's performance in four key areas (financial, customer, internal process, and innovation; Kaplan and Norton 1992)—has been employed in health care quality monitoring to display a core set of measures helpful to a hospital or department and its leadership.

Indicator and Measure Management

Careful management of quality indicators and measures ensures efficiency and avoids waste of resources. A responsible staff member and group/committee oversee this responsibility. This task may be performed by the departmental quality management committee or a similar group. Functions may include 1) establishing a monitoring process for selection of indicators and measures (including review of feedback from staff members whose performance will be assessed by the measure); 2) determining whether key findings from patient satisfaction surveys are being considered for quality measures; 3) maintaining a history of indicators and measures used previously; 4) periodically assessing the current set of measures for value and determining whether any should be discontinued or have a reduced sampling frequency; and 5) maintaining a list of potential indicators and measures that can be prioritized and added to those already in place when resources become available. Any staff member can add suggestions for consideration to the list.

Education

Periodic education of all staff regarding the role of quality indicators and measures is needed. This provides an opportunity to describe current measures and how indicators and measures are managed. If the hospital has residents, medical students as clinical clerks, or other trainees in one of the health care disciplines, this training should be considered for the curriculum. It may be advantageous for residents to participate in quality management committees, groups that manage indicators and measures, and peer review groups that carry out investigations. In addition, providing a brief overview to peer reviewers and attendees at morbidity and mortality conferences or holding staff debriefing sessions after an event involving seclusion and restraint use, with a focus on exploring underlying causes that may have contributed to a specific outcome, may be useful. Sassani (2004) has highlighted the important role of the academic medical center physician in educating medical students and residents in quality improvement.

Additional Resources

The Institute for Healthcare Improvement, founded in 1991, is dedicated to improving health care throughout the world by "cultivating promising concepts for improving patient care and turning those ideas into action" (see http://www.ihi.org/ihi). Its programs include Web-based knowledge exchange programs, conferences, a professional development program, innovation and learning communities, and the IMPACT Network (http://www.ihi.org/IHI/Programs/IMPACTNetwork) for achieving measurable improvement at the system level. Patient safety has been a central focus, and many tools have been developed to assist staff in reducing adverse events. Outcome, process, and balancing measures are shared, the latter being measures to determine whether improvements to one part of the system will lead to adverse effects in other parts of the system. The Institute has developed a Global Trigger Tool for Measuring Adverse Events, which focuses on identification of harm or injury to patients. *Harm* is defined as "unintended physical injury resulting from or contributed to by medical care that requires additional monitoring, treatment or hospitalization, or that results in death." The measure used is adverse events per 1,000 patient days (Griffin and Resar 2007).

The Center for Quality Assessment and Improvement in Mental Health is another good source for information on quality measures in mental health. It maintains a National Inventory of Mental Health Quality Measures and a Directory of Measure Sources in addition to providing a valuable toolkit, "Selecting Process Measures for Quality Improvement in Mental Healthcare" (Hermann et al. 2002).

The American Psychiatric Association (2002) task force report *Quality Indicators: Defining and Measuring Quality in Psychiatric Care for Adults and Children* is another good resource.

The Evaluation Center at the Human Services Research Institute, funded by SAMHSA, provides technical assistance to mental health providers (among others) "for improving the planning, implementation, and operation of adult mental health services" (see http://tecathsri.org). Consultations are available and subsidized by SAMHSA.

Finally, numerous excellent books are available for individuals working in the quality indicator/measurement field (Hermann 2006; Lloyd 2004). Hermann's (2006) book *Improving Mental Health Care: A Guide to Measurement-Based Quality Improvement* is an especially helpful reference.

A Few Closing Observations

The following observations may be helpful in the development and use of quality indicators and measures:

- In development of measure sets, consider all domains/aims of quality for local applicability.
- Ensure that key findings from patient satisfaction/perception surveys are considered for translation into measures.
- Emphasize emerging national core mental health indicators and measures for accountability purposes.
- Accord equal value to hospital-developed and department-developed measures for local quality-of-care issues.
- Learn to identify and respond to passivity in staff interfacing with quality indicators, measures, and their results.
- Value your history of indicators and measures use.
- Feasibility is essential when seriously considering a measure for implementation.
- Design availability of key quality indicators and measures data into the electronic medical record or handwritten records.
- Provide opportunities for review and input by staff prior to implementation of indicators and measures.

References

American Psychiatric Association: Quality Indicators: Defining and Measuring Quality in Psychiatric Care for Adults and Children (Report of the APA Task Force on Quality Indicators). Washington, DC, American Psychiatric Press, 2002

American Psychiatric Association: Practice Guidelines for the Treatment of Psychiatric Disorders: Compendium 2006. Washington, DC, American Psychiatric Press, 2006

Baker DW, Persell SD, Thompson JA, et al: Automated review of electronic health records to assess quality of care for outpatients with heart failure. Ann Intern Med 146:270–277, 2007

Barry R, Murcko A, Brubaker C: The Six Sigma Book for Health Care: Improving Outcomes by Reducing Errors. Chicago, IL, Health Administration Press, 2002

Berghofer G, Lang A, Henkel H: Satisfaction of inpatients and outpatients with staff, environment, and other patients. Psychiatr Serv 52:104–106, 2001

Berwick DM, Godfrey AB, Roessner J: Curing Health Care: New Strategies for Quality Improvement. San Francisco, CA, Jossey-Bass, 1990

Charbonneau A, Rosen AK, Owen RP, et al: Monitoring depression care: in search of an accurate quality indicator. Med Care 42:522–531, 2004

Coleman EA: Transitional care performance measurement (Appendix I: commissioned paper), in Performance Measurement: Accelerating Improvement (Institute of Medicine, Pathways to Quality Health Care Series). Washington, DC, National Academies Press, 2006, pp 250–286

Coleman EA, Mahoney E, Parry C: Assessing the quality of preparation for posthospital care from the patient's perspective: the care transitions measure. Med Care 43:246–255, 2005

Coleman EA, Parry C, Chalmers S, et al: The care transitions intervention: results of a randomized controlled trial. Arch Intern Med 166:1822–1828, 2006

Donabedian A: An Introduction to Quality Assurance in Health Care. Edited by Bashshur R. New York, Oxford University Press, 2003

Druss BG, Miller CL, Rosenheck RA, et al: Mental health care quality under managed care in the United States: a view from the Health Employer Data and Information Set (HEDIS). Am J Psychiatry 159:860–862, 2002

Druss BG, Miller CL, Pincus HA, et al: The volume-quality relationship of mental health care: does practice make perfect? Am J Psychiatry 161:2282–2286, 2004

Frayne SM, Halanych JH, Miller DR, et al: Disparities in diabetes care: impact of mental illness. Arch Intern Med 165:2631–2638, 2005

Goulet JL, Erdos J, Kancir S, et al: Measuring performance directly using the veterans health administration electronic medical record: a comparison with external peer review. Med Care 45:73–79, 2007

Grazier KL: Efficiency/value-based measures for services, defined populations, acute episodes, and chronic conditions (Appendix H), in Performance Measurement: Accelerating Improvement (IOM Pathways to Quality Health Care Series). Washington, DC, National Academies Press, 2006a, pp 222–241

Grazier KL: Table H-1 "Value-based and efficiency metrics," in Efficiency/value-based measures for services, defined populations, acute episodes, and chronic conditions (Appendix H), in Performance Measurement: Accelerating Improvement (IOM Pathways to Quality Health Care Series). Washington, DC, National Academies Press, 2006b, pp 242–249

Greenberg MD, Pincus HA, Ghinassi FA: Of treatment systems and depression: an overview of quality improvement opportunities in hospital-based psychiatric care. Harv Rev Psychiatry 14:195–203, 2006

Griffin FA, Resar RK: IHI Global Trigger Tool for Measuring Adverse Events. Institute for Healthcare Improvement Innovation Series white paper. Cambridge, MA, Institute for Healthcare Improvement, 2007. Available at: http://www.ihi.org/IHI/results/whitepapers. Accessed April 22, 2007.

Hendryx MS, Beigel A, Doucette A: Introduction: risk-adjustment issues in mental health services. J Behav Health Serv Res 28:225–234, 2001

Hermann RC: Improving Mental Health Care: A Guide to Measurement-Based Quality Improvement. Washington, DC, American Psychiatric Publishing, 2006. Available at http://www.cqaimh.org/ImprovingMHcare.htm. Accessed April 20, 2007.

Hermann RC, Palmer RH: Common ground: a framework for selecting core quality measures for mental health and substance abuse care. Psychiatr Serv 53:281–287, 2002

Hermann RC, Provost S: Interpreting measurement data for quality improvement: standards, means, norms, and benchmarks. Psychiatr Serv 54:655–657, 2003

Hermann RC, Rollins CK: Quality measurement in health care: a need for leadership amid a new federalism. Harv Rev Psychiatry 11:215–219, 2003

Hermann RC, Leff HS, Lagodmos G: Selecting Process Measures for Quality Improvement in Mental Healthcare. Cambridge, MA, the Evaluation Center at HSRI, 2002. Available at: http://www.cqaimh.org/quality.html. Accessed March 19, 2007.

Hermann RC, Palmer H, Leff S, et al: Achieving consensus across diverse stakeholders on quality measures for mental health care. Med Care 42:1246–1253, 2004

Hermann RC, Chan JA, Provost SE, et al: Statistical benchmarks for process measures of quality of care for mental and substance use disorders. Psychiatr Serv 57:1461–1467, 2006

Hillemeier MM, Weisman CS, Baker K, et al: Mental health services provided through the national centers of excellence in women's health: do they reach rural women? Womens Health Issues 15:224–229, 2005

Institute of Medicine: To Err Is Human: Building a Safer Health System. Washington, DC, National Academies Press, 2000

Institute of Medicine: Crossing the Quality Chasm: A New Health System for the 21st Century. Washington, DC, National Academies Press, 2001, pp 5–6

Institute of Medicine: Performance Measurement: Accelerating Improvement. Washington, DC, National Academies Press, 2006a, pp 116–117

Institute of Medicine: Improving the Quality of Health Care for Mental and Substance-Use Conditions. Washington, DC, National Academies Press, 2006b

Institute of Medicine: National organizations involved in performance measurement (Appendix B), in Performance Measurement: Accelerating Improvement (Institute of Medicine, Pathways to Quality Health Care Series). Washington, DC, National Academies Press, 2006c, pp 134–143

Joint Commission: Performance Measurement Initiatives: Hospital-Based, Inpatient Psychiatric Services (HBIPS) Candidate Core Measure Set, last updated February 15, 2008. Oakbrook Terrace, IL, The Joint Commission, 2008. Available at: http://www.jointcommission.org/PerformanceMeasurement/PerformanceMeasurement/Hospital+Based+Inpatient+Psychiatric+Services.htm. Accessed April 1, 2008.

Kaplan RS, Norton DP: The balanced scorecard—measures that drive performance. Harv Bus Rev 70:71–79, 1992

Kiefe CI, Allison JJ, Williams OD, et al: Improving quality improvement using achievable benchmarks for physician feedback: a randomized controlled trial. JAMA 285:2871–2879, 2001

Kuosmanen L, Hatonen H, Jyrkinen AR, et al: Patient satisfaction with psychiatric inpatient care. J Adv Nurs 55:655–663, 2006

Lefkovitz PM: Beyond outcomes: benchmarking in behavioral health care. Behav Healthc Tomorrow 13:32–37, 2004

Lloyd R: Quality Health Care: A Guide to Developing and Using Indicators. Sudbury, MA, Jones & Bartlett, 2004

Persell SD, Wright JM, Thompson JA, et al: Assessing the validity of national quality measures for coronary artery disease using an electronic health record. Arch Intern Med 166:2272–2277, 2006

Peytremann-Bridevaux I, Scherer F, Peer L, et al: Satisfaction of patients hospitalized in psychiatric hospitals: a randomized comparison of two psychiatric-specific and one generic satisfaction questionnaires. BMC Health Serv Res 6:108–117, 2006

Sassani JW: Quality care and academic medical centers: the need for physician education, in Portable Health Administration. Edited by Ziegenfuss JT, Sassani JW. San Diego, CA, Elsevier Academic Press, 2004, pp 155–172

Schacht LM, Hines H: Recent applications of risk adjustment for performance measures used by state inpatient psychiatric facilities. Harv Rev Psychiatry 11:220–224, 2003

Sequist T: Automated data from electronic health records is variably accurate in assessing quality of heart failure care. Journal of Clinical Outcomes Management 14:188–193, 2007

Valenstein M, Mitchinson A, Ronis D, et al: Quality indicators and monitoring of mental health services: what do frontline providers think? Am J Psychiatry 161:146–153, 2004

Van den Heuvel J, Does RJ, Bogers AJ, et al: Implementing six sigma in the Netherlands. Jt Comm J Qual Patient Saf 32:393–399, 2006

Varkey P, Reller MK, Resar RK: Basics of quality improvement in health care. Mayo Clin Proc 82:735, 2007

Wahl WL, Talsma A, Dawson C, et al: Use of computerized ICU documentation to capture ICU core measures. Surgery 140:684–690, 2006

Walter LC, Davidowitz NP, Heineken PA, et al: Pitfalls of converting practice guidelines into quality measures: lessons learned from a VA performance measure. JAMA 291:2466–2470, 2004

Weissman N, Allison J, Kiefe C, et al: Achievable benchmarks of care: the ABCs of benchmarking. J Eval Clin Pract 5:269–281, 1999

Williams T, Cerese J, Cuny J: An exploratory project on the state of quality measures in mental health at academic health centers. Harv Rev Psychiatry 15:34–42, 2007

APPENDIX

Online Resources

Agency for Healthcare Research and Quality (AHRQ): http://www.ahrq.hhs.gov

American Academy of Child and Adolescent Psychiatry (AACAP): http://www.aacap.org

American Medical Association (AMA) Physician Consortium for Performance Improvement: http//www.physicianconsortium.org

American Nurses Association (ANA): http://www.nursingquality.org

American Osteopathic Association (AOA): http://www.osteopathic.org

American Psychiatric Association (APA): http://www.psych.org

AQA (formerly called the Ambulatory Care Quality Alliance): http://www.aqaalliance.org/

Center for Quality Assessment and Improvement in Mental Health (CQAIMH): http://www.cqaimh.org

Centers for Medicare and Medicaid Services: http://www.cms.hhs.gov

Evaluation Center at Human Services Research Institute (HSRI): http://tecathsri.org

Failure Modes and Effects Analysis (FMEA): http://www.ihi.org/IHI/Topics/PatientSafety/SafetyGeneral/Measures/Risk+Priority+Number

Institute for Healthcare Improvement (IHI): http://www.ihi.org

Joint Commission: http://www.jointcommission.org

Leapfrog Group: http://www.leapfroggroup.org

National Association of Psychiatric Health Systems (NAPHS): http://www.naphs.org

National Association of State Mental Health Program Directors (NASMHPD): http://nasmhpd.org

National Committee for Quality Assurance (NCQA): http://www.ncqa.org

National Quality Forum (NQF): http://www.qualityforum.org

Quality Indicator Project: http://www.qiproject.org

Quality Measures Management Information System (Centers for Medicare and Medicaid Services): https://www.qualitynet.org/qmis

Substance Abuse and Mental Health Services Administration (SAMHSA): http://www.samhsa.gov

CHAPTER 33

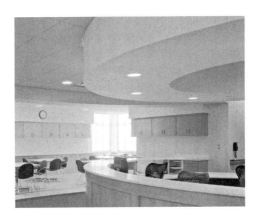

THE ELECTRONIC MEDICAL RECORD

John J. Boronow, M.D.

The field of medicine, which includes psychiatry, has made astonishing strides over the past century. Within this whirlwind of evolving medical science, however, it is equally astonishing to observe that the clinicians who are applying the latest therapeutics in the hospital and clinic are doing so with antiquated tools: free-text handwriting with a pen on paper. Psychiatrists are caring for the most severely ill patients across multiple levels of care with extremely expensive modalities, such as state-of-the-art medications, extended hospitalization and day programs, and sophisticated treatment delivery models (e.g., assertive community treatment teams). Yet despite this, in most instances we simply do not have the clinical information needed at the point of care to make a well-informed, evidence-based decision. The paper chart itself has become an obstacle to evidence-based medicine, limiting our ability to transform anecdotal observations into useful quantitative data that in turn conveys clinically actionable information.

There are numerous specific and practical difficulties that have accrued to the paper chart (Morrissey 2006). Most if not all of these problems pertain to any

medical record, not just a psychiatric chart (where relevant, elements that are unique to behavioral health are highlighted in this chapter). The term *behavioral health* is based on the revolution in health care that is already upon us, which has resulted appropriately in a much wider cadre of behavioral health care providers including psychologists, psychiatric social workers, nurse practitioners, certified addiction counselors, rehabilitation counselors, and vocational counselors, to name but a few. It is extremely important that as we go forward in the development of a true national health information network of medical records, as already envisioned in 2004 by President Bush and presently championed within the U.S. Department of Health and Human Services, the Office of the National Coordinator for Health Information Technology, and the American Health Information Community, that we not be focused narrowly on a single profession within the larger domain of providers. One of the guiding goals of the National Coordinator for Health Information Technology vision is to recognize the value of a patient's clinical information (not limited to just one particular care provider or professional role) across the entire continuum of care—anywhere, anytime.

The challenges of reading handwriting are self-evident, but not trivial. Clinicians can be speeding through a typed summary note from an emergency room, only to come to a crashing halt when they get to the documentation by a nurse regarding dose of medication administered, the details of the use of restraint, or even the phone number of the key contact provided in the critical clinical information ("Is that a 7 or a 1?"). Unfortunately, entire charts of clinical documentation can be literally unreadable, save for the island here and there of a note written by a nurse or a social worker in impeccably clear handwriting. To encounter such a note is to realize just how widespread and serious the problem is.

The handwritten order is an even more problem-prone domain. It is here that the Institute of Medicine made its famous stand in 1999 in its report on accidental deaths and injuries in American hospitals, *To Err is Human* (Kohn et al. 2000). Handwritten orders are open to a wide variety of errors, including errors of omission (time, date, signature, units, route, name [as when a physician's specific idiosyncratic abbreviation is used]) and errors of commission (medications that are unavailable, misspelled, and/or illegibly written; names of medications resulting in transcription errors when a nurse or pharmacist makes the wrong guess as to what the doctor "really meant"; wrong doses by an order of magnitude [as when a zero is left out or a quickly scribbled order makes seeing the tiny little decimal impossible]; wrong number of doses [as when hallowed Latin abbreviations like qd (daily) and qid (four times a day)] are confused with each other; and so forth). Handwritten orders also present a serious problem in terms of data management. In complex cases, just being able to readily review what the current active orders are becomes a major effort. This is particularly challenging for anyone other than the patient's attending physician (who may have a personal memory of the sequence). House officers, cross-covering attending physicians, and consultants all have to somehow re-create the current medication list quickly. And going to the old-fashioned paper medication administration record (MAR), also called a Medex, is often no easier. Hunting through pages and pages of active and inactive MAR entries to determine what is active is time-consuming and error-prone.

So why do most hospital physicians, psychiatrists included, continue to accept and even prefer a paper chart? What are some of the hidden incentives that make transformation to the electronic medical record (EMR) so difficult? Let us begin with productivity. When a physician is overwhelmed with too much to do from the outset, there is only one guiding rule about paperwork: get it done as quickly as possible, irrespective of legibility and content. In this context, the written note is viewed as a personal *aide-mémoire*, and its utility to anyone else is not a primary consideration. The same is true with physician orders. If the physician has already told the nurse what is ordered, actually writing it down legibly and precisely for the pharmacist seems like an avoidable redundancy. In fact, it is precisely because nurses and pharmacists have historically performed so much of these writing tasks that the Joint Commission on Accreditation of Healthcare Organizations recently identified reduction of reliance on verbal orders as a major focus of its safety enhancement program. The move to the EMR actually threatens to radically reorganize the roles not only of the physician but also of the cadre of physician helpers who have enabled the physician to be so productive. Until the physician can feel comfortable with the EMR in effectively replacing such human supports, the old way may seem preferable.

Because fixing the problem of illegibility costs time, and because time represents both the ability to see all of the patients who need to be seen and, of course, money, the consequences of these productivity demands on the physician are also financial. If a busy clinician sees 20 inpatients a day and scrawls illegible notes and careless orders as quickly as possible, he or she will still end up working at least 8 hours (20 patients seen for 25 minutes each). If slowing down to write legible notes and precise orders costs an additional 5 minutes per patient, then 100 fewer minutes a day are available, or 4 fewer patients can be seen, which is a 20% drop in productivity and income, or a nearly 20% increase in the hours a day worked (if the time is simply added to the workday).

Problems with the paper chart transcend illegible handwriting, however. There are many other stories about hospital medical records in which crucial clinical information or communication is corrupted or otherwise made unavailable because of a reliance on chart- and paper-based systems. These would include innumerable kinds of faxing errors, including the frequent omission of every other page when faxing two-sided documents; the misuse or disuse of various mechanical chart flags and associated paper "flag lists" to inform team members of necessary chart management tasks; allergy stickers that detach from the chart and are lost or reaffixed to the wrong chart; and missing charts that may have been misfiled, left carelessly in a variety of places in the nursing station, or taken to an office or the medication room without any way to determine their location. A wasteful search ensues that can easily add 5 minutes a day and nearly half an hour a week to an already very busy work schedule.

But the biggest problem with the paper chart is its failure to organize information reliably, efficiently, and retrievably. The paper page itself is the sole repository of clinical data elements, and it is only as useful as the attributes that define it, such as the patient ID stamp (which validates the medicolegal patient identity), dates (which place data entries into temporal sequence), and chart dividers (which parse related groups of data into clinically meaningful categories). In the bureaucratic world of twenty-first-century American medicine, the amount of paper to be held and ordered for a single hospitalized patient has bloated enormously, thanks to both regulatory and financial demands, as well as the availability of faxing and Xeroxing. There are now pages of preliminary administrative information, financial data, intake and contact data, emergency room records (with their own intake data), assessments, progress notes, consults, lab results, and diagnostic tests. There are outpatient records, school records, immunization records, and documents supplied by family and the patient providing additional history. There are always legal documents in a psychiatric inpatient chart (a signed voluntary admission form, more forms if the admission is involuntary, still more if a clinical review panel is convened to decide on involuntary medication, and yet more again if that panel is appealed). There can be power-of-attorney documentation, guardianship papers, consents of all kinds—including releases of information, permission to reveal the presence of the patient in the hospital, permission to treat an adolescent with a specific medication, and so forth. And we have not yet arrived at the current clinical documentation itself!

The demands of the contemporary regulatory bureaucracy in American medicine have resulted in ever-closer scrutiny of clinical documentation. This has in turn led some organizations to develop specific clinical documentation forms for every discipline to better record what the regulators are looking for and make it easier for the auditors to find such information. The effect has been to increase the number of pages of paper in a chart. A physician's admitting note form can be five pages long; a daily progress note can be three pages long. There are structured fields for data elements that Medicare auditors require to calculate the correct billing code to assign for the service provided as well as to document the medical necessity of that service. There are fields to capture high-risk clinical data requested by Quality Assurance, such as the presence of suicidal or homicidal ideation. And there are fields to capture Joint Commission–driven mandates, such as pain assessments or the rationale for discharging patients who are taking multiple antipsychotic medications. Nursing documentation for seclusion and restraint has become a blizzard of paper, with observations made every 15 minutes, and page after page added if an episode continues for more than a short while. And, of course, all of these forms must be hand-stamped with the patient's ID card, front and back, before they can be filed in the chart.

The result is a very thick and heavy chart compiled within a matter of days in the hospital, with a 3-inch-thick, 10-pound bulk not uncommon after just a 2-week length of stay. The task of maintaining organization of this thick, heavy chart, which is a requisite for any reliable information retrieval, is considerable. Such charts are often dropped and the papers reassembled out of order. Frequent copying and faxing of documents also result in misfiling, both within the correct chart and often within another patient's chart. Similar misfiling or data loss occurs when pages tear from frequent turning. Once again, the result is a very real degradation of clinician efficiency, as the time-pressed doctor either stops to find the missing documents or, worse, just gives up and makes decisions based on memory because the documentation is just not readily available.

Every one of these scenarios is familiar to workers in other sectors of industry that require extensive real-time documentation of industrial or personnel processes and implemented computer-based solutions. Only medicine, a sector representing one-seventh of the total economy, lags behind. Without addressing this shortcoming, medicine cannot hope to achieve Six Sigma quality status (Chassin 1998).

What Added Value Can the Electronic Medical Record Bring to Inpatient Psychiatric Care?

The good news is that the EMR can robustly address every information problem described above qualitatively and efficiently. Legibility problems vanish. Filing accuracy, flagging effectiveness, and information access are vastly enhanced. Data structuring is integrated into the workflow, thus adding to the clinical and quality assurance functions rather than detracting from them. Data integration is performed in seconds, and a current summary of all important clinical parameters is displayed in a single view. The vessel containing and presenting the data thus helps to transform that data into clinically useful *information,* rather than obstruct access to it, as so often happens with paper.

Beyond these improvements on the paper chart, however compelling, there are also new quality-of-care concerns bearing directly on the safety of patients to which the EMR can actually bring added value, even as it performs the onerous task of simple documentation. For example, the EMR allows for documentation and justification of diagnoses and problem lists across levels of care over time. Psychiatric diagnoses have been criterion-based since Robert Spitzer leveraged the groundbreaking work of Research Diagnostic Criteria from 1978 into DSM-III in 1980 (American Psychiatric Association 1980). Yet in spite of extensive and expensive efforts by the American Psychiatric Association to educate psychiatrists in the use of such criterion-based diagnoses, it remains nearly unheard of, except in research settings, to be able to find clear documentation that the criteria were met when a particular diagnosis was made, much less to be able to track these criteria over time, as the patient's illness evolves. By its very nature, however, the EMR can provide a convenient way to maintain a diagnosis and problem list *across episodes of care.* The ability to easily document in a single place the diagnostic criteria met at a given point in time is enormously helpful for the next clinician who may be facing the patient for the first time, along with a confusing array of cross-sectional signs and symptoms. Relying on the old paper chart, which may merely list a diagnostic label without any justification, as we now do so often, is frequently not helpful. But an EMR maintains the diagnosis across episodes of care so that the evidence for the diagnosis can be documented, attached to the diagnosis, and passed along for all to see and add to over time, blog-style. This last functionality is presently an untested promise, awaiting future publications with best-practice guidelines to demonstrate how it might be optimally configured and executed. Here is an example of how technology has opened an exciting window of opportunity. It will be up to clinicians in the next decade to take full advantage of the EMR's power and exploit it for the benefit of excellent patient care.

Computerized physician order entry (CPOE) similarly enhances patient safety and quality of care in many ways (Berger and Kichak 2004; Butler et al. 2006; Kilbridge et al. 2006). To understand the importance of these improvements, one must first analyze the current state of the paper workflow as it typically exists in hospitals. The physician writes orders or gives abbreviated verbal orders to a nurse. The written orders may be "taken off" by a variety of staff members, including the nonmedical unit clerks, nurses, and, in some settings, pharmacists or pharmacist techs. The person who *takes off* the order documents his or her action and must then transcribe the order onto a paper MAR, which is subject to error. The order must also be somehow communicated to the pharmacy. This may be done by faxing, which is problematic if the fax degrades the physician's handwriting legibility. The pharmacist must interpret the physician's order, possibly in a manner different from the nurse or unit clerk who is transcribing the same order onto the MAR, and then manually enter the order into the hospital's pharmacy system. The pharmacy system is typically a standalone computer system exclusively dedicated to keeping track of all medications ordered, dispensed, or returned unused to the pharmacy. The pharmacy system software industry is to some extent parallel to the EMR industry, and only very recently have there been efforts to consolidate these products into a single integrated application—largely because of the major delay in adoption of EMRs by most American hospitals. As a result, it is the pharmacist, not the physician, who has access to the online databases that can and do immediately alert the pharmacist that, for example, an order is in conflict with a patient's known allergy history, exceeds a certain safe dosing threshold, has the potential to interact unsafely with the medications the patient is already receiving, or is a duplicate of a therapeutic treatment already ordered for the patient. Now the pharmacist, who does not usually know the patient, must contact a nurse on the unit (though not necessarily a nurse who had anything to do with *taking off* the original order), and this nurse in turn must track down the doctor and deliver a "callback." But because the nurse is at this point a peripherally related intermediary, the message is often unclear and the physician must make a *second callback* to the pharmacist directly, to clarify the pharmacist's question and make a decision. Having done so, a *third callback* is now needed, this time back to a nurse on the unit who can receive a verbal order to cancel the original order and write a new, revised order.

CPOE changes the dynamics of this complex task dramatically. By placing the physician directly in control of the order entry process, which is now structured by the computer in a way that ensures that all required data elements are present, the initial order is entered—legibly, cleanly, logically, and completely. Just as important, those warnings that only the pharmacist had been receiving now go directly to the physician entering the order. Real-time warnings to the clinician writing the order are more likely to educate a physician about his or her own knowledge base and quality-of-care standards as well as demonstrably improve patient safety (Smith et al. 2006). And the physician can remedy the problem on the spot, thus eliminating all of the callbacks—and saving time for many staff members. The efficiency does not end there, however. The entire process of transcription, faxing, and mailing of orders by others is removed, as are the errors associated with that process. The MAR becomes the eMAR (electronic medication administration record), which is now populated automatically by the EMR, based on the logic associated with the computerized order. Of course, the pharmacist must still verify the order and can delay it if there is a medical or availability concern. But otherwise, once the pharmacist releases the order as verified, the physician's intent is automatically expressed on the eMAR for the next medication administration time. The complexity of the inpatient ordering process, consisting of many error-prone steps, is now managed within three systems: CPOE, pharmacy, and eMAR.

The industry is working toward single-integration systems; in fact, some of these products were already introduced in 2006. The time-saving value of the eMAR to nursing can be huge. In organizations that have increasingly been forced to hire *per diem* or agency staff to cover shortfalls in full-time nurses, a very real increase in medication errors has occurred. A typical response to this problem has been to increase the manual review of the paper MARs and paper orders, often in every shift in settings with high turnover and high volume. The necessity of this quality control effort disappears with the eMAR, freeing the medication nurse to engage in other, more valuable clinical activities, such as actually conducting medication education face-to-face with patients.

The eMAR can become a very medically useful tool for the inpatient psychiatrist. Certain psychiatric inpatients (e.g., acutely psychotic patients) often refuse some or all of their prescribed medications during the early part of an admission and then receive various prn (as needed) medications instead. Keeping track of what is initially refused, what is subsequently taken, and what is taken extra in the form of prn doses adds up to an extremely important information-management activity. It is quite difficult for a busy psychiatrist to track this information quickly with a paper chart when making rounds; such tracking is therefore often not done at all (leading, at times, to serious adverse outcomes) or is delegated to a nurse to research and prepare for the psychiatrist every morning—an expensive and clinically wasteful deployment of resources that might otherwise be put to better use in direct patient contact. A well-configured eMAR can assist the psychiatrist in efficiently keeping track of all the doses of medication a patient receives. In addition, the nursing documentation regarding the efficacy of the prn medications can be readily displayed within the eMAR environment. Duplication of documentation for nursing is thus avoided, and the psychiatrist obtains the valuable clinical information needed to make the next set of treatment decisions.

Another notorious problem universally associated with paper charts and orders is the Joint Commission and Centers for Medicare and Medicaid Services mandate that verbal orders be countersigned by a physician. This requirement, which on the surface might seem innocuous enough, is in fact the focus of a major national effort in American hospitals. How does an organization systematically keep track of all the clinicians who may have given verbal orders but are not based on the patient's unit and therefore not routinely present the next day to see the mechanical flag or receive a paper flagsheet? The EMR addresses this kind of problem brilliantly. Unsigned orders are automatically flagged to the patient list of the original ordering doctor, as well as to the patient lists of any other authorized doctors who may, by virtue of their supervisory role or their membership in a common group practice, sign on behalf of the original doctor, thus eliminating a problem that has consumed countless hours of clinical administrative time. Similar efficiencies accrue in the handling of seclusion and restraint orders, which in recent years have had their oversight ratcheted up to such a degree that reordering must be done every 4 hours and face-to-face reevaluations conducted every 8 hours. The EMR can greatly enhance the efficiency of ensuring that such reordering and reevaluations are done on time, by virtue of the built-in flagging rules, by organizing the patient list in a way that brings focus to select kinds of patients, and, in some scenarios, by automatically paging the doctor should the order renewal time lapse. From the perspective of auditors, monitoring compliance with mandated policies and procedures associated with seclusion and restraint becomes much easier and more reliable, and organizations can routinely self-monitor so much more easily that problems are identified and resolved long before Joint Commission and Centers for Medicare and Medicaid Services auditors visit. We are able to move from a time-sampling methodology delegated to external agencies to a real-time, 100%-sampling methodology owned by the organization itself. In any management system, this counts as a major step forward.

Since deinstitutionalization, inpatient psychiatry has evolved from the isolation of the asylum to a role of equal partner in a continuum of levels of care. The need to communicate—accurately and in real time—the patient's most recent history at the immediately preceding level of care has never been more urgent. The fallback tool has always been the discharge summary.

There was a time when the discharge summary was a serviceable solution. In the current era, there are many problems with this model, however. In many settings today, the discharge summary is often not done by the attending physician and in addition is often incomplete and delayed. Moreover, bureaucratic obstacles imposed by well-intentioned and mandatory privacy rules mean that even if the receiving physician wishes to obtain the discharge summary completed by a social worker 30 days after the fact, he or she will have to take the time to ensure that the patient completes a detailed release-of-information form. The receiving clinician is thus often left with just the patient in front of him or her, having no idea all that was done in the previous level of care.

An EMR by itself cannot solve the discharge summary problem. Some EMRs have been developed with tools that enable clinicians to cut and paste documentation assembled in the EMR during the patient's stay and collect it into a de facto discharge summary. Such a quasi-summary can be quite unsatisfactory. By definition, it is not actually a summary (which intentionally implies a synthesis of a case, with an overall formulation of what was going on, why this or that did or did not work, what the final outcome was, what the recommended aftercare should be, and why). No cut-and-paste technology can create this kind of summary without heavy editing, at which point it is more efficient to just do the whole thing from scratch. And without such editing, one is often left with, at best, a choppy sequential narrative that often fails to reveal the underlying analytical process that is at the heart of the case.

In lieu of a high-quality standard discharge summary, one can imagine an integrated network of health information resources, with all their clinical data pooled into a common system that can be accessed in real time by appropriately authorized clinicians in the service of providing ongoing continuity of care (Markle Foundation 2004).

A full discussion on the vision and progress of the National Health Information Network is well beyond the scope of this chapter, but mention of it is relevant to the extent that such a formal federal focus clearly highlights the increasing urgency with which universal deployment of EMRs in hospitals across the country is being viewed. No network can exist without a preexisting backbone of EMR systems. In 2005, the Office of the National Coordinator for Health Information Technology began the process of standardizing the ambulatory EMR industry with a view toward compatibility within a future National Health Information Network by creating the Certification Commission for Healthcare Information Technology (see http://www.cchit.org).

As always is the case when such global visions meet the daily reality of clinical practice, there are important practical considerations that may have a tremendous impact on the final implementation of a system. Would a busy outpatient psychiatrist ever have the time to peruse an information-packed inpatient EMR, even if he or she did have easy access to it? Would the data be sufficiently standardized, given the current plan, to permit an unlimited number of software vendors to enable outpatient end users to find the same kinds of data from three different hospital EMRs? How would those data be made available to end users? As one considers the potential problems of a global health information network, the traditional physician-dictated discharge summary starts to look better and better. It may in fact be premature to assume that a National Health Information Network will eliminate this important document.

A discussion of discharge summaries necessarily brings up two other often onerous chores of inpatient practice: the writing of discharge prescriptions and the generation of Joint Commission–mandated medication reconciliations at every change in level or location of care. The EMR has the potential to facilitate these tasks enormously. The functionality to generate prescriptions directly from the inpatient orders, with only minor editing needed, already exists. Such prescriptions can be signed electronically and faxed directly to pharmacies. If a small supply of medications must be dispensed directly from the hospital pharmacy to tide the patient over until the outpatient pharmacy fills the prescriptions, this duplicate work can also be speedily handled by the EMR. Medication reconciliations become quite simple when the outpatient medication profile generated at the time of admission by the admitting nurse and doctor is already in the system to populate the reconciliation, and the electronic prescriptions generated at discharge automatically populate the discharge half of the reconciliation. The clinician has saved enough time to actually think about the two lists and ensure that they reconcile as intended.

The EMR offers the possibility of achieving an in-depth knowledge of patients over time. And this, in turn, is a prerequisite for managing risk. A health system with an EMR that spans all levels of care can begin to compete with the managed care industry by acquiring, organizing, and analyzing clinical data on its own, beholden to no corporate agenda. Early efforts at this were made in the 1990s by capitation programs (Braun and Caper 1999). If clinician entrepreneurs were armed with high-quality longitudinal clinical data across all levels of care and perhaps also empowered to take more risk on behalf of the overall care of the patient, we might see a real revolution in patient care that was *truly* managed—in the best interest of the patient, with evidence-based therapeutics. Although such a vision is utopian today, it could only happen with the deployment of EMRs across a large continuum of behavioral health care.

Other examples of improved efficiency from an EMR include automated alerts and automated formulary checking. In the paper world, the nurse, pharmacist, or unit clerk reminds the physician that a task needs to be done by way of a paper flagsheet, phone call, or Post-it note in the physician's mailbox. All of these messages can be easily ignored and have no inherent audit history. The EMR's capacity to support auditable and reportable flag management exposes physicians who routinely ignore reminders to renew orders, sign discharge summaries, and so forth. Ideally, the EMR facilitates the execution of those tasks (e.g., the physician can sign an entire batch of orders from a variety of places with a single click). Formulary checking is computing's solution to managing the proliferation of insurance benefits currently available to our patients. When the consumer advantages of competition in the insurance industry are touted, the providers' struggle to cope with all of the different plans is usually not mentioned. And the consequences of mismanaging formulary benefit information can be worse than just added overhead expense. The fact is, if physicians do not know what formulary a patient's insurance uses at the point of service (in this case, when writing that first order for a new medication that will drive the entire hospitalization), they can make mistakes that result in patients being discharged on medications they cannot pay for, thus having to redo the entire treatment at the worst possible time. Computers are ideally suited to the task of matching benefits to formularies and displaying "allowed" choices to physicians at the point of service if the databases are accurately maintained (no small task in this world of constantly changing benefit structures and insurance choices).

A final example of how the EMR is poised to transform hospital care can be seen in the realm of quality assurance. Joint Commission, Centers for Medicare and Medicaid Services, and state Medicaid authorities all look for evidence that the hospital and its professional staff are providing the highest possible quality of care for patients—not just the highest cost. Assurance methods have been diverse, from the questionable reliance on received "expert" opinion, as solicited by and then published in the *U.S. News & World Report* Annual Rankings, to pseudo-objective scores passed out by site surveys conducted by these agencies. The managed care industry tried briefly and unsuccessfully to force standardized outcome measures on health care in the 1990s, and measures such as the Healthcare Effectiveness Data and Information Set, developed by the National Council on Quality Assurance (Druss 2004), continue to promote this effort. How different might these measures be if the behavioral health community could examine a standardized data set of all of treatments and outcomes based on data-collecting tools embedded in an integrated network of EMRs? Such data could serve multiple purposes. At the macro level, the data could be consolidated from diverse regions to address epidemiological questions. At the systems level, the data could shed light on the differences in patient mix, as well as treatments and outcomes among all programs. At the practitioner level, the information could lift the cover off the shroud of professional secrecy and arouse new interest in a truly exciting and informed peer review process. The EMR can form the backbone of a systematic and transparent data collection system that can reveal what we do so we can do it better. It is an indispensable part of the solution to "crossing the quality chasm" (Chaudhry et al. 2006; Hillestad et al. 2005; Institute of Medicine 2001).

Obstacles to Computerized Records and Computerized Physician Order Entry

Despite the enthusiasm expressed so far for the potential of the EMR, the field is not there yet. The problems associated with current technology, combined with deeply embedded industrywide disincentives, are substantial and worthy of serious analysis (Gesteland 2006). To begin with, the functionality of the utilities described above varies greatly, and discrepancies between the real and the ideal can be downright dismaying. Three examples may suffice to make this point.

The much-vaunted computerized warning alerts, designed to prevent some of the 100,000 accidental and preventable deaths documented by the Institute of Medicine (2001), can be terribly flawed. They can be set to appear for even the most trivial of antacid and diet interactions. They may be displayed in a stunningly arcane format, which can make finding the take-home message an exercise analogous to wading through the PDR. Instead of quickly and efficiently reminding clinicians of the value and importance of remembering a specific aspect of a treatment, the warnings instead irritate doctors and can discourage them from even bothering to read the messages at all. The problem is further compounded when the system does not display the message in large or bold type or requires the user to expand a window or scroll through reams of text to find the relevant nugget of information. Such computer-generated inefficiency can be just as exasperating and debilitating as the problems described regarding the paper chart. Perhaps, however, these difficulties will be reduced by improved and, if necessary, customized programming to meet the needs of specific users and settings.

The problems described earlier with order errors in the paper chart may also unfortunately be supplanted by novel electronic order errors as the bane of Quality Assurance. Although legibility and transcription mistakes vanish instantaneously with the EMR, system- and user-generated errors may create new domains of risk that will require vigilant monitoring (Berger and Kichak 2004). The simplest example is the prn order. In the paper world, prn orders are simply so ingrained that it is virtually inconceivable for a clinician to write an order without the prn included. In the EMR, however, most systems require the prn status to be indicated by checking a prn box. This may seem trivial enough, but we have seen many examples in our setting of problems with this feature in a new EMR. The new user, focused on learning all of the complexities of the EMR and distracted by the novelty of the workflow and the pressure to get the job done quickly and move on, will simply skip the prn checkbox. The consequences of this mistake can be serious: a lorazepam dose of 2 mg every 4 hours can quickly become intoxicating if continued around the clock. The remedy for this problem might be for the pharmacist to verify ev-

ery order before it is released to the eMAR as an active order, or it may be left up to a nurse to question an order because it is unusual or because she sees an obviously sedated patient in front of her. Perhaps the system itself, if sufficiently programmed with dosage-range checking algorithms, may prevent a dangerous error from occurring.

Other examples of novel electronic order mistakes include user errors that occur because of inexperience and unfamiliarity with a complex system: lack of awareness of a previously given dose of medication because the view filter on the eMAR is set incorrectly; failure to dispense a medication because of faulty integration among the EMR, the pharmacy system, and the medication dispensing system; failure to draw a laboratory sample despite timely order entry because of faulty integration with the laboratory workflow and unanticipated requirements for entry of additional defining data in mandatory fields programmed into the routine lab order form. Most of these errors can and are resolved with user experience and ongoing refinements of the system. But they highlight a more general problem associated with the transition to the EMR— namely, the need to recognize the magnitude of the change in daily workflow for all users, not just doctors and nurses, and how many unanticipated complications arise as a consequence of this transition in the initial implementation of a new EMR system.

Perhaps the biggest obstacle to EMR adoption in hospitals, beyond the enormous cost, is physician-user adoption (Audet et al. 2004). Although a hospital can mandate that employees such as nurses, pharmacists, and lab technicians take training classes and learn new technologies, learning new record-keeping techniques often proves quite challenging for medical staff in open-staff hospitals. Doctors who admit to multiple hospitals, especially surgeons or other physicians who do very specialized consulting work, are faced with a daunting prospect of having to master several different systems deployed in the various facilities in which they work. It is hard enough to learn any one system. It is simply unrealistic to expect a busy physician to master two or three different systems, each with its own idiosyncrasies that must be learned through painful trial and error, each with its own logins, passwords, and policies. The process is further compounded by the very real age-dependent variabilities in computer and typing skills across the range of younger to older physicians. The computer revolution and the Internet have literally passed some (but by no means all!) older physicians by in the past two decades. Learning these skills on the job while continuing the frantic pace of clinical work they are used to can simply be unimaginable to some clinicians, young or old, even if they do have previous computer experience. In an open-staff setting, physicians may simply revolt and threaten convincingly to admit their patients somewhere else that does not hassle them with such demands. A medical-surgical hospital in Baltimore implemented CPOE by continuing to allow physicians to write paper orders and paying a technician to pass through each nursing station every 2 hours and enter those orders into the system, with nurses handling any urgent orders on the spot. Thus, the hospital reaps some of the advantages of the EMR order-entry functionality while the physicians perpetuate the timeless handmaiden tradition of yore. This problem has been addressed to some degree by the rise of the *hospitalist model* in the past decade. As managed care has made it increasingly difficult for many ambulatory internists to even afford to do inpatient work, hospitals have come to rely more on a closed staff of employed hospitalists, both in medical-surgical settings and in psychiatry (e.g., the Sheppard Pratt Health System). Such a staffing model facilitates adoption of the EMR, in terms of both training and corporate control, but also because staff members are much more likely to see the value of an EMR if they are focused on the patient care in a single setting, where the functionality of the system is leveraged over the entire patient caseload.

Specific Psychiatric and Behavioral Health Functionality

The EMR has historically been designed for the traditional medical application. Behavioral health imposes its own specialized requirements upon the EMR. As of 2008, the EMR industry has not produced any fully functional product that comprehensively addresses the needs of inpatient behavioral health care. The most prominent example of this need–availability gap is the lack of an electronic product for generating the master treatment plan (MTP), which has been mandated by the Joint Commission, the Centers for Medicare and Medicaid Services, and most state regulatory agencies since the 1960s. The MTP is a major focus of most site visits by regulatory agencies. It is a paper document that has been divorced from routine daily care of patients; it is usually viewed by most clinicians as "paperwork." Although this is not always the case (indeed, first-class MTPs can be developed that truly do advance excellence in patient care), the traditional

model, based as it is on the limitations of the paper chart, is hampered by its status as a onetime exercise subsequently relegated to a section of the chart. The EMR has the power to transform the MTP, however. Beginning with the physician and nursing admission notes, a problem list can be jointly developed, which then populates flowsheets in the EMR and is linked to clinical documentation by nursing. The MTP conference itself becomes a much richer experience because the problem list has already been initiated and documented from the moment of admission and is readily available for incorporation into the MTP itself. A truly "master" treatment plan can thus be developed, because now all relevant data are available in a summary display that includes diagnoses, vital signs, allergies, significant events, and even insurance information, facilitating a comprehensive grasp of the case by all team members. Progress toward objectives can also be tracked in nursing notes linked to the MTP, thereby achieving the Joint Commission "Holy Grail" wherein the MTP finally "drives treatment" as was originally intended.

Documentation of diagnosis in the MTP is greatly simplified by the ability to draw upon the EMR's diagnosis list, which has been added to from the first admission (at any visit) since the EMR was implemented. Tools such as "Significant Event" fields assist the team in focusing on order-specific target problems that the MTP will address. And discharge planning during the MTP may be enhanced by immediate access to insurance benefits contained in the system. The end product is an order of magnitude beyond the scribbled one- or two-line documents that are commonly seen today. Such a document makes competent discussion of the case—by the physician with a colleague, by the utilization reviewer with the managed care reviewer, and by the social worker with the family and the referring agency—possible in a way seldom before realized.

Until now, MTP software has been a standalone product for inpatient applications and has not experienced much user adoption, because of failure to integrate it into a paper chart world. The vision described above of a true EMR-based MTP requires customized forms development and considerable planning by the end-user group during the preparation stage of EMR deployment. In the next generation of EMR software, it is hoped that products will be developed that have such functionality already preconfigured by the developer, requiring only minor final tweaking by the end-user group to accommodate the functionality to the precise needs of its setting.

Another area where the EMR may excel in advancing inpatient behavioral health care is in the domain of behavioral tracking. The paper chart has always valued the narrative note above all else. Graphing has always been the exception. Even in medical-surgical settings, it is the poor medical student who is sent off to laboriously plot the labs over time and then "stick it in the chart." The routine visual display of quantitative data for clinical decision making has not been easy and is thus rarely done.

Behavioral health care often lends itself nicely to semi-quantitative data acquisition and display. Particularly nowadays, with managed care requiring only the highest acuity to justify even a few days within an inpatient setting, there is usually no shortage of readily identifiable target behaviors available for documentation: tearfulness, yelling, refusal to get out of bed, refusal to take medication, refusal to attend groups, attempts to elope, intrusive attention seeking at the nursing station, too-loud talking, touching of other people, defacing of walls, and so forth. The EMR allows the incorporation of a behavioral dictionary of target inpatient behaviors, both pathological and prosocial/adaptive, which can then be coordinated with the MTP and tracked on flowsheets just like vital signs or intakes and outputs (I&Os). Documentation of quantifiable data elements within an integrated electronic flowsheet structure can transform anecdotal impressions ("Sally seemed more agitated when the family visited") into robust quasi-experiments on the fly ("Sally had 2.4 verbal outbursts/day prior to the visit, 6 on the day of the visit, and 2.7 the week after the visit.") The ability to easily plot a single rating scale item such as a Positive and Negative Syndrome Scale hallucinations score or a Montgomery-Åsberg Depression Rating Scale item against a longitudinal display of ongoing medication or other treatments from the moment of admission could rationalize the approach to therapeutics, which, at present, is at risk of being oversimplified by the expediency of managed care demands. One can well imagine the EMR empowering a clinical team with much more actionable data to argue on behalf of their patients when managed care denials threaten inappropriately. These and other possibilities for intelligent and creative improvements to patient care, based on real clinical data, are virtually innumerable with the empowerment of the EMR.

A final example of unique behavioral health care functionality in the EMR is the psychiatric historical time line, which displays the sequence, duration, and severity of psychiatric signs and symptoms over time against other selected relevant parameters such as hospitalizations, medications, stressful life events. In the hospital, especially with the treatment-refractory case, it is often very important to be able to review the course of treatment over time in a way that links the changes in medication to the patient's behavior and mental status. A unique twist in inpatient behavioral health care is that disturbed psychiatric patients often either refuse medication or require significant additional prn medication, thus placing another hurdle before anyone wanting to plot treatment against outcome. The traditional approach to this kind of data display has been to have a nurse or research technician laboriously tally up the total daily doses of medications, by type, on a daily basis, so as to display the total daily dose (i.e., standing medication plus prn medication minus refused doses). This can then be tracked along the X axis over time; as the doses increase or decrease, the medication is changed, or another is added. Therapeutic drug monitoring data can be added to the medication sequence. Above this display one can then plot clinical behavioral data, be it rating scale items or scores, frequency counts of target behaviors, or significant events such as a visit from family. The resulting display can summarize a complex case dramatically, clarifying the extent to which a given medication regimen is indeed helping (or not) and refining the overall understanding of the natural history of a patient's response to treatment. Although no current EMR that we are aware of is quite ready to generate such a display "off the shelf," it is safe to assume that availability of medication data within an eMAR and the structured behavioral data within flowsheets should ultimately allow custom programming to bring these together.

Protection of Patient Privacy

The most visible subject to differentiate behavioral health from the rest of medicine and surgery in every discussion of EMRs is invariably the issue of protecting patient privacy. Since the days of the Pentagon Papers and the burglary of Daniel Ellsberg's psychiatrist's office in 1971, the public has been keenly aware that confidential information disclosed in the privacy of a psychotherapeutic session could potentially be the target of malicious abuse. (Ellsberg had leaked secret documents from the Pentagon about the Vietnam war to the press; to punish him for this, a break-in was authorized by the White House to obtain incriminating evidence against Ellsberg from his psychiatrist's psychotherapy notes.) Psychiatrists, psychologists, and all other behavioral health care providers have traditionally maintained the strictest of confidentiality standards with regard to such information. Most states have endorsed and supported such protections, legislating rules protecting psychotherapy notes as having at least limited privilege, except in a *Tarasoff* situation or in the event of an imminent life-and-death crisis for the patient.

The 1996 Kennedy–Kirshenbaum Health Insurance Portability and Accountability Act (HIPAA) is widely perceived by the lay public as having increased the requirements of medical providers to drastically increase the privacy standards of all patients. However, from the perspective of behavioral health, the act actually lowered the bar. The HIPAA Privacy Rule in fact states that sharing medical information between medical providers on behalf of a patient's medical care, including explicitly psychiatric information, does not demand any HIPAA protection and may include information such as psychiatric diagnosis, psychiatric medications, and past psychiatric hospitalizations (Mosher and Swire 2002). The only explicitly protected behavioral health information in HIPAA is so-called psychotherapy notes (again recalling Ellsberg).

The reason for this brief historical digression is that rules and standards are currently being created that will govern exactly the kind of information that is or is not protected within an EMR and, more broadly, within a national health information network that integrates these EMRs (Terry and Francis 2007). As HIPAA is currently written and construed, there will be no a priori confidentiality protections for a psychiatric diagnosis, psychiatric medication, or history of psychiatric hospitalization. A patient's diagnosis of alcohol or cocaine abuse, a history of amphetamine-treated attention-deficit/hyperactivity disorder (ADHD) in childhood, a hospitalization for postpartum depression—all will be fair game for any health care provider who has a legitimate relationship to the patient's case, including, for example, the plastic surgeon, the dermatologist, the allergist, even the dietitian and physical therapist. The potential for widespread dissemination of personal information that has historically been the privy of only the patient's psychiatrist and perhaps the primary care provider suddenly becomes a very real possibility. Because we focus on inpatient psychiatry, the task of managing this prospect of such widespread exposure is marginally easier than in the ambulatory world. Hospital EMR systems are usually monolithic single entities, within the context of a relatively "closed" system of providers and users, the majority of whom are either employees of the hospital or contractually bound in significant ways to

a hospital's organizational structure and discipline (e.g., the professional medical staff). Even if hospital EMRs are eventually linked to the National Health Information Network as it is envisioned here, it is unlikely, as we have already suggested, that users outside the hospital would have easy access to, or even want, primary source documentation related to a patient's visit. The complexity and volume of data would make such trolling from outsiders quite challenging, if not impossible. However, summary documents or personal health records regarding patient visits will likely be readily available, and if the only thing that protects behavioral health information is an undefined HIPAA standard of medical "need to know," it is clear that many confidential behavioral health secrets may be exposed to the unfettered cyber-breeze of the network. Once information is shared between the source provider and the receiver, there is no guarantee that it will not be *reshared* with third and fourth parties, and beyond. It is for this very reason that psychiatric departments in large academic hospitals can be the last ones to adopt the hospital's EMR.

Solutions to the confidentiality challenge are varied. The most conservative privacy advocates actually demand a nonelectronic alternative to every health care encounter. For those willing to embrace the inevitability of the EMR revolution, options include various integrated software strategies to hide confidential data elements. These safeguards range from the most primitive "confidential" zone (an arbitrary, unstructured password-protected subset of the clinical database populated completely at the discretion of the clinician user) to a more sophisticated behavioral health "lock box" to a highly sophisticated system of granular privacy tags that can link discrete items such as a diagnosis or historical element to a specific set of defined confidentiality rules issued by the patient, controlled by the release of those data elements independently of the clinician who originally elicited the information from the patient. In this last scenario, the tags automatically display certain data to a psychiatrist who has bona fide electronic credentials and also a bona fide current established therapeutic relationship with the patient while hiding that same information from a legitimate but nonbehavioral health provider, such as a surgeon. Clearly, for the present, no EMR is sophisticated enough to stop a clinician from just writing down privileged information inappropriately in a "public" domain, such as an unprotected medical history. So even the most powerful software protections will inevitably only be as strong as the carefulness of the least careful provider.

Standalone behavioral health facilities have a small advantage in this regard, given the built-in barriers of organizational boundaries, which preclude nonbehavioral health care providers from accessing the EMR on a casual or routine basis. All EMRs, however, are vulnerable to security lapses, including stolen laptops and hacking of servers located in distant states that can host a hospital's EMR remotely. Because of numerous recent widely publicized cases of wanton irresponsibility in the breaching of database security, the public is all too aware that no promise of data integrity is foolproof. In fact, it is probably safe to say that the drawbacks of the paper chart also account for its (relative) security in protecting privileged personal health information. As Nixon's plumbers discovered 35 years ago, stealing paper records is difficult and risky, and the chore of writing or copying information by hand is so tedious and costly for the busy clinician that there is a built-in disincentive to share information. Although Ellsberg himself stole other kinds of information and leveraged the then-new photocopying technology to disseminate it publicly to the newsprint media, the power of the Internet to splash personal secrets around the world instantaneously is simply unprecedented. The solution to this dilemma remains in limbo. A national effort is currently under way, under a joint contract by the Agency for Healthcare Research and Quality (AHRQ) and the Office of the National Coordinator for Health Information Technology (ONCHIT), to harmonize HIPAA and the privacy and confidentiality laws of all 50 states to reach a consensus on how to proceed (Dimitropoulos 2007), but many privacy advocates have joined this controversial conversation in a very vocal way. Whatever the outcome, one thing is sure: someday, hospital psychiatry in the United States and Europe will not be using paper records, and one way or the other, we will have made a decision, for better or worse, on how to protect confidential behavioral health personal information within this brave new world.

The Present and Future of the Hospital Electronic Medical Record

Current hospital-based EMR systems are still in a relatively nascent state. Despite the fact that the U.S. Department of Veterans Affairs began to seriously explore computerization of medical information in the 1980s, and the U.S. Department of Defense had a full-blown computerized order entry and results system by 1993, progress in developing a truly user-friendly tool

has been disappointing. The reasons for this are manifold and include the inherent conservatism of physicians as a group, the very real complexity and cost of the task at hand, and the lack of any overarching standards and championship from organized medicine. It is no accident that the most robustly developed systems around the world have evolved in top-down settings such as the Department of Veterans Affairs and the U.S. military or European countries with national health systems. The invention of the personal computer and the Internet, though clearly a net gain for the industry, also confounded it for a time, as products had to be retooled or even reinvented from scratch to fully meet the demands of Windows, graphic user interface displays, and Web-enabled functionality, none of which was even remotely supported by earlier products. The lack of standards and openness continues to hamper the industry, diverting scarce resources to marketing and user support and away from pooled research that might actually produce products that are so successful they do not require an army of technicians to customize, deploy, and debug in the midst of ongoing patient care. Nevertheless, helpful guidelines are available (Amatayakul 2004).

Right now, the EMR continues to be a powerful but cumbersome tool, solving some problems while creating new ones, and always teasing us with the prospect that the best is yet to come (Technology CEO Council 2006).

References

Amatayakul M: Electronic Health Records: A Practical Guide for Professionals and Organizations. Chicago, IL, American Health Information Management Association (AHIMA), 2004

American Psychiatric Association: Diagnostic and Statistical Manual of Mental Disorders, 3rd Edition. Washington, DC, American Psychiatric Association, 1980

Audet AM, Doty MM, Peugh J, et al: Information technologies: when will they make it into physicians' black bags? Med Gen Med 6:2, 2004

Berger RG, Kichak JP: Computerized physician order entry: helpful or harmful? J Am Med Inform Assoc 11:100–103, 2004

Braun P, Caper P: Information needs in a changing health care system: capitation and the need for a population-oriented view. J Ambul Care Manage 22:1–10, 1999

Butler J, Speroff T, Arbogast PG, et al: Improved compliance with quality measures at hospital discharge with a computerized physician order entry system. Am Heart J 151:643–653, 2006

Chassin MR: Is health care ready for Six Sigma quality? Milbank Q 76:565–591, 510, 1998

Chaudhry B, Wang J, Wu S, et al: Systematic review: impact of health information technology on quality, efficiency, and costs of medical care. Ann Intern Med 144:742–752, 2006

Dimitropoulos LL: Privacy and Security Solutions for Interoperable Health Information Exchange [RTI International: Health Information Security and Privacy Collaboration (HISPC) web site]. June 30, 2007. Available at: http://www.rti.org/page.cfm?objectid=09E8D494-C491-42FC-BA13EAD1217245C0. Accessed April 23, 2008.

Druss BG: A review of HEDIS measures and performance for mental disorders. Manag Care 13 (6 suppl):48–51, 2004

Gesteland PH, Nebeker JR, Gardner RM: These are the technologies that try men's souls: common-sense health information technology. Pediatrics 117:216–217, 2006

Hillestad R, Bigelow J, Bower A, et al: Can electronic medical record systems transform health care? Potential health benefits, savings, and costs. Health Aff (Millwood) 24:1103–1117, 2005

Institute of Medicine, Committee on Quality of Health Care in America: Crossing the Quality Chasm: A New Health System for the 21st Century. Washington, DC, National Academies Press, 2001

Kilbridge PM, Welebob EM, Classen DC: Development of the Leapfrog methodology for evaluating hospital-implemented inpatient computerized physician order entry systems. Qual Saf Health Care 15:81–84, 2006

Kohn LT, Corrigan J, Donaldson MS, et al: To Err Is Human: Building a Safer Health System. Washington, DC, National Academies Press, 2000

Markle Foundation: Achieving Electronic Connectivity in Healthcare: A Preliminary Roadmap from the Nation's Public and Private-Sector Healthcare Leaders, 2004. Available at: http://www.connectingforhealth.org. Accessed April 24, 2007.

Morrissey J: A Day in the Life of a Medical Record: Lifting the Veil on the Security of Today's Paper-Based Environment (Hill Briefing). Washington, DC, National Alliance for Health Information Technology, September 2006. Available at: http://www.nahit.org/dl/A_Day_in_the_Life.pdf. Accessed April 24, 2007.

Mosher PW, Swire PP: The ethical and legal implications of Jaffee v Redmond and the HIPAA medical privacy rule for psychotherapy and general psychiatry. Psychiatr Clin North Am 25:575–584, vi–vii, 2002

Smith DH, Perrin N, Feldstein A, et al: The impact of prescribing safety alerts for elderly persons in an electronic medical record: an interrupted time series evaluation. Arch Intern Med 166:1098–1104, 2006

Technology CEO Council: A Healthy System: How Improved Information Management Can Transform the Quality, Efficiency, and Value of Americans' Health Care. Washington, DC, Technology CEO Council, 2006. Available at: http://www.techceocouncil.org. Accessed April 26, 2007.

Terry NP, Francis LP: Ensuring the privacy and confidentiality of electronic health records. University of Illinois Law Review (no volume):681–735, 2007

CHAPTER 34

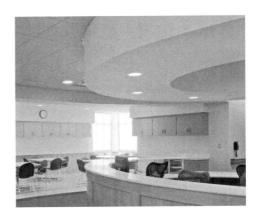

DESIGN AND ARCHITECTURE

Richard C. Lippincott, M.D.
Eugene J. Kuc, M.D.
Todd Hanson, A.I.A.

The environmental design of mental health facilities can facilitate the human interactions essential to treatment and can help in meeting clients' basic needs for safety and security.

V.J. Willis, M.A. (1980)

As described excellently in preceding chapters, mental illness is manifested in many unique, complicated, and challenging ways. Mentally ill individuals often withdraw to make their experiences safer, to control their abnormal thoughts, and to manage significant perceptual distortion of the environment.

Both the older literature and recent writings by evolutionary biologists suggest adaptive traits within human development that identified dangers or harm and led to the recognition of caves as safe; this suggests an image of personal development defined as "one's own internal home." One's environmental perceptions are important and often result in dramatic responses; surroundings that are experienced as harsh, unstimulating, and highly regimented have been shown to promote regression and social withdrawal.

In this chapter, we address the role of specifically designed environments and discuss the importance of special environments for the treatment of mental illness, its recovery, and rehabilitation. We will propose that providing meaningful emancipatory environmental aspects for hospitalized individuals with mental illness is one of the psychiatric hospital's primary tasks; this task also applies to the broader mental health services system. We will propose a design concept and settings that discourage isolation, promote human interaction, and facilitate clear connections to the outside world, as well as the community to which the patient will return; such an orientation facilitates the significant design aspects of hospital treatment.

The chapter will be divided into several separate concepts and variables based on the system and function to which the setting belongs, behavioral patterns and needs, patient age, and proposed length of stay. Psychiatric hospitals, inpatient psychiatric units of a general hospital, geropsychiatry units, and children's units will receive special and specific focus.

History

The earliest institution in America specifically and solely dedicated to the care of mentally ill individuals was Friend's Hospital, which opened in May 1817 in Philadelphia. The facility operated on a spiritual belief that insanity was a temporary impediment and the staff saw it as their mission to help patients out of the darkness. Patients were treated with kindness, respect, and dignity—a concept called "moral treatment."

History shows that for all intents and purposes, the opening of the Pennsylvania Hospital for the Insane in 1841, with Dr. Thomas S. Kirkbride as its chief physician, signaled the real focus on moral treatment and attention to the hospital environment's effect on treatment of the mentally ill (Figure 34–1). When Pennsylvania Hospital for the Insane was completed and opened, it presented an architectural profile that was clearly quite different from any of its predecessors. Many lessons emerged from this early event. First, a congruent group of local citizens, physicians, and individuals who were financial contributors played a developmental role in defining many aspects of this environment, such as location, surroundings, size, and structural design in what today would be called "action research" problem solving (Reason and Bradbury 2001). Further, external concepts were developed to support lawns, gardens, and the impressive size of the asylum building.

Reflected in the design was Dr. Kirkbride's belief in a linear design, which included halls, walking spaces, social meeting rooms, as well as varied accommodations such as comfortable rooms, special accommodations for the dangerous mentally ill, and even apartments for the wealthy.

It is reported that Dr. Kirkbride strived to create a moral architecture that was defined by a set of spatial and social arrangements specifically designed to promote a "generous confidence" in healing. In 1854 he wrote and published a treatise titled *On the Construction, Organization, and General Arrangements of Hospitals for the Insane* (Kirkbride 1854). Contemporary architects such as Joseph Giovanni have acknowledged Dr. Kirkbride's contribution: "The common threads are quality, individuality, and authenticity." Although he was not an architect, Dr. Kirkbride devised the basic

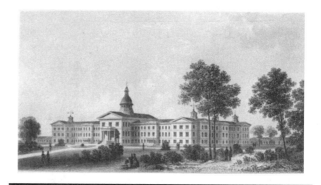

FIGURE 34–1.   Pennsylvania Hospital for the Insane.

floor plans and clarity of the environment. It is important to our understanding of this history to recognize that 38 hospitals of Dr. Kirkbride's design concepts were built and still stand (some are still in use as psychiatric hospitals). As years passed, the numerous psychiatric hospitals built with his design became the model for mental hospitals in American society (Tomes 1984). As Levin (2005) articulated, "If 'architecture manifests scientific knowledge,' as [architecture professor] Carla Yanni (2003) observed, then the crenellated palaces and castles of nineteenth-century insane asylums certainly expressed in brick and stone their vision of psychiatry."

What followed, although not causally linked, was a dark period for mental health services. Involuntary hospitalization, crowding on inpatient units, and ineffective treatments were all that was available. There was limited scientific understanding and confusion about mental illness at this time: Was mental illness a spiritual failing, bad behavior, or a real illness? An example of this uncertainty was reflected by U.S. President Franklin Pierce's veto of a congressional law that would have added mental health services to the functional responsibilities of the newly established Public Health Administration. This veto resulted in state legislatures becoming responsible for services, which led to a variety of treatment approaches. These included varying views of "moral treatment," brain surgery (explored in the United States by Dr. Walter Freeman in California), and the development of electroconvulsive therapy, which was widely used, sometimes inappropriately.

It was not, therefore, until the 1960s and 1970s, when advances in pharmacological treatments became available, that review and redesign of psychiatric hospitals resumed. Fortunately, Dr. Kirkbride's conviction that patients could be treated and possibly "cured" remained respected. In the 1960s, interest and research evidence began to show the important contribution that environmental design made to variance in behaviors, anxiety, and development of hostility. Systematic assessments of hospital environments by Pace and Stern (1958) and Moos and Houts (1968a) showed direct and predictable relationships between the "psychological climate" on psychiatric hospital wards and the patients' reactions to the world.

In 1976, Dr. Rudolf H. Moos published *The Human Context: Environmental Determinants of Behavior,* an extensive study that stimulated significant interest and triggered changes in the approach to architectural design of psychiatric facilities, units, and wards in general hospital structures (Moos 1976). A brief overview of this work demonstrates the importance of various environmental design concepts such as space and distance related to friendship formation (closer is better); closed versus open space in relation to mood and behavior; arrangement of furniture to facilitate social interaction; and amenities such as carpets, pictures, and light to decrease inappropriate behaviors.

Studies show that individuals develop cognitive maps of the environment in which they live and that they use space in ways that are congruent with their needs and images. According to Moos and Houts (1968b), "current personality theories subscribe to the belief that behavior is a joint function of both the person and the environment, representing interaction of individuals' needs and the environment 'press' [Dr. H.A. Murry's term for stress]."

Moos (1968b) summarized his work regarding hospitals as follows: "Since the community environment to which a patient must adapt after hospitalization is crucial, a hospital environment must replicate as much as possible the community into which the patient is to be discharged." And Kandel had this to say about the importance of the environment in his book *In Search of Memory: The Emergence of a New Science of Mind:* "Even though I had been taught that genes of the brain were the 'governors of behavior,' our work showed that in the brain, genes are also 'servants of the environment'" (Kandel 2006, p. 264).

Maintenance of Basic Patient Needs

Willis (1980) examined design considerations for mental health facilities and outlined four basic patient needs:

1. To feel safe in the environment
2. To be secure

3. To feel or develop a sense of self-esteem or self-worth
4. To develop interpersonal skills and management

Within psychiatric hospital environments, especially in the past, research has shown that a poorly designed environment extracts a significant cost, especially for patients with severe and persistent mental illness (Willis 1980). The cost has been reflected in social withdrawal, isolation, inhibitions, poor self-monitoring, poor affect control, and loss of motivation. This is now often defined as loss of "executive function"—a decline in cognitive activities basically intended to achieve one's goals, whether complex or simple. Poor executive function leads to difficulty interacting with others, learning, solving problems of change, or performing self-care; an example of this can be seen when chronically mentally ill patients "forget" to take their medication (Bryan and Luszcz 2000).

Focus group studies have shown that where a psychiatric hospital includes as much as possible of the outside community to which the patient will return and staff facilitate community activity, the loss of executive function is much less pronounced (Kaplan 1977). Pending research by Lippincott and others will address whether the rate of rehospitalization is significantly reduced and length of stay is shortened when patients with severe and persistent mental illness are treated in hospitals in which the therapeutic effects of the environment are included in the design.

It is hoped that the goal of all psychiatric hospital treatment is the return of patients to an active quality of life in their community, where mental health programs can support treatment and rehabilitation. Consistent with this goal is providing treatment in the least restrictive setting possible, especially for individuals with serious mental illness. The data suggest that an organized mental health services system that is integrated and responsive to patients is most effective and, ultimately, least expensive (President's New Freedom Commission on Mental Health 2003).

Nevertheless, outpatient services may not be enough, and patients' symptoms may evolve to the point that an evaluation by general hospital emergency room services may be necessary. Then, based on severity of symptoms and diagnosis, admission to the general hospital's psychiatric unit for stabilization is used; here, length of stay is usually limited (3–10 days).

When patients require more intense, secure, or specialized programming, long-term care or potentially mental health commitment to a specialized psychiatric hospital is needed. These psychiatric hospitals are recognized today based on primary function or purpose. Thus, the patient's needs, legal issues, age, and financial status result in different admission choices. Public psychiatric facilities (e.g., state hospitals) focus on serious and persistent mental disorders that involve disruptive behaviors, specific security needs, legal commitments, and medication use problems. Here, the goal is stabilization, recovery, medication compliance, and, if possible, preservation of the patient's executive function. Individuals with these needs may include many with severe and persistent psychiatric disorders that involve complex Axis I/Axis II comorbidity.

Other specialty psychiatric hospitals have specific populations, such as forensic facilities requiring a specific security and legal focus. Children's facilities obviously also have a special focus and serve unique needs. Psychiatric hospitals designed to provide services for patients with disorders such as borderline personality disorder may have unique goals and environmental needs.

Important in all of these hospital settings is attention to the relationship between the environmental design and the patient population's needs and goals and the role design plays in patients' rehabilitation and return to the community.

Psychiatric Hospital Design Concepts

The cover of the March/April 2007 issue of *Medical Construction and Design Concepts* carries the following caption: "Where the recovery begins: From the warmth of a sun-filled room to the serene views of a green roof, an exterior's design can profoundly impact patient health."

It is essential that all psychiatric hospital designs begin with three essentials: security, safety, and a humane environment. Data to date have shown that it is possible to accomplish such a design with the aforementioned essentials without interfering with the representation of the community environment within the hospital.

Data developed since the mid-1980s point to several overarching concepts that contribute to a successful design. It can be argued that the most significant is that the design must recapitulate within the hospital's controlled environment as much of the patient's community as possible. This would mean that the design incorporates a "community concept," which would include communal, spiritual, and cultural space for meaningful interactions as well as "homelike" living

units with bedrooms, showers, meeting spaces, comfortable living rooms, as well as a nursing station, medication storage, and, as necessary, places for solitude (quiet rooms).

Another important concept is design aimed at minimizing loss of executive function. We have proposed that design facilitate the following objectives (Davis et al. 1979; Osmond 1976):

- Initiating, responding to, and engaging in social interactions
- Engaging in real economic exchanges (for example, shopping in the gift shop)
- Practicing social skills and using new information daily
- Participating in active groups
- Encouraging socially acceptable community behavior

Not unique to the psychiatric hospital design but recommended is the deliberate "one-way in/one-way out" entrance to the facility. This entrance provides access to the community and its functions while remaining open to families, visitors, and staff in a controlled way. The entrance opens into a sizeable community space, which would also have ample available seating, prominently displayed art, and areas that specifically facilitate everyday functions, including access to primary care and dental offices, a hair salon, a library, a general store, a cafeteria, a chapel, and a complete gym, among others. Available to patients on short-term and long-term units would be access from the community space for rehabilitation activities, a greenhouse, and a courtyard garden—all with appropriate security. Another new psychiatric hospital design utilizes a "mall" concept that contains similar multiple community activities down an extended hall looking out onto the courtyard (Figure 34–2).

Natural sunlight and large safety windows result in a continuous interaction with the outside and nature; this feature could serve as a visual metaphor to stimulate the patients' reintegration back into the community. In one facility, this aspect of design is emphasized by a two-floor design and significant skylights covering community space (Figure 34–3). Architectural research has shown that bringing natural light into the hospital has significant benefits: improved attention, reduction of stress, and reduced costs of lighting (Joseph 2006).

The living quarters within these designs have very similar principles of environment, with specific attention to openness, comfortable bedrooms, treatment rooms, medication areas that are integrated, as well as gathering space viewed as living rooms for client inter-

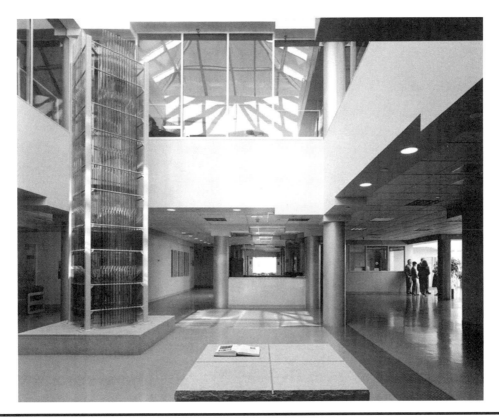

FIGURE 34–2. Entrance and public space, New Hampshire Hospital, Concord, New Hampshire.

The entrance and public space define the hospital's goals and purposes as a recapitulation of the "real" community to which the patient will return.

Source. Image courtesy of JSA, Architects Interiors Planners, Portsmouth, NH; recipient of 1987 Award, Environmental Design Research Association for Institutions.

action and conversation (Figure 34–4). Quiet or seclusion rooms are recommended to facilitate behavioral control (Baum and Koman 1976).

The living quarters can be specifically designed to meet levels of security, intensity of illness, and risk combined with attention to the importance of patient interaction, focus on treatment objectives, and rehabilitation programs. An important design goal is to allow as much freedom as possible to move about and within the hospital based on the assessed risk of each patient. The following design elements are of special importance for the living quarters:

1. Views and visual relief
    *   The availability of "visual relief" to the outdoors is an important element of therapeutic environments. There have been numerous studies that reinforce the benefit of windows and views (Figure 34–5). For example, studies have shown that surgical patients in hospitals recover quicker and use fewer pain medications simply by having a window with natural views. Windows are

critical to comfortable, relaxing, reassuring environments (Ulrich 1984).

2. Lighting—quantity and quality (variety, natural lighting, and appropriateness for the specific use of space)
    *   The quality and quantity of light affect both performance and our health (Joseph 2006). It has been shown to reduce depression, lessen agitation, and improve sleep patterns. The proper quality and quantity can be achieved with a combination of natural and artificial lighting. Poor-quality light can cause poor functional performance. Good lighting design carefully balances natural and artificial sources and provides proper ambient light levels. In psychiatric hospitals, this requires special attention, especially to quiet room design.

3. Acoustic considerations
    *   Noise is perhaps the most overlooked element of hospital design. For example, low-level noise can cause stress, distraction, and sleep loss. Sudden noises such as loud voices, pagers, and

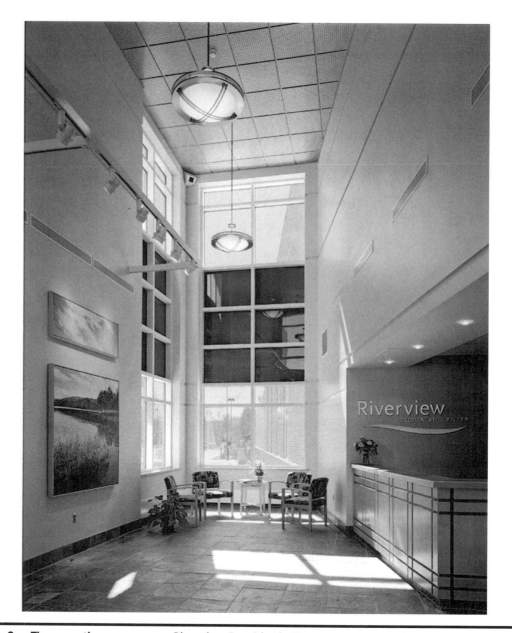

FIGURE 34–3.   Therapeutic group room, Riverview Psychiatric Center, Augusta, Maine.

The therapeutic group room defines the treatment environment while providing light, space, and visual contact with the outside world.

Source.   Image courtesy of JSA, Architects Interiors Planners, Portsmouth, NH.

ringing phones may set off the "fight or flight" response, causing anxiety.

4. Tones and colors
   • Numerous studies have been conducted to ascertain the impact of color on our emotional well-being (Joseph 2006; Moos 1976). Some of the information is conflicting, but the studies' results all indicate clearly that colors and tones can relax, invigorate, or agitate. Most people react in similar ways to warm or cool colors, as well as to light or darker tones. Artwork along hallways also contributes to the mood of the observer.

5. Texture considerations (visual and touch)
   • A textured rug over a shiny floor does more than just dampen sound; it visually softens the environment. Texture is an important element of design for both aesthetic and acoustic reasons. The touch of fabric on the arm of a chair creates a different emotional reaction from that of smooth vinyl. Our senses react to all aspects of our surroundings.

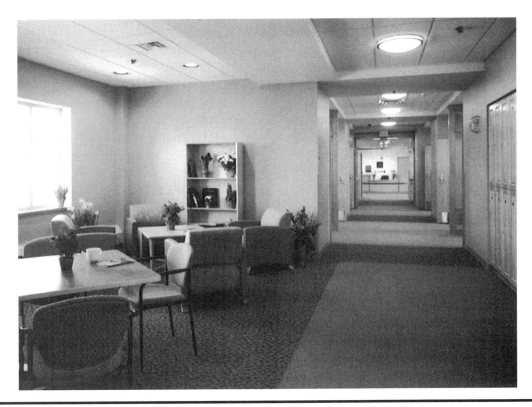

FIGURE 34–4. Group room and hallway, New Hampshire Hospital, Concord, New Hampshire.

An alcove off a hallway frames space for quiet time and social interaction.
Source. Image courtesy of JSA, Architects Interiors Planners, Portsmouth, NH.

6. Temperature and comfort
   - We all have slightly different internal thermostats. The ability to control aspects of our environment, to personalize them to our individual needs, can have positive implications for our sense of empowerment. The best option is to allow people to have some level of control within their private spaces and to rely on each individual dressing in a way that meets his or her comfort needs.

7. Spatial volume (nurturing vs. intimidating, liberating vs. confining)
   - The volume of a room should meet the expectations of the activity it provides. It is appropriate for a public activity room to have width and height to allow activity and action without overwhelming the occupants. A private bedroom or study area should be intimate to nurture, comfort, and reassure the patient.

8. Importance of variation
   - As in nature, our environments should have variation that alters light, temperature, and sounds. Stimulating environments with variation allow us to experience contrasts. Artwork has been shown to have such a positive effect.

Confinement issues are important in the psychiatric hospital. Special considerations should include the following elements:

1. Balance between freedom and control (i.e., allowing choices)
   - The freedom to make personal choices is important to all of us. Opportunities to easily change one's setting should be available. This could mean having the chance to step outdoors into a courtyard, access social activity spaces, or retreat to private zones.
   - Rooms set aside as "quiet space" have been shown to be helpful (Baum and Koman 1976; Moos 1976).

2. Importance of feeling safe (ability to remove bars without compromising safety)
   - Balancing privacy and supervision is extremely important. Patients need to feel safe and secure before they can feel relaxed. In a mental health treatment setting, this is true for both patients and staff. Modern materials have allowed us to create secure environments without using barred windows and block walls, leading to quality therapeutic environments that are safer

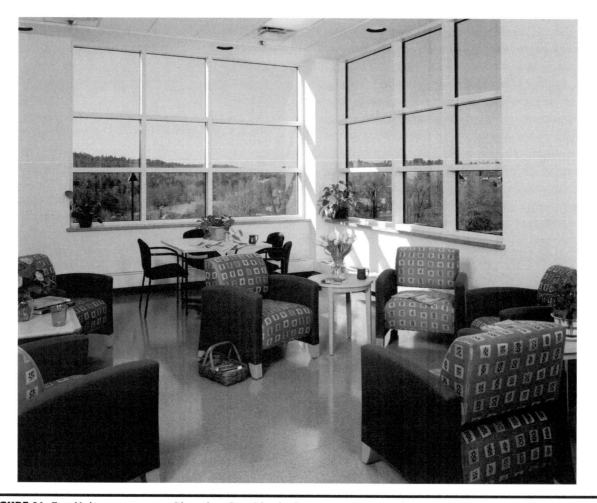

FIGURE 34–5. Unit group room, Riverview Psychiatric Center, Augusta, Maine.

The unit group room offers views of the outdoors as well as quiet space for rest, relaxation, and social interactions.
Source.   Image courtesy of JSA, Architects Interiors Planners, Portsmouth, NH.

than the old institutional settings of the past. Sophisticated electronics improve supervision, allow greater movement, and eliminate the imposing security once required in psychiatric facilities. Advances in glass and plastic technologies have made it possible to eliminate the safety risks of windows and doors.

Family Interaction

Research data and multiple reports indicate that family involvement and visitation for hospitalized patients are crucial in the recovery of the mentally ill (Harbin 1982). Thus, within psychiatric hospital design, family needs must be considered to facilitate their very important role. General concerns should focus on families' comfort, safety, and support to fa-

cilitate appropriate interaction with their ill family member. Families' comfort within the entire hospital environment should be seen as of equal importance to the comfort of the patients. Providing bathrooms for visitors is also an important detail.

Data suggest that families have a complex view of their relative's hospitalization: relief and hope that the hospital staff will provide a cure for the illness may be intertwined with feeling like outsiders to the situation and that nothing in their relationship with their family member will be altered (Harbin 1982). The environmental design is important to altering these perceptions. Studies indicate that family involvement (visits and interaction) with the patient and hospital staff and length of stay are strongly influenced by education, improved family understanding, and meeting in a comfortable homelike environment (Harbin 1982).

Adult Inpatient Units Within the General Hospital

Psychiatric units within the general hospital facilities might best be thought of in two general ways when considering design or architectural structure. One way is to consider how the unit integrates within the local system of mental health services. These units may provide an intermediate treatment role akin to a triage unit functioning between the emergency room and other placement settings, such as a potential transfer to other units or to a psychiatric hospital for more extensive or specialized treatment. Evaluation or commitment may lead to transfer to a psychiatric hospital. Coordination between these settings is thus essential.

The other concept is that the psychiatric unit fits within the "community" provided by the general hospital environment where many patients may be quite active. Patients may frequently leave the unit to visit radiology or laboratories for special consultations, and they may even go to the hospital gift shop after stabilization. Consideration of an integrated design proves helpful in maintaining contact and function. It also makes appropriate security and safety key features, requiring door alarms, voice contact, and staff assessment of risk, given that the patient may be distracted or obtunded by symptoms or treatment.

For many patients, the general hospital unit may be the first setting in which their mental health problems are addressed and thus should be regarded as very important to development of an appropriate attitude and approach to their treatment. It may be easy for providers to underestimate the upheaval that a psychiatric hospitalization causes in the patient's and family's lives. Although the risks and benefits of hospitalization and the decision process involved in choosing to admit a patient to a psychiatric unit are thoroughly discussed throughout this book, the environment clearly influences the transition experience of the patient.

As we consider the elements of architecture and design of an adult unit within a general medical hospital, the values of the system are reflected in decisions made regarding the unit's location. The placement of the unit on the top floor, in the basement, or in a separate building on the campus of the general hospital may speak volumes about how the science of the brain and mind is integrated into the care of the patient. The extent to which psychiatric services are integrated or marginalized may be reflected by its location.

The tasks specific to the adult unit may be summarized as diagnosis and treatment of symptoms of psychiatric illness, relapse prevention, and reconnection to a social support network. As issues of safety precipitate most psychiatric admissions, therapies directed at the reestablishment of safety must be primary concerns on the adult unit. Patients' symptoms such as suicidal or homicidal ideation, disorganization, and difficulty meeting basic needs often result in the collapse of social support networks. Thus, aspects of the hospital environment and treatment directed at these issues, and those that involve the family and other social supports, are paramount.

An inpatient unit is challenged to provide a private nurturing environment while ensuring safety. Technology facilitates monitoring, but the way in which its presence is manifested may either contribute to an oppressive institutional atmosphere or offer significant support. Likewise, the location and access to computer terminals may be such that staff members hide behind their computers and thus distance themselves from patients. Furthermore, computer screens with visible patient information or easy access to protected health information may indicate a dehumanizing environment of disrespect for the privacy of the individual patient. Add to this a location in the basement with no visual relief for the patient, and the inpatient experience could be dreary.

General considerations specific to the adult unit may include numerous special needs: physical access (e.g., wheelchair maneuverability, accommodations for visually impaired patients), falls risk reduction, pregnancy, detoxification, and memory impairment. Even without these complicating issues, the inpatient unit is a novel environment for the patient, and quick orientation to and maneuvering in the space should be easily accomplished.

All of the space on the inpatient unit must reflect concern for visual and lighting elements, acoustic sensitivity, texture, temperature, and spatial proportions. Common areas on the general unit include bedrooms, day rooms, therapy rooms (group, individual, and medical treatment), as well as spaces for staff offices and meeting areas.

Bedrooms

Allocation of space within the hospital and general structural considerations often limit the arrangement of rooms; thus, the layout of the unit is often similar to a general surgical or medical unit, with patient bedrooms opening onto rather long hallways. Such a configuration can be an obstacle for psychiatric patients, who need and benefit from interaction with and support from the community. A layout that accentuates the sleeping quarters can only diminish this focus. Bedrooms should be arranged so that their presence is not a hindrance to community and therapy activity. The layout should promote safety and limit intrusions—physically, visually, or acoustically—of patients or staff.

Day Rooms

For better or worse, the location of the television on a unit will invariably be a place for congregation of patients. Also, group meetings, meals, and individual sessions will likely take place in this area. Because people are often territorial, conflict will invariably occur in these spaces. The elements of design are critical when considering that these spaces need to provide varied settings in which patients can choose to conduct their work yet not be isolated from staff or the community. Because patients will be struggling with symptoms and may be experiencing side effects of medications, attention to issues of comfort—visual, auditory, personal space, and so on—will be tremendously helpful.

Therapy Rooms

Therapy that takes place on the adult unit can be individual psychotherapy, group therapy, psychoeducation, self-help groups (such as Alcoholics Anonymous), education groups, and medical treatment, including physical exams, repetitive transcranial magnetic stimulation, or other physical treatments. These rooms are invariably multifunctional; therefore, the ease with which a room can be converted is largely a function of the furniture and other devices in the room. The basic elements of privacy, aesthetics, and lack of distraction from other activities on the unit or outside of the unit should be considered.

Although each unit will develop its own particular philosophy, space for occupational therapy, music therapy, art therapy, pet therapy, and other adjunctive therapies should be considered for availability.

Staff Spaces

The nurses' station has evolved from a walled-off room that patients would access through a window to largely open areas. This transition, although very useful to the development of a less institutional environment, presents limitations, especially in the area of privacy of patient information—either printed records, computer screens, or telephone conversations. Staff need places to congregate, to conduct work-related activities, and to disengage from the unit to eat meals and have breaks. Offices on the units must be both accessible and safe so that staff and patients are not sequestered in an unsafe manner. The design

should be inviting and should include all of the elements already described.

Smoking Areas

Although no responsible medical professional would encourage smoking, smoking is often a major area of focus on inpatient units. Some facilities accommodate this with independent access to smoking areas outside of the facility or in facility courtyards; increasingly, hospitals adopt a strict no-smoking stance anywhere on campus.

Geropsychiatry Units

As medicine becomes more successful at treating medical illnesses, people survive longer and need to adapt to sequelae of diseases, aging, and treatments. Medicine has made significant strides in the treatment of cardiovascular diseases, neurological disorders, dementia, and cerebrovascular accidents; advances in neurosurgery have produced the need for better rehabilitation techniques and facilities in which to conduct them.

Design and architecture have special impact on safety, a major function of the unit. Patients often have cognitive deficits, and their resiliencies for dealing with these deficits are frequently overloaded because of their medical and neurological needs. The units should be designed to facilitate medical and neurological treatment—easy access for patients to use wheelchairs, walkers, and other similar equipment, and space for patients to walk about in an unrestricted way. Patients respond well to direct contact, and staffing is largely responsible for ensuring adequate contact. Design can place staff in places that optimize that contact—especially at special times of the day such as at meals and early evening (the time at highest risk for "sundowning").

Mobility issues deserve additional attention. Patients will exhibit wandering or attempts at mobility. Often these behaviors are dangerous for the patient due to, for example, instability of gait. Sometimes previously agile patients are trying to adjust to neural insults such as cerebrovascular accidents or the side effects of medications (e.g., anticholinergic side effects) and need special attention when arising.

Present within the unit and the patient's private area should be soothing elements of sight, sound, and touch, with orienting objects related to date and time, family photos, and other accents. Color or colored markings may be used to guide or to help orient patients to specific spaces on the unit.

Pediatric Units

Pediatric units offer a variety of issues to consider such as age range and specific therapeutic and developmental tasks important for a particular age range. Furthermore, the elements of design appropriate for one age group may be countertherapeutic for another age group. As noted previously, family engagement, interaction, and visitation comfort are important concepts that need to be realized and accommodated within the space of the pediatric unit.

Bedrooms

Given that the goal of the therapeutic environment is to foster reintegration with the patient's nonhospital environment, living areas must approximate in furniture, light, texture, and accents and decorations what would be expected at his or her home. Also important are independent work areas for schoolwork, play, crafts, socialization, and other age-specific activities.

Day Rooms

As with the case of the general adult unit, location and access to television, radio, and telephone are important design elements. Their location will lead to areas of congregation and potential behavioral acting out.

Therapy Rooms

As with the general adult unit, therapy rooms will be utilized in a variety of ways. In addition to the tasks already described, functions unique to pediatric units will include more teaching and mentoring activities and more family sessions and play areas.

Unit Layout

Normal child development involves exploration and experimentation, and the pediatric unit should accommodate normal activities of childhood in addition to specific therapeutic areas. Staff will be challenged to shift the use of a space from one activity to another. Therefore, another design challenge is to be able to quickly convert the space from one function to the next.

Other Design Considerations

Every element of design on psychiatric units deserves discussion, and every unit will have specialized needs of specific elements. For example, special considerations might include placement of mirrors on an eating disorder unit, ability of patients to safely bring personal objects from home to help alleviate trauma and stress, inclusion of or access to areas for spiritual reflection and rituals, whether the unit is to be locked or open, location of seclusion or restraint rooms, whether bedrooms are to be single- or multiple-occupancy, ability to shop for snacks (e.g., at a canteen) or other personal care products, and access to laundry facilities.

In addition to some of the overarching principles already outlined, attempts should be made to include quiet, pleasant colors for walls, a view if possible, art for the walls, and a small "library space" containing newspapers, magazines, books (including those that deal with mental health), and places for patients to write. The goal is to facilitate a positive outlook, good mood, and maintenance of the patients' executive functioning.

Conclusion

Design and architecture are very important aspects of the inpatient psychiatric treatment experience and, as described throughout this chapter, offer important issues for consideration. We propose that it is the responsibility of all staff to define and construct the environment to best facilitate the therapeutic work of the psychiatric unit.

References

Baum A, Koman S: Differential response to architectural crowding: psychological effects of social and spatial density. J Pers Soc Psychol 34:526–536, 1976

Bryan J, Luszcz MA: Measurement of executive function: considerations for detecting adult age differences. J Clin Exp Neuropsychol 22:40–55, 2000

Davis C, Glick ID, Rosow I: Architectural design of a psychotherapeutic milieu. Hosp Community Psychiatry 30:453–460, 1979

Harbin HT (ed): The Psychiatric Hospital and the Family. New York, SP Medical & Scientific Books, 1982

Joseph A: The Impact of Light on Outcomes in Healthcare Settings. Concord, CA, The Center for Health Design, 2006

Kandel ER: A dialogue between genes and synapses, in In Search of Memory: The Emergence of a New Science of Mind. New York, WW Norton, 2006, pp 261–264

Kaplan S: Participation in the design process: a cognitive approach, in Perspectives on Environment and Behavior: Theory, Research, and Application. Edited by Stokols S. New York, Plenum, 1977, pp 221–233

Kirkbride TS: On the Construction, Organization, and General Arrangements of Hospitals for the Insane. Philadelphia, PA, Lippincott Press, 1854

Levin A: Rational buildings designed to calm the disorderly mind. Psychiatric News 40(17):24, 2005

Levin A: Psychiatric hospital design reflects treatment trends. Psychiatric News 42(2):9, 2007

Moos RH: Coping with environmental impact, in The Human Context: Environmental Determinants of Behavior. New York, Wiley, 1976, pp 394–427

Moos RH, Houts PS: Assessments of the social atmospheres of psychiatric wards. J Abnorm Psychol 73:595–604, 1968a

Moos RH, Houts PS: Differential effects of the social atmosphere of psychiatric wards. Hum Relat 23:47–60, 1968b

Osmond H: The psychological dimension of architectural space. Progressive Architecture 46:159–167, 1976

Pace CR, Stern GG: An approach to the measurement of psychological characteristics of college environments. J Educ Psychol 12:269–277, 1958

President's New Freedom Commission on Mental Health: Achieving the Promise: Transforming Mental Health Care in America, Final Report (DHHS Pub No SMA-03-3832). Rockville, MD, U.S. Department of Health and Human Services, 2003

Reason P, Bradbury H: Handbook of Action Research: Participative Inquiry and Practice. London, Sage, 2001

Tomes N: A Generous Confidence: Thomas Story Kirkbride and the Art of Asylum-Keeping 1845–1883. New York, Cambridge University Press, 1984

Ulrich RS: View through a window may influence recovery from surgery. Science 224:420–442, 1984

Willis VJ: Design considerations for mental health facilities. Hosp Community Psychiatry 31:483–490, 1980

Yanni C: The linear plan for insane asylums in the United States to 1866. Journal of the Society of Architectural Historians 62:24–49, 2003

Part V

THE FUTURE OF HOSPITAL PSYCHIATRY

CHAPTER 35

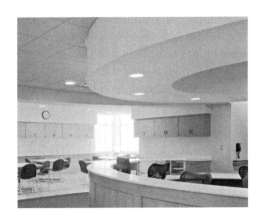

HOSPITAL PSYCHIATRY FOR THE FUTURE

Steven S. Sharfstein, M.D., M.P.A.

"I proceed, gentlemen, to briefly to call your attention to the present state of insane persons confined within this commonwealth in cages, closets, stalls, pens! Chained, naked, beaten with rods, and lashed into obedience" (Gollaher 1995). From the time that Dorothea Dix wrote those impassioned words to members of the Massachusetts legislature, we have struggled in this country with how best to manage the ravages of acute and chronic psychotic illness in hospitals and community settings. The asylum movement of the nineteenth century, led by Ms. Dix and her allies, embodied many humane principles such as moral treatment. It led, however, to the growth of large, impersonal, custodial institutions funded by state treasuries (see Chapter 1, "History of Hospital Psychiatry and Lessons Learned," by Geller). With deinstitutionalization following the introduction of antipsychotic medications in state hospitals in the 1950s, which accelerated throughout the 1960s and 1970s, states sought the opportunity to save money by downsizing public institutions and shifting support to federal programs. Patients were moved to community settings.

Every state in America experienced the influx of chronically and acutely ill patients into communities without adequate resources to treat them. Homelessness, incarceration of the mentally ill, and concerns about public safety inevitably followed and became major public health and public policy questions that continue today and will persist into the future. Beginning in the late 1980s, the for-profit managed care effort to control the cost of public and private third-party payments further downsized inpatient treatment in private psychiatric hospitals and general hospitals (see Chapter 30, "Financing of Care," by Liptzin and Summergrad). The question of the day became What, if ever, is the "medical necessity" of hospitalizing an individual with acute psychosis or other mental illness?

This chapter emphasizes and summarizes the major theme of this book—hospital psychiatry is here to stay. Hospitalization is always based on the need for 24-hour nursing care in high-technology settings. The hospital stay provides an opportunity to evaluate, diagnose, and stabilize complex and comorbid mental illness. In addition, involvement of the family in the process of hospital care is essential. Further, the community at large has a need for respite from an individual in severe crisis. In relation to the continuing shortfall in adequate community-based services, all of these issues make a compelling case for inpatient care and the need for inpatient care to be an integral and critical part of a continuum of comprehensive community-based care. Inpatient treatment is an important solution to the national disgrace of the neglect of persons with mental illness who are, once again, homeless, incarcerated, and, in the words of Dorothea Dix, living "in deplorable conditions" (Gollaher 1995).

Important demographic trends reinforce the rationale for psychiatric hospitalization, even as the differentiating and changing boundaries of hospital treatment raise a basic question, "What is a hospital?" The hospital of the future will be a hub for a comprehensive system of care that is highly subspecialized and, at the same time, integrated with general medical and community-based social services.

Trends in the Twenty-First Century

The U.S. population is aging, and the number of individuals who suffer from dementias and other psychiatric conditions of old age is rising dramatically. Co-occurring serious medical and psychiatric conditions have increased. The premature death of individuals with serious mental illness (by at least 10 years) underscores the consequences of these comorbidities (Parks et al. 2006). Another major comorbidity is that of serious psychiatric illness and substance use disorders. The HIV/AIDS epidemic is both a major cause and consequence of this and other comorbidities. The strong linkage of poverty and mental illness makes a solid case for the public financing of psychiatric care. Although treatment continues to improve, patients are "better but not well" (Frank and Glied 2006). We will continue, for the foreseeable future, to deal with halfway technologies, that is, treatments (both medical and psychosocial) that help, that stabilize, that may prevent relapse but that do not cure. The chronicity of many psychiatric conditions, especially schizophrenia, schizoaffective disorder, bipolar illness, pervasive developmental disorders, major depressive disorder, severe personality disorders, and some severe anxiety syndromes, will be with us for some time.

In addition to key demographic changes and the growth of comorbid psychiatric conditions, there are other trends in the wider world of hospital treatment that will have a major impact on psychiatric care into the twenty-first century.

Stigma has plagued and continues to plague psychiatric hospital treatment across the world. In this country, films such as *The Snake Pit* and *One Flew Over the Cuckoo's Nest* exemplified and exaggerated the gothic horror of insane asylums. Stigma about hospital treatment is changing today in large part because of the nature of treatment. Brief inpatient stays similar to stays for other medical or surgical conditions contribute strongly to the lessening of stigma. Modern facilities with private rooms, baths, and other amenities normalize a psychiatric admission as similar to any medical or surgical admission. This is especially true in general hospital psychiatric units but is also increasingly true in modern psychiatric hospitals such as the new hospital at Sheppard Pratt, the Menninger Clinic, McLean Hospital, the Institute of Living, New York–Presbyterian Hospital, and Butler Hospital. Even with these changes, there may always be some stigma attached to being hospitalized for a psychiatric illness. The design of units to be safe requires certain physical restrictions and constraints that remind patients that they are on a psychiatric ward. The facts that many units are locked and, depending on the hospital and the nature of the unit, that many personal items are not allowed serve to remind psychiatric patients that patient and staff safety are paramount. When patients require safety interventions such as seclusion or restraint, it is an additional reminder of the different nature of a psychiatric hospital stay, and this can be quite anxiety provoking for many patients and their families.

Involvement of families in all phases of treatment (see Chapter 17, "Working With Families," by Dixon et al.) and efforts to reduce, if not eliminate, the use of seclusion and restraint (see Chapter 18, "Improving Safety in Mental Health Treatment Settings," by Huckshorn and LeBel) help to alleviate the alienating experience of a psychiatric inpatient stay. The facts that treatment is effective, that symptoms can be stabilized well enough for rapid discharge, that medications are key to the treatment experience, and that medical insurance typically pays for the inpatient stay all help to reduce stigma. These days, we even see a reduction in stigma for electroconvulsive therapy, not only because it is effective but also because it is carried out as a medical procedure with anesthesia and muscle relaxants, in titrated and localized doses adjusted on the basis of new research findings. The fact that more and more health insurance offers "parity" of psychiatric treatment with general medical/surgical treatment also reduces stigma. Consumers and families are now better informed and, in the process of collaboration with psychiatric professionals, have a much more sophisticated view of what a psychiatric hospital stay should be and what they should demand and expect. Diagnosis is much more of a collaborative process, and with publication of the Fifth Edition of the *Diagnostic and Statistical Manual of Mental Disorders*, there will be even more consumer input into the diagnostic process. Overall, the trend toward more transparency and accountability will continue to grow.

A major trend for which there is growing concern is the lack of access to acute psychiatric inpatient care. Demand for care is high, again in large part due to the perception that treatment is effective and efficient. But in many areas of the country today, there are serious bed shortages. Patients can remain for days in emergency rooms waiting for a psychiatric bed. Lack of access to a bed is mostly a cost-driven phenomenon. Psychiatric inpatient care competes with medical and surgical inpatient care. With various efforts to contain costs, including managed care, there are likely to be continuing bed shortages throughout the country.

Trends in Settings for Care

The vertically integrated comprehensive general hospital today is being disaggregated into subspecialty areas and units, as well as subspecialty hospitals. Medicine has become extremely subspecialized, and psychiatry is a leader in subspecialization. As this book makes clear, subspecialties (such as care for children, adolescents, and geriatrics, as well as for key diagnostic categories including psychoses, eating disorders, trauma, and neuropsychiatry) rely on the state-of-the-art techniques in the biological as well as the psychosocial aspects of care for each of these subspecialty areas (see Chapters 3–12). As psychiatric patients move from general hospital wards to specialized psychiatric units in general hospitals, we are seeing (and we will continue to see) difficult-to-treat patients move from units in general hospitals to specialty hospitals. Improvements in treatment throughout the life span will require highly specialized physicians and clinicians (see Chapter 27, "Psychiatrists and Psychologists," by Roca and Magid), social workers (see Chapter 28, "Social Work and Rehabilitation Therapies," by Ramsay et al.), and nurses (see Chapter 29, "Psychiatric Nursing," by Delaney et al.) to deliver these services. We can expect future breakthroughs in the treatment of psychoses. We can anticipate third and fourth generations of antipsychotic medications that will be free of the serious medical comorbidities of the first- and second-generation medications; when that happens, it will, once again, transform the prospects for care, especially in the outpatient continuum of treat-

ment (see Chapter 24, "Outpatient Community Mental Health Services," by Cournos and LeMelle).

The President's New Freedom Commission Report called for system "transformation" with the goal of "recovery for everyone" (President's New Freedom Commission on Mental Health 2003). As community-based services are increasingly consumer centered, so will the acute phase of inpatient hospitalization become more consumer informed and directed (see Chapter 16, "From Within: A Consumer Perspective on Psychiatric Hospitals," by Halpern et al.). Self-directed care requires the consumer's and family's abilities to understand and be educated about illness and self-management through early symptom identification and rapid treatment. Many psychosocial services in community settings are a key part of the effort to build resiliency in individuals with long-term illness. Individualized and specialized plans of care are critical as we engage consumers and families as full partners in the enterprise called hospital treatment.

The President's New Freedom Commission Report and its recommendations were reinforced by the groundbreaking Institute of Medicine study, *Crossing the Quality Chasm* (Institute of Medicine Committee on Quality 2001). This report, which was a clarion call for culture change in all health care organizations, recommends health services characterized by 1) continuous healing relationships, 2) customization of care to individual needs and values, 3) consumers as the source of control of care, 4) free flow of information and transparency of information, 5) anticipation of needs, and 6) use of best practices. The Institute of Medicine has applied these principles specifically to the treatment of mental illness and substance use disorders in its recent report (Institute of Medicine 2006). The report underscores the need for the integration of psychiatric care with the rest of medicine, even as much of that care is subspecialized and often delegated into subspecialty arenas.

The revolution in genetics and information systems may have a profound effect on psychiatric hospital care as psychiatric treatment is integrated more fully with somatic medicine. Advancements in genetics may allow psychiatric treatment to be tailored to the genetic profiles of patients. For example, medication strategies may be focused on the most effective and efficient approach for affective disorders and schizophrenia as we better understand the genetic substrates of these conditions. The electronic medical record (see Chapter 33, "The Electronic Medical Record," by Boronow) will revolutionize psychiatric treatment, allowing that treatment to better integrate with general medicine because many, if not most, psychiatric patients are comorbidly medically ill and require good medical care in addition to their psychiatric treatment. The field of consultation–liaison psychiatry (see Chapter 15 by Epstein and Muskin) will be a growing component of psychiatric care in the future. The subspecialty of psychosomatics will expand, and many patients subjected to high-technology medicine will increasingly have psychiatric consultation as part of their comprehensive medical treatment. As the population ages and dementias and delirium become more prevalent, psychiatrists will become even more strategic within general medicine. Neuroimaging will continue to grow and may become more sophisticated in the diagnosis and treatment of a variety of psychiatric and medical conditions that are interrelated.

What Is the Hospital of the Future?

As this book clearly demonstrates, the hospital is much more than a collection of 24-hour beds. Both clinical and financial concerns require hospital-based treatment from day one to be part of a community-based strategy to return patients, young or old, back to community settings. It is in those settings that treatment can expand and continue. Expensive acute hospital care must take place in a matter of days; then patients must be moved to less expensive alternative settings, including day treatment, intensive outpatient care, home-based care, and other outpatient services. This is and will be the challenge of the hospital today and in the future. With the evolution and implementation of the electronic medical record linking home and hospital, we can imagine today's treatments continuing at home with careful monitoring and oversight by the hospital. The hospital must be the hub of a comprehensive continuum of care. Rapid intervention becomes possible when concerns about safety such as suicide or homicide become apparent. A major challenge will continue to be to integrate the various subspecialties with the general medical comorbidities and problems of substance use and homelessness.

Principles for the Hospital of the Future

A roundtable was recently convened by the Joint Commission on the future of the hospital (see http://www.jointcommission.org/PublicPolicy/future.htm). This roundtable focused on possible futures of hospitals and developed principles to guide all hospitals— not just psychiatric hospitals or psychiatric units—for the future. The roundtable proposed that hospitals of the future abide by the following principles: 1) patient and family centeredness; 2) recovery as the ultimate goal; 3) use of evidence-based designs to improve patient safety, including single rooms and decentralized nursing stations; 4) development of workplace cultures that attract and retain key personnel, including physicians, psychologists, nurses, social workers, occupational therapists, and others; and 5) development of high-technology-based knowledge and delivery skills on the part of health professionals with the ability to use the electronic medical record as an organizing technology to put forward appropriate treatment plans and follow-up care.

There is renewed emphasis and acceptance that the patient and the family should be and are at the center of care. How can patients in the psychiatric setting be respected as equal partners in their care, especially in the context of acute psychotic illness? The Institute for Family Centered Care (http://www.familycenteredcare.org/faq.html) has developed core concepts for patient-centered care, which include 1) conveying dignity and respect, and listening to and honoring patient and family perspectives in the context of varied cultural backgrounds and differences in values and beliefs in the ongoing delivery of care and the planning for treatment; 2) sharing information in a complete and unbiased manner, as a key for patients and their families to receive timely, complete, and accurate information to effectively participate in care and decision making, especially in the context of the stabilization of patients in the inpatient setting and rapid discharge; 3) including patients and families on an institutionwide basis; 4) collaborating with patients and families in program development, implementation, and evaluation; and 5) emphasizing patient safety.

Who will staff the hospital of the future? We currently confront a serious shortage of nurses in the United States, and for this reason, we must think creatively to sustain the critical 24-hour nursing function essential for the acute inpatient stay. High-touch and high-technology care, including the use of the electronic medical record, are essential. The challenge is the handoff to community-based psychiatrists for the medical aspects of treatment and to community mental health centers or outpatient providers for psychosocial care. There will also be an even greater need for a person on staff—perhaps a social worker specialist—who knows how to obtain financing of treatment and who can help move patients through the system.

Who will lead psychiatric inpatient care in the future? The psychiatrist administrator will be someone intimately familiar with the mission of helping patients and families achieve outcomes that not only meet the treatment goals of the acute stay but also provide for care in a continuum of services. Whether the administrative leader is a physician or not, he or she must have an informed fiscal sense so that the hospital can achieve its mission within the competitive medical marketplace. Above all, the administrative leader will need to see the "big picture" and have the vision to anticipate and provide new programs and services that will define the next chapter of service delivery (see Chapter 26, "Administration and Leadership," by Schwartz and Sharfstein).

Design Trends

What should be the future design considerations for hospitals? How can we provide for flexibility and comfort and, at the same time, safety? How do we deal with the need for patient privacy and confidential discussions, the need for team-based treatment, and the involvement of numerous individuals in the care of acutely ill patients?

For psychiatric hospitals and units in general hospitals, design is a very important part of the future (see Chapter 34, "Design and Architecture," by Lippincott et al.). The use of natural light, considerations related to privacy, provision of private patient rooms and bathrooms that address safety and security challenges, minimization of the use of seclusion and restraint, need for various fixtures throughout the institution to be very durable and safe, and use of color to create warmth and soften the institutional experience of the hospital (Davis et al. 1979) are all vital for the psychiatric hospital of the future.

Reimbursement Trends

Although health costs are rising around the world, no country has costs climbing at the rate of the United States. Overall, U.S. per capita health spending is more than 50% higher than in any other country. We pay much more for pharmaceuticals, hospital stays, and physician visits, and this is a major contributor to our high cost of care. Despite all this investment, however, we do not receive a more favorable rate of return in terms of higher-quality care, greater patient satisfaction, or increased breadth of access to care. Recently, the number of uninsured in the United States has topped 46 million (Dubay et al. 2007).

These high health care costs, which are borne by government, employers, private payers, and consumers themselves, have become untenable. It is crucial that health care plans proposed by future governmental administrators contain initiatives that will change the economics and entire landscape for the delivery of medical care in this country.

More and more stakeholders are demanding transparency in the cost and quality of health care. The emergence of price-sensitive consumers in parallel with very price-sensitive purchasers will likely depress costs of various parts of health care and diminish the opportunity for cross-subsidization to cover money-losing procedures and patient care. These economic trends, I believe, will boost the market position of specialty hospitals. The opportunity to be very effective and efficient "focused health systems" serving the subspecialized needs of patients is happening today in cardiology and orthopedics and, to some extent, psychiatry. High volumes and focused expertise are the hallmarks of our specialty hospitals and units; their market advantages will likely lead to their further growth.

Many psychiatric patients are poor, under- or uninsured, and chronically ill. This makes it very difficult to deliver effective psychiatric hospital care as lower reimbursement rates and shorter lengths of stay often push these patients out of the hospital sooner than might be desirable. Looking at outcomes of hospital treatment will, in part, force a reevaluation of very short hospital stays. New payment schemes, such as pay-for-performance, will push back managed care–driven discharge directives as economic incentives will need to better match quality goals and results. The psychiatric hospital needs to fulfill its social mission in an environment of increasingly constrained payments. The best way to accomplish this is through a linking of inpatient treatment to a continuum of care aided by new technologies such as evidence-based treatments, the electronic health record, and telepsychiatry. The use of the computer and home monitoring, which has already had an impact, especially through the Department of Veterans Affairs model for highly specialized medical care such as heart disease, has its application in psychiatry as well. Here is the concept of the migration of care from the inpatient hospital bed and the physician's office to the patient's home in the context of a new technology such as a tie-in to the hospital via a home computer. Through the home monitoring system, symptoms that indicate early relapse will lead to rapid intervention.

In the future, psychiatric treatment will be an even more strategic partner with the rest of medicine than it is today. This will be especially apparent in the payment for care, as the movement and trend toward parity in public programs (such as Medicare) and private insurance will be an accepted fact rather than the controversial issue it is today. Consumers especially will not accept that their treatment for cancer or heart disease is at all different from their treatment for depression, anxiety, or schizophrenia. Inpatient hospitalization is lifesaving and life enhancing. In a society like ours, which values humane care, psychiatric treatment in and out of the hospital will be an essential and enduring fact of life.

References

Davis C, Glick ID, Rosow I: The architectural design of a psychotherapeutic milieu. Hosp Community Psychiatry 30:453–460, 1979

Dubay L, Holahan J, Cook A: The uninsured and the affordability of health insurance coverage. Health Affairs Web Exclusives, 21 November 2006–1 May 2007: A Supplement to Health Aff w22–w30, 2007

Frank RG, Glied SA: Mental Health Policy in the United States Since 1950. Baltimore, MD, Johns Hopkins University Press, 2006

Gollaher D: Voice for the Mad: The Life of Dorothea Dix. New York, Free Press, 1995

Institute of Medicine: Improving the Quality of Health Care for Mental and Substance-Use Conditions. Washington, DC, National Academies Press, 2006

Institute of Medicine Committee on Quality: Crossing the Quality Chasm. Washington, DC, National Academies Press, 2001

Parks J, Svendsen D, Singer P, et al. (eds): Morbidity and mortality in people with serious mental illness (13th technical report). Alexandria, VA, National Association of State Mental Health Program Directors Medical Directors Council, October 2006

President's New Freedom Commission on Mental Health: Achieving the Promise: Transforming Mental Health Care in America, final report (DHHS Publ No SMA-03-3832). Rockville, MD, New Freedom Commission on Mental Health, 2003

INDEX

*Page numbers in **boldface** type refer to figures or tables.*